COMMUNICATION SCIENCES AND DISORDERS

A Contemporary Perspective

COMMUNICATION SCIENCES AND DISORDERS

A Contemporary Perspective

SECOND EDITION

Laura M. Justice

The Ohio State University

Allyn & Bacon

Boston   New York   San Francisco   Mexico City
Montreal   Toronto   London   Madrid   Munich   Paris
Hong Kong   Singapore   Tokyo   Cape Town   Sydney

Executive Editor and Publisher:
   Stephen D. Dragin
Editorial Assistant: Anne Whittaker
Marketing Manager: Amanda Stedke
Managing Editor, Production: Joe Sweeney
Editorial Production Service: Progressive
   Publishing Alternatives

Manufacturing Buyer: Megan Cochran
Electronic Composition: Progressive
   Information Technologies
Interior Design: Progressive Publishing
   Alternatives
Photo Researcher: Annie Pickert
Cover Designer: Linda Knowles

For related titles and support materials, visit our online catalog at www.pearsonhighered.com.

Between the time website information is gathered and then published, it is not unusual for some sites to have closed. Also, the transcription of URLs can result in typographical errors. The publisher would appreciate notification where these errors occur so that they may be corrected in subsequent editions.

Library of Congress Cataloging-in-Publication Data

Justice, Laura M.
    Communication sciences and disorders : a contemporary perspective / Laura M. Justice.—2nd ed.
        p. cm.
    Includes bibliographical references and index.
    ISBN-13: 978-0-13-502280-1
    ISBN-10: 0-13-502280-0
  1. Communicative disorders.   2. Speech disorders.   3. Language disorders.   I. Title.
    RC423.J87 2009
    362.196'855—dc22

                                                                    2009007596

Printed in the United States of America

Credits appear on page vi, which constitutes an extension of the copyright page.

10 9 8 7 6 5 4 3   EB   13 12 11 10

**Allyn & Bacon
is an imprint of**

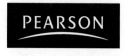

www.pearsonhighered.com

ISBN-10: 0-13-502280-0
ISBN-13: 978-0-13-502280-1

This book is for Griffin . . . whose uncanny abilities
to communicate
with joy and love make every day a delight.

BRIEF CONTENTS

CONTENTS

PREFACE

A CONTEMPORARY PERSPECTIVE ●

In the summer of 2008, the American Speech-Language-Hearing Association's Schools Conference took place at the Disney Contemporary Resort in Orlando, Florida. I was delighted, as always, to participate in this annual conference, as it offers me the opportunity to keep pace with the numerous scientific and theoretical advances affecting the field of school-based speech-language pathology. For this particular year, the conference was especially enjoyable because of the truly "contemporary" setting in which it took place. I happen to appreciate a contemporary look, and to stay at a resort that is all things contemporary (from the faucets to the lighting) was a special treat for me.

My appreciation for the contemporary is apparent throughout this book, from the title to the text itself. The importance of providing readers with the most contemporary perspective of the study of communication sciences and disorders has never been so critical, given perpetual advances in technology, ongoing revisions to education and health care policies, dramatic shifts in population demographics, and rapidly accumulating scientific literature on health and wellbeing, as well as disease and disability. Readers will find that this innovative and contemporary textbook is not only up-to-date in its substantive content concerning both theory and research, but also is designed to bring the field to life for the introductory student.

Communication Sciences and Disorders: A Contemporary Perspective introduces students to the field in a clear and succinct manner that allows access to the most current theories, research, and practices through rich examples and anecdotes. It employs a clinical case-based, lifespan approach with special attention given to certain areas:

- The application of knowledge, skills, and concepts through comprehensive case studies, which include evaluation and treatment plans and multimedia samples

- The use of technologies to better understand communication development and to assess and treat disorders of communication

- Literacy development, to include attention to dyslexia (reading disability)

- Multicultural issues, emphasizing the interactions among culture, communication ability, and communication disability as relevant to topics addressed throughout the text

- Research-based practices in assessment and intervention

ORGANIZATION OF THE TEXT: A UNIQUE PERSPECTIVE ●

The organization of this textbook provides a useful framework to ensure students' understanding of basic concepts and principles in Part I. Then, in Part II students can apply these concepts and principles to each disorder presented. Within Part II each disorder appears in a self-contained chapter. Thus, instructors can follow the suggested order of presentation or adopt an order based on their own preferences.

Part I includes five chapters that introduce the key principles and theories in communication sciences and disorders that are needed to understand disordered communication. Chapter 1 defines communication, provides an overview of different types of communication disorders, and identifies those professionals who work most closely with persons with communication disorders. Chapter 2 describes communication development across the lifespan, including major milestones from birth through adolescence. Chapter 3 describes the anatomical and physiological bases of communication and communication disorders, including key terms and concepts required to understand the structures and functions of the human body involved with speech, hearing, language, and swallowing. Chapter 4 discusses general principles and practices of communication assessment and intervention, laying a foundation for concepts such as psychometric terminology, categories of common tests and measures, and prevalent intervention approaches. Chapter 5 discusses complex communication needs and the use of augmentative and alternative communication devices (AAC) as a means to address these.

Part II includes ten chapters, each surveying a particular disorder of communication and following a similar organization to provide coherence to the discussion. Each chapter addresses a set of key questions concerning the definition, classification, defining characteristics, identification, and treatment of a disorder. Chapters 6 and 7 describe disorders of language, with Chapter 6 focusing on disorders affecting children and adolescents and Chapter 7 addressing acquired disorders and other cognitive-based dysfunctions in adults. Chapter 8 is new to this text and provides an introduction to reading disabilities. The inclusion of this chapter reflects the increasing recognition that reading disabilities often reflect underlying difficulties with language skill. Chapters 9 through 12 address disorders of speech-sound production; Chapter 9 is devoted to phonological disorders, Chapter 10 to fluency disorders, Chapter 11 to voice disorders, and Chapter 12 to the motor speech disorders of apraxia and dysarthria. Chapters 13 and 14 examine hearing loss, with Chapter 13 focusing on pediatric populations and Chapter 14 focusing on the adult population. Chapter 15 addresses disorders of feeding and swallowing.

KEY FEATURES OF THE TEXT: BRINGING THE FIELD TO LIFE ●

In preparing this work, an important goal was to bring the field to life for students. Therefore, throughout all of the chapters in the text, students receive ample opportunities to build and extend their knowledge. Each feature is designed not only to facilitate students' comprehension of key topics, but also to entice their interest in the field through clinical case-based connection and active learning opportunities.

- *Case examples:* Each of the 10 disorders chapters (Chapters 6 through 15) features two authentic case examples at the opening of the chapter. These vignettes provide examples of how disorders of communication affect children and adults in various ways, enabling students to draw connections among research, theory, and practice through discussion and reflection.

- *Discussion points:* Throughout the text, students will find a number of discussion points that elaborate upon specific topics addressed within the text. These discussion points are meant to provoke discussions among students to foster their active engagement with the text.

- *Spotlights:* Each chapter features a special boxed insert that spotlights individuals currently working as researchers and practitioners in the field of communication sciences and disorders. These special inserts introduce students to the wealth of possibilities available in both research and clinical practice. Chapter 2, for instance, spotlights Jennifer Anderson, a program manager at Microsoft who works to develop speech recognition software. Speaking in their own words, researchers and practitioners tell what they are currently doing in the field.

SUPPLEMENTARY MATERIALS: A WEALTH OF RESOURCES FOR STUDENTS AND PROFESSORS ●

The text itself is designed to support learning and facilitate better understanding of chapter concepts through the features discussed here. In addition, both students and professors can benefit from a wealth of supplementary materials.

COMPANION WEBSITE

Located at **www.pearsonhighered.com/justice2e,** the Companion Website for this text includes a wealth of resources such as chapter overviews, reflection questions, suggested readings, several updated clinical cases, and interactive self-assessments (multiple choice, true/false, and short-answer quizzes).

COMMUNICATION SCIENCES AND DISORDERS: AN INTERACTIVE MULTIMEDIA INTRODUCTION CD-ROM

The CD-ROM that accompanies the text provides immediate access to clinical case examples of the communication disorders presented in the text. Each of the five cases on the CD contains nine video clips, which give students an opportunity to hear directly from individuals experiencing communicative impairments and to observe authentic assessment and treatment activities. These video snapshots provide a means for the instructor to bring the field to life for students—through observation, discussion, and reflection.

Instructor's Manual with Test Items and TestGen Software

Instructors will find a wealth of resources to support their introductory course within the text itself. Each chapter contains focus questions, key terms, chapter summaries, and numerous discussion questions to be infused throughout lectures and to engage students' interest. Beyond the text, instructors receive a manual also available online at the Instructor Resource Center located at **www.pearsonhighered.com,** which includes chapter overviews, chapter outlines and instructional guides, key terms, discussion questions, suggested readings and resources, and a list of PowerPoint slides and transparency masters. Test items include multiple choice, true/false, short answer, and essay (40–45 questions per chapter). The computerized version of these test items (TestGen) is available in both Windows and Macintosh format, along with assessment software allowing professors to create and customize exams and track student progress.

Overhead Transparencies/PowerPoints

The transparencies—available in PowerPoint slide format by going to the Instructor Resource Center, described next, at **www.pearsonhighered.com**—highlight key concepts and summarize content from the text.

Instructor Resource Center

The Instructor Resource Center at **www.pearsonhighered.com** has a variety of print and media resources available in downloadable, digital format—all in one location. As a registered faculty member, you can access and download passcode protected resource files, course management content, and other premium online content directly to your computer.

Digital resources available for *Communication Sciences and Disorders: A Contemporary Perspective* include:

- Text-specific PowerPoint lectures
- An online version of the Instructor's Manual

To access these items online, go to **www.pearsonhighered.com** and click on the Instructor Support button; then go to the Download Supplements section. Here you will be able to log in or complete a one-time registration for a user name and password. If you have any questions regarding this process or the materials available online, please contact your local Pearson sales representative.

ACKNOWLEDGMENTS

As with the first edition of this book, I must explicitly recognize my spouse, Ian Mykel, for his unwavering and unequivocal support of my extracurricular writing activities. Heather Doyle Fraser, development editor at Merrill/Prentice Hall, also deserves a special and sincere thank you for guiding me through the first edition of this book, as many of the features she advocated for are maintained in this second edition. I would also like to commend Steve Dragin for his guidance as we considered how to improve upon the book in its revision; his focused advice based on considerable experience and knowledge of the field have made this book more effective.

Finally, a number of experts served as reviewers of this manuscript in its various stages of development. I am very grateful for their constructive input.

REVIEWERS

Matthew Gillispie, University of Kansas

Julia Rademacher, Indiana University

H.S. Venkatagiri, Iowa State University

Gary Cottrell, University of Wisconsin, River Falls

Marilyn Nippold, University of Oregon

Michael Trudeau, Ohio State University

A. Lynn Williams, East Tennessee State University

Jennifer Garrett, University of Northern Iowa

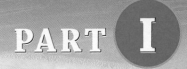
Foundations of Communication Sciences and Disorders

FUNDAMENTALS OF COMMUNICATION SCIENCES AND DISORDERS

FOCUS QUESTIONS

This chapter answers the following questions:

1. What is communication?
2. How does communication relate to language, speech, and hearing?
3. What is a communication disorder?
4. What careers are available in the field of communication sciences and disorders?

CHAPTER 1

INTRODUCTION

How important is communication to you? If you give this question serious consideration, you will likely realize that your ability to communicate is essential to who you are and is something you would never want to do without. Your understanding of the importance of communication is likely what drew you to this textbook. All of us have at some time been in a situation in which we had difficulty communicating. Perhaps you were visiting another country and did not know the language. Perhaps you were at the dentist, mouth numb from anesthesia, and you could not articulate well. Perhaps you had a panic attack and were too nervous to talk. Or perhaps you had laryngitis and temporarily lost your voice. It is usually times like these that remind us how important our ability to communicate is to us and how unpleasant and challenging it is to lose this ability.

While experiences like losing your voice or having your mouth numbed from anesthesia are inconvenient, they are temporary. Many other types of communication difficulties are more long lasting, such as those resulting from vocal nodules (calluses on the vocal cords), aphasia (loss of language skill following a brain injury), dysarthria (imprecise speech due to nervous system dysfunction), or noise-induced hearing loss (hearing loss from noise exposure). People experiencing these significant communication challenges need medical or therapeutic interventions, or both, to improve their experiences of and to increase their enjoyment of life at home, at work, in school, and in the community. These people do not take their communication skills for granted. Indeed, they realize that communication is "the heart of life's experience" (American Speech-Language-Hearing Association [ASHA], 2008a).

Communication disorders are relatively common. The National Institutes of Health estimate that 42 million Americans, or one out of every six persons, have a communication disorder (National Institute on Deafness and Other Communication Disorders [NIDCD], 2006). It is likely that everyone reading this book knows someone who has a disorder of communication or has experienced a significant communication disorder themselves. Perhaps you know someone who stutters, a communication disorder that hinders the fluency of speech and that affects about 3 million individuals in the United States (NIDCD, 2006). Or, perhaps you have a family member who has a hearing loss, a condition that affects as many as 28 million individuals in the United States. If you do not know someone directly who has experienced a communication disorder, you have likely heard of instances of it within the media. For instance, the media provided a great deal of coverage on Bob Woodruff's recovery after he sustained a traumatic brain injury while working as a news correspondent in Iraq. After 7 weeks in a coma, Woodruff received intensive speech-language therapy coupled with

DISCUSSION POINT:
Can you think of a book you've read or a movie you've seen that featured an individual with a communication disorder? One example is the book *Schuyler's Monster: A Father's Journey with his Wordless Daughter* by Robert Rummel-Hudson, in which the author describes his experiences raising a daughter who is unable to speak.

a range of additional medical interventions. He returned to television 13 months after his injury, in an hour-long documentary on his recovery process (National Public Radio, 2007).

This chapter defines *communication,* provides an overview of different types of communication disorders, and identifies those professionals who work most closely with people with communication disorders. As you read this chapter, think about the role of communication in your life and the importance of communication in our society. Let me also encourage you to use this introduction to the study of communication sciences and disorders as a springboard to a future career helping people with communication disorders—as a teacher, a clinician, a researcher, or a public-policy advocate. ●●●

| CASE STUDY 1.1 | **Communication Disorders Across the Life Span: Case Examples** |

Ten weeks premature and weighing 2 pounds, 1 ounce, **ANIKA** was born on August 14, 2003, to single parent Lina Roster. Her prematurity and low birth weight were attributed to lack of prenatal care and prenatal exposure to high carbon monoxide levels—Anika's mother smoked two packs of cigarettes daily throughout her pregnancy. The neonatal intensive care unit attempted to feed Anika orally using maternal breast milk for 1 week, at which time Anika was diagnosed by her neonatal specialist as severely undernourished and too weak to be fed orally. Anika was then placed on a nasogastric tube (NG tube), fed through her nose to her stomach. NG tube feedings were supplemented three times daily with oral feeding of breast milk by her mother. A neonatal intensive care nurse trained Ms. Roster to give Anika the tube feedings and to replace the tube each week. At 4 weeks of age, Anika is consistently gaining weight but is no longer interested in breast-feeding or in any type of oral activity. A speech-language pathologist has been called in to consult with Ms. Roster and the medical team on ways to promote Anika's oral interest and oral intake.

Internet research

1 What is the general developmental prognosis for infants born at very low birth weights?

2 How common are feeding problems in infants?

3 What supports are available for families when babies are born prematurely or with significant medical concerns?

Brainstorm and discussion

1 What are some strategies that the speech-language pathologist might use to promote Anika's interest in oral exploration?

2 What types of supports should be provided to Ms. Roster to help her cope with the challenges of giving birth to a medically fragile infant?

● ● ●

JAN SHEN is a 62-year-old man who has worked in a print shop at a local community college for the last 35 years. His hearing has been steadily decreasing, and during the last several years, Mr. Shen has been unable to actively participate in most conversations. He recently was in a car accident that his wife believes was caused by his inability to hear what was happening around him. In the weeks since the accident, Mr. Shen has been very depressed, refusing to participate in many activities that previously gave him pleasure (e.g., walking each morning, talking on the phone to his daughter). At his wife's request, Mr. Shen received a comprehensive audiological evaluation last week, which showed a severe hearing loss, likely due to ongoing exposure to noise. The audiologist recommended use of a hearing aid but also indicated that because of the type and the nature of the hearing loss, the hearing aid would not fully restore Mr. Shen's hearing to the level Mr. Shen would like. The audiologist also asked Mr. Shen to participate in a hearing-loss support group and has recommended he receive auditory rehabilitation therapy to help him best use his residual hearing and hearing aid. Mr. Shen has told his wife that he will not be returning to the audiologist, and he does not think that the hearing aid, the support group, or the therapies are needed.

WHAT IS COMMUNICATION? ●

DEFINITION

Understanding the meaning of the term *communication* is, of course, critical for the study of human communication sciences and disorders. **Communication** refers to the process of sharing information between two or more persons, or more specifically, "the transmission of thoughts or feelings from the mind of a speaker to the mind of a listener" (Borden, Harris, & Raphael, 1994, p. 174). People share their thoughts and feelings for many reasons, the three most basic being to request ("I need some coffee."), to reject ("This coffee is awful!"), and to comment ("Ah, that's much better."). Even children as young as 1 year are able to communicate for these three basic purposes ("Milk?" "Milk!" "Milk.").

Communication involves two main players—a sender and a receiver—and four processes: formulation, transmission, reception, and comprehension. The sender formulates and then transmits the information being conveyed, and the receiver receives and then comprehends the information. **Formulation** is the process of pulling together one's thoughts or ideas for sharing with another: What is the thought or feeling I want to share? **Transmission** is the process of conveying those ideas to another person, often by speaking but also by signing, gesturing, or writing. **Reception** is the process of receiving the information from another person, and **comprehension** is the process of making sense of that message.

Although speaking is one of the most frequent modes of communication, communication need not be spoken. A person can reject by turning away, a baby can comment by smiling, and a dog can request by panting at the door. Persons who use sign language as their native language do not use speech at all to communicate. However, what is particularly unique about human communication is our use of language. Much of this text, and indeed much of the study of human communication science and disorders, emphasizes the use and breakdown of this uniquely human process for communication.

Modality describes the manner in which information conveyed via communication is transmitted and received. Speech is the most common modality of communication for humans. For people who cannot speak, hear, or both, sign language is a prevalent modality for communication, particularly among members of the deaf and hard-of-hearing community. In literate cultures, reading and writing are also common means of communication. People who cannot read or write—who are illiterate—cannot participate in this communication modality. Individuals who have reading and writing disabilities may have

DISCUSSION POINT: We communicate not only through speech, but also through such modalities as gesture, sign, and writing. View Clip 5 for Diana (Study 1) on the companion CD and identify the primary modalities through which she communicates.

profound challenges using these modalities to communicate at work, school, home, or in the community.

Obviously just being able to speak, hear, read, write, and sign does not ensure effective communication. For instance, if I wrote *¿Qué crees que esto dice aquí?* and you did not know Spanish, our communication would not be successful. Why? Although we are both able to participate in the modality (reading and writing), we do not fully share the symbolic system being used. For communication between two individuals to be effective, they must have an agreement as to the symbol system to be used to communicate, and they must be proficient in that system. Language is one symbol system with many variations (e.g., Spanish, English, Chinese, Swahili, American Sign Language [ASL]); it is also the most sophisticated symbol system used for communication. Other, less sophisticated symbol systems include gestures, pictures, and facial expressions.

A Model of Communication

Figure 1.1 provides a basic model of communication that includes three essential components: (1) a sender to formulate and transmit a message, (2) a receiver to receive and comprehend the message, and (3) a shared symbolic system. An additional component, feedback, is also included in this model. **Feedback** is information provided by the receiver to the sender. In effective communication, feedback is continually provided by the receiver, and the sender responds to this feedback to maintain the effectiveness of the communication process. This feedback system is what makes communication active and dynamic. Communication is active because both sender and receiver must be fully engaged. It is dynamic because the receiver is constantly sending feedback that is interpreted and used by the sender to modulate the flow of communication.

Feedback is provided in numerous ways by the receiver. **Linguistic feedback** includes speaking, such as saying, "I totally agree," "I hear what you are saying," or "Wait, I don't get it." It also includes vocalizing, such as saying "mmm-hmm" or "uh-oh." **Nonlinguistic** or **extralinguistic feedback** refers to the use of eye contact, facial expression, posture, and proximity. This type of feedback may supplement linguistic feedback, or it may stand alone. **Paralinguistic feedback** refers to the use of pitch, loudness, and pausing, all of which are superimposed over linguistic feedback. These linguistic and nonlinguistic forms of feedback keep communication flowing and provide the speaker with valuable information concerning the receiver's comprehension.

You can probably think of a time when you were trying to communicate something and you got the impression the receiver was not getting it. What kind of feedback was the receiver using to give you this message? Perhaps they looked

---

FIGURE 1.1

Model of communication.

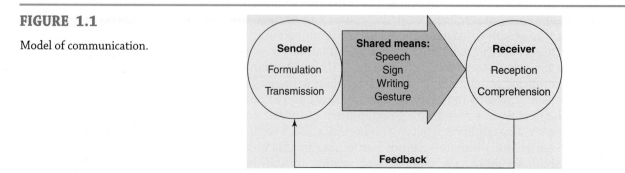

away while you were talking or interrupted you frequently for clarification. You can also probably think of a time when you were on the receiving end and your feedback was not being attended to. Perhaps you were having a difficult time understanding what someone was telling you. What kind of feedback did you give to the sender? Perhaps a few linguistic cues ("Well, this is all very interesting, but . . .") and some paralinguistic cues too (e.g., looking at your watch).

For communication to be effective, feedback from the receiver is just as important as the information the sender provides. Feedback is used by the sender and receiver to prevent a **communication breakdown** from occurring:

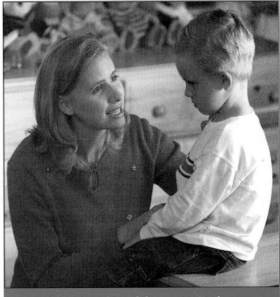

We communicate through linguistic, nonlinguistic, and paralinguistic ways.

SENDER: His whole demeanor is totally insouciant. It drives me crazy.

Receiver furrows her brow in confusion.

SENDER: I mean, he is so indifferent! How can he not care about this stuff?

RECEIVER (NODDING): Oh, I totally know what you mean. Like the other day . . .

If you look closely at this snippet of conversation, you should be able to find a communication breakdown. It centered on the word *insouciant,* which the sender used but the receiver did not understand. By giving the speaker prompt feedback (a furrowed brow, which is a type of nonlinguistic feedback), the sender was able to repair the breakdown by indicating that *insouciant* means "indifferent." This is called a *conversational repair.* Minor communication breakdowns happen in every conversation but are easily recognized and repaired if the receiver is sending ongoing feedback and the sender is closely monitoring that feedback. More serious communication breakdowns occur when receivers do not send appropriate types or amounts of feedback or when senders do not attend to the feedback. In such cases, the communication interaction is ineffective, as it does not meet the purposes of the participants.

THE PURPOSE OF COMMUNICATION

The main purpose of communication is to provide and solicit information. We communicate to provide information about our feelings ("I love you.") and to get information from others ("Do you love me?"). We communicate to share information about trivial ("Ouch! I stubbed my toe.") and exciting events ("Today I won a new car!") and to describe our needs and desires ("Won't you please lend me $5.00 for lunch?"). Halliday (1975) differentiated the purposes of communication into seven categories, or **communication functions:**

1. *Instrumental communication:* used to ask for something ("I would like the shrimp, please.")

2. *Regulatory communication:* used to give directions and to direct others ("You need to take a right here.")

3. *Interactional communication:* used to interact and converse with others in a social way ("What did you think of the game yesterday?")

4. *Personal communication:* used to express a state of mind or feelings about something ("I am just furious about this!")

5. *Heuristic communication:* used to find out information and to inquire ("Do you know when this dam was built?")

6. *Imaginative communication:* used to tell stories and to role-play ("If I had a million dollars, I would . . .")

7. *Informative communication:* used to provide an organized description of an event or object ("What happened was, we got to the game, and then it began to rain. . . .")

All of these purposes are vitally important to developing and maintaining social relationships with other people and for meeting our own basic needs and desires. These diverse functions are used by effective communicators every day in various ecological contexts, including home, school, work, and community. Use of communication to meet these many different purposes begins early in life, typically within the first year, and these purposes serve our many needs in life across the life span. Consider for which purposes you have used communication in the last 24 hours. Which ones have you used? Which ones have you not?

People who have a restricted range of communication functions face significant challenges and frustrations. As will be discussed later in this chapter, a communication disorder is present when a person experiences a substantial impairment in his or her ability to communicate. Often, a restricted range of communication functions is one of the first signs of a communication disorder. This is the case for very young children who develop communication skills more slowly than their peers, as commonly happens with children who have an intellectual disability. Children who are unable to use communication for diverse purposes feel great frustration, as do their caregivers. Adults who have experienced neurological injury, such as a stroke, may lose the ability to communicate for diverse purposes, such as asking for a prescription at the pharmacy or telling a friend how much they enjoy their company, and may feel similar frustration.

DISCUSSION POINT:
We communicate for many different purposes. Consider the case of Mr. Shen in Case Study 1.1. What communication purposes may be impacted by his hearing loss?

Effective Communication

We can all think of instances when we did not communicate as effectively as we needed to. For instance, I can think of a recent example where my communication was completely ineffective. Traveling in a central European country in which few persons speak English, I needed to register my passport at the police station within 48 hours of arrival. At the police station with passport in hand, I found myself completely illiterate (unable to read information on signs posted around me) and unable to ask for help. Effective communication occurs when information is successfully shared between a sender and a receiver; there is no breakdown in formulation, transmission, reception, or comprehension. An effective communicator is one whose communications with others are effective most of the time. They communicate through a modality that is shared by important people in their lives and communities, such as speaking and hearing, reading and writing, or signing. Effective communicators avoid communication breakdowns by responding to and giving feedback during conversations. They use communication for diverse purposes: to ask for things, to direct others, to interact with others in a social way, to express their own feelings, to find out information, and to tell stories. Additionally, effective communicators abide by four principles known as **Grice's maxims** (Grice, 1975): (1) quantity, (2) quality, (3) relevance, and (4) manner. These principles refer specifically to the way in which senders formulate and transmit information, as described by Damico (1991):

1. *Principle of quantity:* The sender provides the right amount and type of information needed by the receiver, uses clear and concise vocabulary, and is not redundant. The following breakdown results from the speaker's lack of adherence to this principle:

   Speaker: He is not coming! Can you believe it?
   Receiver: Who is "he"? What are you talking about?

2. *Principle of quality:* The sender shares information that is accurate. The following breakdown results from a speaker ignoring this principle:

   Speaker: I am *not* angry at you.
   Receiver: Why are you shouting at me?

3. *Principle of relevance:* The sender maintains the topic and uses appropriate transitions as needed; the sender communicates in a way that is appropriate to the situation and to their relationship with the receiver. The following speaker is not abiding by this principle:

   Speaker: I am so worried about the test tomorrow. This is such crazy weather! What do you think?
   Receiver: It is kind of hot.
   Speaker: I was asking you about the test!

4. *Principle of manner:* The sender speaks fluently without frequent hesitations or revisions, takes appropriate turns, pauses as needed but does not delay responses longer than called for, uses appropriate loudness and pitch, and engages in eye contact as expected by cultural norms. The following communication exchange breaks down by inordinate pauses, going against this principle of manner:

   Speaker: You want to know what time it is? Um . . . um . . . uh (pauses for 10 seconds). I don't have a watch.

HOW DOES COMMUNICATION RELATE TO LANGUAGE, SPEECH, AND HEARING?

Language, speech, and hearing are the essential ingredients of human communication. The sophisticated use of these three processes for communication is what makes the human species unique. This textbook focuses on language, speech, and hearing as key communication tools and on how difficulties in these areas can result in disorders of communication.

Language, speech, and hearing are used for the formulation, transmission, reception, and comprehension of information using spoken channels (see Figure 1.2). Language is used for formulation and comprehension. Speech is used for transmission. Hearing is used for reception. Although the terms *language, speech,* and *communication* are often used synonymously, they describe very different processes.

The term *language* describes the cognitive process by which we formulate ideas and thoughts. Once these ideas and thoughts are formulated, we can orally communicate them to others through speech. We can also choose to keep these thoughts and ideas to ourselves (inner language) or to write them down (written language).

FIGURE 1.2

Key processes in spoken communication.

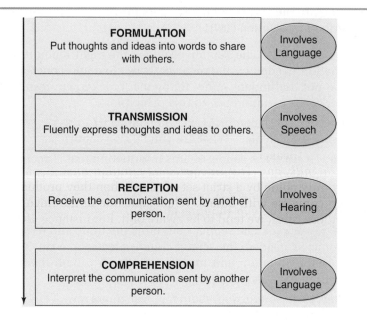

FORMULATION	Involves Language
Put thoughts and ideas into words to share with others.	

TRANSMISSION	Involves Speech
Fluently express thoughts and ideas to others.	

RECEPTION	Involves Hearing
Receive the communication sent by another person.	

COMPREHENSION	Involves Language
Interpret the communication sent by another person.	

The term *speech* describes the neuromuscular process by which we turn language into a sound signal that is transmitted through the air (or other medium, like a telephone line) to a receiver. Speech involves using voice and articulators (e.g., tongue, lips, palate) to make the sounds that produce words and sentences.

Why do humans have speech and language? These evolved for only one purpose: to communicate. The information shared through communication is language, and speech is a primary means by which language is transmitted. Although many other species are able to communicate, only humans have speech and language. The capacities for speech and language allow humans to share remarkably complex ideas and thoughts with one another, a feat that is not possible for other species.

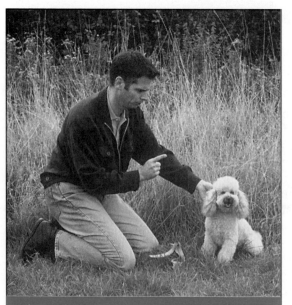

Other species are able to communicate, but only humans have the capacity for speech and language.

LANGUAGE

Definition

Language is the "socially shared code that uses a conventional system of arbitrary symbols to represent ideas about the world that are meaningful to others who know the same code" (Nelson, 1998, p. 26). The key elements of this definition are:

1. *Language is* socially shared: A community of speakers shares the same system for communicating their ideas. For example, everyone reading this textbook shares the English language as a means for communicating ideas about communication sciences and disorders.

2. *Language is a* code: Ideas about the world are communicated using a set of symbols. The symbols used in language are words, which are made up of sounds that are combined in various ways. The code for what you

are holding in your hand right now involves three sounds—b + oo + k—blended together to form a word (*book*). Those of us who speak English and therefore know this particular code are a linguistic community. The word itself (in this case, *book*) is completely arbitrary; the thing in your hand could just as well be called a *trift*, formed by blending five sounds—t + r + i + f + t.

3. *Language is* conventional: Language follows specific, systematic conventions; it is a rule-governed code. Strict rules govern the way a linguistic community organizes words into sentences, the way word units are put together, and the way sounds are combined to make words. The rules of English constrain English speakers from saying things like *Sat cat the the on hat, He drankeding the milk,* and *Thit rinches shug gfmiiikn nink.* Speakers in a linguistic community abide by a strict set of rules when they produce words and sentences and converse with others. When someone in the linguistic community violates those rules, we tend to be aware of it. For instance, if a doctor said to you, "Need prescription store go," you would be aware that some linguistic rules were being violated. If a young child said, "He goed to the store," you would also probably recognize that a rule was being violated, but you would be more accepting, knowing that the child was still learning the rules of language and would shortly figure out that the past tense of *go* is *went.*

4. *Language is a* representational tool: Language allows us to represent our thoughts and ideas to others. Language is a tool for communication, and the only reason humans evolved language was to communicate with one another. In addition to allowing us to represent our ideas to others for communication purposes, language enables our brains to store information and to carry out many cognitive processes, such as reasoning, hypothesizing, and planning (Bickerton, 1995). Although the relationship between thought and language continues to spur controversy (Can we think without using language?), we do know that much of human thought uses the code of language.

Remarkable Features of Language

Language is undoubtedly one of the most remarkable capacities of the human species. It is what makes us human and what makes us uniquely different from other species. Language is studied by more disciplines than any other subject. It commands the interest of psychologists, speech-language pathologists, audiologists, linguists, sociologists, philosophers, biologists, anthropologists, childhood educators, special educators, neuroscientists, nurses, physicians, mathematicians, and musicians, among others. Several of the remarkable features of language that attract scholars include its universality, species specificity, semanticity, productivity, and rate of acquisition.

Universality.   Language is ubiquitous. Every human culture has one and sometimes many languages, and all languages are equally complex. The **universality** of language, as Steven Pinker wrote in *The Language Instinct* (1994, p. 26),

> fills linguists with awe, and is the first reason to suspect that language is not just any cultural invention but the product of a special human instinct. . . . Cultural inventions vary widely in their sophistication from society to society. . . . language, however, ruins this correlation. There are Stone Age societies, but there is no such thing as a Stone Age language.

Species Specificity.   Language is a human capacity, and no other animals share this aptitude. The **species specificity** of language recognizes that while many nonhuman species are able to communicate, their communication abilities are wholly iconic (Bickerton, 1995). Iconic communication systems are those for which there is a transparent relation between what is being communicated and how it is being communicated. For instance, the purring of a cat is a fairly transparent way to say "I like your petting." If the purring goes up a notch to a veritable roar, it says, "I *really* like your petting. Keep it up." All nonhuman communication systems are more or less iconic, whereas there is little that is iconic about human language.

Semanticity.   Human language allows us to represent events that are decontextualized, or removed from the present—what happened before this moment or what may happen after this moment. We need not talk only about what is concrete and in the here and now; rather, language allows us to talk about things that are decidedly not concrete, that are intangible, abstract, hypothetical, complex, and far removed from the present. **Semanticity** is this unique aspect of language, and it relates to the noniconic aspect of human language. Because the relations between our language and what we are talking about are not tied together, we have an immensely powerful tool for use.

Productivity.   **Productivity** is the principle of combination, specifically the combination of a small number of discrete units into seemingly infinite novel creations. Productivity is a phenomenon that applies to other human activities—such as mathematics and music—as well as to language. With a relatively small set of rules governing language, humans are capable of producing an endless number of ideas and new constructions. For instance, humans use only a small set of sounds (for speakers of Standard American English, there are about 40 or so), and we can combine these small units on the basis of a set of rules we intuitively know (e.g., /g/ does not typically follow /l/) into an infinite number of words and syllables. Similarly, with a relatively small number of words, humans are capable of creating an infinite variety of sentences, the majority of which no one has ever heard before. If you desired, right now, you could produce a sentence that no person has ever uttered before because of the remarkable principle of productivity.

This principle is inherent to language in its earliest stages of acquisition. Children who are 18 months of age and who have about 50 words in their vocabulary begin to combine and recombine this small set of words to produce sentences that express a range of needs. The productivity feature of language is unique to humans, as the units of nonhuman communication systems cannot be recombined to make new meanings. For instance, night monkeys have 16 communication units. These 16 units cannot be recombined to make more than 16 possible ways to communicate, as the principle of productivity is not operating (Bickerton, 1995).

Rate of Acquisition.   Hoff-Ginsberg (1997, p. 3) has stated that language development "reveals the genius in all children. . . . It is remarkable that 3-year-olds who can't tie their shoes or cross the street alone have vocabularies of thousands of words and can produce sentences with relative clauses." For many of us who are researchers of child language, this is the remarkable feature of language that drew us to the field—the sheer rate of acquisition, the marvelous feat of children in learning so much so fast. Children go from using perhaps 5 words at 12 months, to 2-word sentences and about 50 words at 18 months, to thousands of words and complex sentences by 5 years. Spend a few minutes with a 3-year-old child in the next week, and it is likely that you will be amazed by the language you hear. The rate of language acquisition is a key achievement of early childhood, and many scholars view language development as fairly complete by about 5 years of age, although the system is continually refined during middle and later childhood (e.g., new words are added to the vocabulary). Thus the first 5 years of life are a critical period for language development; after this period, the rate of language development slows, and never again will so many linguistic achievements be possible in such a short period of time.

Language Domains

Language consists of three rule-governed domains that together reflect an integrated whole: content, form, and use (Lahey, 1988). **Content** refers to the meaning of language—the words we use and the meaning behind them. Content is conveyed through our vocabulary system, or lexicon, as we select and organize words to express our ideas or to understand what others are saying. **Form** is how words, sentences, and sounds are organized and arranged to convey content. **Use** is how language is used functionally for meeting personal and social needs.

Let's take, for instance, the two-word sentence spoken by 2-year-old Dakota: "Daddy's cup." This sentence can be analyzed for its content, form, and use. The content is the words Dakota selected from her vocabulary and the meaning behind those words; concepts expressed here include Daddy's ownership and an object used to hold liquid and to drink from. Form is how these concepts are conveyed by organizing sounds (eight sounds are used), by manipulating word structure ('s is added to *Daddy* to convey possession), and by organizing words in a particular order (*cup* comes after *Daddy's*). Use is how the content and forms function within a social routine. In this case, Dakota says "daddy's cup" while pointing to a cup sitting on a table. Although there are many possible functions for Dakota's utterance, in this case she appears simply to be commenting, possibly to initiate a conversation with her mother.

DAKOTA: Daddy's cup.

MOTHER (LOOKING UP): Yes, that is Daddy's cup.

DAKOTA: Mommy's cup.

MOTHER: You're right. This is my cup.

DAKOTA: That Mommy.

MOTHER: Yep, this one's mine. Where's your cup?

DAKOTA: My cup.

Content, form, and use thus constitute a three-domain system used to represent and organize the major dimensions of language. A five-domain system is also often used to provide a slightly more refined description of language dimensions (see Figure 1.3): semantics, syntax, morphology, phonology, and pragmatics. The domains of semantics and pragmatics are synonymous with the domains of content and use, respectively. The domains of syntax, morphology, and phonology reflect three elements of form.

1. **Semantics** (content): The rules of language governing the meaning of individual words and word combinations. For instance, we know that a *culprit* is someone who has done something wrong and that *green* and *blue* go together meaningfully. Our knowledge of semantics tells us that something is wrong with the sentence *Colorless green ideas sleep furiously,* a sentence produced by the linguist Noam Chomsky to differentiate semantics and syntax (Pinker, 1994).

2. **Syntax** (form): The rules of language governing the internal organization of sentences. The sentence *Colorless green ideas sleep furiously* abides

FIGURE 1.3

The domains of language.

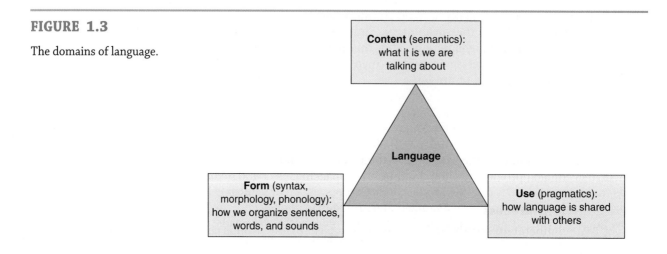

by conventional rules of syntax: its word order is acceptable despite its lack of meaning.

3. **Morphology** (form): The rules of language governing the internal organization of words. Words can be morphed (manipulated) to change their meanings; for instance, -*ed* can be added to *walk* to show that this activity happened in the past (*walked*), or -*er* can be added to turn the verb *walk* into a noun to describe a person who is walking (*walker*).

4. **Phonology** (form): The rules of language governing the sounds we use to make syllables and words. Every language has a relatively small number of sounds, called *phonemes*. Standard American English (SAE) uses about 40 phonemes (depending on the dialect), as shown in Figure 1.4. SAE relies on the combination of 15 vowels and 25 consonants to create some 100,000 words. Some languages use more phonemes, and others use less (for instance, the Lakhota language, a Sioux language, uses 34 phonemes [Rood & Taylor, 1996], many of which would be unfamiliar to speakers of Standard American English).

FIGURE 1.4

The phonemes of Standard American English.

Consonants						Vowels			
/p/	pat	/t/	tip	/g/	go	/i/	feet	/ɪ/	fit
/b/	bat	/d/	dip	/ŋ/	sing	/e/	fate	/ɛ/	fret
/m/	mat	/n/	not	/h/	hop	/u/	food	/ʊ/	foot
/f/	fit	/s/	sun	/ʔ/	uh-oh	/o/	phone	/ɔ/	fought
/v/	vat	/z/	zoo	/l/	lose	/æ/	fan	/a/	hot
/θ/	think	/tʃ/	chew	/r/	rose	/ʌ/	cut	/ə/	bathtub
/ð/	those	/dʒ/	jeep	/j/	young	/aɪ/	fight	/au/	found
/ʃ/	shop	/k/	kiln	/w/	week	/ɔɪ/	toy		
/ʒ/	measure								

In addition, each language has rules governing how sounds are organized in words, called *phonotactics.* In English, for instance, the sound /g/ never follows /s/ or /l/ at the beginning of a word.

5. **Pragmatics** (use): The rules of language governing how language is used for social purposes. Pragmatics governs three important aspects of the social use of language: (1) using language for different purposes (communication functions), (2) organizing language for discourse (conversation) (Lahey, 1988), and (3) knowing what to say and when and how to say it (social conventions). In using language for social purposes, pragmatic rules govern linguistic, extralinguistic, and paralinguistic aspects of communication, to include word choice, turn taking, posture, gestures, eye contact, proximity, pitch, loudness, and pausing.

DISCUSSION POINT:
Language consists of five domains. View Clip 1 for Mr. Johnson (Study 4) and try to identify which domains of language have been affected by his hearing loss.

Metalinguistic Awareness

The ability to deliberately scrutinize language as an object of attention is called **metalinguistic awareness.** Because language is a highly abstract concept, working at a metalinguistic level can be challenging. For instance, if you were asked to find the first article in this paragraph, you would have to think about the meaning of the linguistic term *article* before doing so. Then, starting at the beginning of the paragraph, you would look at each word and consider whether it was an article. Thinking about the various parts of speech and then analyzing words for their linguistic category (article, noun, etc.) is a metalinguistic act, and a certain degree of metalinguistic awareness is needed to be successful at this task.

Each domain of language can be the object of metalinguistic scrutiny. Semantic awareness is needed to analyze words or concepts explicitly. For example, asking, "What does *shipwreck* mean?" makes the word *shipwreck* an object of scrutiny much as asking, "What is the cat doing?" makes the cat an object of scrutiny. Obviously, the *shipwreck* task is more challenging, as it involves working at an abstract level to analyze a word in one's lexicon rather than a cat sitting nearby. When a person says, "I can't come up with the right word," this, too, is a metalinguistic comment. Syntactic awareness is needed to analyze sentence grammar explicitly, as in analyzing what is wrong with the sentence *Her did it.* Morphological awareness is needed to analyze the structure of words in a deliberate way, as in asking, "What do I add to the word *walk* to show that it already happened?" Phonological awareness involves analyzing the sound structure of language, as in asking, "What is the first sound in the word *bottle*?" Pragmatic awareness involves analyzing language use in social situations, as in asking a child, "How could you phrase that to be more polite?" or "Why do we not talk loudly in libraries?"

SPEECH

Definition

Speech is the neuromuscular process that allows humans to express language as a vocal product. In spoken communication, after our ideas are formulated (language), they must be transmitted. Speech involves the very precise activation of muscles in three systems to transmit ideas: respiration, phonation, and articulation. These three systems represent the remarkable coordination of a breath of air that begins in the lungs (respiration), travels up through the trachea, or windpipe, over the vocal cords, and into the oral and nasal cavities (phonation), and then is manipulated by the oral articulators—tongue, teeth, and jaw (articulation)—to

FIGURE 1.5

Systems involved with speech.

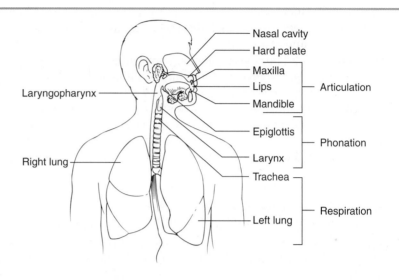

Nasal cavity
Hard palate
Maxilla — Articulation
Lips
Mandible
Epiglottis — Phonation
Larynx
Trachea — Respiration
Left lung
Right lung
Laryngopharynx

come out as a series of speech sounds that another person can understand and attribute meaning to (see Figure 1.5).

To better understand the processes involved with speech, say the word *eat* slowly and deliberately and think about the process as you do so. You will see that the speech process begins with the intake of a breath which is then exhaled; this is the basic fuel needed for all speech. The exhalation travels up from the lungs through the windpipe (trachea) and over the vocal cords (within the larynx), which begin to vibrate and create the "eeeee" sound. This "eeeee" sound is then sent into the oral cavity, which is open and marked by a big, toothy smile with the lips pulled wide. Notice that the upper and lower jaws (maxilla and mandible) are held fairly close together but are not closed; the tongue sits low in the mouth, with the tip tucked behind the lower row of teeth and the middle rounded up on the sides to touch the upper teeth. Once the "eeee" sound is in the oral cavity, a brief "ea" escapes, and then the tongue comes quickly up behind the teeth to produce the "t" sound following the "ea."

The complete neuromuscular and neuroanatomical description of this process is provided in later chapters. For now, it is important to recognize that speech is a neuromuscular act involving precise coordination of three systems. It is also important to appreciate how highly complex speech is. As a neuromuscular activity requiring considerable accuracy across a number of biological systems, there are many sites of possible breakdowns. Breakdowns in these systems, if serious enough, can result in a variety of communication disorders. Go ahead and produce the word *eat* again; as you do so, think about each stage of the speech-production process and consider where breakdowns might occur.

The systems used by humans for speech—respiration, phonation, and articulation—did not evolve for the purpose of speech. Rather, speech as an evolutionary capacity superimposed itself on systems that were already in place. The structures of the respiratory and phonatory systems allow us to breathe, and the structures of the articulatory system allow us to eat and drink. Although when and how humans first began to use speech is the subject of considerable popular, philosophical, and scientific debate, it is generally accepted that speech became the mode for language expression because of its advantages over other possible modalities. Unlike gestured, signed, or

DISCUSSION POINT:
The concepts of speech and language are often confused and considered synonyms. Describe in your own words how to differentiate between speech and language.

written communication, speech can be used with much less constraint—effective in the dark, across relatively large distances, and even across time when storage media are used.

Model of Speech Production

How a human being is able to go from an idea ("I am hungry.") to a clearly articulated spoken product ("Let's eat!") is a question that has yet to be fully answered. This question is interesting to scientists in diverse disciplines, because speech is one of several critical capacities that make humans human.

Figure 1.6 presents a basic model of speech production. A model is a way to represent an unknown event based on the current best evidence governing that event. This model shows speech production as a three-stage process (Raphael, Borden, & Harris, 2007) initiated with an abstract mental representation of the speech stream to be produced. This perceptual target is a cognitively based conceptualization of a series of individual sounds, or phonemes. A **phoneme** is the smallest unit of sound. The word *mama,* for instance, is made up of four phonemes strung together. These phonemes are represented in Figure 1.6 as /m/ /a/ /m/ /a/. (Phonemic representations are usually bounded by slashes.) The symbols of the International Phonetic Alphabet (see Figure 1.4) are used to represent individual phonemes.

The next stage is development of a motor schema to represent this sound sequence. The motor schema is a rough motor plan based on the abstract representation of the perceptual target. The rough plan organizes the phonemes into syllable chunks; *mama* is represented as two syllables to be executed—/ma/ /ma/. The rough plan is sent forward to the major muscle groups involved with speech production. These include muscle groups in the respiratory system, which will initiate and modulate the flow of air; the larynx, which contains the vocal cords; and the muscle groups of the oral cavity, which govern the movement of the tongue and the positioning of the upper and lower jaws and lips.

Sending forward the motor schema stimulates the production of speech, or speech output. The flow of air, vibration of the vocal cords, and movements of the oral cavity are all finely manipulated to carry out the motor schema and to create speech. Ongoing feedback relays information about the timing, delivery, and

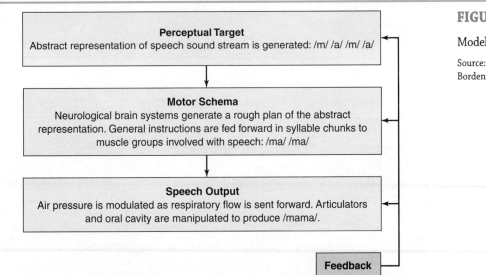

FIGURE 1.6

Model of speech production.

Source: Adapted from Raphael, Borden, & Harris (2007).

precision of speech output back to the origin of the perceptual target and motor schema. This feedback, occurring in the speaker's unconscious, provides information about what is to come next at the perceptual and motor levels. Occasionally, feedback occurs at a conscious level—for example, when we are aware that we are stumbling over our words and thus become more deliberate in our speech.

Building Blocks of Effective Speech

Speech is a representational tool for the sharing of language. Language is not dependent on speech, as it can be shared via other means (e.g., writing, sign language) or can be kept to ourselves as a tool for thinking. However, speech is wholly dependent on language; speech is a tool for language. Without language, speech is just a series of grunts and groans. Language gives speech its meaning.

Speech is functional when we are able to use it to accurately translate our thoughts as language for other people to hear. We want our speech to be as clear and fluent as possible to serve this purpose. Speech that is unclear and is dysfluent is a barrier to sharing our language and may signify the presence of a speech disorder. A person can have a speech disorder and still have excellent language and communication skills, as speech is itself a process that is distinct from communication and language.

For instance, Stephen Hawking, the famous theoretical physicist at Cambridge University, has a profound speech disorder resulting from amyotrophic lateral sclerosis (ALS), a disease of the motor neurons. Hawking was diagnosed with ALS while completing his doctorate at Oxford University. Over the next decade, the disease progressed to the point that Hawking had serious difficulties with any motor task, and eventually he was no longer able to produce functional speech. However, Hawking's language and communication skills are as intact as ever. Like many people who have a severe or profound speech disorder, Hawking uses augmentative/alternative communication (AAC) to express

DISCUSSION POINT:

Some situations can compromise the fluency of one's speech. Identify a situation in which your speech was dysfluent. In what ways did your dysfluent speech sound differ from your fluent speech?

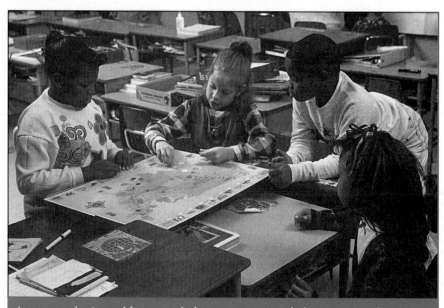

A person who is unable to speak does not necessarily have impaired language abilities.

himself. Although he is satisfied with the speech synthesizer he uses, Hawking has complained that it gives him an American accent (Hawking, 2003).

There are four essential building blocks of normal speech: (1) breathstream, (2) voice, (3) articulation, and (4) fluency.

1. *Breathstream:* Speech begins with the exhalation of breath. A speaker must have an adequate breathstream that is exhaled consistently and evenly for good speech to occur. A speech disorder can result from an inability to produce or maintain a strong breathstream.

2. *Voice:* Speech requires a strong and even voice. Voice quality can affect speech significantly; a breathy, hoarse, broken, or nasal voice can distract a listener and undermine the functionality of speech. Likewise, a voice that is too loud, too soft, too high, or too low can also undermine speech quality. *Loud* and *soft* describe vocal loudness, whereas *high* and *low* describe vocal pitch.

3. *Articulation:* Speech requires precision in phoneme production. In Standard American English, roughly 40 phonemes are used and reused to produce a seemingly endless supply of words. The difference between two words—like *bat* and *pat,* or *pin* and *pen*—may be only one phoneme. Phonemes must be produced accurately and consistently for effective speech. There is room for some minor variation in how particular phonemes in a language are produced, as in dialects, which are the systematic variations of a particular language that arise in social or geographic communities. However, consistent omission (e.g., saying "tee" for *tree*) or distortion (e.g., saying "bark" for *park*) of phonemes can lead to significant problems in using speech to encode language.

4. *Fluency:* Speech is most functional when it is produced effortlessly and smoothly, with few hesitations, interjections, and circumlocutions. Hesitations are long pauses. Interjections are the use of filler words (*um, er*) and phrases (*I mean, like, you know*). Circumlocution is talking around a word by describing features of it (e.g., "That thing you keep dishes in") and is accompanied by hesitations and interjections ("I put it on the, on the, uh, you know . . . the thing you keep dishes in."). Speech is fluent when all the elements of good delivery come together.

HEARING

Definition

In the spoken communication process, there is a sender and a receiver. The receiver's job includes reception and comprehension of the information being conveyed—namely, language via speech. Hearing is essential to reception and comprehension. Hearing, or **audition,** is the perception of sound; applied to the communication process, audition involves specifically the perception of speech.

Sound Fundamentals

To understand hearing, it is important to have a general sense of **acoustics,** which is the study of sound (Raphael et al., 2007). To understand acoustics, we'll use a demonstration. Clap your hands. Your clap creates a sound, which is subsequently registered in the auditory portion of your brain. There are four essential steps that get the clap sound from your hands to your brain, where

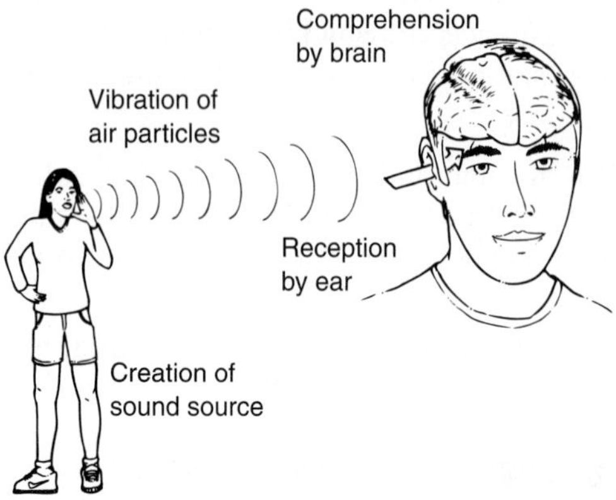

FIGURE 1.7

Role of hearing in spoken communication.

the sound is processed, as shown in Figure 1.7: creation of sound source, vibration of air particles, reception by ear, and comprehension by brain (Champlin, 2000).

1. *Creation of sound source:* A sound source sets in motion a series of events. It creates a disturbance, a set of vibrations, in the surrounding air particles. When you bring your hands together to clap, this sets the air particles near the sound source into a complex vibratory pattern.

2. *Vibration of air particles:* Sound is, fundamentally, the movement or vibration of air particles. The air particles, set in motion by the sound source, move back and forth through the air (or other medium, such as water). How fast the particles move back and forth is the sound **frequency,** which corresponds to the perception of pitch. How far apart the particles move when going back and forth relates to **intensity,** or the perceived loudness of the sound. When you clap your hands, you set the air particles around the sound source into a vibratory pattern, and how the particles move carries information about frequency and intensity; this information is carried through the air to the receiver's ear. Note that *frequency* and *intensity* are terms used to describe physical properties of sound. In contrast, *pitch* and *loudness* describe our perceptions of frequency and intensity, respectively.

3. *Reception by ear:* The ear is specially designed to channel information carried by the air particle vibrations into the human body. The ear is a complex structure with three chambers. The outer chamber (outer ear) captures the sound and channels it to the middle chamber (middle ear). The third chamber then receives the sound information (inner ear); this chamber is connected to a nerve that leads to the brain. Information from the air-particle vibrations—and particularly information about frequency and intensity—is sent through these three chambers and then along the auditory nerve to the audition centers of the brain.

4. *Comprehension by brain:* The auditory centers of the brain, located in the left hemisphere, translate frequency and intensity information sent through the ear and along the auditory nerve. If the information that arrives at the brain involves speech sounds, the speech and language centers of the brain help in the comprehension process. If the information that arrives at the brain is not a speech sound—as is the case with a clap—the speech and language centers are not involved. Sound information is differentiated by the human brain as speech or nonspeech. The human ear and brain are designed to be "remarkably responsive" to processing the sounds that humans use for speech (Borden, Harris, & Raphael, 1994, p. 176).

Speech Perception

Speech perception is the processing of human speech and is different from auditory perception, a more general term that describes the brain's processing of any type of auditory information. The processing of a clap or an insect's buzz involves auditory perception, but processing the word *Help!* requires speech

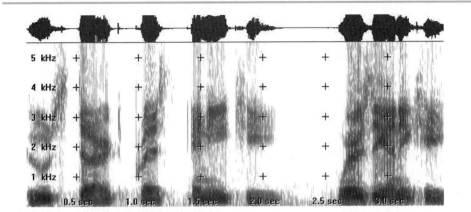

FIGURE 1.8

Spectrogram depicting human speech.

Source: Spectrogram produced using Spectrogram Version 16 (www.visualizationsoftware.com), Courtesy of Richard Horne.

perception. As sound information is sent from the ear and auditory nerve to the brain, the brain differentiates between general auditory information and speech sounds. Speech perception involves specialized processors in the brain that have evolved specifically to make sense of human speech.

A spectrogram is a three-dimensional depiction of the speech signal that is carried by the movement of air particles into the human ear. The dimensions represented include frequency/pitch (on the vertical *y*-axis), time (on the horizontal *x*-axis), and intensity/loudness (darkness of the shadings). The spectrogram is included here to provide a general sense of the information that is translated by the human brain in the speech-perception process. It also shows how complicated this information is, which is most apparent when we compare the speech spectrogram to other types of sounds in our environment.

Sometimes analogies are made between reading a spectrogram and reading the alphabet, suggesting that we can read a sequence of phonemes (e.g., /ʤ/ + /ʌ/ + /ʤ/ = /ʤ ʌ ʤ /) just as we can read a series of letters (e.g., j + u + d + g + e = judge). Scientists have shown that this analogy is incorrect. When humans produce phonemes, the phonemes overlap, or "smear," with one another, a process called *co-articulation*. For instance, say the word *judge* and think closely about your production of the first /ʤ/ sound. You will realize that it carries information about the next sound—the /ʌ/. Hold the /ʤ/ for a moment or two before releasing to the vowel, and notice that your lips are jutting forward in a rounded position, as if you are about to give your pet a kiss. Now note how this initial /ʤ/ in *judge* is quite different from the final /ʤ/, in which the lips are not rounded in anticipation of the vowel.

The articulators (lips, tongue, etc.) co-articulate speech sounds because it is much quicker than producing just one sound at a time, and the brain has evolved to make sense of co-articulated speech sounds. The production and processing of co-articulated phonemes are what allow humans to produce words at incredibly rapid rates and what undermine the notion of speech as a sort of spoken alphabet.

DISCUSSION POINT:
Produce the words *zoo* and *zebra*, focusing your attention on how the initial sound /z/ is produced in each word. In what ways does your production of the two /z/ sounds differ for these two different words? Why does this happen?

WHAT IS A COMMUNICATION DISORDER? ●

NORMAL AND DISORDERED COMMUNICATION

Whether communication occurs via speech and hearing, writing and reading, or sign or other manual means, individuals are functional and effective communicators when they are able to successfully formulate, transmit, receive, and comprehend information from other individuals. A communication disorder or impairment is present when a person has significant difficulty in one or more of these aspects of communication when compared with other people sharing the same language, dialect, and culture. Formulation and comprehension difficulties usually signal a language impairment; problems with transmission usually suggest a speech impairment; and problems with reception usually signal a hearing loss. The term *significant* means that the communication difficulty is serious enough to adversely impact an individual's ability to participate in the home, school, work, or community environment.

The process of communication is remarkably complex and involves many biological systems. For instance, spoken communication involves the hearing apparatus, the visual system, the articulators, the left and right hemispheres of the brain, the larynx, and the respiratory system. (The way in which these systems are used for communication will be described in Chapter 3.) Given the many systems involved, there are many possible points at which a breakdown can occur, resulting in communication impairment. For instance, a stroke can cause damage to the brain regions governing language comprehension, which can affect the communication process to the extent that the person might not be able to understand spoken language. Traumatic brain injuries, developmental disabilities, hearing loss, and aging are other factors that can adversely influence communication and can result in significant communication impairment.

There are four key points at which a breakdown in communication may occur (see Figure 1.2):

1. *Formulation:* Difficulty in effectively formulating a message for communication. Aphasia is a type of communication disorder resulting from stroke in which people can have significant problems formulating their thoughts and ideas into words. Aphasia is described in Chapter 7.

2. *Transmission:* Difficulty in effectively transmitting a message for communication. Motor speech disorders are a type of communication disorder affecting the neuromuscular systems governing the articulators, such as the tongue, lips, and palate. People with cerebral palsy, for instance, may experience a motor speech disorder resulting in difficulty in effectively transmitting their thoughts and ideas through speech, even if these ideas are formulated well. Motor speech disorders are described in Chapter 12.

3. *Reception:* Difficulty in effectively receiving a message being communicated. Noise-induced hearing loss, a type of communication disorder in which significant hearing loss is caused by prolonged exposure to loud noise, can result in a problem with reception. Noise-induced hearing loss is described in Chapter 14.

4. *Comprehension:* Difficulty in effectively decoding or comprehending a message being communicated. Intellectual disability is a developmental disorder characterized by mild to severe cognitive impairment. Individuals with moderate to profound levels of intellectual disability often have problems comprehending what others are saying, even though their reception is intact. Intellectual disability is discussed in Chapter 6.

COMMUNICATION DISORDERS AND COMMUNICATION DIFFERENCES

The way an individual communicates with others is highly influenced by the individual's culture. *Culture* describes a system of knowledge comprising beliefs, behavior, and values that are shared by a particular community (Battle, 2002, p. 3).

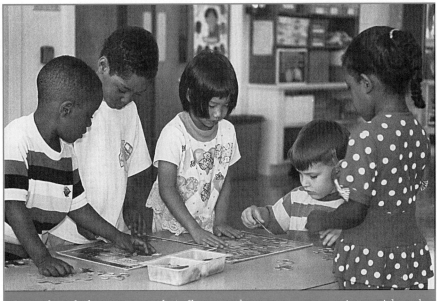

Our cultural identity strongly influences the way we communicate with each other.

The community may be defined by many diverse parameters, including language (speakers of African American English), religion (people who are Catholic), geography (inhabitants of Brooklyn), ethnicity (people who are Hispanic), race (people who are Asian), health status (people with diabetes), sexual identity (people who are heterosexual), marital status (unmarried people), and so forth. Any one person's cultural identity is likely to be influenced by these many dimensions as well as others. Likewise, the way a person communicates is also influenced by these diverse dimensions, and there is no one way to communicate that is better than others. Rather, "speech, language and communication are embedded in culture" (Battle, 2002, p. 3). Accordingly, culture influences communication, and communication influences culture. The two cannot be separated.

Being aware of how culture influences communication patterns is important in nations characterized by high levels of cultural diversity. The United States is one of the most culturally diverse countries in the world. Consider, for instance, that 10% of the current U.S. population are immigrants, and in some states (California, New York, Florida, Hawaii, Nevada, and New Jersey), immigrants comprise more than 15% of the population (Camarota, 2001). Immigrants arriving to the United States bring the cultural values and practices of their home countries, such as Mexico, China, Haiti, and Russia, with them. Linguistic diversity is also remarkable in the United States. Today, nearly 20% of people in the United States speak a language other than English at home, corresponding to an estimated 47 million people (U.S. Census Bureau, 2003). Table 1.1 presents the 20 languages most frequently spoken at home by people within the United States.

Because communication is so heavily influenced by one's linguistic background and culture, it is important when trying to identify a communication disorder to first rule out the presence of a communication difference. In our increasingly diverse country, communication differences are common. Consider two kindergarten children on a playground in Charlottesville, Virginia. One child, JaJuan, lives in a Latino household in which only Spanish is spoken. The family recently immigrated to the United States from Cuba. JaJuan knows very few words

TABLE 1.1 Twenty languages most frequently spoken at home in the United States (Census, 2000)	
Language Spoken at Home	**Number of Speakers**
English Only	198,600,798
Non-English	46,951,595
1. Spanish	28,101,052
2. Chinese	2,022,143
3. French	1,643,838
4. German	1,382,613
5. Tagalog	1,224,241
6. Vietnamese	1,009,627
7. Italian	1,008,370
8. Korean	894,063
9. Russian	706,242
10. Polish	667,414
11. Arabic	614,582
12. Portuguese	564,630
13. Japanese	477,997
14. French Creole	453,368
15. Greek	365,436
16. Hindi	317,057
17. Persian	312,085
18. Urdu	262,900
19. Gujarati	235,988
20. Armenian	202,708

Source: From U.S. Census Bureau. (2003). Language use and English-speaking ability (Census 2000 Brief). Copyright 2003 by U.S. Census Bureau. Reprinted with permission.

in English and tends to be unresponsive to the communication of adults and children in his classroom. The other child, Gabrielle, has lived in central Virginia her whole life. She is African American, speaks the local dialect of African American English, and is one of the more communicative children in her classroom, often persistently asking questions of her teachers and initiating conversations with her peers. The communication skills of these two children are very different. An observer might view JaJuan as having poor communication skills—on the playground, he doesn't understand what others are saying, he doesn't initiate conversations with his peers, and he has a difficult time getting his needs met.

Could we say that JaJuan has a communication disorder? After all, earlier in this chapter, a communication disorder was defined as significant difficulties in formulation, transmission, reception, and/or comprehension. Clearly JaJuan has difficulties in all four of these areas, at least on this English-speaking playground. However, in identifying communication disorders, an individual's communication skills must be significantly discrepant when compared with those of others who have the same language, dialect, and cultural background.

Thus it would be inappropriate to view JaJuan's communication skills as anything more than simply different from those of the children around him.

A communication difference is present when an individual's communication patterns differ substantially from those of the person or persons with whom he or she is communicating. The differences between speakers may be relatively minor, as in the case of people using different dialects of English. Dialects are the variations of a language shared by a particular group of speakers; dialectical variations of a language affect all domains of language, including content, form, and use. In many cases, however, the communication differences among speakers may be significant, particularly when they do not share the same language or when they speak distinct dialects of one language. Having spent a year in a Chinese-speaking country without speaking Chinese, I can attest to the frustration that can result from communication differences. While it would not be appropriate to say that I had a communication disorder during that year in Taiwan, significant communication differences made some daily living activities challenging indeed.

For professionals working in the fields of communication sciences and disorders, understanding the distinction between a communication disorder and a communication difference is not a light matter. Mistaking a communication difference as a disorder has likely contributed to the overrepresentation of children from minority populations, such as Native Americans, among those receiving special education services in U.S. schools (Battle, 2002). Professionals who diagnose or treat communication disorders must study an individual's communication performance within the context of the indigenous culture or language group. A communication disorder is present only when an individual's communication ability

1. operates outside the minimal norms of acceptability of one's culture or language group;
2. is considered disordered by one's culture or language group; and
3. interferes with communication or calls attention to itself within one's culture or language group (Taylor, 1986, p. 13).

CLASSIFICATION OF COMMUNICATION DISORDERS

Language, speech, and hearing are the fundamental elements of spoken communication. A breakdown in any one of these three areas can result in a communication disorder. Communication disorders are generally differentiated into three broad categories: disorders of language, disorders of speech, and hearing loss. An additional category of communication disorder is discussed in this textbook: disorders of feeding and swallowing. Because the feeding and swallowing processes are so intricately tied to the communication system— particularly the areas involved with speech—feeding and swallowing problems are increasingly considered under the communication disorders umbrella. The entire umbrella is presented in Figure 1.9.

Disorders of Language

A language disorder refers to a significant breakdown in the linguistic system that has an impact on one or more of the following domains: semantics, syntax, morphology, phonology, or pragmatics. Language disorders can affect children or adults. Language disorders that significantly compromise reading development are called reading disabilities.

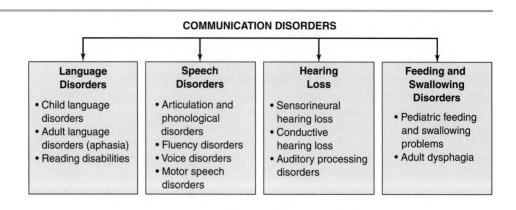

FIGURE 1.9

The communication disorders umbrella.

Child Language Disorders.   Child language disorders are one of the most common disorders of early childhood. Children with language disorders have problems communicating with others because of difficulties in the development of semantics, syntax, morphology, phonology, or pragmatics. Language disorders in children may be developmental or acquired. Developmental disorders are present at or soon after birth, and symptoms are manifested as children develop. Acquired disorders are experienced after birth, usually as a result of an injury. One of the most prevalent types of child language disorders is specific language impairment (SLI), which affects about 7% of children (Tomblin et al., 1997). SLI refers to a significant disorder of language in the absence of any other developmental disability. Language disorders are also common in children who have intellectual disability, autism, and traumatic brain injury. Altogether, about 12% of young children exhibit a language disorder (Johnson, 2007).

Adult Language Disorders.   Adult language disorders comprise a diverse range of developmental (present since birth, e.g., adult SLI) and acquired disorders. Aphasia is a prevalent adult language disorder that results from damage to the brain, particularly the language areas of the left hemisphere. Aphasia is a frequent consequence of stroke, but it can also result from traumatic brain injuries, such as would be caused by a gunshot wound or car accident. Aphasia takes different forms, depending on the location and severity of the brain injury. Some people with aphasia have problems only with complex language tasks, such as reading and writing or following complicated directions, whereas others are unable to produce or understand any language at all. Approximately 80,000 people are diagnosed with aphasia each year. While this disorder can affect adults of any age, the majority of people with aphasia are 65 or older (NIDCD, 2006). Acquired brain injuries, including those resulting from stroke or neurological disease, also can result in general cognitive-based dysfunctions, such as difficulties with remembering, problem-solving, reasoning, and planning. Because of the close anatomical and physiological interrelationships between language and cognition in the human nervous system, the treatment of adult language disorders also typically includes attention to cognitive-based dysfunction.

Reading Disabilities.   Reading disabilities (RD) are types of learning disabilities (LD) in which reading skills are significantly impaired. Severe reading disability, also called *dyslexia,* is among the most common types of LD, affecting approximately 2.2% of school-aged children (U.S. Department of Education, 2002), and many of these children also exhibit writing and spelling problems.

SPOTLIGHT ON LITERACY

Reading Psychology Meets Speech Science

In 2001, the American Speech-Language-Hearing Association (ASHA) broadened the scope of practice of speech-language pathologists to include an explicit focus on reading and writing (ASHA, 2001b) when working with children, adolescents, and adults. The scope of practice as it concerns reading and writing encompasses

- designing and implementing prevention programs (programs designed to reduce children's risks for reading and writing problems),
- identifying children who are at risk for reading and writing problems,
- assessing reading and writing abilities,
- designing and delivering intervention programs devised to address reading and writing problems.

Historically, speech-language pathologists have not taken a direct role in addressing reading and writing problems. Largely, this was due to limited knowledge of the role that language plays in the reading process, as understanding of the reading process through the 1960s and 1970s primarily focused on the visual processes involved. One of the more important advances in our knowledge of the linguistic processes involved in reading occurred in the 1960s at Haskins Laboratories by Isabelle and Alvin Liberman. A reading psychologist and speech scientist, respectively, the Libermans were among the first scientists to emphasize the important role that phonemic awareness plays in the reading process.

Phonemic awareness, considered an oral language skill, refers to the awareness of the individual speech sounds that make up syllables and words (e.g., the three sounds comprising the word *soap*— /s/ + /o/ + /p/). This awareness provides an important scaffold to a child's learning of the systematic letter-sound correspondences that are essential to understanding the alphabetic principle (e.g., that the letter S corresponds to the sound "s"). The Libermans' research and that of others showed that achieving phonemic awareness is a necessary precursor to becoming a skilled reader. This discovery also made it clear that reading development involves language skills.

The Libermans' work was essential for igniting a great body of scientific work extending from the 1970s to the present and for creating a better understanding of the relationships among specific language, reading, and writing abilities. Indeed, we might view the 2001 ASHA enhancement to the scope of practice of speech-language pathologists to include a focus on reading and writing as a direct result of the Libermans' research.

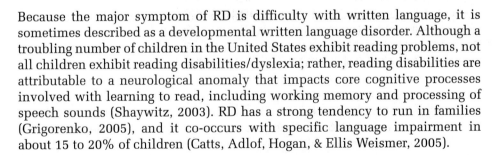

Because the major symptom of RD is difficulty with written language, it is sometimes described as a developmental written language disorder. Although a troubling number of children in the United States exhibit reading problems, not all children exhibit reading disabilities/dyslexia; rather, reading disabilities are attributable to a neurological anomaly that impacts core cognitive processes involved with learning to read, including working memory and processing of speech sounds (Shaywitz, 2003). RD has a strong tendency to run in families (Grigorenko, 2005), and it co-occurs with specific language impairment in about 15 to 20% of children (Catts, Adlof, Hogan, & Ellis Weismer, 2005).

Disorders of Speech

A speech disorder refers to a breakdown in one or more of the systems involved with speech production: respiration, phonation, and articulation.

Articulation and Phonological Disorders. Articulation and phonological disorders are speech-production impairments characterized by distortions, substitutions, and omissions of speech sounds. Speech-production impairments are most common in young children, affecting about 10% of youngsters (Gierut, 1998). An articulation or phonological impairment is present when a child fails to use speech sounds at a level appropriate for their age and cultural and linguistic background.

Disorders of articulation occur at the site of speech output, shown in the speech-production model in Figure 1.6, and are usually attributed to some sort of structural problem or problem with articulatory placement. Articulation disorders are a common consequence of cleft palate, which is a congenital malformation of the lip and/or palate. Disorders of phonology occur at the site of the perceptual representation of speech sounds (see Figure 1.6), resulting in underdeveloped or faulty representations of speech sounds, which undermines production of those sounds. Although the point of breakdown differs in these two varieties of speech disorders, the manifestation is similar in that the child has difficulties with the production of speech sounds. Technically, phonological disorders are best viewed as disorders of language, but because the disorder is evidenced as a problem with speech sound production, they are typically viewed under the umbrella of speech disorders.

Fluency Disorders. Communication difficulties that are characterized by an abnormally high rate or duration of breaks in the continuity of producing spoken language are referred to as *fluency disorders* (ASHA, 1999). Their most common characteristics are repetition and prolongation of sounds and complete blockages of airflow, usually accompanied by body movements (e.g., head nods, blinking) in an attempt to stop or reduce these disfluencies. As might be expected, many people with disorders of fluency have tense, negative feelings about speaking. Many young children go through a stage of normal dysfluency, which should be differentiated from true fluency disorders. Current estimates of the incidence of stuttering come from an examination of stuttering among the entire population of children on the Danish island of Bornhold born over a 2-year period (Månsson, 2000). This study found that about 5% of children (51 out of 1,021) exhibited stuttering at age 3 years, and the majority of these children (71%) resolved their stuttering by the age of 5 years. At age 5, only 15 children (1.4%) were stuttering, and at 8 to 9 years, 0.8% of children were stuttering. These findings show that stuttering affects a relatively large percentage of children in the early years, yet the number of children who will exhibit persistent stuttering is actually quite small.

Voice Disorders. Communication difficulties characterized by difficulties with the voice are voice disorders. An underlying difficulty with voice production usually manifests itself as either a complete lack of voice (aphonia) or a hoarse voice (dysphonia). Aphonia and dysphonia affect nearly everyone at some point, as they can result from illness or isolated overuse of the voice (e.g., cheering at a football game). However, chronic aphonia or dysphonia due to ongoing overuse or misuse of the voice or that results from an underlying pathology, such as cancer of the vocal folds, can seriously affect one's life.

Severe voice disorders, including a complete lack of voice, can result from injuries or illnesses to the vocal folds or the surrounding tissues or organs. One of the most common reasons for a complete loss of voice is laryngeal cancer. The larynx is the cartilaginous container that holds the vocal folds. The vocal folds vibrate to produce voice. Cancer of the vocal folds, a risk for smokers, particularly older men, may necessitate surgery to remove vocal fold growths or, in some cases, to remove the larynx. In such cases, a loss of voice is the trade-off for survival.

Motor Speech Disorders. Like the speech-production impairments previously described, motor speech disorders are communication disorders characterized

SPOTLIGHT ON TECHNOLOGY

Real-Time Spectrograms

A spectrogram is a three-dimensional representation of the speech signal (or any other sound). The three dimensions are time (horizontal axis), frequency (pitch, on the vertical axis), and intensity (loudness, represented in coloring). A real-time spectrogram shows changes in time, frequency, and intensity as the speech signal unfolds over a period of time. Spectrograms are used for a range of clinical applications. For instance, clinicians might use it as a way to document pre- and postintervention speech characteristics for clients, or they might use them as visual aids to train clients to use their voice in certain ways (Ertmer, 2004).

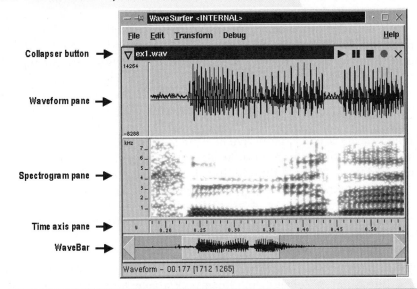

Source: From WaveSurfer User Manual. Retrieved February 10, 2008, from www.speech.kth.se/wavesurfer/man.html. Copyright 2006 by Kåre Sjölander and Jonas Beskow. Reprinted with permission.

FIGURE 1.10

Historically, the clinical use of spectrograms has required expensive and highly specialized software and hardware technologies (McGuire, Lorang, & Hoffman, 2006). However, in this age of technology, with personal computers typically featuring relatively good digital sound capabilities, an increasing number of low-cost and no-cost options are available for conducting spectrographic analysis. For example, WaveSurfer is a free open-source software download available at no cost from the Centre for Speech Technology at KTH in Sweden (www.speech.kth.se/wavesurfer/). Figure 1.10 depicts a spectrogram generated with the WaveSurfer software; note that the middle pane is the spectrogram. (The upper pane and lower pane present basic waveforms.) Additional options for no-cost software downloads permitting spectrographic analyses include the Speech Filing Systems at the University College London's Department of Phonetics and Linguistics (www.phon.ucl.ac.uk/resource/software.html) and PRAAT from the Institute of Phonetic Sciences at the University of Amsterdam (www.phon.ucl.ac.uk/resource/software.html).

by distortions, substitutions, and omissions of speech sounds. However, with motor speech disorders, the pathology is attributed to a dysfunction with the nervous system that controls motor output of the speech stream. Motor speech disorders are also often referred to as *neurogenic speech disorders* to emphasize their neurological underpinnings. There are two major types of motor speech disorders, apraxia and dysarthria, both of which affect children and adults.

DISCUSSION POINT:
Hearing loss can impact the quality of one's voice. Study the video clips of Ashley (Study 3) and discuss how hearing loss has impacted the quality of her voice.

Hearing Loss

Hearing loss occurs when there is a breakdown in the reception or transmission of sound along the auditory pathways traveling from the ear to the brain. Hearing loss can be present at birth or acquired sometime thereafter. When loss occurs (e.g., early in life vs. during adulthood) impacts on how it is identified and treated. Therefore, in this text, we discuss hearing loss in pediatric populations and hearing loss in adults separately.

Sensorineural Hearing Loss.   Sensorineural hearing loss refers to a breakdown in the hearing system in the inner ear or in the auditory nerve that runs from the inner ear to the brain centers. Sensorineural hearing loss can be congenital (present at birth) or acquired, as in the case of noise-induced hearing loss, in which the hair cells of the inner ear are damaged and become less sensitive to sound. Sensorineural hearing loss can range from mild, requiring no or minimal treatment, to profound. Cochlear implants are a late-twentieth-century cutting-edge treatment used to enhance or restore hearing ability in people with profound sensorineural loss, also referred to as *deafness.*

DISCUSSION POINT:

Consider the case of Jan Shen presented in Case Study 1.1. Is Mr. Shen's hearing loss conductive or sensorineural? What is the difference between the two types?

Conductive Hearing Loss.   Conductive hearing loss describes a breakdown in the hearing system in the outer or middle ear. Malformation of the outer ear, a torn eardrum, and the buildup of fluid in the middle ear (associated with middle-ear infections) are common causes of conductive hearing loss, particularly in children. Middle-ear infections, or otitis media, are increasingly common in young children. One study conducted with 2,253 infants in Pittsburgh found that 91% of children experienced otitis media between birth and 2 years of age (Paradise et al., 1999). Chronic otitis media during the first few years of life has been linked (although not definitively) to delays in communication development (Roberts, Burchinal, & Zeisel, 2002; Roberts, Wallace, & Henderson, 1997).

Auditory Processing Disorder.   An auditory processing disorder (APD) is a breakdown in the processing of speech sounds in the auditory center in the brain. This center is responsible for localizing sounds, discriminating sounds, and recognizing auditory patterns. Auditory processing disorders have been linked to specific nervous system disorders, such as Alzheimer's disease; however, in many cases, no neuropathology can be identified (ASHA, 2005a). Symptoms of APD overlap with those of other learning and attentional difficulties, making it challenging to accurately diagnose this disorder. Symptoms include difficulty paying attention, poor listening skills, difficulty following multistep directions, slow processing time, and impaired language and literacy development (ASHA, 2005a).

Disorders of Feeding and Swallowing

Feeding and swallowing problems are considered within the spectrum of communication disorders because of the functional overlap of the neurological systems that control feeding and swallowing functions and those that control communication. Historically, the treatment of feeding and swallowing problems has received little attention. Traditional treatment for children and adults who could not eat or swallow focused on bypassing the feeding/swallowing systems (e.g., putting the person on a feeding tube) with little attempt to improve or restore feeding and swallowing. The recognition that the ability to eat and drink is a critical aspect of quality of life for people of all ages has brought changes in the last two decades, and there has been significant progress in the design and delivery of treatments focused on improving or restoring feeding and swallowing functions.

Pediatric Feeding and Swallowing Problems.   Pediatric feeding and swallowing problems tend to be associated with specific developmental disorders, such as cleft palate or cerebral palsy, and prematurity or low birth weight. In addition to undermining the child's growth and development, feeding and swallowing disorders may bring adverse behavioral reactions to feeding and may compromise the caregiver–child relationship. Children with structural impairments, such as cleft palate, may not be able to feed or to swallow because of lip or palate malformations. Children with neurological impairments, as in the case of cerebral palsy, may not be able to manage the precise motor control needed to feed and to swallow. Children who are born prematurely or who are of a low birth weight may not have the neurological maturity to handle the complexities of the feeding/swallowing process. Children with chronic reflux, or regurgitation of stomach acids into the oral cavities, may resist eating altogether. Pediatric feeding and swallowing problems can also result from traumatic events, such as brain injuries, stroke, and infections (Arvedson & Rogers, 1997). When children are unable to feed or swallow, it is critical that their nutritional needs be met in other ways. One common method is tube feeding, as when a nasogastric tube is run through the nose down into the stomach. It is important to provide therapies to children who are being tube fed to promote feeding and swallowing skills so that they can later be transitioned to oral means of nutrition.

Adult Dysphagia.   Dysphagia refers to a swallowing disorder. Often the result of a nervous system dysfunction, such as that resulting from stroke or a progressive ailment like Alzheimer's disease, dysphagia experienced among adults includes such problems as difficulty with chewing or managing food orally and difficulty with triggering or maintaining a swallow. Symptoms of these difficulties include choking and coughing while eating, repetitive swallows or throat clearing, regurgitation of food after eating, pain while swallowing, loss of weight or energy, and change in appetite (Schulze-Delrieu & Miller, 1997). Swallowing problems should always be treated quickly and aggressively, as people with dysphagia are at risk for choking and for malnourishment, both of which can have fatal consequences.

> **DISCUSSION POINT:**
> Consider the case of Anika presented in Case Study 1-1. Why was Anika placed on a feeding tube? How did its use influence her oral activity?

WHAT CAREERS ARE AVAILABLE IN THE FIELD OF COMMUNICATION SCIENCES AND DISORDERS? ⬤

As a broad discipline that brings together psychology, education, health, technology, and linguistics, the field of communication science and disorders attracts many people from diverse backgrounds. The disciplines most closely aligned with the study and treatment of communication disorders are speech-language pathology and audiology. Within these disciplines, specialization is available in many areas, among them speech science, hearing science, multicultural issues, geriatrics, child language, phonology, and neurogenics. Increasingly, treatment of communication disorders involves a multidisciplinary, team-based approach involving many educational, medical, and allied health professionals, such as special educators, pediatricians, occupational therapists, physical therapists, and nurses. A foundation in communication sciences and disorders will be advantageous to many career paths.

SPEECH-LANGUAGE PATHOLOGY

Speech-language pathologists, or SLPs, are frequently the lead service providers for people with speech and language disorders and are also key members of the treatment team for people with hearing, swallowing, and feeding disorders. The scope of practice for speech-language pathologists is presented in Figure 1.11. These professionals have diverse responsibilities, from evaluating infant feeding and swallowing problems to identifying alternative communication techniques

---

FIGURE 1.11

Scope of practice for speech-language pathology.

Professional Roles and Activities

Speech-language pathologists serve individuals, families, and groups from diverse linguistic and cultural backgrounds. Services are provided based on applying the best available research evidence, using expert clinical judgments, and considering clients' individual preferences and values. Speech-language pathologists address typical and atypical communication and swallowing in the following areas:

- Speech sound production
- Resonance
- Voice
- Fluency
- Language (comprehension and expression)
- Cognition
- Feeding and swallowing

Clinical Services

Speech-language pathologists provide clinical services that include the following:

- Prevention and prereferral
- Screening
- Assessment/evaluation
- Consultation
- Diagnosis
- Treatment, intervention, management
- Counseling
- Collaboration
- Documentation
- Referral

Examples of these clinical services include

1. using data to guide clinical decision making and determine the effectiveness of services;
2. making service delivery decisions (e.g., admission/eligibility, frequency, duration, location, discharge/dismissal) across the life span;
3. determining appropriate context(s) for service delivery (e.g., home, school, telepractice, community);
4. documenting provision of services in accordance with accepted procedures appropriate for the practice setting;
5. collaborating with other professionals (e.g., identifying neonates and infants at risk for hearing loss, participating in palliative care teams, planning lessons with educators, serving on student-assistance teams);
6. screening individuals for hearing loss or middle-ear pathology using conventional pure-tone air-conduction methods (including otoscopic inspection), otoacoustic emissions screening, and/or screening tympanometry;

7. providing intervention and support services for children and adults diagnosed with speech and language disorders;
8. providing intervention and support services for children and adults diagnosed with auditory processing disorders;
9. using instrumentation (e.g., videofluoroscopy, electromyography, nasendoscopy, stroboscopy, endoscopy, nasometry, computer technology) to observe, collect data, and measure parameters of communication and swallowing or other upper-aerodigestive functions;
10. counseling individuals, families, coworkers, educators, and other persons in the community regarding acceptance, adaptation, and decision making about communication and swallowing.

Source: Excerpts from *Scope of practice in speech-language pathology* [Scope of Practice] (2007a), published by the American Speech and Hearing Association (ASHA), are reprinted by permission. Readers are directed to the ASHA website (www.asha.org) to access the position statement (and any updates) in its entirety.

for people who have severe communicative difficulties. Speech-language pathology assistants (SLPAs) are paraprofessionals who work under the supervision of SLPs to conduct speech-language screenings, assist in assessment, and implement treatment plans with clients. The roles and responsibilities of SLPAs, as well as training avenues, are still evolving, and the extent to which SLPAs are involved in speech-language services can vary significantly across states.

Employment Contexts

Speech-language pathologists work in a variety of settings, including public and private schools, hospitals, rehabilitation facilities, home health agencies, community and university clinics, private practices, group homes, state agencies, universities, and corporations (ASHA, 2007a). Currently more than 110,000 speech-language pathologists in the United States are certified by the American Speech-Language-Hearing Association (ASHA), yet there remains a significant shortage of speech-language pathologists in most regions of North America. Reports from the U.S. Bureau of Labor Statistics describe the job outlook for speech-language pathologists as "excellent" with anticipated growth of 11% from 2006–2016 (U.S. Bureau of Labor Statistics, 2008). Reasons for the continued growth of this profession include (1) an increased awareness of the importance of early intervention, (2) greater success in life-saving measures for children born with significant health impairments, (3) the aging of the U.S. population, (4) an increased awareness of health promotion and disease prevention, (5) a nationwide increase in implementation of newborn hearing-screening measures, and (6) the passage of federal laws focused on improving the rights and addressing the needs of people with disabilities (e.g., Individuals with Disability Education Act, Medicare, and Medicaid). In addition, there is great demand for doctoral-level speech-language pathologists to fulfill university research and teaching positions in part because of the overall growth of the profession and in part because of the retirement of baby boomers holding faculty positions.

Employment benefits, including overall job satisfaction as well as compensation, are high for speech-language pathologists. The median annual salary for speech-language pathologists in 2006 was about $58,000, with the middle 50% of speech-language pathologists earning between $46,000 and $72,000 annually (U.S. Bureau of Labor Statistics, 2008). Those working in nursing care facilities reported the highest annual earnings (average of $70,180), whereas those working in schools reported the lowest annual earnings (average of $53,110), although the latter figures likely represent a 10-month work year (U. S. Bureau of Labor Statistics, 2008). In a recent survey of more than 500 speech-language pathologists, the majority reported high satisfaction with their work and low overall job stress levels (Blood, Thomas, Ridenour, Qualls, & Hammer, 2002). On the other hand, like many other professionals in the education and health disciplines, SLPs currently face many challenges in effectively executing their jobs. In education, some SLPs encounter inappropriately high caseloads, excessive paperwork, isolation from other professionals, lack of support for collaboration, inadequate access to up-to-date materials, and the like. In health care, SLPs have many of the same challenges, compounded by constantly changing federal and state regulations regarding reimbursement for therapies. To address these challenges, speech-language pathologists organize themselves through state-level associations, such as the Speech and Hearing Association of Virginia (SHAV), and national organizations, such as the American Speech-Language-Hearing Association (ASHA), to lobby for improved working conditions.

Credentials

The entry-level credential for a speech-language pathologist (SLP) is a master's degree from an ASHA-accredited training program. The degree typically requires completion of a 2-year postbaccalaureate specialized program involving intensive training in diagnosis and treatment of speech, language, and swallowing disorders. At least 36 semester hours of graduate-level coursework are required, as well as 400 hours of supervised clinical fieldwork. Of these 400 hours, 375 must involve direct contact with clients/patients. Accredited graduate programs typically offer a systematic scope and sequence of graduate-level courses designed to ensure that students meet a comprehensive set of knowledge and skills (KASA:

FIGURE 1.12

So you want to become a certified speech-language pathologist or audiologist? Here's how.

Adapted from: American Speech-Language-Hearing Association (2005b, 2007a, 2007b).

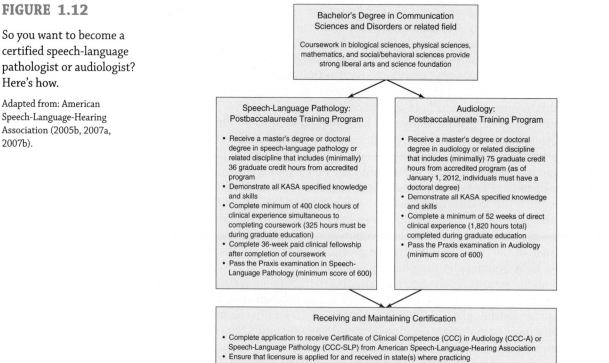

Knowledge and Skills Acquisition Standards) required to achieve certification in speech-language pathology by ASHA. This includes knowledge of ethics as well as evidence-based practice. For national certification, SLPs must pass a national examination in speech-language pathology and complete a supervised 9-month clinical fellowship. Figure 1.12 presents the steps for clinical certification by ASHA. The entry-level credential for a research or faculty-level position in speech-language pathology is typically a research doctorate (Ph.D.) in speech and hearing sciences, speech-language pathology, or a related field (e.g., psychology).

AUDIOLOGY

Audiologists are specialists in identifying, assessing, and managing disorders of the auditory, balance, and other neural systems (ASHA, 2007b). Primary roles involve prevention, identification, and management of hearing and balance system dysfunction. The scope of practice for audiologists is presented in Figure 1.13. These professionals work closely with SLPs when hearing affects an individual's communicative ability.

FIGURE 1.13

Scope of practice in audiology: Professional roles and activities.

Audiologists serve a diverse population and may function in one or more of a variety of activities. The practice of audiology includes the following:

A. Prevention
   Example activity: Promotion of hearing wellness and the prevention of hearing loss and protection of hearing function by designing, implementing, and coordinating occupational, school, and community hearing conservation and identification programs
B. Identification
   Example activity: Identification of populations and individuals with, or at risk for, hearing loss and other auditory dysfunction, balance impairments, tinnitus, and associated communication impairments as well as of those with normal hearing
C. Assessment
   Example activity: The conduct and interpretation of behavioral, electroacoustic, and/or electrophysiologic methods to assess hearing, auditory function, balance, and related systems
D. Rehabilitation
   Example activity: Provision of comprehensive audiologic rehabilitation services, including management procedures for speech and language habilitation and/or rehabilitation for persons with hearing loss or other auditory dysfunction, including but not exclusive to speechreading, auditory training, communication strategies, manual communication, and counseling for psychosocial adjustment for persons with hearing loss or other auditory dysfunction and their families/caregivers
E. Advocacy/Consultation
   Example activity: Consultation in development of an Individual Education Program (IEP) for school-age children or an Individual Family Service Plan (IFSP) for children from birth to 36 months old
F. Education/ Research/Administration
   Example activity: Education, supervision, and administration for audiology graduate and other professional education programs

Source: Excerpts from *Scope of practice in audiology* [Scope of Practice] (2004a, 2007b), published by the American Speech and Hearing Association (ASHA), are reprinted by permission. Readers are directed to the ASHA website (www.asha.org) to access the Position Statement (and any updates) in its entirety.

Employment Contexts

Audiologists work in many of the same settings as speech-language pathologists, including schools, hospitals, rehabilitation facilities, community and university clinics, private practices, and universities (ASHA, 2007b). There are more than 12,000 audiologists currently working in the United States.

For the first decade of the twenty-first century, the occupational outlook for audiology is strong, and job prospects are favorable, particularly for those with the clinical doctorate (Doctor of Audiology/Au.D.) (U.S. Bureau of Labor Statistics, 2008).

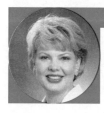

SPOTLIGHT ON RESEARCH AND PRACTICE

Name: Ann W. Kummer, PhD, CCC-SLP, ASHA-F

Profession/Title

Senior Director of Speech Pathology, Cincinnati Children's Hospital Medical Center and

Professor of Clinical Pediatrics, University of Cincinnati Medical Center

Professional Responsibilities

I have a job that involves all four of my interests: management, teaching, research, and clinical services. I manage a large department of over 120 people who provide services at 11 locations. Our program includes inpatient, outpatient, rehabilitation, and home care. We serve 19 interdisciplinary programs and have a variety of specialty teams. I also present regular lectures within the medical center and travel to do seminars on cleft palate and craniofacial anomalies. I occasionally have a research study on my own, but more frequently, I supervise graduate students in their research endeavors. Finally, I see patients through our Craniofacial Anomaly Team and Velopharyngeal Insufficiency Clinic.

A Day at Work

One thing that I like about my job is that no two days are exactly alike. A day at work can include several meetings regarding our "business" or one of our programs. I might meet with a few staff members or spend time working on our strategic plan. Many days, I see patients in clinic, or I do a lecture.

Academic Degrees/Training

1986	PhD University of Cincinnati
1973	MAT Indiana University
1972	BA Indiana University

How Interests in Communication Sciences and Disorders Began

My dad was an otolaryngologist. When I was in high school, I worked in his office on Saturdays and in the summers. I noticed that he referred many of his patients to a speech pathologist, so I decided to check out the field. After one observation, I was hooked.

Current Research and Practice Interests

My clinical and research interests are in the areas of cleft palate, craniofacial anomalies, and velopharyngeal dysfunction. I am also very interested in leadership and business practices.

Most Exciting/Interesting Professional Accomplishment in CSD

Completing a textbook has given me gratification in sharing what I've learned with others. It's also nice to know that when I die, at least some of the knowledge in my brain will be preserved for others to use. The development of a large, well-respected speech-pathology department has also been gratifying. It's fun to create programs, lead innovative projects, and nurture staff in their professional growth.

Future Trends in CSD

I think that the demand for our services will continue to grow. My concern is that if we do not actively educate consumers in the value of our services, funding and reimbursement can be affected in future.

A 10% increase in jobs is anticipated from 2006 to 2016. The reasons for this growth include advances in hearing technologies as well as the involvement of audiologists in providing services to a rapidly increasing older population.

The median annual salary for audiologists in 2006 was about $57,120, with a salary range of about $38,000 to $90,000 (U.S. Bureau of Labor Statistics, 2008). There is currently a shortage of practitioners and researchers in the audiology field. Like SLPs, audiologists also face challenges in the current health care climate, in which professionals are asked to do more with less, and regulations governing reimbursement change frequently. Audiologists advocate for their profession through their affiliation with state-level and national organizations, including the American Academy of Audiology (AAA, or Triple A) and ASHA.

Credentials

The entry-level credential for a clinical audiologist is a master's degree from an ASHA-accredited graduate training program. The steps for becoming a certified audiologist are presented in Figure 1.12. The requirements for becoming a certified audiologist have recently changed, most noticeably with the requirement that individuals applying for certification after January 1, 2012, have a doctoral degree. To achieve certification, individuals need 75 postbaccalaureate semester credit hours as well as the equivalent of 12 months full-time supervised clinical practicum. A number of Au.D. (doctor of audiology) programs have been developed across the United States to address these shifts in graduate training requirements and to replace the traditional master's degree in audiology. Largely, this doctorate is designed to be clinical in nature, similar to clinical doctorates available in other disciplines (e.g., Pharm.D. in pharmacy, N.D. in nursing). For individuals seeking to conduct primarily research or to serve in faculty-level positions in university audiology programs, the traditional research doctorate (Ph.D.) in speech and hearing sciences or audiology typically serves as the entry-level credential.

ALLIED PROFESSIONS

Key partners in the assessment and treatment of communication disorders include special educators and many medical and allied health professionals, such as neurologists, occupational therapists, otorhinolaryngologists, pediatricians, and psychologists. Although the diagnosis and treatment of a communication disorder is usually the primary responsibility of speech-language pathologists and audiologists, these additional players have critical roles.

Special Educators

Special educators support the educational progress of children with communication disorders and often work closely with speech-language pathologists and audiologists. There are nearly 500,000 special educators in U.S. schools (U.S. Bureau of Labor Statistics, 2008). Serving primarily in public and private educational settings, special educators worked with nearly 6 million students in the year 2000 (Individuals with Disabilities Education Act [IDEA] Data, 2006). Early childhood special educators typically work with children who are 3 to 5 years of age, whereas special educators work with those between 6 and 21 years of age and tend to specialize in a particular area (e.g., learning disabilities or behavioral disorders). More than 1.3 million 3- to 21-year-old children in U.S. public schools were identified as requiring speech-language services in 2000 (IDEA Data, 2006). Special educators are critical team members in designing special services for these children and in coordinating service delivery with parents, regular educators, and specialists. Special educators often collaborate with speech-language pathologists and other educators on eligibility, program, and placement decisions for students with communication disorders (Council for Exceptional Children, 2001). In working with families of children with communication disorders, special educators are often involved with activities associated with behavior management; career, vocational, and transitional planning; technology utilization; and promotion of independent living and community participation.

The field of special education is rapidly growing. In the next 10 years, growth will average about 15%, with the largest growth typically among those special educators who work with younger children (preschool to elementary grades). Licensure for special educators varies by state. The minimal requirement is typically a bachelor's degree from an accredited program, which involves specialized coursework in the characteristics of learners, individual learning differences, strategies for individualizing instruction, typical and atypical communication development, assessment, instructional planning, and collaboration. Almost 50% of special educators hold a graduate degree, and the majority are specially certified for their specific assignment (Boyer & Mainzer, 2003).

Occupational Therapists

Occupational therapists (OTs) deliver interventions to help people with disabilities, illnesses, or injuries develop or regain the activities of daily living (ADL), such as grooming, eating, and writing. OTs often work closely with infants, toddlers, and elderly people who are experiencing problems with feeding and swallowing. There are presently about 100,000 occupational therapists working in the United States, most in hospital settings. The employment outlook for these professionals is strong, with about 20% growth in the number of positions anticipated for the next decade (U.S. Bureau of Labor Statistics, 2008).

Otorhinolaryngologists

Otorhinolaryngologists, or ear-nose-throat physicians (ENTs), collaborate with speech-language pathologists and audiologists in the diagnosis and management of communication disorders. ENTs work closely with people who have injury or illness of the ear, nose, or throat, performing surgery, prescribing medication, and conducting diagnostic investigations.

Neurologists

Neurologists help to identify the etiology of many communication disorders, particularly those involving nervous system dysfunction, such as autism, cerebral palsy, stroke, Alzheimer's disease, and Parkinson's disease.

Pediatricians

Pediatricians play an important role in early identification and ongoing treatment of communication disorders in children of all ages. Pediatricians, in collaboration with parents, provide referrals to speech-language pathologists and audiologists for speech, language, feeding, swallowing, and hearing assessments when warning signs are present.

DISCUSSION POINT:
Consider the cases of Anika and Mr. Shen presented in Case Study 1.1. What is the role of the speech-language pathologist and audiologist in each of these cases?

Psychologists

Psychologists are often involved in the evaluation and treatment of people with communication disorders, particularly when educational, behavioral, and emotional complications exist. Psychologists may complete diagnostic evaluations to include speech-language assessment and can help families cope with the challenges associated with communicative impairments.

CHAPTER SUMMARY

Communication is the sharing of information between two or more people. Humans communicate to achieve instrumental, regulatory, personal, heuristic, imaginative, and informative purposes. An effective communicator uses communication for these diverse purposes and is able to avoid communication breakdowns by providing and attending to feedback during the communication process.

Language, speech, and hearing are the essential ingredients of communication. Language is a socially shared, rule-governed symbol system used by humans to represent ideas about the world. Five domains of language include semantics, syntax, morphology, phonology, and pragmatics. Speech is a complex neuromuscular process that turns language into a sound medium that is transmitted to another person. Speech involves a three-stage process: conceptualization of a perceptual target, development of a motor schema, and speech output. Hearing is the perception of sound, and when applied to the communication process, refers specifically to the perception of speech. The acoustic process involves the creation of a sound source, the vibration of air particles, reception by the ear, and comprehension by the brain.

Significant, ongoing communication breakdowns may signal a communication disorder. Communication disorders are differentiated as language disorders (child language disorders, adult language disorders, reading disabilities), speech disorders (articulation and phonology disorders, fluency disorders, voice disorders, motor speech disorders), hearing disorders (sensorineural hearing loss, conductive hearing loss, auditory processing disorders), and feeding and swallowing disorders (pediatric feeding and swallowing disorders, adult dysphagia).

The primary professionals who work with people who have communication disorders are speech-language pathologists and audiologists, both of whom are certified by the American Speech-Language-Hearing Association. Special educators, medical professionals, and members of the allied health professions also play key roles in diagnosis and remediation of communication disorders.

KEY TERMS

acoustics, p. 19
audition, p. 19
communication, p. 5
communication breakdown, p. 7
communication functions, p. 7
comprehension, p. 5
content, p. 13
extralinguistic feedback, p. 6
feedback, p. 6
form, p. 13
formulation, p. 5

frequency, p. 20
Grice's maxims, p. 8
intensity, p. 20
linguistic feedback, p. 6
metalinguistic awareness, p. 15
modality, p. 5
morphology, p. 14
nonlinguistic feedback, p. 6
paralinguistic feedback, p. 6
phoneme, p. 17
phonology, p. 14

pragmatics, p. 15
productivity, p. 12
reception, p. 5
semanticity, p. 12
semantics, p. 13
species specificity, p. 11
speech perception, p. 20
syntax, p. 13
transmission, p. 5
universality, p. 11
use, p. 13

ON THE WEB

Check out the Companion Website at www
.pearsonhighered.com/justice2e! On it, you will
find the following:

• Suggested readings
• Reflection questions

• A self-study quiz
• Additional cases
• Links to additional online resources, including information about current technologies in communication sciences and disorders

AN OVERVIEW OF COMMUNICATION DEVELOPMENT

Khara L. Pence Turnbull, Ph.D.

FOCUS QUESTIONS

This chapter answers the following questions:

1. What is communicative competence?

2. What is the foundation for communicative competence?

3. What are major communicative milestones in infancy and toddlerhood?

4. What are major communicative milestones in preschool and school-age children?

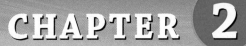

CHAPTER 2

INTRODUCTION

Before we learn more about disorders of communication, it is important to first understand how communication abilities typically develop. This chapter provides an overview of communication development in typical populations. It defines communicative competence, describes the foundation for communicative competence, details some of the major milestones in language and speech development that take place between birth and adolescence, and considers some important multicultural issues relevant to language and speech development. As you read this chapter, think about the development of communicative competence in some of the people you know—your children, nieces and nephews, brothers and sisters, or children you see on a regular basis. After reading this chapter, you may be surprised by the many capabilities we possess at birth, and you will gain a deeper appreciation for the rapid pace of communicative development and the qualitative differences in communication skills that humans exhibit at various stages across the life span. ●●●

WHAT IS COMMUNICATIVE COMPETENCE? ●

DEFINITION

Communicative competence is the knowledge and implicit awareness that speakers of a language possess and utilize to communicate effectively in that language. Communicative competence entails much more than speaking in grammatically well-formed sentences; it is the speaker's skilled navigation of both linguistic and pragmatic elements of language that enable them to communicate successfully with other members of their speech community (Hymes, 2001). A speaker with communicative competence knows how, where, when, and with whom to speak in a global sense.

Communicative competence should be distinguished from **communicative performance,** which describes a speaker's *actual* speech behavior. Some people may associate the term *communicative performance* with *performance errors.* Although we tend to ignore our own performance errors and those of others, speakers routinely pause, stutter, repeat words, repair words and sentences, swap sounds from one word to another, and make slips of the tongue. By some accounts, we make performance blunders about once for every ten words we speak (Erard, 2007). It is important to note that speakers can demonstrate communicative competence even when they make performance errors. In fact, you would be hard pressed to find a speaker with flawless communicative performance!

DISCUSSION POINT:
Think about the infant-directed speech that you have heard others use. How does infant-directed speech differ from the speech you use with your friends?

To further demonstrate the meaning of communicative competence, consider, for example, how a speaker carefully modifies his or her vocabulary choices, sentence structure, pitch, volume, and body posture to simplify speech for an infant: "Addie go bye-bye!" Consider how this speech differs from speech to a peer: "Are you planning on taking Adelaide with you to the picnic?" The former is an example of infant-directed speech, or the speech that we use when addressing young language learners, and it illustrates how communicative competence does not necessarily equate to using grammatically well-formed sentences. Instead, communicative competence allows a speaker to fine-tune language across different contexts and with different speakers to communicate most effectively.

CASE STUDY 2.1   Communication Disorders Across the Life Span

LA'KORI is a 2-year-old boy whose mother, Angie, works in a daycare center. (You can meet La'Kori on the companion CD-ROM, Study 5.) Angie has noticed that at 2 years of age, La'Kori is not saying as many different words as some of the other young children his age at the daycare center. He has been using the words *mommy, daddy, eat,* and *cup,* but he hasn't been using words for other common objects, such as *juice, blocks,* or *doll,* nor has he been combining multiple words into sentences. Angie is becoming concerned that La'Kori's language is developing more slowly than that of his peers. On a visit to the hospital when La'Kori is ill, Angie makes a point to speak with the doctor about her concern that La'Kori is not using as many words as she thinks he should be at his age. Angie also talks with a friend, who is a speech-language pathologist, to determine whether there is anything she can do to help with La'Kori's language development and whether he might be a "late talker."

Internet research

1 See what sources are available on the Internet concerning language milestones in young children. Evaluate the reputability of the resources you find.

2 Use the Internet to see what you can find out about strategies that parents might use to help children who could be late talkers. What are some common strategies suggested?

Brainstorm and discussion

1 What are some possible reasons for why La'Kori might not be saying as many words as the other children his age?

2 Because word use is only one of several aspects of a child's language development, what other areas might a doctor or speech-language pathologist talk about with Angie in regard to La'Kori's language to better understand her concerns?

● ● ●

RESTON is an 8-year-old boy who has struggled with speech and language development since he was a toddler. He is currently in the third grade at a public elementary school in northern Virginia. He receives speech and language therapy at his school for a language disorder, and he works with the learning disabilities specialist to help him with reading and writing. Reston still has difficulty recognizing how combinations of letters correspond to certain sounds in English. For example, he tries to decode, or sound out, words such as *weigh* and *neighbor.* Reston also struggles with reading sentences fluently, because he devotes so much of his attention to sounding out words. Reston's parents are concerned, because at the end of the year, Reston will be required to take the third-grade state-mandated achievement test. They do not think he will pass; moreover, they do not think he should have to take the test. Reston's parents are organizing a parent meeting at the school to discuss what they call "high-stakes testing" and whether it is appropriate for third graders in general and for those with disabilities.

Internet research

1. What is a third-grade state-mandated achievement test?

2. Do all students have to take state-mandated achievement tests?

3. Why are these tests called "high-stakes tests"?

Brainstorm and discussion

1. Should all students in public schools be required to take state-mandated achievement tests? Why or why not?

2. Should their tests be modified for students with disabilities? If so, what kinds of modifications would be appropriate?

Recall from Chapter 1 that successful communication requires a sender to formulate and transmit a message and a receiver to take in and comprehend the message in the context of four communication processes (formulation, transmission, reception, and comprehension). Two aspects of communicative competence—linguistic and pragmatic—enable humans to engage successfully in all four of these communication processes. Figure 2.1 provides a description of the different types of linguistic and pragmatic competencies that provide for successful communication.

Linguistic Aspects of Communicative Competence

Linguistic aspects of communicative competence relate to the nature and structure of language and include phonological competence, grammatical competence, lexical competence, and discourse competence.

Phonological Competence. Phonological competence is the ability to recognize and produce the distinctive, meaningful sounds of a language, or phonemes. For

> **DISCUSSION POINT:**
> Explain why it is so difficult to learn to speak a new language without an accent in light of what you now know about phonological competence.

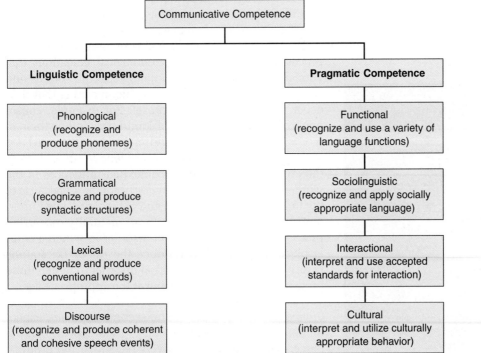

FIGURE 2.1

Linguistic and pragmatic aspects of communicative competence.

English speakers, the consonant sounds /r/ and /l/ are phonemes, and changing these sounds in the context of other sounds would produce a change in meaning (*rip* and *lip* have different meanings, as do *rot* and *lot*). For speakers of some other languages, including Japanese, the consonant sounds /r/ and /l/ are not phonemic, which means that substituting one sound for the other would not produce a change in meaning. As anyone who has studied another language knows, learning to distinguish and pronounce sounds that are not part of your native language's inventory is extremely challenging, such as the rolling or trilling features of sounds in the Spanish word *ferrocarril* or the sequencing of three consonants in the Croatian word *trg.* Luckily, infants learning language for the first time are experts at dealing with fine phonemic contrasts.

Infants arrive in the world ready to distinguish among the sounds of all languages. Over the first few years of life, however, infants become attuned to the sounds they hear on a regular basis, and their ability to distinguish among sounds that are not in the phonemic repertoire of their own language diminishes (Werker & Tees, 2002). By the time infants reach their first birthday, they have become proficient in the sounds of their native language(s). At this time, children enter a period of vocabulary explosion; they begin to devote precious resources to the task of learning new words, perhaps at the expense of being able to make finer distinctions among sounds.

Although children achieve receptive phonological competence within their first year, competence in producing individual phonemes for purposes of spoken communication comes at a slower pace, because it depends heavily on the development of the articulators. An infant's vocal tract is not a miniature version of an adult vocal tract; rather, infants' vocal tracts more closely resemble those of nonhuman primates. The infant vocal tract is very small, and the larynx sits high in the throat. Only with development and time does the larynx drop lower to approximate its location in human adults.

Even as the vocal tract takes on its more adultlike shape, phonological competence does not magically appear. Although the articulators may be in place for children to produce the sounds of their native language, phonological errors that characterize children's expressive phonology often mask competence. In the field of language development, we call these errors **phonological processes.** Phonological processes are the normal phonological deviations that young children make in producing specific sounds and words, and thus are context-specific, meaning that they occur in certain speech contexts. For example, consonants often take on features of sounds that follow them in words; thus, many young children produce the word *dog* as "gog," *cat* as "tat," or *yellow* as "lellow." In each case, the error occurs because of contextual influences in the word—for instance, the /d/ in *dog* becomes /g/ because of the influence of the /g/ at the end of the word. It is important that we not confuse these naturally occurring processes with an articulation disorder in which a child is physically unable to produce the /d/ or /k/ sounds in any context, or a phonological disorder in which these processes do not stop occurring at the appropriate age.

Grammatical Competence. The second linguistic aspect of communicative competence, grammatical competence, is the ability to effectively recognize and produce

DISCUSSION POINT:
Consider the case of La'Kori in Case Study 2.1. What evidence suggests that he is having difficulty in the area of lexical competence?

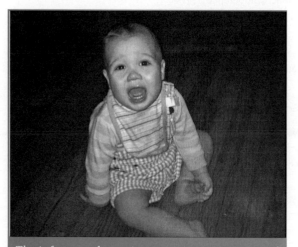

The infant vocal tract is not a miniature version of the adult vocal tract.

the syntactic and morphological structures of a language. For example, using their knowledge of word order, English speakers understand the sentence "Jim is hitting Bob" to mean that Bob is the recipient of Jim's unwelcome actions, and not the other way around. By around 2 years of age, children have an understanding of the word order to which their language adheres (Gertner, Fisher, & Eisengart, 2006) and can thus understand the difference between "Jim is hitting Bob" and "Bob is hitting Jim." In addition to using their knowledge of word order, English speakers use their knowledge of morphological structures to infer meaning. For example, they understand that in the sentence "Jim is hitting Bob," the description of hitting and the act of hitting occur simultaneously, because they recognize that /ing/ denotes ongoing or continuous action. By about 18 months of age, English-learning infants process these small but telling grammatical morphemes separately from the verbs on which they appear (Addy et al., 2003).

Children's comprehension emerges prior to production for grammatical competence. Although children understand the difference between "Jim is hitting Bob" and "Bob is hitting Jim" prior to 2 years of age, they might not produce such sentences until between 2 and 3 years of age. Likewise, by 18 months, children understand the meaning that the morpheme /ing/ conveys, but they do not produce this morpheme until about 24 months of age (Brown, 1973).

Lexical Competence.   The third linguistic aspect of communicative competence is lexical competence—the ability to recognize and produce the conventional words that the speakers of a language use. Developments in this area occur early in the life of the language learner: infants usually understand their own names by about 4 months of age, they understand the names of salient figures in their lives (e.g., *Mommy, Daddy*) by 6 months of age, and they begin to comprehend other words shortly thereafter (e.g., *bottle, hug*). Interestingly, infants as young as 6 months who recognize their own names (or other highly salient and familiar names, such as *Mommy*) use this ability to their own advantage to learn new words. When infants hear their name embedded in continuous speech, they are able to segment the word that follows it from the speech stream (Bortfeld, Rathbun, Morgan, & Golinkoff, 2003). So, an infant whose name is Annie and who hears "Annie up" can segment the *up* that follows *Annie,* which helps her to learn this new word. This early example of lexical competence shows how infants use their own names to get a foot in the door—once they learn to recognize their names as a unit of speech, they infer that the speech following it begins a new unit.

At all stages of life, lexical comprehension precedes lexical production. For instance, although infants may understand a number of words at a very young age, they do not generally produce their first true word until 12 months of age. There are several possible reasons for why comprehension outpaces production (Golinkoff & Hirsh-Pasek, 1999). First, language comprehension requires only that we retrieve words, whereas language production requires that we assemble and pronounce words. Second, with language comprehension, sentences are preorganized with lexical items, a syntactic structure, and intonation. Language production, however, requires that the speaker search for words, organize the words, and place stress and emphasis in the proper places. Third, at least for infants and toddlers, much of the language that others direct toward them is highly contextualized, with many clues to aid comprehension. Children are generally at an advantage for comprehension, because in most cases the words that others speak to them have referents that are immediately available in the environment. In production, however, children must construct a match between the context and language in order to express meaning.

> **DISCUSSION POINT:**
> Throughout this chapter, you have read that comprehension precedes production in several areas of communicative competence. What are some ways to test whether a child comprehends a word that he or she is not yet producing?

Discourse Competence.   Discourse competence, the fourth and final linguistic aspect of communicative competence, refers to the ability to relay information to others fluently and coherently. The speech event, rather than individual words or sounds, is the unit of analysis for discourse competence. People possessing discourse competence understand how to navigate ideas expressed across entire speech events when interpreting and producing extended conversation. For example, discourse competence allows listeners to assign reference to pronouns. Consider the following passage:

> My friend Jen once took a trip to the island of Corfu in Greece. While *there*, *she* joined her friends in swimming through a dark cave, which *they* later learned was called the "Canal D'Amour," because legend says that if a woman swims through *it* and passes a man swimming in the opposite direction, *they* will fall in love.

In order to successfully interpret each of the italicized words in the passage, the listener must rely on information given previously in the discourse. The word *there* refers to the island of Corfu, *she* refers to Jen, *they* refers to Jen's friends, and so forth. Likewise, the speaker navigates the expression of meaning over multiple sentences. For instance, the speaker identifies his or her friend Jen in the first sentence and then reverts to the pronoun *she* in future references.

As with phonological, grammatical, and lexical competence, comprehension precedes production in discourse competence. Children who have not yet acquired discourse competence may not understand, for example, how to take the listener's perspective into account when using pronouns. Preschool teachers frequently hear such exclamations as "He won't share with me," when the child speaking does not realize that he or she must introduce the conversational topic (in this case, name the offending child) prior to voicing the complaint.

Pragmatic Aspects of Communicative Competence

Pragmatic aspects of communicative competence relate to the social contexts in which we use language. People who possess competence in pragmatics take their conversational partner's attitudes, values, and beliefs into account when communicating. They also take the context of language into account and recognize that they can use language for a variety of purposes. Pragmatic aspects of communicative competence include functional competence, sociolinguistic competence, interactional competence, and cultural competence.

Functional Competence.   Functional competence refers to the ability to communicate for a variety of purposes in a language. Recall from Chapter 1 that people share their thoughts and feelings for a variety of reasons; the three most basic functions are to request ("I'd like to try the red ones."), to reject ("No, thanks, these are too small."), and to comment ("I'll see if another store has my size."). As children develop, they communicate for an increasingly large set of purposes, such as to reason, predict, problem-solve, and explain.

Sociolinguistic Competence.   Sociolinguistic competence is the ability to interpret the social meaning that language conveys and to choose language that is socially appropriate for communicative situations. One important aspect of sociolinguistic competence is speech **register,** or the variety of speech appropriate to a particular speech situation. When talking with friends and family, informal registers are suitable ("Hey, how's it going?"), whereas conversations with a prospective employer call for a more formal register ("It is a pleasure to meet you."). The ability to switch among registers—for instance, to use a colloquial dialect with friends and a standard dialect with employers—is called *code switching.*

Interactional Competence.   Interactional competence involves the ability to understand and apply implicit rules for interaction in various communication situations. Initiating and managing conversations appropriately are important skills for interactional competence, as is adhering to accepted standards for body language, eye contact, and physical proximity. Such standards vary from culture to culture and even within cultures according to the communicative situation. To see how standards vary between cultures, we can compare two forms of interactional competence—initiating conversations and eye contact—in Japan and the United States. In Japan, children do not typically initiate conversations with adults, and people of all ages avoid direct eye contact. Conversely, in the United States, children frequently initiate conversation with adults, and Americans generally consider eye contact a sign of sincerity or confidence. To illustrate how standards for interactional competence differ within a culture according to the social context in which communication occurs, consider a new recruit in U.S. Army boot camp. It would be considered rude for the recruit to initiate conversation with the drill sergeant without first requesting permission to speak. Likewise, it would be considered inappropriate for the recruit to look the drill sergeant directly in the eye. Although these actions would be perfectly acceptable in other situations in American culture, the rules for this specific social situation dictate otherwise.

Cultural Competence.   Cultural competence is the ability to function effectively in cultural contexts, both by interpreting behavior correctly and by behaving in a way that would be considered appropriate by the members of the culture. Cultural competence encompasses a wide variety of cultural understandings, including the attitudes, values, and beliefs of a culture's people. One mark of cultural competence is the ability to recognize expressions of emotion. For example, if we were to observe two people in close proximity to each other speaking in raised voices, we might infer that they were angry with each other or that they disagreed about something.

WHAT IS THE FOUNDATION FOR COMMUNICATIVE COMPETENCE? ⬤

The previous sections described the many areas of competence needed to achieve effective communication. This section describes the developmental pathways for these achievements from infancy to adulthood.

EARLIEST FOUNDATIONS

We are not born with communicative competence. Rather, it takes time to acquire, and it builds on a number of early foundations. Several important early foundations characterize the infant's first year, including joint reference and attention, rituals of infancy, and caregiver responsiveness.

Joint Reference and Attention

There are three developmental phases that characterize infancy (Adamson & Chance, 1998): (1) attend to social partners, (2) emergence and coordination of joint attention, and (3) transition to language.

Phase One: Birth to 6 Months.   In the first phase, spanning from birth to about 6 months, infants develop patterns of attending to their social partners. In these early months of life, infants come to value and participate in interpersonal

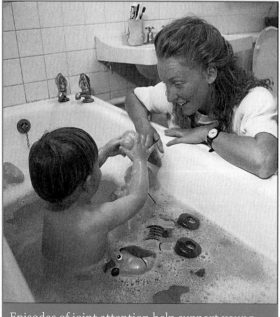

Episodes of joint attention help support young children's learning of new words.

interactions as they learn how to maintain attention within sustained periods of engagement. Caregiver responsiveness is an important feature of this first phase; caregivers who are warm, sensitive, and responsive to their infants promote their children's ability and desire to sustain long periods of joint attention.

Phase Two: 6 Months to 1 Year.   In the second phase, spanning from 5 or 6 months of age through about 1 year, children learn to navigate their attention between an object of interest and another person (Adamson & Chance, 1998, p. 18). This type of event signals the emergence of joint attention. **Joint attention** is the simultaneous engagement of two or more individuals in mental focus on a single external object or event. For example, audience members at a movie theater engage in joint attention as they focus on the movie. A baby and mother engage in joint attention as they look at storybooks together, as one example of a common early routine. This seemingly simple activity symbolizes a critical avenue for early communication development, as periods of joint attention are the context in which children develop important communicative abilities. Children who initiate and respond to bids for joint attention have relatively larger vocabularies at 24 months compared with children whose joint attention abilities are not as strong (Mundy, Fox, & Card, 2003). Often, caregivers take on much of the burden in sustaining periods of joint attention through a variety of techniques, such as using an animated voice and introducing novel objects; this is called *supported joint engagement.* In supported joint engagement, the adult attempts to sustain the child's participation in a period of joint focus.

Why is joint attention so important? Without it, infants may miss out on word-learning opportunities and world-to-word mappings. Imagine a mother pushing her infant down the sidewalk in a stroller as she points upward and exclaims, "Look at the birdie!" Suppose the infant misses his mother's pointing gesture and hears the word *birdie* while he is focused intently on his new shoes. In this situation, mother and son are not jointly attending to the same entity in the world, making it unlikely that the baby will learn what the word *birdie* refers to. In the worst-case scenario, the baby might associate the word *birdie* with his new shoes. Infants do not tend to associate the sounds they hear with the objects and events on which they themselves are focused, unless the speaker provides some social cues that would support such an association.

Before infants can use cues to infer another's intentions, however, they must possess **intersubjective awareness,** or the recognition of when one shares a mental focus on some external object or action with another person. Only after infants realize that they can share a mental focus with other humans do they begin to interpret others' referential actions as intentional and use their own referential actions to call attention to objects and events that interest them. An infant's attempt at deliberate communication with others is called **intentional communication,** which typically emerges around 9–10 months. Identifying when an infant's communicative behaviors are intentional or preintentional can be difficult unless you are familiar with some established guidelines. Indicators of intentionality include the following: (1) the infant is able to follow another person's line of regard (gaze) and pointing gestures at a distance (i.e., the infant is able to respond to another person's bid for joint attention); (2) the infant is able to use gestures or voice to direct another person's attention to an object of interest; (3) the infant is able to use gestures or voice to request or protest an object of interest; (4) the infant is able to use gestures or voice to get another person to look at, notice, or comfort him or her; and (5) the infant is able to use some gestures to communicate his or her intentions (Watt, Wetherby, & Shumway, 2006).

Phase Three: 1 Year and Beyond.   In phase three, children transition to using language within communicative interactions with others. Once children are adept at soliciting bids for joint attention with others, they shift to being able to engage socially with others by using language to represent events and objects within these interactions.

Rituals of Infancy

Infants' lives center around the routines of feeding, bathing, dressing, and sleeping. These routines provide a sense of comfort and predictability, and they also provide early opportunities for language learning. Consider dressing, for example. During this routine, parents often provide a commentary for their infants not unlike that of a sports commentator giving a play-by-play during a baseball or football game. Babies hear such things as "Okay, let's put your right arm in. Now your left arm. Good job. Let's get these snaps. Snap! Snap! All done!" Although infants are much too young to learn about the concepts of right and left, they benefit from hearing the same words and phrases that others repeat to them each day. Infants are adept at computing and making sense of the statistical patterns they hear in speech. By hearing words and phrases over and over again, they become attuned to where pauses occur, which helps them to segment phrases, clauses, and eventually words from the speech stream. They also learn about **phonotactics,** or the combinations of sounds that are acceptable in their language. For example, English-learning infants quickly come to recognize that when they hear /ft/, as in the word *left,* the sounds preceding it (/lɛ/) belong to the same unit, because they never hear /ft/ preceded by a pause.

> **DISCUSSION POINT:**
> What are some rituals from infancy that you think would be particularly important to support early language and communication development?

In addition to the many linguistic patterns infants encounter in routines, they also have many opportunities to engage in episodes of joint attention with their caregivers. At bath time, for example, infants may look back and forth between their bathtub toys and the person who is bathing them, creating periods of joint attention where baby and adult are focused on the same entity in the world.

Caregiver Responsiveness

Caregiver responsiveness refers to caregivers' attention and sensitivity to infants' vocalizations and communicative attempts. Caregiver responsiveness helps teach infants that others value their behaviors and communicative attempts. Both the quality and the quantity of responsiveness by caregivers play a large role in early language development. Parents who are responsive and follow their children's lead foster greater occasions of joint attention and increase children's motivation to communicate, which results in more frequent initiations and bids for attention by children. More responsive language input by mothers is linked to children's language milestones, including saying the first word and producing two-word sentences (Nicely, Tamis-LeMonda, & Bornstein, 1999). Researchers

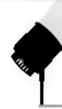

SPOTLIGHT ON LITERACY

Emergent Literacy and the Science of Prevention

Prior to becoming readers and writers, children develop a range of precursory knowledge concerning reading and writing, referred to as *emergent literacy knowledge.* The importance of emergent literacy knowledge to children's later success in reading and reading was not recognized until relatively recently, with historical models of reading and writing development largely absent in their attention to emergent literacy.

Today, there is much interest among policymakers, practitioners, and researchers regarding emergent literacy development among young children. Largely, this interest concerns the important relations between emergent literacy knowledge and later reading and writing success, and the potential for improving children's outcomes in these areas by building their emergent literacy foundation. Unfortunately, in the United States today, too many children do not fare well in reading achievement. Educational statistics from the National Center for Educational Statistics of the U.S. Department of Education (2003) indicate that more than one-third of fourth graders do not exhibit minimal levels of competency on standardized measures of reading ability. In some states, like New Mexico, Louisiana, and Mississippi, one-half of fourth graders do not exhibit minimal levels of competency. Educational experts suggest that we can use the science of prevention to address these alarming statistics and increase the number of children within the United States who are proficient readers in fourth grade and beyond (Snow, Burns, & Griffin, 1998).

Adherence to the science of prevention suggests that early detection of reading and writing difficulties in conjunction with early intervention focused on those difficulties can reduce the incidence of reading and writing problems. Presently, reading and writing difficulties are typically detected in the early primary grades when children exhibit problems in this area. Experts say that this approach, referred to as "wait to fail," is too slow and that we must identify children at risk for reading and writing problems much earlier, ideally before they enter formal schooling. Indeed, recent scientific findings suggest that we can reliably identify children who are at risk for reading and writing difficulties by examining their progress in developing emergent literacy knowledge (Catts, Fey, Zhang, & Tomblin, 2001a) and that early intervention directed toward increasing emergent literacy knowledge can reduce children's later risks for reading and writing difficulties (Gillon, 2000).

Girolametto, Weitzman, and Greenberg (2000) described the following characteristics as several key indicators of caregiver responsiveness:

1. *Waiting and listening:* Parents wait expectantly for initiations, use a slow pace to allow for initiations, and listen to allow the child to complete messages.

2. *Following the child's lead:* When a child initiates either verbally or nonverbally, parents follow the child's lead by responding verbally to the initiation, using animation, and avoiding vague acknowledgments.

3. *Joining in and playing:* Parents build on their child's focus of interest and play without dominating.

4. *Being face-to-face:* Parents adjust their physical level by sitting on the floor, leaning forward to facilitate face-to-face interaction, and bending toward the child when above the child's level.

WHAT ARE MAJOR COMMUNICATIVE MILESTONES IN INFANCY AND TODDLERHOOD?

Chapter 1 described the universal nature of children's communicative achievements as a remarkable feature of language. Children achieve certain language and communication milestones at roughly the same age and in roughly the same order across the communities of the world. The sections that follow chronicle these achievements in a developmental fashion, beginning with infancy.

INFANCY

Infancy spans the period from birth to about 2 years of age, during which some of the most dramatic developments in communicative competence occur. We enter infancy essentially as helpless beings, unable to express anything beyond the most rudimentary calls for assistance. We leave infancy as intentional beings, well on our way to being competent communicators and able to express "No! Me do it!" with force and clarity. Infancy is a period of exploration and discovery.

Stages of Vocal Development

Young children follow a fairly predictable pattern in their early use of vocalizations—the sounds children produce. These are different from verbalizations, which refer to the words children use. One way to think about the emergence of vocalizations is by using a stage model, whereby children's vocalizations emerge in an observable and sequential pattern. These stages are presented in Figure 2.2 and are adapted from Vihman's (2004) writing on this topic.

Phonation Stage (0–1 Month).   The very first kinds of sounds infants produce are called **reflexive sounds.** These include sounds of distress (crying, fussing) and vegetative sounds produced during feeding (burping, coughing). Although neonates have no control for the most part over reflexive sounds, adults tend to respond as if these reflexes were true communication attempts. We hurry to babies' cribs when we hear them cry and use soothing voices in an attempt to alleviate their distress. It is only natural to interpret these early sounds as intentional. We might even ask, "Are you hungry? Does your diaper need to be changed?" although the child's vocalizations could mean something entirely different.

Gooing and Cooing Stage (2–3 Months).   By 2 or 3 months, infants begin to produce gooing and **cooing sounds.** These are consonant-like sounds that infants produce when they are content ("kooooh," "gaaaa"). Infants typically begin by producing

---

FIGURE 2.2

Stages of vocal development.

Phonation Stage (0–1 month)	• Infants produce reflexive (e.g., crying) and vegetative sounds (e.g., coughs)
Gooing and Cooing Stage (2–3 months)	• Infants produce consonant-like and vowel-like sounds
Expansion Stage (4–6 months)	• Infants produce yells, growls, squeals, trills, raspberries
	• Infants produce marginal babbling, an early form of babbling
Canonical Babbling (6+ months) and Variegated Babbling (9+ months)	• Infants use true consonants and true vowels in various combinations
	• No true words at this stage
	• Jargon emerges at end of this stage (about 1 year)

Sources: Oller (1980); Vihman (2004).

/g/ and /k/ sounds, which are consonant sounds we make far back in the oral cavity. These sounds are easier for infants to produce than other sounds that require more precise manipulation of the tongue, lips, or teeth (/t/ and /v/, for instance).

Expansion Stage (4–6 Months).   In the expansion stage, infants gain more control over the articulators. Their vocal repertoire increases as they begin to manipulate the loudness and pitch of their voices and to play with sounds. Infants at this stage begin to yell, growl, squeal, and make raspberries and trills. Also, marginal babbling emerges, an early type of babbling containing short strings of consonant-like and vowel-like sounds.

Canonical Babbling (6+ Months) and Variegated Babbling (9+ months).   True babbling, which appears sometime about or after 6 months, is distinguished from the earlier cooing, gooing, and marginal babbling by the child's production of authentic syllables. These vocalizations have a true consonant combined with a true vowel and are strung together to form chains: *ma-ma, di-di,* and *guh-guh,* for example. Often, parents view their children as beginning to talk when they begin to babble because of the resemblance of these syllable strings to the native language of the child. Canonical babbling consists of the single production or repetition of consonant-vowel sequences in which the same consonant-vowel sequence is repeated (*da-da-da-da*). Sequences of these canonical consonant-vowel repetitions are called **reduplicative babbling.** A mother should not fret when at 6 months her infant produces constant streams of *da-da-da-da.* It is not that the infant is favoring one parent over the other; it is more likely that the baby is just experimenting with sounds.

Variegated babbling emerges soon after infants begin to produce canonical babbling at about 9 months. Infants begin to use a wider range of sounds than in reduplicative babbling and begin to string together different consonant and vowel sequences (*da-bi, da-ma*). Across many languages, infants prefer the nasal consonants (*m, n,* and *ng*) and the stop consonants (*p, b, t, d*) in the variegated stage (Locke, 1993), combining these variously with vowels to produce long vocalized sequences. Many of the infant's early words, such as *Mommy* and *Daddy,* emerge directly from these variegated strings.

Jargon is a special type of babbling in which infants use the melodic patterns of their native language through a combination of rhythm, rate, stress, and intonation contours. Babies using jargon may sound as if they are producing questions, exclamations, or commands even in the absence of true words. Although the vocalizations that infants make while babbling or when producing jargon may sound like short words or syllables, they are not true words, because they are not referential, nor do they convey meaning.

Interestingly, babbling does not necessarily refer only to the specific types of sounds that infants make. Deaf babies and hearing babies born to profoundly deaf parents babble silently with their hands. In the same way that the vocalizations of babies exposed to oral language show sensitivity to specific rhythmic patterns that bind syllables, so, too, do the hand movements of babies born to deaf parents. Their hand movements have a slower rhythm than ordinary gestures, and they produce these movements within a tightly restricted space in front of the body (Petitto, Holowka, Sergio, & Ostry, 2001).

Emergence of Intentionality

Between 7 and 12 months, infants begin to communicate their intentions more clearly than before. Prior to this period, we consider children to be preintentional.

Although infants may do things that are considered intentional (e.g., cry out in a certain way, babble), adults bear the burden of inferring their intentions in these acts, as in the following:

INFANT: (*squeal, smile*)

FATHER: Oh, you liked that!

INFANT: (*burp*) Maa.

FATHER: You want more? You do, don't you? Yes, you do.

In this interaction, the infant produces preintentional behaviors that are ambiguous at best, but the father views these as intentional. The infant's intentionality comes not from within, but rather from the adult with whom the infant is interacting.

In the latter half of the first year of life, infants become increasingly interested in the people and objects around them, and they also become interested in intentionally communicating to people about objects and events. During this stage of development, infants become attuned to the referential signals of others (e.g., pointing, eye gaze, line of regard), and they begin to incorporate their own intentional gestures to direct others' attention. This transition to intentionality is a particularly important event in the communication achievements of young children. With intentionality, children are well on their way to being able to deliberately describe their needs, interests, and thoughts to the world around them as in the following interaction:

INFANT: Mama (looks at mother and raises arms).

MOTHER: Oh, you want me to pick you up?

Infants demonstrate evidence of intentionality through their communicative efforts toward others, by pointing to objects, showing objects, gesturing, and using eye contact.

Transition to Symbolic Representations

A word is a symbol, as it stands for and represents something else in the world. As infants approach their first birthday, they become aware of how sequences of sounds symbolize concepts in the world. Words are arbitrary symbols; with the exception of some onomatopoeic words (words, like *buzz* and *coo,* that sound like the concept they represent), they do not directly signal the concepts they represent. As infants develop, their **lexicons,** or mental dictionaries, develop as well. For each word they learn, infants create an entry in their lexicon, similar to the boldfaced words in dictionaries. The lexical entries are essentially a series of symbols. Each entry comprises the word, the word's sound, the word's meaning, and the word's part of speech (Pinker, 1999). Figure 2.3 shows the lexical representation for the word *money.*

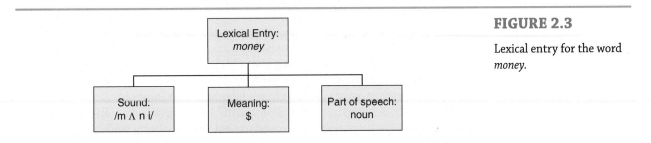

FIGURE 2.3

Lexical entry for the word *money.*

At roughly 1 year of age, children transition from using intentional communicative behaviors, including eye contact, gesture, and vocalizations, to using symbols, including words and gestures, to communicate. This 1-year mark signals an important and exciting transition for developing children. Although children at 1 year likely understand only a few words, parents often are quite gleeful when their children begin to use these words expressively.

Words are not the only types of symbols children use as they transition from nonsymbolic to symbolic communication. Children begin to use referential gestures at roughly the same time that they begin to use words. A referential gesture is that which carries a fixed meaning, such as flapping the arms to refer to a bird (Iverson & Thal, 1998). Referential gestures are different from deictic gestures, such as pointing or waving, which are used to indicate or call attention to something. Referential gestures are symbolic and function much like words for young children; for instance, a young child waving her hand a particular way can clearly communicate to her parents her disdain for a particular food. As children develop their initial lexicons, it is important to recognize the contributions of referential gestures. Young children's use of referential gestures provides them a much larger communicative repertoire in their transition to symbolic communication than is possible with spoken words alone (Iverson & Thal, 1998).

We know from Chapter 1 that adults communicate for three main reasons: to request, to reject, and to comment. Once intentionality emerges in infants, they, too, communicate for these same reasons, although the methods they employ are somewhat different. Prelinguistic infants may request a favorite toy by pointing to it. They may reject a not-so-favorite toy by pushing it away or hurling it across the room, and they may comment on a toy by holding it up for another person to see or even offering it to someone. When children begin to produce words, they use their first words for these same three communicative functions.

The First Word.   Of all the communicative milestones infants reach, parents, grandparents, and other family members tend to be the most excited about an infant's first word. On average, infants utter their first true word at 12 months. First words usually refer to salient people and objects in infants' everyday lives, such as *mama, dada, doggie,* and the like. Researchers consider a vocalization a true word if it meets three important criteria.

First, an infant needs to utter the word with a clear intention and purpose. When a baby says "doggie" while petting a dog, the baby undoubtedly has a clear intention and purpose of referring to the pet. If, however, a parent tells his or her child to "say doggie, say doggie" and the baby does so, the utterance is an imitation or repetition rather than a true word.

Second, a true word has a recognizable pronunciation. Obviously, 12-month-olds are not capable of producing all sounds accurately, but their first word should be a close approximation of the adult form, and others should be able to recognize the word. Thus, the child's "doddie" for *doggie* is a close enough approximation that this can be considered a true word. However, if a child produces *doggie* as "oo-na"—even consistently and while clearly using "oo-na" to refer to the family doggie—it is not considered a true word, because it does not closely approximate the form adults use. The term *phonetically consistent form,* or *PCF,* describes these idiosyncratic, wordlike productions that children use consistently and meaningfully but do not approximate forms used by adults. Although not true words, these forms are important aspects of children's language development.

Third, a true word is one that a child uses consistently and in contexts beyond the original context. We would expect the baby who said "doggie" while petting the dog to use this word not only with that particular dog, but also for other people's dogs, pictures of dogs, and possibly even when hearing dogs barking in the distance. The extension of words across various contexts is related to the symbolic aspect of words and how one word can have many diverse referents across time and place. Children demonstrate the symbolic element of word use when they take a word and apply it to diverse contexts of use, even incorrectly, as in the child who calls every man "daddy" or all furry animals "cats."

TODDLERHOOD

The word *toddlerhood* takes its name from children learning to walk, who take short, unsteady steps. Coincidentally, toddlers' achievements in communicative competence might also sound a bit clumsy to the naive listener. Have you ever heard a toddler say, "I am do it!" or "I have two mouses."? During this stage, toddlers experiment with form, content, and use as they continue to acquire communicative competence.

Achievements in Form

From roughly 1 year to 18 months of age, children acquire an expressive lexicon of about 50 words. For approximately 6 months after toddlers reach the 50-word mark (roughly from 18 months to 24 months), significant changes in children's communicative competence are evident. Children begin to show evidence of a rudimentary use of syntax, or language form, and begin to inflect words with grammatical morphemes. A grammatical morpheme is an inflection added to words to indicate aspects of grammar, such as the plural *s*, the possessive *'s,* the past tense *-ed,* and the present progressive *-ing.* These morphemes are an important aspect of grammatical development.

Children typically begin to move from single-word to multiword utterances between the ages of 18 and 24 months. During this time, parents begin to hear phrases such as "go bye-bye?" and "Mommy ball." It is at the two-word stage that children begin to acquire a sense of syntax, or language structure. They see the value that combining words has over using single words and can begin to use language for a greater variety of communicative functions. Some simple functions that children express during the two-word stage include commenting ("Daddy go"), negating ("No juice"), requesting ("More juice"), and questioning ("What that?").

When children move beyond one-word utterances to produce two- and three-word utterances, they begin to have a distinct grammar that governs the order of words. Recall from Chapter 1 that grammar, or syntax, refers to the rule system that governs the internal organization of sentences. When children produce only one-word utterances, there is no internal organization to consider. However, once children begin to link words to express ideas and desires ("Want go!" "Me do it!"), then syntax emerges to govern how these words are organized.

Grammatical morphemes appear in children's speech when children are between 18 and 24 months of age, which is when expressive morphology can first be documented. When grammatical morphemes first emerge, language exhibits a *telegraphic* quality that results from the omission of key grammatical markers. For instance, the toddler's "Mommy no go" and "Daddy walking" are telegraphic reductions of "Mommy, don't go" and "Daddy is walking." The emerging use of grammatical morphemes signals the development of morphology and the child's gradual increase in grammatical precision.

Roger Brown, a pioneer in early morphological development, isolated 14 grammatical morphemes and documented the ages at which children master these

TABLE 2.1	Acquisition of Brown's 14 grammatical morphemes	
Grammatical Morpheme	**Age (in months)**	**Example**
Present progressive -*ing*	19–28	*doggie running*
Plural -*s*	27–30	*shoes*
Preposition *in*	27–30	*milk in cup*
Preposition *on*	31–34	*cat on couch*
Possessive *'s*	31–34	*kitty's bowl*
Regular past tense -*ed*	43–46	*froggy jumped*
Irregular past tense	43–46	*Dad broke it*
Regular third-person singular -*s*	43–46	*birdy eats*
Articles *a, the, an*	43–46	*the car*
Contractible copula *be*	43–46	*she's tall*
Contractible auxiliary	47–50	*she's cooking*
Uncontractible copula *be*	47–50	*we were [we were busy]*
Uncontractible auxiliary	47–50	*she was [she was working]*
Irregular third person	47–50	*she made it*

Source: Brown (1973).

common morphemes as well as their order of acquisition (See Table 2.1 for a list of grammatical morphemes, the approximate ages when they appear, and examples of how we might use these morphemes.) These grammatical morphemes develop in the same order and emerge at roughly the same time in all English-speaking children. The first grammatical morpheme that children use expressively is the present progressive form -*ing,* as in *doggie running.* Children begin to use this morpheme at around 18 or 19 months of age, with mastery by 28 months. Additional morphemes that appear during toddlerhood include the prepositions *in* and *on,* which children start to use at about 2 years of age (*in cup, on table*), the regular plural *s (babies eating),* the possessive *'s (kitty's bowl),* and the irregular past-tense verb (*Dad broke it.*). Irregular past-tense verbs, of which there are between 150 and 180, are verbs that children must memorize rather than form by adding -*ed* (e.g., *eat/ate,* not *eat/eated*). Once children have acquired the regular past-tense rule, they often overgeneralize its use to irregular verbs until they have had sufficient exposure to and practice with what Steven Pinker (1999) calls "words" (e.g., the irregular form of a verb) and "rules" (e.g., applying the past tense ending of a regular verb, -*ed*). There are other cases in language where children learn words and rules differently. For example, with contractions, children generally learn the word *won't* as a unit, rather than by combining the words *will not.* This likely occurs because the sound of the root (*will*) is not the same in the contracted form (*won't*).

Sentence forms appear awkward for the most part during the toddler years. Toddlers tend to use uninflected verb forms ("Kitty eat") and to misuse or omit pronouns ("Me go," "Her do it"). Despite these awkward constructions, toddlers begin to use more adultlike forms for a variety of sentence types, including the yes/no question ("Are we going, Mommy?"), *wh*- questions ("What's that?"), commands ("You do it."), and negatives ("Me no want that.")

In addition to documenting grammatical morpheme usage, Roger Brown also created Brown's stages of language development, which characterize children's

TABLE 2.2 Brown's stages of language development

Stage	Age (upper limit)	MLU	MLU Range	Major Achievements
I	18 months	1.31	.99–1.64	• Single-word sentences • Uninflected nouns and verbs (*mommy, eat*)
II	24 months	1.92	1.47–2.37	• Two-element sentences • True clauses not evident (*Mommy up; Eat cookie*)
III	30 months	2.54	1.97–3.11	• Three-element sentences • Independent clauses emerge (*Baby want cookie*)
IV	36 months	3.16	2.47–3.85	• Four-element sentences • Independent clauses continue to emerge (*The teacher gave it to me*)
V	42 months	3.78	2.96–4.60	• Recursive elements predominate
Post V	54 months	5.02	3.96–6.08	• Complex syntactic patterns • Connecting devices emerge (*and, because*) • Subordination and coordination continue to emerge • Complement clauses used (*She's not feeling well*)

Source: Adapted from R. D. Kent. (1994). Reference manual for communicative sciences and disorders: Speech and language. Austin, TX: Pro-Ed; and L. M. Justice & H. K. Ezell. (2002). The syntax handbook. Eau Claire, WI: Thinking Publications.

language achievements based on their ability to produce utterances of varying syntactic complexity (see Table 2.2). One of the defining characteristics of preschoolers' increasing language complexity is their **mean length of utterance (MLU).** MLU refers to the average length of children's sentence units, or utterances. Each utterance a child produces contains one or more morphemes, which are the smallest units of meaning. We can calculate MLU by counting the total number of morphemes in a sample of 50 to 100 spontaneous utterances that a child produces and then dividing the total number of morphemes by the total number of utterances. The calculation is *MLU = total number of morphemes/total number of utterances.*

During the toddler and preschool years, children's MLU increases systematically, as shown in Figure 2.4. Calculating MLU is a common way to evaluate children's language skills against the expectations for their age. In order to achieve consistency in morpheme counts, researchers and practitioners generally use

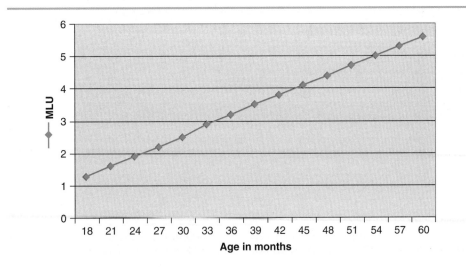

FIGURE 2.4

Age-related progression in mean length of utterance.

Source: Adapted from J. F. Miller & R. Chapman. (1981). The relation between age and mean length of utterance in morphemes. *Journal of Speech and Hearing Research, 24*, 154–161. Reprinted with permission.

Brown's rules for counting morphemes (see Brown, 1973), although other protocols exist for this procedure. Using Brown's rules, we could calculate a child's MLU using a language sample of at least 50 utterances to increase the chances that the sample is valid and represents how a child usually uses language. For the sake of explanation, however, we use a short sample to demonstrate how to calculate the MLU for a 2-year-old.

	Utterance	Morphemes
1	Me do it.	3
2	No, me do it.	4
3	Eli want it.	3
4	Me go outside.	3
5	Outside.	1
6	What that?	2
7	Mommy do.	2
8	What that?	2

In this very brief transcript, the child produced eight utterances and a total of 20 morphemes, resulting in an MLU of 2.5. The norms presented in Table 2.3 show that the predicted MLU for a 2-year-old is 1.92. Sixty-eight percent of children have scores within one standard deviation of 1.92, or between 1.47 and 2.37. If our sample is accurate, this child's MLU is slightly higher than expected for his or her age.

TABLE 2.3 Normative references for interpreting MLU

Age (in months)	Predicted MLU	Predicted MLU +/– One Standard Deviation (68% of Population)
18	1.31	0.99–1.64
21	1.62	1.23–2.01
24	1.92	1.47–2.37
27	2.23	1.72–2.74
30	2.54	1.97–3.11
33	2.85	2.22–3.48
36	3.16	2.47–3.85
39	3.47	2.71–4.23
42	3.78	2.96–4.60
45	4.09	3.21–4.97
48	4.40	3.46–5.34
51	4.71	3.71–5.71
54	5.02	3.96–6.08
57	5.32	4.20–6.45
60	5.63	4.44–6.82

Source: Adapted from J. F. Miller & R. Chapman. (1981). The relation between age and mean length of utterance in morphemes. Journal of Speech and Hearing Research, *24, 154–161. Reprinted with permission.*

Achievements in Content

Have you ever known parents who keep a diary or a list of words that their children produce? Parents who keep track of their children's new words generally begin to have trouble keeping up with the word-learning pace when their children are between 18 and 24 months of age. During the second half of the second year, or around the time when children have acquired 50 words, they often experience a **vocabulary spurt,** or word spurt (also called *naming explosion*), a remarkable increase in the rate of vocabulary acquisition. During the vocabulary spurt, children learn an average of 7 to 9 new words per day. Many parents of toddlers report that their children use new words out of the blue, such as *plenty, vent, dangerous, steep,* and so on.

During toddlerhood, substantial growth occurs in both the receptive and expressive lexicons. The receptive lexicon encompasses the words a person can comprehend, whereas the expressive lexicon refers to the words a person can produce. As we described earlier in this chapter, comprehension generally precedes production in language learning; this pattern holds as well for the receptive and expressive lexicons. For example, girls who are 18 months of age have an average of 65 words in their receptive vocabularies but only 27 words in their expressive vocabularies; in comparison, boys of the same age understand an average of 56 words and produce an average of 18 (Fenson et al., 2000). The trend for a disparity between the size of receptive and expressive lexicons continues throughout toddlerhood, the school years, and into adulthood.

Although children learn about 7 to 9 new words per day between the ages of 18 and 24 months, they do not always use these words the way adults do. Children tend to use a new word cautiously at first. They apply newly learned words to specific referents rather than to a category of referents. This practice is called an **underextension.** For instance, children who have just learned the word *doggie* might use it only to refer to the family pet; or children might use their new word *cup* to refer only to their green sippy cup. A child might learn the word *yellow* for a specific shade of yellow and stoically refuse to apply this word to other variants of yellow.

Children also engage in a process called **overextension,** which is the opposite of underextension and is when children use words in a wider set of contexts than adults would consider appropriate. Toddlers tend to overgeneralize about one-third of new words (Rescorla, 1980) on the basis of categorical, analogical, and relational similarities. A categorical overextension is when a child extends a known word to other referents because they are in the same category. For instance, a child may learn the color green and then call all colors by the word *green.* Likewise, a child may call all animals by the word *cat,* all liquids by the word *juice,* or all actions that involve clothing (buttoning, zippering, folding, etc.) by the word *snap.* An analogical overextension is when a child extends a known word to other referents because they have perceptual similarities. For instance, a child may use the word *ball* to describe anything that is round (e.g., a tire) or may use the word *ladder* to describe anything tall (e.g., a flagpole). A relational overextension is when a child extends a known word to other semantically related referents. For instance, the child may use the word *bird* to refer to both a bird feeder and birdseed.

Achievements in Use

In addition to acquiring new grammar and words as they transition from the single-word to the multiword stage, children acquire important new language functions and conversational skills. By the time children enter the multiword stage, they are capable of using a variety of language functions, including instrumental, regulatory, personal interactional, heuristic, imaginative, and informative functions (Halliday, 1978). Children can use requests to satisfy their own needs (instrumental), use directives to control the behaviors of others (regulatory), tell information about themselves and share feelings (personal interactional), request information and ask questions to learn and investigate the world (heuristic), tell stories to make-believe and pretend (imaginative), and give information to communicate with others (informative). Children's success at using communication for a variety of purposes is one of the most important aspects of communicative development during toddlerhood. With their growing lexicon and sophisticated grammar, children use these resources for many purposes. When children's internal demand for speech—their desire to communicate various functions or intentions—exceeds their capacity, they can become frustrated.

One area in which toddlers are not highly skilled is conversation. Conversational skill requires being able to initiate a conversational topic, sustain a topic for several turns, and then appropriately take leave of the conversation. Those of us who have recently attempted to have a conversation with a young child know it is not usually very sophisticated:

> PARENT: What did you do at school today?
>
> TODDLER: Miss Sarah, Eli, Lila.

Toddlers may demonstrate some skill in starting a conversation but cannot usually sustain one for more than one or two turns. Typically, the adult has to provide a great deal of assistance to maintain a particular topic. Toddlers also have difficulty keeping their audience's needs in mind: They may use pronouns without appropriately defining to whom they refer, and they may discuss topics without ensuring that the listener has a frame of reference within which to understand them (Owens, 2001). Additionally, when adults ask toddlers a specific question or give them an explicit opportunity to take a turn, toddlers do not always take advantage of the opportunity. They may simply not respond, or they may respond noncontingently (off the topic). Toddlers are not proficient at realizing when they are not following along in a conversation and thus are not likely to seek clarification.

Achievements in Speech

In the infancy period, children's vocal development undergoes considerable change as they move from reflexive sounds, like burping and coughing, to variegated babbling that sounds more like the language of their community. During the toddler years, children's development of phonology—their knowledge of the rules concerning the sound system—grows rapidly.

Expressive phonology refers to the observable sounds and sound patterns children use when producing syllables and words. When they speak, toddlers tend to use the sounds with which they are most skilled; because of this tendency, 2-year-olds correctly produce about 70% of the sounds they use (Stoel-Gammon & Dunn, 1985). Underlying every sound or sound pattern that a child produces is a *phonological representation,* a mental representation of a particular phoneme or sound pattern. These internal representations differentiate each phoneme in the child's repertoire from all the other phonemes and provide children with the rules for combining sounds into different patterns. Together, these underlying representations form a child's phonological repertoire, or phonological system.

Attainment of Specific Phonemes.   Published norms for phoneme acquisition are a common source for representing phonemic attainment in young children. Norm references consider when children master certain phonemes, as well as the order in which they master them. We interpret norm references with respect to the phonemic attainment of other children, rather than to an agreed criterion score. These references are derived from published studies that investigate the acquisition of phonology in large groups of children. Table 2.4 presents five sets of norms for the English consonants. These norms show the ages at which children typically acquire particular phonemes, providing a point of comparison for children of the same age. As shown in Table 2.4, however, these norms vary widely, depending on whether researchers elect to chart average ages of achievement of particular phonemes or to chart upper ages of achievement (e.g., the age at which 90% or 100% of a given sample produces adultlike phonemes). The data in the table show, for instance, that children acquire /m/ sometime between 2 and 3 years of age.

TABLE 2.4 Normative references for phoneme acquisition				
Consonant	Wellman et al. (1931)	Poole (1934)	Templin (1957)	Sander (1972)	Prather et al. (1975)
m	3	3 1/2	3	Before 2	2
n	3	4 1/2	3	Before 2	2
h	3	3 1/2	3	Before 2	2
p	4	3 1/2	3	Before 2	2
f	3	5 1/2	3	3	2–4
w	3	3 1/2	3	Before 2	2–8
b	3	3 1/2	4	Before 2	2–8
ŋ		4 1/2	3	2	2
j	4	4 1/2	3 1/2	3	2–4
k	4	4 1/2	4	2	2–4
g	4	4 1/2	4	2	2–4
l	4	6 1/2	6	3	3–4
d	5	4 1/2	4	2	2–4
t	5	4 1/2	6	2	2–8
s	5	7 1/2	4 1/2	3	3
r	5	7 1/2	4	3	3–4
tʃ	5		4 1/2	4	3–8
v	5	6 1/2	6	4	4
z	5	7 1/2	7	4	4
ʒ	6	6 1/2	7	6	4
θ		7 1/2	6	5	4
dʒ			7	4	4
ʃ		6 1/2	4 1/2	4	3–8
ð		6 1/2	7	5	4

Source: From Creaghead, Newman, & Secord. (1985). Assessment and remediation of articulatory and phonological disorders *(2nd ed.). Boston: Allyn & Bacon. Copyright © by Pearson Education. Reprinted/adapted by permission of the publisher.*

FIGURE 2.5

Sander's norms for age ranges of consonant development.

Source: From E. K. Sander. (1972). When are speech sounds learned? *Journal of Speech and Hearing Disorders*, 37, 62. Reprinted with permission.

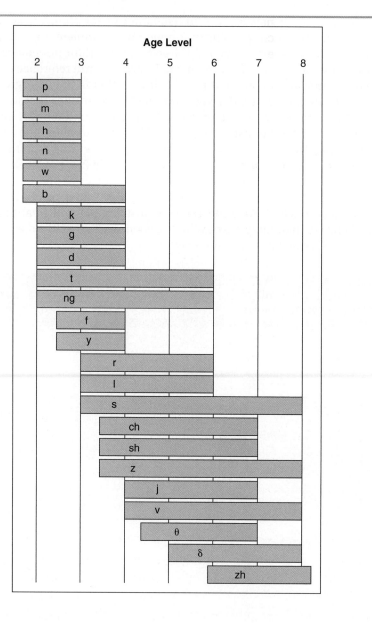

The data in Figure 2.5 are probably the most widely used for determining when children can be expected to produce a particular sound correctly more often than they misarticulate or omit it (Sander, 1972); this is known as the customary age of production and differs from age of mastery, which is represented in Figure 2.5 as the right edge of the blue bars; this is the point at which 90% of all children are customarily using the phoneme.

Children are said to have mastered a consonant once they can produce the sound correctly in three different positions: in the initial position of a syllable (syllable initial, *b* in *bear*), in the middle position of a syllable (syllable medial, *r* in *berry*), and in the final position of a syllable (syllable final, *d* in *bread*). However, determining mastery is not as simple as it might seem, because the consonants and vowels that surround a particular sound may influence how a child produces that sound. For example, producing the syllable initial /t/ in the word *tip* differs from the initial /t/ in *trip*, because we utter the latter with slight affrication (sounds more

DISCUSSION POINT:
What are some factors that contribute to a sound being acquired earlier than other sounds? For instance, children master /b/ long before they master /r/ in English. What are some possible explanations for this?

like "chrip"). A child may be able to produce syllable initial /t/ accurately in *tip* but not in *trip,* and so we could arrive at different conclusions about a child's mastery of /t/ depending on the word we have the child say.

Although the exact age by which children can produce a particular phoneme varies across the norms, the order in which children tend to acquire the phonemes is generally the same across the normative samples. As shown in Figure 2.5, /m/, /n/, /h/, and /p/ are early acquired phonemes, and /v/, /z/, and /θ/ (as in *th*ink) are later-acquired phonemes. The data in Figure 2.5 identify the age range for attainment of the consonant phonemes; the left side of the bar shows when 50% of children use a consonant, and the right side of the bar shows when 90% of children use it.

Phonological Processes.   As children develop their phonological prowess, they make a number of adjustments to the production of specific sounds and sound classes. These natural adjustments are called *phonological processes;* they are processes of sound change that children apply to words and syllables to simplify the phonological production. These processes reflect normal patterns of deviation from the adult phonology that will change as the child matures. These patterns are fairly universal across children. For instance, many preschool children say "doddie" for *doggie* and "tee" for *tree.* They say "jamas" for *pajamas* and "tum" for *thumb.* Adults who work often with young children expect to hear these systematic phonological patterns, or processes, in their speech.

Toddlers' expressive phonology exhibits a large variety of phonological processes. Common ones include the following:

1. *Final consonant deletion:* The final consonant of a word is omitted ("ca" for *cat*).
2. *Reduplication.* The first syllable in a word is repeated ("wa-wa" for *water*).
3. *Consonant harmony:* One consonant in a word takes on features of another consonant ("doddie" for *doggie*).
4. *Weak syllable deletion:* The unstressed syllable in a word is omitted ("jamas" for *pajamas*).
5. *Diminutization:* The second syllable in a word is changed to "ee" ("mommy" for *mother* and "blankie" for *blanket*).
6. *Cluster reduction:* A consonant cluster (two or more consonants that occur together, as in *st*ick or *cr*ayon) is reduced to a single consonant ("tick" or "cayon").
7. *Liquid gliding:* The consonants /l/ and /r/ are changed to *w* and *y* ("wabbit" for *rabbit* and "yove" for *love*) (Vihman, 2004).

These and many other types of phonological processes represent the systematic substitutions, omissions, and additions that young children make as they acquire the phonology of their language (Vihman, 2004). Gradually, as children's phonology matures, these processes undergo suppression, meaning that children exchange the immature production (e.g., liquid gliding) for the mature, adultlike production.

The suppression of processes tends to follow a general age-related pattern. For instance, of the processes listed previously, children tend to suppress the first five processes (final consonant deletion, reduplication, consonant harmony, weak syllable deletion, and diminutization) by age 3 (Stoel-Gammon & Dunn, 1985). Thus, although these processes may occur frequently in toddlers, they become less frequent as children age from 2 to 3 years. The last two processes, cluster reduction and liquid gliding, are suppressed later.

SPOTLIGHT ON TECHNOLOGY

Child Language Data Exchange System: CHILDES

The CHILDES project, which began in 1984, is the largest effort to date to develop an international database of child language samples using common transcription protocols. CHILDES technically involves three integrated components (MacWhinney, 1996):

- *CHAT.* CHAT is a highly explicit and detailed system for preparing written records of language and speech samples. In addition to detailing how transcripts are to be prepared, CHAT specifies how to transcribe such common speech behaviors as interruptions, exclamations, dialectical variations of words, baby talk, pauses, and so forth. The screenshot below illustrates how a sample is transcribed following the CHAT conventions. In this example, a record is made of a 47-year-old male's descriptions of three pictures (MacWhinney, 1996). The entire CHAT manual can be downloaded free of charge at http://childes.psy.cmu.edu/manuals/chat.pdf.
- *CLAN.* CLAN (**C**omputerized **L**anguage **An**alysis) is computer software that allows users to analyze language transcripts prepared using CHAT conventions. The software is designed to conduct such basic analyses as counting the number of words produced by a speaker or determining the average length of utterances (mean length of utterance). A group of transcripts can be analyzed simultaneously to develop normative profiles of individuals (e.g., to determine if certain children produced fewer words than the group, on average). The software can be downloaded at no cost at http://childes.psy.cmu.edu/, as can the CLAN manual specifying how to use the software, at http://childes.psy.cmu.edu/manuals/clan.pdf.
- *CHILDES Databases.* Perhaps the most unique feature of CHILDES is the availability of databases containing numerous corpora of transcribed language samples from across the world; these submitted by research teams and are prepared using the CHAT protocols. The Slavic Languages database, for example, contains five sets of transcripts representing children acquiring different Slavic languages (Croatian, Polish, and Russian). Additional databases are available for American English, British English, Germanic, Romance, East Asian, and Celtic languages (as well as Other, which includes Farsi, Greek, and Hebrew, among others); specialized databases also focus on bilingual acquisition, language disorders, and narratives. Researchers can use these in many ways; they may access existing databases to research specific topics, or they may collect language samples of their own and compare aspects of these to samples available in the databases. The databases are publicly available at http://childes.psy.cmu.edu/manuals/.

```
@g:        3c = bunny is eating banana
*PAT:      rabbits [*].
%mor:      DET|0 N|rabbit-*PL
%err:      rabbits = rabbit $SUB;
@g:        3b = squirrel eating banana
*PAT:      squirrel.
%mor:      DET|0 N|squirrel
@g:        3a = monkey eating banana
*PAT:      monkeys [*].
%mor:      DET|0 N|monkey-*PL.
%err:      monkeys = monkey $SUB ;
```

Source: From B. MacWhinney. (1996). The CHILDES system. *American Journal of Speech-Language Pathology, 5*, 5–14. Reprinted with permission.

WHAT ARE MAJOR COMMUNICATIVE MILESTONES IN PRESCHOOL AND SCHOOL-AGE CHILDREN? ⬤

PRESCHOOL ACCOMPLISHMENTS

The preschool period, when children are between 3 and 5 years old, precedes formal schooling. During the preschool years, children overcome much of the language toddling of the experimenting phase of toddlerhood and truly begin to master form, content, and use in their development of communicative competence. By many accounts, language acquisition is nearly complete by the time children leave preschool. Those of you who have recently had a conversation with a 5-year-old realize how true this is. The 5-year-old has an amazingly large vocabulary, demonstrates skill (relatively speaking) in holding a conversation, and uses the syntax of an adult. From kindergarten on, achievements in language are subtle and protracted relative to the remarkable and rapid advances of the infancy, toddlerhood, and preschool years.

Achievements in Form

During the preschool years, children refine their syntax and morphology in significant ways. Noteworthy advances occur in children's use of grammatical and derivational morphology. Grammatical morphemes, discussed earlier, are the modifications to words that provide additional grammatical precision, such as pluralizing words (*cat/cats*) and inflecting verbs (*go/is going*). Grammatical morphemes do not really carry meaning; rather, they provide grammatical detail. Derivational morphology is similar to grammatical morphology in that it modifies words structurally. However, derivational morphology refers to the addition of prefixes and suffixes that carry meaning and thus change a word's meaning and sometimes its part of speech. For instance, we can add the suffix *-er* to *work* to change its meaning and its part of speech from a verb to a noun (*worker*). We can also add the prefix *un-* to *happy* to change its meaning. Additional common derivational morphemes include *pre- (preschool), super- (supernatural), -est (fullest), -ness (freshness),* and *-ly (slowly).* Morphological development is the ability to manipulate word structure by adding these and other prefixes and suffixes, allowing children to become increasingly precise and specific in their communication. Morphology allows children to magnify their basic word repertoire exponentially; for instance, from the word root *run,* the child with well-developed morphology has access to numerous variations (*rerun, ran, running, runner,* etc.).

During the preschool years, children acquire additional grammatical morphemes, described by Brown (1973). For instance, children begin to use the articles *a, an,* and *the* to elaborate nouns (*a horse, an ant, the house*). The greatest area of development at this time is in verb morphology. Speakers of English inflect verbs to provide information about time (e.g., past, present, future). Often, the verb *be* serves as an important marker of time. When the verb *be* or one of its derivatives (*am, is, are, was, were*) is the main verb in a sentence, it is called a *copula,* as in *I am Paul.* When the verb *be* or one of its derivatives serves as a helping verb in a sentence, it is called an *auxiliary,* as in *I am hugging Paul.* The *be* copula and auxiliary forms can be contracted (*He's happy; I'm going*) or uncontracted (*He is happy; I am going*). During the preschool years, children acquire many of the nuances about verb morphology, including mastering the variations of *be* as both copula and auxiliary. Delayed development of verb morphology is one of the major signs of a language disorder (Brackenbury & Fey, 2003). Major achievements in verb morphology that occur in children between the ages of 3 and 5 include mastering

> *Uncontractible copula (27 to 39 months):* be copula that cannot be contracted, as in *Here she is* and *We were happy.*
>
> *Contractible copula (29 to 49 months):* be copula that can be contracted, as in *Debbie's here.*
>
> *Uncontractible auxiliary (29 to 49 months):* be auxiliary that cannot be contracted, as in *They were going* (note that if *were* were contracted, it would change the meaning).
>
> *Contractible auxiliary (30 to 50 months):* be auxiliary that can be contracted, as in *Mommy's working.* (Owens, 2001)

In addition to major achievements in morphology, the preschool years shepherd in significant advances in sentence complexity. Preschoolers move from simple declarative subject-verb-object constructions (*Daddy drives a truck.*) and subject-verb-complement constructions (*Truck is big*) to more elaborate sentence patterns, such as

- Subject-verb-object-adverb (*Daddy's hitting the hammer outside.*)
- Subject-verb-complement-adverb (*Baby is sleepy now.*)
- Subject-auxiliary-verb-adverb (*Baby is eating now.*)

Children at this time begin to embed phrases and clauses in their sentences to create complex and compound sentences. Children also use coordinating (e.g., *and, or, but*) and subordinating conjunctions (e.g., *then, when, because*) to connect clauses. By the end of the preschool period, children produce compound sentences, as in *I told Daddy, and Daddy told Mommy,* as well as complex sentences with embedded clauses, as in *I told Daddy, who told Mommy* (see Justice & Ezell, 2002).

Achievements in Content

The preschool period represents an active and rich period of lexical development in which children build the content of their language. Two areas of preschool content achievements warrant discussion. First, preschoolers show rapid expansion of their receptive and expressive lexicons. Second, preschoolers increase their ability to use decontextualized language.

The Lexicon.   By some accounts, children understand about 10,000 words by first grade (Anglin, Miller, & Wakefield, 1993)! Children learn new words during the preschool period through *incidental exposures,* or situations in which children informally experience new words within contexts of use. Preschool children show remarkable talent in their ability to effectively and efficiently acquire new words within a variety of daily activities (Brackenbury & Fey, 2003).

A single exposure is often adequate for giving children a general sense of a novel word's meaning. However, children's vocabulary acquisition is a gradual process. Their initial word representations progress from immature and incomplete to mature and accurate. The initial exposure to a word accompanied by the rapid acquisition of a general sense of its meaning is called *fast mapping* (Carey & Bartlett, 1978; McGregor, Friedman, Reilly, & Newman, 2002). These initial representations are then refined over time with repeated exposure to the concept over multiple contexts.

Curtis (2005) describes vocabulary development (as it applies both to children and to adults) as a four-stage process. In stage 1, a child has no knowledge of a word ("I've never heard it"); in stage 2, a child has emergent knowledge of a word ("I've heard of it, but I don't know what it means"); in stage 3, a child has contextual knowledge of the word ("I recognize it in context. It has something to do with . . . "); and in stage 4, a child has full knowledge of the word ("I know it") (p. 43). During the preschool period, children's vocabularies include words at each of these stages: some are quite familiar and consistent with full knowledge, whereas others are fairly rudimentary, with emergent and contextual knowledge.

Decontextualized Language Skills. Preschool-age children begin to make an important shift from being highly contextualized in their language skills to being decontextualized. Contextualized language is rooted in the immediate context: the here and now. It aids understanding through the incorporation of and reliance on shared knowledge, gestures, intonation, and immediately present situational cues. A child using contextualized language might say, "Gimme that" while pointing to something in the listener's hands or might refer to a "Superman cake" in the context of a birthday party.

Decontextualized language is appropriate and necessary for discussing events and concepts beyond the here and now. These events may have occurred long ago or might occur in the future; they may be occurring in the next room or only in an abstract realm. Sometime during the preschool years, children become able to use language in a decontextualized manner. Decontextualized discourse relies heavily on the language itself in the construction of meaning. Decontextualized language may not contain context cues and does not assume shared background knowledge or context in the same way contextualized language does. A child using decontextualized language might ask a parent for something in another room of the house ("Can you get the blocks down from my bookshelf?") or might describe a Superman cake to someone after the birthday party has taken place ("My mom made a Superman cake for my birthday party."). In the first example, the child cannot rely on context to help in the communication with the mother; as with all types of decontextualized discourse, the child must use highly precise syntax and vocabulary to represent events that are beyond the here and now.

> **DISCUSSION POINT:**
> Children of lower socioeconomic status generally have a more difficult time producing decontextualized language. Why do you think this is?

The ability to engage in decontextualized discourse is fundamental to academic success, as nearly all the learning that occurs in schools focuses on events and concepts beyond the classroom walls. This ability develops during the preschool years as children learn to use grammar and vocabulary in a highly precise manner.

ACHIEVEMENTS IN USE

Use describes how we apply language functionally for meeting our personal and social needs. During the preschool years, children begin to master several new discourse functions, improve their conversational skills, and use narratives.

Recall that as toddlers enter the two-word stage, they are already capable of using language to satisfy six different communicative functions (instrumental, regulatory, personal interactional, heuristic, imaginative, and informational). Preschoolers begin to use language for an even greater variety of discourse functions, including interpretive, logical, participatory, and organizing functions (Halliday, 1975, 1977, 1978). Interpretive functions are those that interpret the whole of one's experience. Logical functions express logical relations between ideas. Participatory functions express wishes, feelings, attitudes, and judgments. Organizing functions organize discourse. As the number of discourse functions grows, so, too, do preschoolers' conversational skills.

One mark of an effective conversationalist is the ability to take turns in a conversation. Preschool-age children quickly become adept at turn taking. They can maintain a conversation for two or more turns, particularly when the topic is their favorite: themselves! Although they still have some difficulties understanding when communication breakdowns occur and giving listeners the appropriate amount of information to facilitate understanding, preschoolers are increasingly sophisticated conversationalists. They understand that they should respond to questions, and they discover that speaking at the same time as another person makes for ineffective communication.

Children also begin to hone their narrative skills in the preschool years. "Hey, Mom, guess what happened on the bus today?" is one way in which a preschooler might begin a narrative. Narratives are essentially decontextualized monologues, in that rather than describing the here and now, they often focus on people or characters not immediately present or on events removed from the current context. Narratives are monologues in that they are largely uninterrupted streams of language, unlike conversations, in which two or more people share the linguistic load.

In a narrative, the speaker presents a topic and organizes the information pertaining to that topic in such a way that the listener can assume a relatively passive role, providing only minimal support to the speaker. Two important types of narratives are (1) personal, in which an individual shares a factual event of his or her life, and (2) fictional, in which an individual shares a made-up event. Usually, both types of narratives are threaded by an explicit sequence of events that are either causally or temporally related. A causal sequence unfolds following a cause-and-effect chain of events (e.g., Jesse didn't want to go to school . . . so Jesse told his mom he was sick.). A temporal sequence unfolds over time (e.g., First we went to the store. Then we told the clerk what we wanted.). In producing narrative—whether personal or fictional—the speaker must negotiate a complex set of linguistic skills, including syntax for ordering words and ideas, verb morphology for signaling the time of events, vocabulary for precisely representing events and people, and pragmatics for knowing how much information to share with the listener.

Although narrative skills begin to develop as early as age 2, most children are not able to construct true narratives until around age 4. Children's early narratives may include only a minimal description of the participants, time, and location relevant to the event. In some cases, they may omit this information altogether. So, for example, when listening to a 3-year-old narrate a story, it may be necessary to ask such questions as "You said Dominick scratched you—is he your brother or your cat?" and "Did that happen on TV?" to get a better picture of what the child is trying to express. Importantly, narratives become clearer for the listener as children's ability to consider the listener's perspective emerges. Children's repertoire of linguistic devices, including adverbial time phrases (e.g., *yesterday, this morning*) and verb morphology (signaling the time of activities) also grows, thus increasing the comprehensibility of their narratives.

Narrative skills are an important area of mastery for preschoolers and have been found to be one of the best predictors of children's later school outcomes (Roth, Speece, & Cooper, 2002). The decontextualized language inherent in narratives may be the critical link to the acquisition of early literacy skills and subsequent school achievement (Peterson, Jesso, & McCabe, 1999). Table 2.5 summarizes these major achievements in narrative and shows how children move from "heaps" and descriptive sequences to well-rounded, complex stories ("true narratives") in the elementary years.

| TABLE 2.5 Major achievements in narrative |||
Approximate Age of Emergence	Narrative Stage	Characteristics
2 years	Heaps	• Few links from one sentence to another • Organization based on immediate perception
2–3 years	Sequences	• Superficial but arbitrary time sequences • No causal links between events
3–4 years	Primitive Narratives	• Have a concrete core surrounded by a set of clarifying or amplifying attributes
4–4 1/2 years	Unfocused Chains	• Story as a whole loses its point and drifts off
5 years	Focused Chains	• A main character experiences a series of events, but no true concept is present
5–7 years	True Narratives	• Has a theme or moral • Concrete, perceptual, or abstract bonds hold the story together

Source: Adapted with permission from D. Hughes, L. McGillivray, & M. Schmidek. (1997). Guide to narrative language: Procedures for assessment. Eau Claire, WI: Thinking Publications.

Achievements in Speech

During the preschool years, children continue to expand and stabilize their sound repertoires. By the end of the preschool period, children are likely to have mastered nearly all of the phonemes in their native language. Four- and 5-year-olds typically exhibit only lingering difficulties with a few of the later-developing phonemes, including r (row), l (low), s (sun), ch (cheese), sh (shy), z (z_oo), and th (think, though). Difficulties with some of the earlier acquired sounds may persist in complex multisyllabic words (daffodil) or in words with consonant clusters (split). However, by the end of the preschool period, children are highly intelligible, and their expressive phonemic repertoire is nearly as extensive as an adult's.

As mentioned earlier, phonological processes refer to the systematic deviations children make in their expressive phonology. In the preschool years, nearly all processes are suppressed as children's phonological systems stabilize. The greatest rate of suppression occurs at 3 to 4 years of age (Haelsig & Madison, 1986). Weak syllable deletion and cluster reduction may occur with 4-year-olds but are usually suppressed by 5 years of age. Two patterns that may persist past the fifth birthday include liquid gliding (substituting y and w for l and r) and th substitution (substituting d and t for th).

Receptive phonology also continues to develop during the preschool years. The achievement of strong internal phonological representations is very important. Reading development—discussed later in this chapter—requires that a child have robust phonological representations in order to make sense of the alphabetic principle, or the relationship between letters (graphemes) and sounds (phonemes). Environmental and biological factors can impact the development of adequate phonological representations. For instance, children who receive little linguistic stimulation and children who have ongoing middle-ear infections are at risk for delays in the development of solid phonological representations (Nittrouer, 1996). The quality and quantity of phonological stimulation relates to children's development of robust phonological representations.

Achievements in Emergent Literacy

The preschool period marks several critical achievements in young children's development of literacy. Between ages 3 and 5, children begin to make sense of reading and writing in a rudimentary way (Justice & Ezell, 2001). They learn how print works, they begin to play with the sound units that make up words, and they develop an interest in reading and writing. Researchers refer to this earliest period of learning about reading and writing as *emergent literacy.* Emergent literacy encompasses children's developing knowledge about reading and writing conventions. Although children at this time are not yet reading and writing in a conventional sense, their emerging knowledge about print and sounds forms an important foundation for the reading instruction that commences in kindergarten (Justice & Pullen, 2003).

Emergent literacy achievements depend largely on metalinguistic ability, or the child's ability to view language as an object of attention. Emergent literacy involves the child's engagement in activities in which oral or written language is the object of scrutiny, such as pretending to write, looking at words in a storybook, or making up rhyming patterns (Chaney, 1998). The two most important achievements in emergent literacy for preschoolers are print awareness and phonological awareness. **Print awareness** describes the young child's understanding of the form and functions of written language. **Phonological awareness** describes the young child's understanding of and sensitivity to the sound units of oral language, namely the series of larger and smaller units that make up speech (phonemes, syllables, words).

Print awareness includes a number of specific achievements that children generally acquire along a developmental continuum (Justice & Ezell, 2004): (1) print interest, (2) print functions, (3) print conventions, (4) print forms, and (5) print part-to-whole relationships (see Figure 2.6). First, young children develop an interest in and appreciation for print. Children recognize that print is a specific type of stimulus in the environment and in books. Second, they

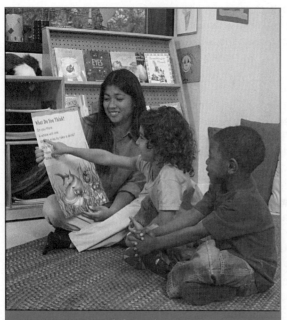

Pointing to print while reading to preschoolers can help foster print awareness.

begin to understand that print conveys meaning, that it has a specific type of function. Third, children develop an understanding of specific print conventions, such as how print moves left to right and top to bottom. Fourth, children learn the language that describes specific print units, such as words and letters. Fifth, children learn the relationship among different print units, such as how letters combine to form words. Influences on children's development of these abilities include their home environment and their general oral language ability (Boudreau & Hedberg, 1999).

Phonological awareness is the child's sensitivity and access to the sound structure of spoken words. Phonological awareness emerges incrementally, beginning around 2 years of age, moving from a shallow level of awareness to a deep level of awareness (Stanovich, 2000). Children possessing shallow levels of phonological awareness show an implicit and rudimentary sensitivity to large units of sound structure. They are able to hear and produce rhymes, segment sentences into words and words into syllables, and detect beginning sound similarities across words (e.g., *sing, sack, sun*). Children develop these shallow sensitivities during the preschool

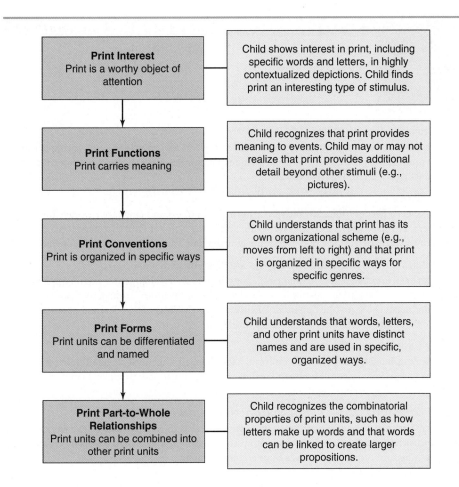

FIGURE 2.6

Major achievements in print awareness during the preschool years.

Source: L. M. Justice & H. K. Ezell. (2004). Print referencing: An emergent literacy enhancement technique and its clinical applications. *Language, Speech, and Hearing Services in Schools, 35*, 185–193. Reprinted with permission.

years, from roughly 3 to 5 years of age. Children with a deep level of phonological awareness demonstrate an explicit and analytical knowledge of the smallest phonological segments of speech, representing the phoneme. They are able to count the number of phonemes in words (e.g., *wig* has three sounds, and *spray* has four sounds), segment words into their constituent phonemes (e.g., *big* can be broken into /b/+ /I/+ /g/), and manipulate the phonological segments contained within words (e.g., deleting the first sound in *spray* and moving it to the end of the word, for *prays*) (Justice & Schuele, 2004).

DISCUSSION POINT:
How good are your phoneme segmentation skills? Say the following words aloud and identify how many sounds (not letters!) are in each: *nothing, wheat, elephant, ostrich, fantastic.* (Answers: 5, 3, 7, 6, 9)

SCHOOL-AGE ACCOMPLISHMENTS

You may wonder what language and communication achievements remain for school-age children to master. So much of the research concerning language development focuses on the achievements of infants and young children that it is tempting to equate language development with the very young child, overlooking the accomplishments of older children. Yet substantial development and refinement in the areas of syntax, pragmatics, and semantics occur throughout the school-age years and adolescence. The following sections discuss the most important aspects of communicative development among school-aged children, which include functional flexibility, reading and writing, literate language, and form and content refinements.

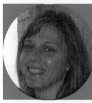

SPOTLIGHT ON RESEARCH AND PRACTICE

NAME: JEN ANDERSON
PROFESSION/TITLE
Program Manager, Microsoft

PROFESSIONAL RESPONSIBILITIES

I oversee projects—setting project requirements and priorities, timelines, and writing specifications for product design. I also mediate between teams, oversee work we do with other companies, and conduct customer and market research.

A DAY AT WORK

I work in Speech Recognition, currently in acquiring data to expand language coverage for various recognizers. I oversee the collections and setup, define the types of data that need to be collected, set deadlines and expectations, and determine how the data should be validated before use.

HOW INTERESTS IN COMMUNICATION SCIENCES AND DISORDERS BEGAN

I've always been interested in math and psychology, especially development. I was an Applied Math major in college and took a linguistics course and discovered the intersection of math and language. During my master's degree in Cognitive Science at Brown University, I learned about language acquisition and was able to combine all of my interests.

CURRENT RESEARCH AND PRACTICE INTERESTS

Since I work in industry, my research interests have changed. Currently, I spend time researching differences (especially cultural) between languages and their use. Additionally, I conduct research on how people use speech recognition.

MOST EXCITING/INTERESTING PROFESSIONAL ACCOMPLISHMENT IN CSD

Having my first experiment in graduate school work—it was mirroring some of the work done by Janet Werker but was the first time I had set up an experiment and analyzed data by myself. Having everything turn out correctly was a huge accomplishment.

FUTURE TRENDS IN CSD

Better understanding of developmental disorders, multilingual acquisition.

Functional Flexibility

Functional flexibility refers to the ability to use language for a variety of communicative purposes, or functions. This flexibility is increasingly important for school-age children who must compare and contrast, persuade, hypothesize, explain, classify, and predict in the context of classroom activities and projects. Figure 2.7 provides a more complete list of language functions that are extremely relevant to school-age children, attesting to the importance of flexibility in language for children of this age.

Each of the language functions requires a distinct set of linguistic, social, and cognitive competencies, all of which develop over the school-age years and must be integrated by the child for communicative competence. For example, according to Nippold (1998), students must integrate seven skills in order to use language to persuade:

1. Adjust to listener characteristics (e.g., age, authority, familiarity)
2. State advantages as a reason to comply
3. Anticipate and reply to counterarguments

FIGURE 2.7

Language functions required of school-age children.

1. *To instruct:* To provide specific sequential directions
2. *To inquire:* To seek understanding through asking questions
3. *To test:* To investigate the logic of a statement
4. *To describe:* To tell about, giving necessary information to identify
5. *To compare and contrast:* To show how things are similar and different
6. *To explain:* To define terms by providing specific examples
7. *To analyze:* To break down a statement into its component parts, telling what each means and how they are related
8. *To hypothesize:* To test a statement's logical or empirical consequences
9. *To deduce:* To arrive at a conclusion by reasoning; to infer
10. *To evaluate:* To weigh and judge the relative importance of an idea

Source: From C. Bereiter & S. Engelmann. (1966). *Teaching disadvantaged children in the preschool.* Boston: Allyn & Bacon. Copyright © 1996 by Pearson Education. Reprinted/adapted by permission of the publisher.

4. Use positive techniques such as politeness and bargaining as strategies to increase compliance

5. Avoid negative strategies such as whining and begging

6. Generate a large number and variety of different arguments

7. Control the discourse assertively

Students who cannot use language flexibly are more likely than other students to have difficulty with the academic and social demands of elementary, middle, and high schools.

Related to children's development of functional flexibility is their development of conversational abilities. During the school-age years, and particularly throughout adolescence, children's conversational abilities improve dramatically. Key developments occur in the following areas: staying on topic for longer periods of time, participating in extended dialogues with others that last for several conversational turns, including an increasing number of relevant and factual statements and comments in conversations, making smooth transitions from one conversational topic to another, and adjusting the content and style of one's speech according to the listener's feelings and ideas (Nippold, 1998).

Reading and Writing

Reading and writing are two major achievements that take place during the school-age years. Success at learning to read requires the child's unlocking of the alphabetic principle, meaning that children must learn how the orthography of letters (graphemes) corresponds to the phonology of sounds (phonemes). Children's success with grapheme–phoneme correspondence rests on their achievement of print awareness and phonological awareness in the preschool period. Children who enter school with skills in these areas are more likely than others to succeed at beginning reading instruction (Chaney, 1998).

Children learning to read generally progress through a predictable series of stages that span the period between preschool and adulthood (Chall, 1996). The preschool years correspond to an emergent literacy or prereading stage, during which the most critical developments consist of oral language, print awareness,

DISCUSSION POINT:
Using what you know about Reston, introduced in Case Study 2.1, do you predict that he would also exhibit difficulties with reading comprehension? Why or why not?

and phonological awareness. Children then progress through five stages that build on this early foundation, as presented by Chall (1996).

Stage 1, *initial reading, or decoding,* covers the period between kindergarten and first grade, when children are between 5 and 7 years of age. During this stage, children learn to associate letters with the sounds they represent and attend to sound–spelling relationships as they begin to decode words. The focus at this stage is learning to read, or the development of decoding skills and the untangling of the alphabetic principle.

Stage 2, *confirmation, fluency, and ungluing from print,* covers the period between second and third grade, when children are between 7 and 8 years of age. During this stage, children hone their decoding skills and develop strategies for comprehending what they read. Children gradually transition from learning to read to reading to learn.

Stage 3, *reading for learning the new,* lasts from grades 4 to 8, when children are between 9 and 13 years of age. Children read to gain new information and are solidly reading to learn. Reading during this stage helps expand children's vocabularies, build background and world knowledge, and develop strategic reading habits.

Stage 4, *multiple viewpoints: high school,* covers the high school period from the age of 14 to the age of 18. During stage 4, students learn to handle increasingly difficult concepts and to read the texts that describe them. Students learn to analyze texts critically and to understand multiple points of view.

Stage 5, *construction and reconstruction—a world view: college,* occurs from age 18 on. During this stage, the linguistic and cognitive demands placed on readers continue to increase, and readers are able to construct understanding by analyzing and synthesizing text.

Literate Language

DISCUSSION POINT:

Describe in writing what you did last night. Document the use of literate language features in this written sample. Which features occur most frequently? Least frequently?

An earlier section of this chapter described the difference between contextualized and decontextualized language. When children enter school, language becomes increasingly decontextualized—removed from the here and now. *Literate language* is the term used to describe language that is highly decontextualized. The literate language style characterizes language that is used to "monitor and reflect on experience, and reason about, plan, and predict experiences" (Westby, 1985, p. 181). Literate language refers to the child's ability to use language without the aid of context cues for supporting meaning; the child must rely on language itself to make meaning. Developing a literate language style, or progressing from contextualized to decontextualized language, is crucial for children's participation in the type of discourse that occurs in school settings. Imagine the following conversation taking place between 4-year-old Amber and her 8-year-old sister, Kristy:

AMBER: I want that crayon!

KRISTY: No way! You wrote on the wall with my crayons the other day while I was at school, and I got in trouble.

Discourse development lies along a continuum, reflecting oral language on one end and literate language on the other (Westby, 1991). In our example, Amber's and Kristy's utterances represent opposite ends of this continuum. At the lower level of the discourse continuum is *oral language,* or the linguistic aspects of communicative competence necessary for communicating very basic desires and needs (phonology, syntax, morphology, and semantics). Westby describes children at this end of the continuum as "learning to talk." Children learning to talk are able to satisfy some basic language functions, including requesting and greeting. They can also produce simple syntactic structures. English speakers, for example, can form yes or no questions by inserting *do* before the subject (*You like ice cream* becomes *Do you like ice cream?*) and can mark the past tense by adding -*ed* or by retrieving the appropriate irregular past-tense verb. The most salient characteristic of oral language is its highly contextualized style. Highly contextualized language is that which depends heavily on the immediate context and environment. Markers of highly contextualized language include referential pronouns, or pronouns that refer to something physically available to the speaker ("I want *that*."), as well as gestures and facial expressions. Only when children have mastered oral language can they begin to "talk to learn," or to use language to reflect on past experiences and to reason about, predict, and plan for future experiences using decontextualized language (Westby, 1991).

Children who talk to learn represent the literate language end of the continuum. At this end, children use language chiefly as a way to communicate higher-order cognitive functions (e.g., reflecting, reasoning, and planning). Highly specific vocabulary and complex syntax that express ideas, events, and objects beyond those of the present typify literate language. Some specific features of literate language that children learn to use include the following (Curenton & Justice, 2004):

1. *Elaborated noun phrases:* Groups of words consisting of a noun and one or more modifiers that provide additional information about the noun, including articles (e.g., *a, an, the*), possessives (e.g., *my, his, their*), demonstratives (e.g., *this, that, those*), quantifiers (e.g., *every, each, some*), *wh-* words (e.g., *what, which, whichever*), and adjectives (e.g., *tall, long, ugly*).

2. *Adverbs:* Syntactic forms used to modify verbs, which enhance the explicitness of action and event descriptions. Adverbs provide additional information about time (e.g., *suddenly, again, now*), manner (e.g., *somehow, well, slowly*), degree (e.g., *almost, barely, much*), place (*here, outside, above*), reason (*therefore, consequently, so*), and affirmation or negation (e.g., *definitely, really, never*). Adverbial conjuncts used to link two sentences together (e.g., *conversely, similarly*) are particularly important to engaging in analogical reasoning (Nippold, 2007).

3. *Conjunctions:* Words or phrases that organize information and clarify relationships among elements. Coordinating conjunctions include *and, for, or, yet, but, nor,* and *so.* Subordinating conjunctions are more numerous and include *after, although, as, because,* and *for,* among others.

4. *Metacognitive and metalinguistic verbs:* These verbs refer to various acts of thinking and speaking. Metacognitive verbs include *think, know, believe, imagine, feel, consider, suppose, decide, forget,* and *remember.* Metalinguistic verbs include *say, tell, speak, shout, answer, call, reply,* and *yell.*

Consider these structures in the following example of decontextualized language:

> Last night, after I got home, I was wondering how to occupy myself when I decided that I would rearrange my kitchen cabinets. You see, I was quite bored, given all that had transpired. I started to pull cans off the top shelf, at which point I came upon something quite odd. Now, before I tell you what I found . . .

This author paints a picture for the listener by using a variety of techniques that transcend vocabulary and syntax. Specificity is provided lexically by elaborated noun phrases (*my kitchen cabinets, the top shelf*), adverbs (*last night, now*), and metacognitive/metalinguistic verbs (*wondering, decided, tell*). Conjunctions and conjunctive adverbs are spread liberally across the story to weave together events in a causal and temporal manner (e.g., *at which point, now*). These devices provide context that is not otherwise available to the listener, or in this case, the reader. As children move through the elementary grades into adolescence and high school, we expect them to be able to use literate language structures to create context for readers and listeners.

Form and Content Refinements

Form Refinements.   As students move through the elementary grades into high school, form achievements progress slowly and subtly. Because many of the syntactic skills that children exhibit are only rarely used in conversation, such as the passive voice, these form accomplishments can be hard to witness. The most important achievements in form for school-age children are in the area of complex syntax, or developmentally advanced grammatical structures that mark a literate language style (Paul, 1995). These structures occur relatively infrequently in spoken language, but when used in written language indicate more advanced levels of grammar. Examples of complex syntax include noun phrase postmodification with past participles (*a tree called the willow*), complex verb phrases using the perfective aspect (*They have driven a long way*), and adverbial conjuncts (e.g., *consequently, similarly, however*).

The development of syntax over the school-age years is most easily visible in students' writing. Persuasive writing in particular is a vehicle for the expression of more complex syntax. Persuasive writing, according to Nippold (2000), is a challenging communicative task, yet it is an important skill that children develop in the school-age period. Persuasive writing requires an awareness of what others believe and value and the ability to present one's ideas in a logical sequence. Syntactic complexities arise in persuasive writing as children must produce "longer sentences that contain greater amounts of subordination and stronger linkages between sentences, attainments that are partially achieved through the proper use of adverbial connectors" (Nippold, 2000, p. 20).

School-age children also continue to experience development in morphology. One important area of morphological development is children's use of derivational prefixes and suffixes. Derivational prefixes are morphemes that we add to the beginnings of words to change their meanings, such as *dis- (disallow)*, *non- (noncompliant)*, and *ir- (irreversible)*. Derivational suffixes are morphemes that we add to the ends of words to change their form class, or part of speech (i.e., to change a verb to a noun or to change an adjective to an adverb), such as *-hood (sisterhood)*, *-ment (encouragement)*, *-er (faster)*, and *-ly (happily)*. Some of the later-learned derivational suffixes include *-y*, which is used to form an adjective, and *-ly*, which is used to form an adverb.

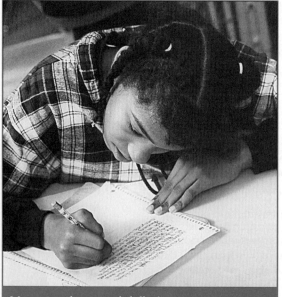

Mastering the art and skill of persuasive writing is one linguistic challenge school-age children face.

Context Refinements.   The typical school-age child makes considerable gains in developing the lexicon. These gains occur primarily from reading books, an activity that provides students with access to words and concepts that are not typically the topic of everyday conversations. The receptive and expressive vocabularies of school-age children continue to expand; by the time they graduate from high school, they will have command of over 60,000 words (Pinker, 1994).

Three areas of notable content development for school-age students are (1) understanding multiple meanings, (2) understanding lexical ambiguity, and (3) understanding figurative language. As children's lexicons grow and they encounter more and more words, they realize that many words have more than one meaning. Students become able to provide multiple definitions for words that have several common meanings. Doing this requires lexical knowledge and metalinguistic knowledge, both of which are necessary to achieve full competence at the literate end of the oral–literate language continuum.

The understanding of lexical ambiguity is a second and related area of notable content achievement for school-age children. Lexical ambiguity occurs for words with multiple meanings, as in "That was a real bear," in which the meaning of "bear" is ambiguous. Lexical ambiguity regularly fuels the humor in jokes, riddles, comic strips, newspaper headlines, and advertisements (Nippold, 1998), as in the joke "Is your refrigerator running?" ("You'd better go catch it!"). When students encounter words that are ambiguous, they must first notice the ambiguity, and then they must scrutinize the words to arrive at the appropriate meaning. Students with weak oral-language skills are often not very adept at noticing lexical ambiguities and are less likely than other students to seek clarification for an ambiguity when they do notice one. The result can be a communication breakdown (Paul, 1995).

A third semantic refinement that occurs over the school-age years is the ability to use and understand figurative language, or the use of words, phrases, symbols, and ideas in a nonliteral and often abstract way to evoke mental images and sense impressions. Of the different types of figurative language, including similes, metaphors, oxymorons, hyperboles, and proverbs, Nippold (2000) reports that proverbs are one of the most difficult types to master. Proverbs serve a variety of communicative functions, such as

- commenting (Blood is thicker than water.);
- interpreting (His bark is worse than his bite.);
- advising (Don't count your chickens before they hatch.);
- warning (Better safe than sorry.); and
- encouraging (Every cloud has a silver lining.) (Nippold, 2000).

Nippold reports that proverb understanding improves gradually during the adolescent years and that the presence of a supportive linguistic environment can facilitate the process. Proverb understanding has been correlated with measures of academic success in literature and mathematics in adolescents (Nippold, 2000), likely because proverb understanding reveals a student's ability to contend with abstract and metalinguistic aspects of language.

LANGUAGE DIVERSITY CONSIDERATIONS

It is estimated that between 60 and 75% of people in the world speak more than a single language (Baker, 2000). According to the 2000 U.S. Census, within the United States, 47 million people aged 5 and over (18% of those sampled) reported speaking a language other than English in the home. This figure represents an increase from the 1990 and 1980 U.S. Census, in which 31.8 million (14%) and 23.1 million (11%) people, respectively, reported speaking a language other than English in the home. Because many young American children speak languages other than English in the home, teaching English as a second language (ESL) becomes an important consideration as children enter formal schooling and remains an important consideration throughout the school-age years.

In the 2003–2004 school year, some 3.8 million students (11% of all students) participated in English language learner (ELL) services in U.S. schools (U.S. Department of Education, National Center for Education Statistics, 2006). Although the number of children learning ESL in American schools may present practical and logistical challenges for schools that use English as the language of instruction, it is important to recognize that the majority of ELLs do not have a communication disorder. In fact, they most likely exhibit communicative competence in the same areas (linguistic, phonological, grammatical, lexical, and discourse) as their English-speaking peers, within their own speech community (e.g., at home). However, within the English-speaking educational environment, children who do not have communicative competence in the English language may face particular challenges in learning; consequently, many current policy initiatives support teaching ESL in public schools in order to ensure that students can acquire communicative competence in the English-speaking community as well (e.g., No Child Left Behind Act of 2001, Title III administered by the Office of English Language Acquisition, Language Enhancement and Academic Achievement for Limited English Proficient Students).

School-age students who arrive in the classroom with little or no proficiency in the English language may experience four stages of language development as they learn a second language in the classroom (see Genesee, Paradis, & Crago, 2004). The first stage is called the *home language stage.* In this stage, students tend to speak their home language (e.g., Spanish, Arabic) with other students and adults in the classroom who also speak their home language. Younger children may even use their home language when speaking to others who do not speak that language until they realize that such a strategy does not make for effective communication. In the second stage, the *nonverbal period,* students focus on understanding rather than speaking English. They may use some gestures to communicate but tend to listen more and say less during this period. During the third stage of *telegraphic and formulaic* use, students use single words (recall the earlier discussion of telegraphic speech in this chapter), repeat words and phrases that others use, and use simple phrases that they are able to memorize ("See you later," "Where is the restroom?"). During the fourth stage, *language productivity,* students continue to expand their lexical and grammatical repertoire. They may construct simple sentences, rather than use memorized phrases, using the subject-verb-object pattern (e.g., "I go home," "She make breakfast"). Students in the stage of language productivity may also use verbs with multiple meanings (e.g., *make, do, go*) to express a wide variety of language functions.

It is worth repeating that although school-age children learning ESL may experience communication challenges in the classroom, they do not necessarily have a communication disorder. Chapter 1 describes the difference between communication disorders, in which one's communication skills are discrepant in comparison to others who share the same language, cultural background, and dialect, and communication differences, in which one's communication patterns differ from the communication patterns with whom the individual is speaking.

CHAPTER SUMMARY

Communicative competence refers to the understandings and abilities that speakers of a language must possess and utilize in order to communicate effectively in that language. Communicative competence is acquired at two main levels—linguistic and pragmatic. Linguistic aspects include phonological competence, grammatical competence, lexical competence, and discourse competence and are related directly to the nature and structure of language. Pragmatic aspects of communicative competence include functional competence, sociolinguistic competence, interactional competence, and cultural competence and relate to the social contexts in which language is used. Communicative competence develops along a fairly predictable trajectory across the life span, with major milestones achieved in roughly the same order and at roughly the same ages across cultures. Communicative competence is constructed on some innately given abilities and early foundations and continues to develop throughout toddlerhood, the preschool years, the school-age years, and into adulthood.

KEY TERMS

communicative competence, p. 41

communicative performance, p. 41

cooing sounds, p. 51

intentional communication, p. 48

intersubjective awareness, p. 48

jargon, p. 52

joint attention, p. 48

lexicon, p. 53

mean length of utterance (MLU), p. 57

overextension, p. 59

phonological awareness, p. 70

phonological processes, p. 44

phonotactics, p. 49

print awareness, p. 70

reduplicative babbling, p. 52

reflexive sounds, p. 51

register, p. 46

underextension, p. 59

variegated babbling, p. 52

vocabulary spurt, p. 59

ON THE WEB

Check out the Companion Website at www.pearsonhighered.com/justice2e! On it, you will find

- suggested readings;
- reflection questions;
- a self-study quiz; and
- links to additional online resources, including information about current technologies in communication sciences and disorders.

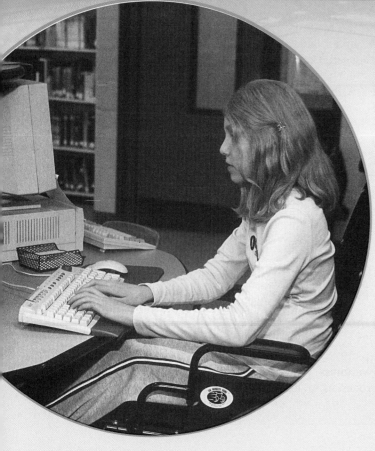

ANATOMICAL AND PHYSIOLOGICAL BASES OF COMMUNICATION AND COMMUNICATION DISORDERS

FOCUS QUESTIONS

This chapter addresses the following topics:

1. Neuroscience and human communication
2. Anatomy and physiology of speech
3. Anatomy and physiology of hearing
4. Anatomy and physiology of swallowing

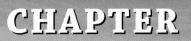
INTRODUCTION

Human communication involves the complex interaction of many systems of the human body. People involved in the assessment and treatment of communication disorders require a sophisticated understanding of the functions and structures of these systems. This chapter provides a basic introduction to the anatomy, physiology, and neuroscience involved with speech, language, hearing, and swallowing.

Anatomy and physiology together form the branch of science concerning the description of body structures (anatomy) and the functions of those structures (physiology) (Marieb, 2005). To understand the process of human communication, we need to consider both structure and function—to understand the specifics of a particular anatomical structure, including how it relates to other structures and forms an anatomical system, and how a structure works both by itself and in concert with other structures as a physiological system.

Anatomy and physiology are ancient sciences dating back many centuries. The Greek physician Hippocrates (c. 460–377 B.C.E.) is considered the father of medicine and of anatomy as a science. Hippocrates' work provided an important impetus for centuries of inquiry into how the human body is organized and how its parts work (or do not work) when in a state of health or disease. Inquiries into the anatomy and physiology of speech, language, hearing, and swallowing date back hundreds of years.

Neuroscience is a particular branch of science that focuses on the anatomy and physiology of the nervous system, including the brain (Bhatnagar, 2007). It is a relatively new science characterized by rapid and remarkable advances in new technologies, such as magnetic resonance imaging (MRI), positron emission tomography (PET), and computed tomography scan (CT Scan). These technologies are able to provide detailed images of both the anatomy and the physiology of the brain. The brain is the mediator of the body's sensory and motor systems, including those involved with speech, language, hearing, and swallowing. Therefore, interest in how the brain works has consumed many researchers and practitioners in the discipline of communication sciences and disorders in recent decades. ●●●

CASE STUDY 3.1   Communication Disorders Across the Life Span

Timmy Sullivan is a 60-year-old, thrice-divorced man living in Washington, D.C. Timmy is a Vietnam veteran who, near the end of his 2-year tour of duty in 1968, experienced a severe head injury, for which he received a silver star. Specifically, during combat, shrapnel pierced Timmy's left forehead and lodged in his frontal lobe. Surgery was performed within hours to remove the shrapnel, and after a 1-month rehabilitation and recuperation period, Timmy was discharged from active service. Timmy has not sought any additional rehabilitation for his injury in the years since discharge, and he does not feel that he shows any symptoms related to his 35-year-old brain injury. Timmy has not had a regular job in the last 10 years but brings in some income by doing odd jobs in his neighborhood. His friends and ex-wives describe Timmy as fun-loving, energetic, and warm, but erratic, irresponsible, and disorganized in his behavior.

Internet research

1 What kind of assistance is available for military personnel who have experienced brain injuries?

2 How common are brain injuries among active-duty military personnel today? How do these figures compare with corresponding figures from the Vietnam era?

3 What is the Vietnam Head Injury Study?

Brainstorm and discussion

1 Brainstorm some possible short- and long-term repercussions of a serious injury to the frontal lobe.

2 What kinds of supports should be made available to military personnel who experience brain injuries during active duty?

● ● ●

Patricia is a 3-year-old girl recently adopted by Mr. and Dr. Franklin of Cincinnati, Ohio. Patricia's birth parents died in a car accident when she was only 12 weeks old. From the age of 12 weeks to the age of 18 months, Patricia lived with a foster family, where she was allegedly physically and mentally abused by two older foster siblings. Patricia was removed from this foster home and lived in a second foster home until she was 3 years old, when she was adopted by the Franklins. Mr. and Dr. Franklin are concerned about Patricia's history of abuse, although she appears to have no symptoms associated with abuse and seems to be a well-adjusted and happy child. Mr. Franklin is a stay-at-home dad; Dr. Franklin is a neuroscientist who studies the effects of early maltreatment on the brain development of rodents at the University of Cincinnati. She is familiar with research showing that early abuse and maltreatment can affect brain physiology in rodents. The Franklins are thus seeking assistance through an early intervention program in Cincinnati to have Patricia comprehensively evaluated for social, emotional, cognitive, and linguistic development.

However, the early intervention program is balking at covering the cost of the assessment, given that Patricia shows no apparent signs of developmental difficulties due to abuse.

Internet research

1 What is early intervention?

2 How common are maltreatment and abuse among young children in the United States?

3 Is there evidence showing that early childhood abuse can have a negative impact on brain development?

Brainstorm and discussion

1 Should a developmental assessment be provided to Patricia even if she displays no outward signs of developmental difficulties?

2 What are some possible repercussions of early abuse on brain development?

NEUROSCIENCE AND HUMAN COMMUNICATION ●

TERMINOLOGY

Descriptions of anatomy and physiology often utilize a specific terminology, or nomenclature. Much of this terminology has its roots in ancient Latin and Greek. It is essential for the student of communication sciences and disorders to be familiar with the terminology associated with positions and directions. Common positional terms used to describe aspects of anatomy and physiology include **anterior** (toward the front) and **posterior** (toward the back); **ventral** (toward the abdomen) and **dorsal** (toward the back); **superior** (toward the top) and **inferior** (toward the bottom); **external** (toward the outside) and **internal** (toward the inside); **proximal** (toward the body) and **distal** (away from the body); and **medial** (toward the middle) and **lateral** (toward the side) (Zemlin, 1997). Two directional terms often used to describe organization of the nervous system and neuroscience include **afferent** (toward the nervous system) and **efferent** (away from the nervous system).

Becoming knowledgeable about neuroscience and, specifically, neuroanatomy, can be challenging. Many of the terms and concepts may be new to students. Nonetheless, this knowledge is crucial both for professionals who work with people who have communication disorders and for those who conduct research in speech, language, hearing, and swallowing disorders. This knowledge base helps professionals and researchers to (1) better understand and identify the neurological causes of communication disorders, (2) recognize signs and symptoms associated with specific neurological pathologies, and (3) find solutions to neurological problems, resulting in improved interventions for children and adults (Bhatnagar & Andy, 1995).

THE NERVOUS SYSTEM

The human nervous systems mediate nearly all aspects of human behavior. The human body has two major nervous systems: the central nervous system (CNS) and the peripheral nervous system (PNS). The CNS consists of the brain and the spinal cord. The PNS consists of the nerves that emerge from the brain and the spinal cord to innervate the rest of the body. In neuroscience, the term *innervate* describes the supply of nerves to a particular region or part of the body. The 12 pairs of nerves that emerge from the brain are the **cranial nerves.** The 31 pairs of nerves that emerge from the spinal cord are called **spinal nerves.** The cranial and spinal nerves carry information back and forth between the brain, the spine, and the rest of the body. This information includes sensory information carried to the brain and motor information carried away from the brain. Figure 3.1 illustrates the major structures in the CNS and PNS.

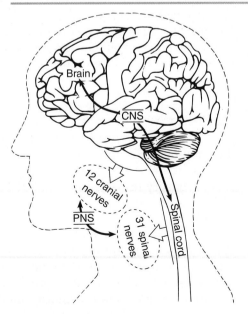

FIGURE 3.1

The central and peripheral nervous systems.

FIGURE 3.2

The neuron.

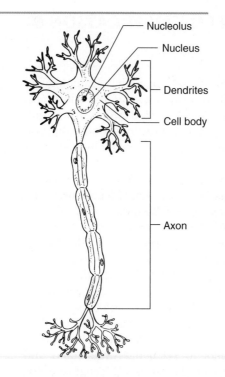

- Nucleolus
- Nucleus
- Dendrites
- Cell body
- Axon

Neurons

The highly specialized cells that make up the nervous system and carry its sensory and motor information are **neurons.** The brain is made up of billions of neurons. A neuron consists of a cell body and two extensions that receive and transmit information in the form of electrical-chemical nerve impulses to and from the cell body, as shown in Figure 3.2. The two types of neural extensions are dendrites and axons. **Dendrites** are afferent extensions, meaning that they bring nerve impulses into the cell body. **Axons** are efferent extensions, meaning that they take nerve impulses away from the cell body. Electrical-chemical nerve impulses move from one neuron to another, traveling down one neuron's dendrite and into its cell body, and then along the axon to another neuron's dendrite. The **synapse** is the space where two neurons meet. For the two neurons to communicate, the nerve impulse must cross the synapse. **Neurotransmitters** are chemical agents that help to carry information across the synaptic cleft, which is the minute space between the axon of the transmitting neuron and the dendrite of the receiving neuron.

Most neurons are sheathed in a coating called **myelin.** The myelin sheath contributes importantly to the rapid relay of nerve impulses; this sheath also helps to protect the neuron. Myelinization, the growth of the myelin sheath, is a slow process that is not complete until late in childhood. Incomplete myelinization or the loss of myelin can result in serious neurological problems. For instance, multiple sclerosis (MS), an autoimmune neurological disease affecting the CNS, results from the loss of myelin. With MS, the body's immune system attacks the myelin sheath covering the nerve cells, which may cause a buildup of sclerosis, or scar tissue. Consequently, the nerve cells malfunction or do not function efficiently, resulting in a variety of symptoms associated with MS, such as slurred speech, balance problems, numbness, and blurred vision (Cook, 2001).

Central Nervous System

The CNS consists of the brain and the spinal cord. The brain is essentially the chief operator of the entire CNS: The brain initiates and regulates virtually all motor, sensory, and cognitive processes (Bhatnagar, 2007). The CNS carries sensory information from the body to the brain via afferent pathways and carries motor commands from the brain to the rest of the body via efferent pathways.

The CNS is what makes humans human. Accordingly, damage to the CNS—the brain or spinal cord—can result in grave consequences. Damage to the brain, as occurs with a traumatic brain injury, can completely alter a person's personality, because the brain is where all the components of personality are stored. Serious brain damage can also disable many of the cognitive acts that make humans what they are—rational and thoughtful problem solvers. Damage to the spinal cord can severely restrict a person's ability to perform both essential and nonessential physical functions, such as breathing, swallowing, walking, and writing.

Many of us know or know of a person who has experienced significant damage to the CNS. Christopher Reeve, an actor who played Superman in several movies, is one such well-known person. Reeve sustained serious spinal cord injury in 1995 in a horse-riding accident and passed away in 2004 due to complications from this injury. He worked tirelessly to find a cure for paralysis. Our familiarity with such cases may make it seem as though the CNS is particularly vulnerable to injury. To the contrary, the CNS is designed to be resistant to damage. Think of all the times you have hit your head or fallen on your back without sustaining serious injury. This is possible because the CNS has a series of three protective shields that help keep it from being damaged.

The first shield is bone. Both the brain and the spinal cord are protected by bone; the skull covers the brain, and the vertebral column covers the spinal cord. The second shield is a series of three layered membranes, the **meninges,** that completely encase the CNS. The inside layer of membrane, called the *pia mater,* tightly wraps around the brain and spinal cord and holds the blood vessels that serve the brain. It is a thin, transparent shield that gives the brain its bright pink color. The second layer is the arachnoid mater. The third and outermost layer is the dura mater (literally, "hard mother"), which consists of thick fibrous tissue that completely encases the brain and the spinal cord. Finally, the third shield protecting the CNS is a layer of fluid, specifically, cerebrospinal fluid (CSF). CSF circulates between the innermost two layers of the meninges, the pia mater and the arachnoid mater. CSF carries chemicals important to metabolic processes, but it also serves as an important buffer for any jolts to the CNS.

> **DISCUSSION POINT:**
> What are some common activities in which persons engage that could result in CNS injuries?

Brain

The brain is the commander in chief, or mediator, of the entire human body. Of all the structures of the human body, the human brain has changed the most in our recent evolutionary history. The most marked change has been in its size and weight. Our ancestor of approximately 3.5 million years ago, *Australopithecus africanus,* had a brain vault roughly the size of a chimpanzee's, weighing about 14 ounces. At that time in our history, the brain was approximately 1% of our body weight. In comparison, the modern human brain averages about 46 to 49 ounces in weight (about 3 pounds), constituting roughly 2.5% of our body weight (Sears, 2003). The greatest change in the human brain, accounting for these increases in weight and mass, has been the enlargement of the cerebrum. The cerebrum is one of three major parts of the brain. The two other major parts are the brain stem and the cerebellum (see Figure 3.3).

Brain Stem. The **brain stem** sits directly on top of the spinal cord and serves as a conduit between the rest of the brain and the spinal cord. The brain stem consists primarily of nerve tracts that carry sensory information to the brain and motor information away from the brain. It is a major relay station for nerves supplying the head and face and for controlling the visual and auditory reflexes. The brain stem structures and functions are also associated with metabolism and arousal. Three major reflex centers are located in the brain stem: the cardiac center, which controls the heart; the vasomotor center, which controls the blood vessels; and the respiratory center, which controls breathing.

FIGURE 3.3

The human brain.

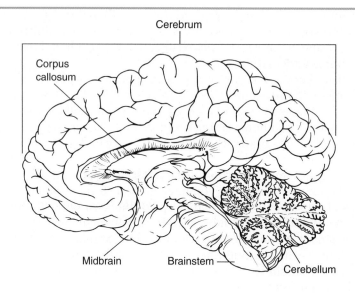

Cerebrum

Corpus callosum

Midbrain   Brainstem   Cerebellum

DISCUSSION POINT:

Consider the case of Timmy in Case Study 3.1. To what extent do you think it likely that his brain damage is linked to the personality qualities his friends describe?

Cerebellum.   The **cerebellum** is an oval-shaped "little brain" that sits posterior to the brain stem. It is primarily responsible for regulating motor and muscular activity. The motor-monitoring functions of the cerebellum include coordination of motor movements, maintenance of muscle tone, monitoring of movement range and strength, and maintenance of posture and equilibrium (Bhatnagar & Andy, 1995). Historically, the cerebellum was seen to have little involvement or association with the brain's cognitive processes, including language and speech. Findings from recent research have challenged this presumption. For instance, a study of 19 preschool-aged children following surgical removal of cerebellar tumors found that more than one-half exhibited expressive language disorders (11 of the 19 children); a similar percentage also had significant problems with short-term memory (Levisohn, Cronin-Golomb, & Schmahmann, 2000). Similarly, results of a study of 20 adults with diseases of the cerebellum (e.g., stroke, tumor, infection) also found that the majority had problems with expressive language (13 of 20 patients); additionally, 15 of the 20 patients exhibited problems modulating their own behavior, and 14 had problems performing arithmetic calculations (Schmahmann & Sherman, 1998). The presence of such cognitive deficits in children and adults with cerebellar injury provide evidence that the cerebellum is physiologically and anatomically linked to the neural circuitry involved with higher-order cognitive functions.

Cerebrum.   The **cerebrum,** or cerebral cortex, is the part of the brain that governs the unique human qualities of thinking, problem solving, planning, creating, and rationalizing. Of the three major divisions of the brain—brain stem, cerebellum, and cerebrum—the cerebrum is the largest. It consists of two mirror-image hemispheres, the right and the left. The two hemispheres are separated by a long cerebral crevice, or fissure, called the *longitudinal fissure.* The **corpus callosum** is a band of fibers that connects the two hemispheres, serving as a conduit for communication between the hemispheres.

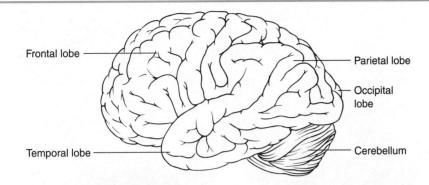

FIGURE 3.4

Lobes of the brain.

The cerebrum contains four lobes: the frontal lobe, the temporal lobe, the parietal lobe, and the occipital lobe. Figure 3.4 shows the lobe locations. Each lobe is represented in both the left and right hemisphere of the cerebral cortex (e.g., left temporal lobe, right temporal lobe). The insular cortex (also called the *insula* or the *Island of Reil*) is considered by some experts to be a fifth lobe; the insula sits deep within the brain within a sulcus (i.e., depression) separating the temporal and parietal lobes. It can only be seen by retracting the frontal and temporal lobes (Flynn, Benson, & Ardila, 1999). The insula contains many cortical projections to other parts of the brain, from the brain stem to the frontal, parietal, and temporal lobes, and plays a role in integrating information from all five senses. The insula also may play a role in linking language processing to the limbic system, modulating the emotional and motivational responses to language stimuli (Flynn et al., 1999).

The **frontal lobe** is the largest lobe; it sits in the most anterior part of the brain, behind the forehead. Two key functions of the frontal lobe are (1) activating and controlling both fine and complex motor activities, including the control of speech output, and (2) controlling human executive functions. **Executive functions** include problem solving, planning, creating, reasoning, decision making, social awareness, and rationalizing. These unique and important human qualities represent executive functions, because they describe the organized, goal-directed, and controlled execution of critical human behaviors. The executive functions are what allow humans to "override or augment reflexive and habitual reactions in order to orchestrate behavior in accord with our intentions" (Miller, 2000, p. 59). Executive functions are what allow you to keep your arm from reaching for a second piece of chocolate cake (if you really want to)!

Within the frontal lobe sits the prefrontal cortex, which is the part of the brain that has evolved most recently and that is most developed in humans relative to other species (Miller, 2000). The prefrontal cortex is connected with all other sensory and motor systems of the brain, allowing it to synthesize the vast stores of information needed for complex, goal-directed human behavior (Miller, 2000). As noted by Miller, people with damage to the prefrontal cortex may superficially appear quite normal (e.g., they can carry on a conversation or can perform well on perceptual and memory tests) but can have profound difficulties with organization, self-control, and goal-oriented tasks. Accordingly, the prefrontal cortex represents the seat of the executive functions.

The frontal lobe is also the home to **Broca's area,** an important region of the brain for communication. Situated in the left hemisphere of the frontal lobe, Broca's area is responsible for the fine coordination of speech output. It is named after the French physician Paul Broca, who was among the first to recognize the functional specializations of the brain in the mid-1800s. Broca's

DISCUSSION POINT:
Consider the case of Timmy in Case Study 3.1. If he did have serious frontal lobe damage, what might be some characteristics of this damage?

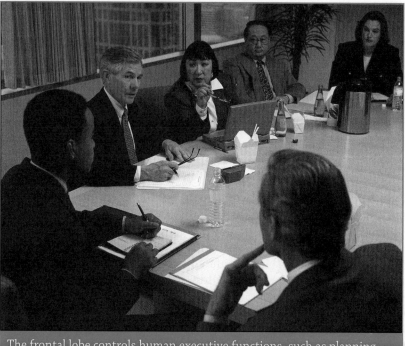

The frontal lobe controls human executive functions, such as planning, reasoning, and decision making.

discovery stemmed from his curiosity about a patient who lost the ability to speak following brain damage. When he performed an autopsy on the patient, Broca found damage to the area subsequently named after him.

The **parietal lobe** sits posterior to the frontal lobe on the left and right sides, above the ears. Key functions of the parietal lobes include (1) perceiving and integrating sensory and perceptual information and (2) comprehending oral and written language and calculation for mathematics.

The **temporal lobe** also sits posterior to the frontal lobe but inferior to the parietal lobe (medial to the ears). The temporal lobe is a particularly important site for human communication. To start, it contains the auditory cortex (represented bilaterally in the left and right hemispheres), also known as **Heschl's gyrus.** The auditory cortex conducts fine-grained analysis of the frequency spectrum, temporal properties, and periodicity of sounds received from the auditory pathways (Schneider et al., 2005). Frequency is represented tonotopically within the auditory cortex, with particular regions processing particular aspects and frequencies of incoming sounds. For instance, the "pitch processing center" within Heschl's gyrus is specialized for processing the complexities of pitch (e.g., pitch sequences, pitch direction). The auditory cortices of the right and left hemispheres show some hemispheric specialization for processing different elements of incoming auditory stimuli (Schneider et al., 2005). For instance, the left auditory cortex appears highly specialized toward processing the fine-grained temporal features of rapidly varying acoustic information, as is characteristic of human speech. This is termed *temporal processing.* The right auditory cortex, by contrast, shows specialization for processing melody, prosody, and certain aspects of pitch (Schneider et al., 2005). Interestingly, persons who have a clear affinity for processing auditory information, such as musicians, show enlarged Heschl's gyri compared to others (Schneider et al., 2002).

The temporal lobe also contains **Wernicke's area** within the left hemisphere, which is a highly specialized site for language comprehension. Heschl's gyrus first processes the sounds of spoken language, and then Wernicke's area (connected via a range of pathways) takes over for further linguistic processing. Damage to these regions of the left temporal lobe can impact aspects of speech and language processing. For instance, damage to Wernicke's area can significantly affect one's ability to comprehend spoken and written language. If damage to this area occurs, it is possible for language comprehension processes to functionally reorganize to the right hemisphere (Liégeois et al., 2004), particularly in instances when brain damage is relatively widespread and occurs early in one's life. Deficits in the left auditory cortex can affect the fine-grained temporal processing of speech. However, the auditory cortex is represented bilaterally in the two hemispheres, and as a result, damage to Heschl's gyrus will not necessarily affect language processing, although some more general aspects of auditory processing may be impacted (Zatorre & Penhume, 2001).

The **occipital lobe** sits at the rear of the cerebral cortex, in front of and above the cerebellum. The occipital lobe receives and processes visual information.

Organizational Principles of the Human Brain.   To help you understand how the human brain works and make sense of its critical role in communication function and dysfunction, this section presents five key principles governing the brain's organization. These principles are derived from Bhatnagar and Andy's text on neuroscience (1995).

1. *Interconnectedness.* The brain functions and structures are highly interconnected. The two hemispheres and their combined lobes constantly interact via a rich weaving of brain fibers. Thus, while one area of the brain might be recognized as critical for a particular brain function (e.g., Wernicke's area for language comprehension), the reality is that brain activity reflects the ongoing and intricate integration of information from across the brain's regions.

2. *Hierarchy.* The central nervous system is organized hierarchically. Although all human behavior passes through the central nervous system—and indeed no two body parts are able to communicate without involvement of the CNS—lower-level functions can be directed by the spinal cord, whereas higher-level functions require mediation by the brain's cerebral cortex. The more sophisticated or complex the behavior, the greater the involvement of the brain.

3. *Specialization.* The brain is organized into two hemispheres that communicate via the corpus callosum. Although the two brain hemispheres are mirror images in appearance, they are quite different functionally. In fact, each area of the brain is highly specialized for particular functions. The nerve cells within specific brain areas are specialized to process particular types of information—for example, about touch, temperature, incoming auditory information, or outgoing motor movement. All areas of the brain are connected by highly specialized motor and sensory pathways, which are designed to carry very specific types of information.

4. *Plasticity.* **Plasticity** refers to change, and in neuroscience this term describes the remarkable ability of the brain "to reorganize and modify functions and adapt to internal and external changes" (Bhatnagar & Andy, 1995, p. 5). From birth, the human brain has the important capacity to organize and reorganize itself as a result of experience. Because of plasticity, children who lose their sight early in life become able to process auditory information better than children with sight as the brain reorganizes itself to compensate for the visual

deprivation (Bavelier & Neville, 2002). However, plasticity describes not only changes in the brain following accidents or injuries, but also all changes that occur in the brain. Developmental plasticity describes neural organization that is stimulated by sensory experiences in the environment, as when young children hear the language of their parents. Learning plasticity describes the way the brain changes as a result of instruction and learning. Learning plasticity explains why the auditory cortex of musicians is better tuned than that of nonmusicians to complex harmonic sounds (Münte, Altenmüller, & Jäncke, 2002). Injury-induced plasticity describes the way the brain reorganizes and even regenerates itself following injury (Kandel, Schwartz, & Jessell, 2001). Similar processes underlie all three types of plasticity. Furthermore, the human brain demonstrates plasticity across its life span, which has important implications for the promise of therapeutic interventions for restoring communicative abilities following injury.

   5. *Critical period.* A critical period is a period of time during which growth in a particular function or structure in the developing brain is most rapid. During a critical period, specific neurons grow rapidly and forge important neural pathways. In the earliest critical period of brain development, 3 to 4 weeks after conception, neurons migrate from their place of origin through a process called *neural migration* to form the inner structures and functions of the brain. Neurons glide along pathways to their final destiny, at which point they forge connections associated with their ultimate function. During this early critical period of brain development, various prenatal influences, such as drug abuse by a mother, can impact neural migration and misplace neurons, resulting in significant developmental disabilities, such as epilepsy.

   The critical period for the development of language, extending from the prenatal period approximately through puberty, is well established (Moskovsky, 2001) and involves three phases:

   1. *Sensory learning:* developing an internal representation (or template) of one's native language through exposure

   2. *Sensorimotor output:* producing language and gradually matching one's own performance to a stored template of mature language through internal and external feedback

   3. *Stabilization:* stabilizing of mature language patterns due to loss of plasticity and maintenance through use (Brainard & Doupe, 2000)

The critical period for development of speech and language in humans corresponds to that in many other species as well. For instance, songbirds must be exposed to the songs of their own species, even if it is via audiotape, during a critical period early in life in order to be able to produce those songs themselves later (Brainard & Doupe, 2000).

DISCUSSION POINT:
The critical period is an important concept in language acquisition. What have you heard about it? How does this concept apply to the case of Patricia in Case Study 3.1?

Contralaterality.   Contralateral organization describes the architectural organization whereby bodily senses and functions are processed in the opposite side of the brain. For instance, the sensation resulting from a pinprick to one's left index finger or a light touch to one's left foot is processed in the right hemisphere of the brain (although the ipsilateral/same hemisphere will exhibit some processing of this sensation, the contralateral response is far greater; Hagen & Pardo, 2002). Nearly all of the human sensory system exhibits contralateral representation. For instance, information that is heard in the right ear is processed in the auditory cortex of the left hemisphere, and vice versa. The contralateral organization of the auditory system can be tested using dichotic listening tasks, in which two different sounds are played into a listener's ears simultaneously. The right-ear advantage (REA) is a well-studied phenomenon that describes the tendency for individuals for whom language is left-lateralized to provide better accuracy in describing linguistic stimuli (e.g., words, syllables) presented to the right ear versus the left ear. Interestingly, for nonlanguage stimuli, such as environmental sounds or tones, individuals typically will show a right-ear advantage (Mildner, Stankovic, & Petkovic, 2005).

Understanding the principle of contralateral organization is important to assess and treat human communication disorders. For instance, Nakajima and colleagues (2005) recently described the case of a 53-year-old man who experienced damage to the left side of a brain-stem region (the medulla). Subsequently, he had a "heaviness" of the right extremities (arms, legs) and weakness to the lower right part of the face. He also had persistent paralysis of the muscle innervating the right side of the pharynx, resulting in minor problems with speech and swallowing.

Speech and Language in the Human Brain.   The brain contains the essential architecture of human communication. Key centers of the brain involved in communication include Broca's area, Heschl's gyrus, and Wernicke's area, as shown in Figure 3.5.

These three sites sit near to one another in the left hemisphere of the brain, allowing for close communication among the centers. Broca's area is the primary center for fluent expression of speech and language. It is located in the posterior portion of the left frontal lobe. Heschl's gyrus is the primary center for auditory perception and sensation. Located in the superior portion of the left temporal lobe, Heschl's gyrus is responsible for the interpretation of all types of sounds, not just speech and language. It is connected via a band of fibers to Wernicke's area, the primary center for language comprehension, which is located just posterior to Heschl's gyrus in the left temporal lobe. In Wernicke's area, meaning is attributed to the linguistic stimuli sent forth from Heschl's gyrus. Thus, Wernicke's area is where language comprehension takes place.

These three centers for communicative processes share information with many other parts of the brain during the processes associated with speech, language, and hearing. For instance, in comprehending linguistic information, Wernicke's area corresponds with regions of the frontal lobe involved with higher-order functions, such as problem solving, reasoning, and planning. Likewise, in interpreting auditory information, Heschl's gyrus utilizes memory stores from throughout the brain. Thus, while it is important to understand

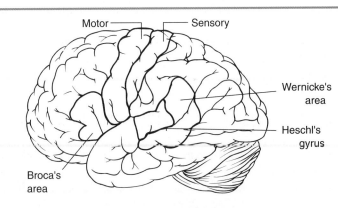

Motor — Sensory
Wernicke's area
Heschl's gyrus
Broca's area

FIGURE 3.5

Communication centers of the brain.

brain specializations in speech, language, and hearing, it is also necessary to recognize the integrative linkages across the brain that are critical in human communication.

Peripheral Nervous System

The peripheral nervous system, or PNS, is the system of nerves connected to the brain stem and the spinal cord. The PNS carries sensory information to the CNS and motor commands away from the CNS, controlling both voluntary and involuntary activity.

SPOTLIGHT ON LITERACY

Reading by Touch

Reading, as you are doing right now, involves the visual and linguistic processing of written letters and words. For individuals who cannot see, an alternative means for accessing written letters and words is provided through braille. Braille, like written English, is a rule-governed system based on systematic correspondences between sounds and letters (called *characters*). In this case, however, the letters are represented with an arrangement of one to six raised dots, discernible by touch. Braille also has characters to depict punctuation, numbers, and so forth. The dots are presented in a 2 by 3 cell—two dots horizontally by three dots vertically. (The first ten letters are presented below.) The presence or absence of dots within each space in the cell is used to decode the character. Because a braille character is physically larger than its letter counterpart, fewer words are printed on a page of braille; a standard braille page has only about 25 lines of text that each contains about 43 characters. Consequently, many words are abbreviated to save space and increase reading fluency; this is called *contracted braille* or *grade 2 braille* (Herzberg, Stough, & Clark, 2004). (By contrast, uncontracted braille, in which every letter in a word is represented by a character, is called *alphabetic braille*.) As an example of contracted braille, a set of 23 words (e.g., *but, can, do, every*) form a set of "one-cell whole-word contractions"; each of these words is represented using a single letter of the alphabet (e.g., *b/but, c/can, d/do, e/every;* Risjord, Wilkinson, & Stark, 2000). Although there are benefits to using the contracted form, experts believe that its prevalence has resulted in a decline in braille literacy, as learning it is too cognitively demanding for young children (Herzberg et al., 2004); additionally, some research has shown that readers of braille appear to be more fluent and accurate when reading uncontracted braille than contracted braille (Troughton, 1992).

There is a great shortage of teachers of braille; some estimates suggest that 5,000 teachers of braille are needed right now to meet the needs of students with vision impairments. As a result, too many children with significant visual impairments are not learning to read braille fluently or at all, and in some cases, the educational interventions provided to them by schools are wholly inappropriate (e.g., giving them large-print texts instead of teaching them to read by an alternative and more appropriate method; see Smith, Geruschat, & Huebner, 2004).

While it may not be easy to learn braille, becoming literate in the braille system would greatly broaden one's professional opportunities and potential contributions to improving the literacy achievements of individuals with visual impairment. A self-study correspondence course is available from the Library of Congress that can lead to certification as a braille transcriber; the materials for the course are available for download at no charge at http://loc.gov/nls/bds/manual/.

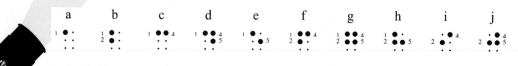

Reprinted with permission from *Instruction manual for braille transcribing* (Risjord, Wilkinson, & Stark, 2000). The Library of Congress, Copyright 2000.

The PNS consists of cranial nerves and spinal nerves. The 12 pairs of cranial nerves run between the brain stem and the facial and neck regions and are particularly important for speech, language, hearing, and swallowing. The cranial nerves carry information concerning four of the five senses to the brain: vision, hearing, smell, and taste. Importantly, the cranial nerves also carry the motor impulses from the brain to the muscles of the face and neck, including those activating the tongue and the jaw, both of which are involved with speech. The seven cranial nerves most closely involved with communicative functions and the functions they are related to are the following:

- Trigeminal (V): Facial sensation; jaw movements, including chewing
- Facial (VII): Taste sensation; facial movements, including smiling
- Acoustic (VIII): Hearing and balance
- Glossopharyngeal (IX): Tongue sensation; palatal and pharyngeal movement, including gagging
- Vagus (X): Taste sensation; palatal, pharyngeal, and laryngeal movement, including voicing
- Accessory (XI): Palatal, pharyngeal, laryngeal, head, and shoulder movement
- Hypoglossal (XII): Tongue movement

The additional five sets of cranial nerves include the olfactory (I, smell sensation), optic (II, visual information), oculomotor (III, eye movement), trochlear (IV, eye movement), and abducens (VI, eye movement).

The 31 pairs of spinal nerves run between the spinal cord and all peripheral areas of the human body, including the arms and legs. These spinal nerves mediate reflexes and volitional sensory and motor activity.

ANATOMY AND PHYSIOLOGY OF SPEECH ●

The production of spoken language involves the complex interaction of three interrelated systems of human anatomy and physiology: respiration, phonation, and articulation (see Figure 3.6).

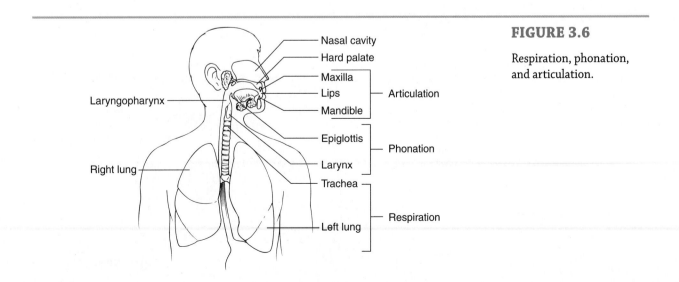

FIGURE 3.6

Respiration, phonation, and articulation.

RESPIRATION

The evolution of spoken language as the essential act of being human did not require the creation of any new body structures. Rather, the evolution of spoken language efficiently made use of many body structures that had already been developed to serve other purposes. Respiration is an excellent example. Respiration is the system of the human body that controls breathing; its purpose is to draw oxygen from the air into the blood and to exchange it with carbon dioxide. The major respiratory organs are the lungs. The human respiratory system has undergone few modifications in the several million years of our existence, with the exception of its being borrowed to serve as the power supply for speech.

Many key structures are involved in the respiratory process and, therefore, in human speech production (see Figure 3.7). The respiratory system is divided into a lower and upper respiratory system. The lower respiratory system comprises the lungs, bronchi, and alveoli; the upper respiratory system comprises the trachea, larynx, and oral and nasal cavities.

The thorax is the skeleton of the chest, which houses the structures of the lower respiratory system. The thoracic skeleton consists of the rib cage in the front connected to the vertebral column in the rear. The thoracic skeleton creates a thoracic cavity, housing the heart and lungs, which work in concert to exchange oxygen from the air and carbon dioxide from the blood. The diaphragm, a large muscle that contracts and expands with breathing, forms the bottom of the thoracic cavity. The lungs—of which there are two, a right and a left—sit within the **pleura,** a thin sac that attaches to the inner side of the thorax and the outer side of the lungs. Both lungs contain an intricate web of bronchi and alveoli. Air enters the lungs through two main bronchi, one for each lung. The bronchi divide into smaller and smaller tubes, ending in small sacs called *alveoli.* Oxygen from the air and carbon dioxide from the blood are exchanged in the alveoli.

Respiration is controlled in the brain stem and is typically an involuntary activity. However, respiratory control can be voluntary, as in using deep breathing as a relaxation technique.

The respiratory system serves as the power supply for speech production through the inhalation and exhalation of air during breathing. To produce speech, one inhales and then exhales air. The exhaled airflow is sent up through the larynx, over the vocal folds, and into the oral and nasal cavities, where it is manipulated

FIGURE 3.7

The respiratory system.

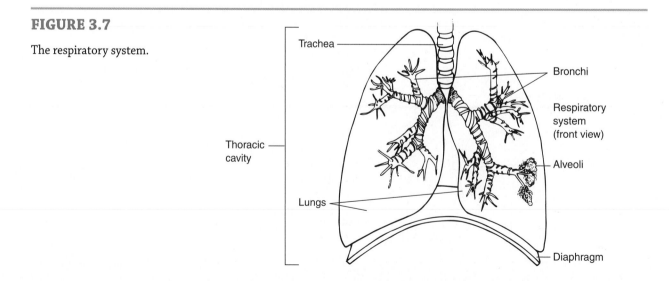

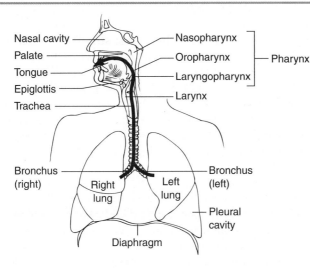

FIGURE 3.8

Exhalation for speech.

to make different speech sounds (see Figure 3.8). Good speech requires a strong energy source: inhalation must bring an adequate supply of air into the lungs, and exhalation must be strong enough to propel this supply upward and outward.

The muscles of respiration are involved with the processes of inspiration and expiration. The inspiratory muscles are differentiated into the primary muscles and the secondary, or accessory, muscles. The primary muscles are involved with quiet restful breathing, whereas the secondary muscles are involved with active forced inspiration—such as with lifting something, yelling, or singing—along with the primary muscles. The primary inspiratory muscles include the diaphragm and the intercostals, which fill the spaces between the ribs and sit on the outside and inside of the rib casing. The intercostals are particularly important for inspiration: as they contract, they raise the ribs to increase the volume of the lungs, which, in turn, creates a negative pressure vacuum. For more active inspiration, a number of additional muscles of the neck, back, and abdomen (e.g., pectoralis major and minor) are involved.

The muscles of expiration are also differentiated into primary and secondary muscles. Largely, expiration during quiet restful breathing is a passive act that involves the elastic recoiling of the muscles after a period of constriction. The external intercostals and diaphragm recoil into their relaxed state. Also involved are a specific set of internal intercostal muscles (the interosseous intercostals) that contract to bring the ribs closer together and create a positive pressure difference between the lungs and the outside air, causing expiration. As with forced inspiration, a number of additional muscles of the neck, back, and abdomen (e.g., external and internal obliques) are involved with active forced expiration.

Respiration for breathing, or passive respiration, differs from respiration for speaking in several key ways (Borden et al., 1994). First, more air is inhaled and then exhaled for speech respiration than for passive respiration. To illustrate, speak the sentence, "Hi, my name is Alfred Peterson, and I am a college student." You will note that you inhale and exhale a greater volume of air than you do when simply breathing for the purpose of staying alive. Second, the inhalation-exhalation process involved in speech is subject to greater voluntary control than the process involved in normal breathing. Passive respiration is controlled reflexively—we usually don't think too much about it. In contrast, when we are usurping respiration for speech production, we take greater

DISCUSSION POINT:

How long is a typical breath cycle in passive respiration? Work with a partner and a stopwatch to find out. Then, contrast your finding with a breath cycle in speech: Tell what you did last night using just one breath cycle, and calculate the length of exhalation.

control of the activity, manipulating inhalation and exhalation to serve the dynamics of speech. For instance, in responding to the query, "Can I have the rest of your chocolate brownie?" the breath supply to produce a vehement "Absolutely not!" is manipulated in a particular way to get the unequivocal message across. Third, speech respiration differs from passive respiration in the ratio of inhalation to exhalation in one respiratory cycle. A respiratory cycle comprises one inhalation and one exhalation. In respiration for breathing, a cycle is about 40% inhalation and 60% exhalation. During speech, the ratio is about 10% inhalation to 90% exhalation—exhalation dominates the cycle because it is the part that is used for producing speech.

PHONATION

The energy source provided by the respiratory system must be converted to speech; otherwise, it is just another breath of air. The phonatory and articulatory systems carry out this process. The phonatory system takes the energy that is sent upward from the lungs and further modulates the airflow to convert the energy into sound.

Key structures in phonation include the pharynx, the trachea, and the larynx. The **pharynx** is a mucosa-lined muscular tube that runs from the nasal cavity, through the rear of the oral cavity, to the entrance of the larynx and the esophagus. The pharynx can be divided into three sections: the nasopharynx, the oropharynx, and the laryngopharynx, as depicted in Figure 3.8. The **nasopharynx** is a posterior continuation of the nasal cavity. The **oropharynx,** or throat, is the length of the pharynx that connects with the oral cavity. The **laryngopharynx** is the most inferior portion of the pharynx, a small portion of tube that opens in the anterior to the larynx and in the posterior to the esophagus.

The **larynx** is a cartilaginous box that sits at the front of the neck on top of the trachea, or windpipe. The trachea leads from the larynx to the lungs. The primary function of the larynx is to protect the trachea by keeping out everything but air. Within the laryngeal box sit the vocal folds, which close tightly to prevent foreign matter from descending into the trachea. In addition to serving as a protective seal, the vocal folds vibrate to produce the voice; hence the larynx—home to the vocal folds—is also known as the *voice box.*

The larynx is suspended from the **hyoid bone,** a horseshoe-shaped bone that floats horizontally at the base of the neck. The larynx is made up of cartilages that are connected through muscle and ligament: one cricoid cartilage, one thyroid cartilage, two arytenoid cartilages, and the epiglottis cartilage (see Figure 3.9). The cricoid cartilage is a ring of cartilage that forms the base of the larynx and sits at the top of the trachea. Superior to the cricoid cartilage is the thyroid cartilage, the largest of the laryngeal cartilages. The thyroid cartilage looks like two shields fused together; you can feel the two shields by pressing your fingers softly against the front of your neck. The ridge where the two shields come together is sometimes called the Adam's apple; the V-shaped opening above it is the thyroid notch. Two tiny arytenoid cartilages, small, pyramid-shaped structures, attach to the top posterior portion of the cricoid cartilage and form anchors for the vocal folds. The epiglottis, a leaf-shaped cartilage, is attached anteriorly to the top of the thyroid cartilage, running up against the hyoid bone and to the back of the tongue. The epiglottis is able to drop over the larynx, helping to protect it from penetration by unwelcome substances.

The movements of the larynx and the vocal folds contained within it are controlled by two sets of muscles. The extrinsic laryngeal muscles extend

SPOTLIGHT ON TECHNOLOGY

Functional Magnetic Resonance Imaging: fMRI

Functional magnetic resonance imaging (fMRI) is an important technology used to study neural activity within the brain. fMRI permits the direct examination of specific brain structures and the activity within those structures, given the physiological phenomenon concerning the increase in blood flow to and volume in a specific brain region that accompanies neural activity. The advantages of fMRI over prior technologies used to study brain activity are considerable: It requires no injections into the blood (e.g., radioactive isotopes), the time needed to collect a scan is relatively short, and the resolution is quite good (Functional MRI Research Center, 2008). To collect data on how the brain functions in a specific neural processing task, an individual is positioned within the scanner. Then, a series of 30 images are collected in about 90 seconds. The first 10 images are collected to provide a baseline (prestimulation) index of neural activity, typically as the individual is engaged in some sort of neutral activity (e.g., looking at a picture). The next 10 images (stimulation activity) are collected during a specific activity, such as listening to a particular speech sound. The final 10 images repeat the baseline procedure (poststimulation; Functional MRI Research Center, 2008).

The use of fMRI has been particularly informative to understanding the human brain's functional specializations for speech, language, hearing, and communication. Additionally, fMRI data have proven important to treating some communication disorders. Seidman and colleagues (2008) recently described use of fMRI with two patients with debilitating tinnitus (persistent ringing in the ears) to identify the specific sites within the auditory cortex that corresponded to the pitch and loudness of their tinnitus symptoms (the fMRI data for one patient is presented below). Implants were then placed at these specific sites as a way to reduce the symptoms.

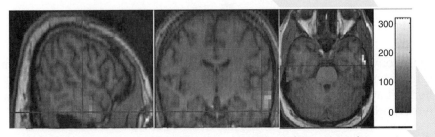

Functional magnetic resonance imaging activation of the auditory cortex from patient one during music stimulation presented binaurally. Note the entire auditory cortex in the right hemisphere is seen in these images. Z-score scale is shown at right.

Reprinted from: Seidman, M. D., Ridder, D. D., Elisevich, K., Bowyer, S. M., Darrat, I., et al. (2008). Direct electrical stimulation of Heschl's gyrus for tinnitus treatment. *Laryngoscope, 118*, 491–500.

externally from the larynx to the hyoid bone or other nearby structures. They keep the larynx in its midline position while also controlling its vertical movements for purposes of speech and swallowing (Fucci & Lass, 1999). The intrinsic laryngeal muscles, situated within the larynx itself, control the movements of the vocal folds.

The extrinsic laryngeal muscles are typically differentiated into the suprahyoids, as they run from the larynx to the region superior to the hyoid bone, and the infrahyoids, as they run from the larynx to the region below the hyoid bone (Fucci & Lass, 1999). The four suprahyoids, which are also called *laryngeal elevators* for their role in elevating the larynx, are the digastricus, stylohyoid, geniohyoid, and mylohyoid muscles. These are presented in Figures 3.10 and 3.11. The four infrahyoids are the omohyoid, sternohyoid, sternothyroid,

FIGURE 3.9

The larynx.

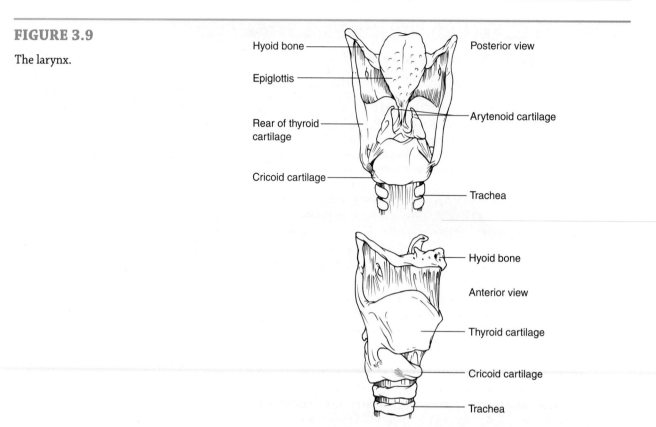

Posterior view

Hyoid bone

Epiglottis

Rear of thyroid cartilage

Arytenoid cartilage

Cricoid cartilage

Trachea

Hyoid bone

Anterior view

Thyroid cartilage

Cricoid cartilage

Trachea

and thyrohyoid muscles. The infrahyoids serve as laryngeal depressors, depressing the larynx and hyoid bone after they have elevated for swallowing or speech. The thyrohyoid muscle is also able to serve as a laryngeal elevator, pulling the thyroid cartilage up behind the hyoid bone (Gray, 1918/2000).

FIGURE 3.10

Muscles of the neck—lateral view.

Source: Gray, H. *Anatomy of the Human Body*. Philadelphia: Lea & Febiger, 1918; Bartleby.com, 2000. www.bartleby.com/107/. [Online Edition, Figure 385.] Reprinted with permission.

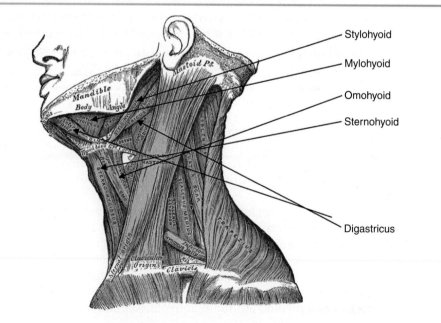

Stylohyoid

Mylohyoid

Omohyoid

Sternohyoid

Digastricus

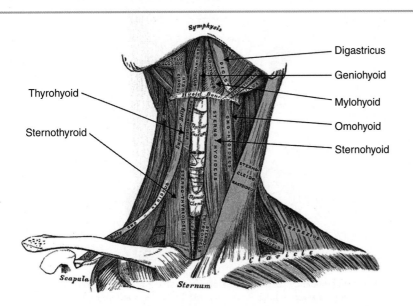

FIGURE 3.11

Muscles of the neck—anterior view.

Source: Gray, H. *Anatomy of the Human Body.* Philadelphia: Lea & Febiger, 1918; Bartleby.com, 2000. www.bartleby.com/107/. [Online Edition, Figure 386.] Reprinted with permission.

The intrinsic laryngeal muscles govern the movements of the vocal folds for purposes of speech and respiration and are confined entirely within the larynx. There are five in total (three of which come as a set of pairs). The cricothyroid muscle runs between the front of the cricoid cartilage to the posterior part of the thyroid cartilage; it contracts to lengthen the vocal folds. The posterior cricoarytenoid muscles (a pair) run from the front of the cricoid cartilage to insert into the back of each of the arytenoid cartileges; they contract to pull the arytenoid cartileges apart, therefore opening the vocal folds. The lateral cricoarytenoid muscles (also coming as a pair) run from the sides of the cricoid cartileges into the fronts of the arytenoids; they contract to pull the arytenoid cartileges together, therefore closing the vocal folds. The arytenoid muscles (a pair) run between the two arytenoid cartileges, forming a sort of cross as each member of the pair runs from the base of one cartilage to the apex of the other. These also help to close the vocal folds, particularly at the back. The thyroarytenoid muscles, or the vocalis, comprise a broad but thin set of small muscles that run from the front of the thyroid cartilage to insert into the base of the arytenoid cartileges. The thyroarytenoid muscles help to shorten and relax the vocal folds as well as to bring the two vocal folds together for voicing (Gray, 1918/2000).

The vocal folds stretch horizontally from the arytenoid cartilages in the back to the thyroid cartilage in front. The **vocal folds,** or vocal cords, are two thin sheets of tissue connected on their outer edge to the inside of the thyroid cartilage. Figure 3.12 provides a sketch of the vocal folds looking down into the larynx. Lying within the tissue of the vocal folds is a thin layer of muscle sometimes called the vocalis muscle, and along the

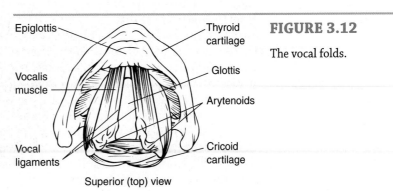

Superior (top) view

FIGURE 3.12

The vocal folds.

FIGURE 3.13

Vocal fold movement.

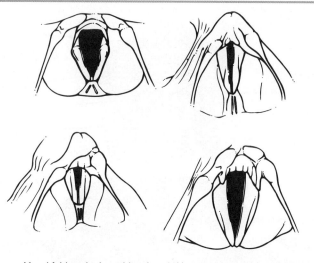

Vocal fold cycle: breathing (*top left*), start of phonation (*top right*),
end of phonation (*bottom left*), and breathing (*bottom right*).

internal edge of each tissue is a vocal ligament. As noted, the vocal folds can close tightly to protect the trachea and lungs from foreign matter. When the vocal folds are brought together, they are said to be approximated. The sequence in Figure 3.13 shows the vocal folds open for breathing (top left and bottom right) and approximated for voicing (top right and bottom left).

At some point in the evolution of humans, the vocal folds began to be utilized for creating voice. **Voice** is the creation of sound by vocal fold vibration. When air is exhaled from the lungs and sent up through the larynx, the vocal folds can be set into rapid vibration to create voice. Humans can speak without voicing, by whispering, but using one's voice has clear advantages, as anyone knows who has experienced laryngitis, in which the ability to produce voicing is lost.

The **trachea** is the cartilaginous tube that runs from the oral cavity down to the lungs, where it separates into the two bronchi. The trachea is about 28 centimeters (cm; 11 in.) long and 5 cm (2 in.) wide. The trachea's principal function is to transport air between the environment and the lungs. The trachea should not be confused with the esophagus, another tube that sits behind the trachea and transports food and water from the oral cavity to the stomach. Air, water, and food all enter via the same cavity—the mouth—and need to be directed to the appropriate channel: the trachea for air to the lungs, or the esophagus for water and food to the stomach.

The pharynx, larynx, and trachea constitute the phonatory system, which plays three important roles in speech production. First, these structures together form the essential pathway for the energy supply of speech. They channel the air supply from the lungs into the oral and nasal cavities.

Second, the vocal folds in the larynx turn the airflow into voice through their vibration. The number of times the vocal folds vibrate in a second (the cycles per second) relates to the frequency of a person's voice. Female vocal folds vibrate roughly 240 times per second, translating to a fundamental frequency of 240 hertz (or Hz, cycles per second). The fundamental frequency is the lowest, or base, frequency of a complex sound wave. Male vocal folds vibrate at a slower rate, roughly 130 hertz. These differences relate to the mass of the vocal folds; women's vocal folds are smaller and shorter than those of men, and thus they vibrate at a higher rate.

Third, the pharynx provides a resonating chamber for the airflow. *Resonance* describes the airflow's ongoing vibration as it moves through the pharyngeal tract. Airflow resonates along the laryngopharynx, oropharynx, and nasopharynx and provides an added fullness to speech. To understand resonance and its influence on vocal quality, think about the last time you had a stuffy nose. When the nose is stuffed up, the nasopharynx is not available as a resonating chamber for the airflow, which impacts the quality of speech.

DISCUSSION POINT:
Sometimes a girl's voice may be indistinguishable from her mother's or sister's voice. What is the explanation for this?

ARTICULATION

The column of air that is channeled through the phonatory system is further modulated by the articulatory system. The role of the articulators is best illustrated by an activity:

Produce a continuous "ahhhh."

After 3 seconds, change "ahhh" to "eeee."

After 3 more seconds, change "eeee" to "seee."

How does "ah" become "ee" and "ee" become "see"? Articulation. Articulation is the act of manipulating the airflow submitted by the phonatory system to create highly precise speech sounds. In Standard American English, there are around 40 speech sounds, or phonemes, depending on the particular dialect. The chief manipulators—or articulators—involved with the precise production of these phonemes include the maxilla and mandible, lips, teeth, hard and soft palates, and tongue (see Figure 3.14). These articulatory structures were not evolved for the purpose of speech; rather, they are principle organs for tasting, chewing, and swallowing. However, in developing the capacity for speech, humans have usurped the articulators for key and critical functions.

The maxilla and mandible are the upper and lower jaws, respectively. Although the maxilla does not move during speech production, the mandible is able to open and close and move side to side, actions important for producing specific speech sounds. To illustrate, note the position of the mandible when you produce the sound "ee," as in *meet,* and then when you produce the sound "ah,"

FIGURE 3.14

The articulators.

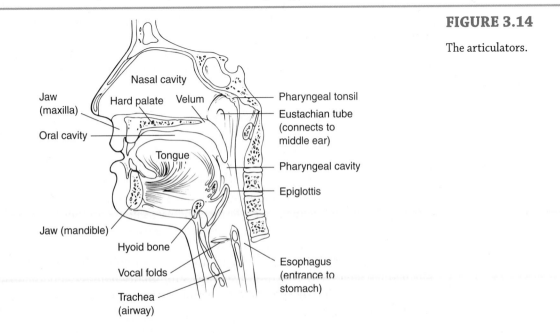

as in *hot.* The lips are also important for articulation. For some sounds, the lips are brought tightly together (e.g., /b/) and then are popped open, and for other sounds (e.g., /m/) the lips are pressed together. The teeth are articulators used for the production of several sounds (e.g., /ʃ/ and /s/), although for other sounds (e.g., /m/) they have little articulatory role. The palate, or roof of the mouth, is another articulatory structure. The palate includes the hard palate and the soft palate. The hard palate spans from the alveolar ridge (the hard bump right behind the upper teeth) back to the end of the bony part of the roof of the mouth. (Draw your tongue back from the alveolar ridge until the roof of your mouth becomes soft. This signals the end of the hard palate.) The soft palate, or velum, is the roof of the mouth that extends from the hard palate back to the uvula—the portion of the soft palate that hangs like a teardrop in the back of the oral cavity. The hard and soft palates play important roles for a number of speech sounds. For instance, /t/ and /d/ are made by striking the tip of the tongue against the alveolar ridge of the hard palate; /k/ and /g/ are made by lifting the root of the tongue up against the soft palate. Additionally, for several sounds (e.g., /n/ and /ŋ/), the soft palate is raised to block off the oral cavity and channel air into the nasal cavity. Of all the articulators, the tongue is probably the most important, as it is manipulated in some principal way for all sounds. The tongue consists of the tip, blade, and root. The tip is the endmost portion (apex) of the tongue; the blade is the front body of the tongue that sits under the palates; and the root, or dorsum, is the part of the tongue that sits deep within the mandible.

Although each speech sound has a shared source of energy, each also has its own distinct articulatory gesture, or pattern, that describes how the airflow is manipulated within the oral and nasal cavity to produce the sound. For instance, the gesture for the speech sound /b/ involves a complete closure of the lips followed by an opening of the lips in which the sound is forced out. The gesture for /b/ is the same gesture as that for /p/; /b/ and /p/ are distinct speech sounds, because they differ in their voicing. In the production of /b/, the vocal folds vibrate, whereas in the production of /p/, the vocal folds do not vibrate. Each sound, or phoneme, that we use in speech has its own unique articulatory pattern. Take a moment to think about how the following pairs of sounds are different: "ee," as in *beet,* versus "ai," as in *bait;* "t," as in *tan,* and "f," as in fan; and "sh," as in *ship* and "ch," as in *chip.* Think about whether the energy source for each sound is unvoiced or voiced; also think about how the articulators are positioned for the production of each sound. (Chapter 9 presents an in-depth description of the articulatory pattern that characterizes each English speech sound.)

ANATOMY AND PHYSIOLOGY OF HEARING ●

The human ear plays an essential role in communication involving spoken language. While the sense of hearing, or audition, provides humans access to diverse auditory stimuli from the environment—from the rustle of leaves to the cry of a baby to the thunderous boom of jet engines—it also provides the means for spoken language to enter the sensory system and then to be delivered to the brain. Spoken language is essentially a series of rapidly changing, complex sound waves. These sound waves—acoustic energy—are received by the outer portion of the hearing apparatus and subsequently transformed into mechanical energy, then hydraulic energy, and finally neural energy. The neural energy is interpreted by specific brain centers to identify the linguistic meaning of spoken language.

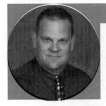

SPOTLIGHT ON RESEARCH AND PRACTICE

NAME: R. KEVIN MANNING, PH.D., CCC-SLP

PROFESSION/TITLE
Speech-Language Pathologist
Traumatic Brain Injury Service
Brooke Army Medical Center

PROFESSIONAL RESPONSIBILITIES
Assess and treat soldiers with acquired brain injury.

A DAY AT WORK
I attend daily multidisciplinary (e.g., physiatrists, neurologists, physician assistants, nurse practitioners, neuropsychologists, psychologists, physical therapists, and occupational therapists) staffings and conduct assessments and treatments throughout each day.

ACADEMIC DEGREES/TRAINING
I received my doctorate in Speech and Hearing Sciences from Ohio University in 2002; prior degrees including an M.A. in Speech-Language Pathology from University of North Texas and a B.A. in Government from University of Texas at Austin.

HOW INTERESTS IN COMMUNICATION SCIENCES AND DISORDERS BEGAN
I am "tongue-tied" and received speech-language pathology services in my childhood. It had a profound impact on my life.

CURRENT RESEARCH AND PRACTICE INTERESTS
Acquired brain injury, cognitive rehabilitation, neurologic stuttering, psychogenic stuttering.

MOST EXCITING/INTERESTING PROFESSIONAL ACCOMPLISHMENT IN CSD
I think my most exciting accomplishment is being asked to join the Traumatic Brain Injury Service at Brooke Army Medical Center. On a daily basis, I have the opportunity to improve the quality of life for injured soldiers. I am humbled by the opportunity to work with these American heroes.

FUTURE TRENDS IN CSD
I think future trends in CSD will include more attention to assessment and treatments for men and women injured in war. We will need to be innovative in our approaches to assessment and treatment due to the unusual types of needs for many of these young men and women.

To accommodate all these energy transformations, the human ear is a complex organ. The portion of the ear that sticks out from both sides of our head belies the complexities of the ear inside. The human ear consists of three distinct sections: the outer ear, the middle ear, and the inner ear. The auditory nerve runs from the inner ear to the auditory centers of the brain, where auditory stimuli are interpreted. Figure 3.15 depicts major structures along the pathway of audition: outer ear, middle ear, inner ear, auditory nerve, and auditory brain center.

OUTER EAR

The **outer ear** is the outermost portion of the human ear. It comprises the auricle, the external auditory canal, and the tympanic membrane. The outer ear serves as the entry point into the human hearing apparatus for sound waves. The funnel shape of the outer ear helps gather sound waves and channel them inward. The outer ear also helps protect the interior of the hearing apparatus from damage.

The visible portion of the outer ear is the **auricle,** sometimes referred to as the *pinna.* The auricle consists of cartilage covered by skin. Key parts of the

FIGURE 3.15

The auditory pathway.

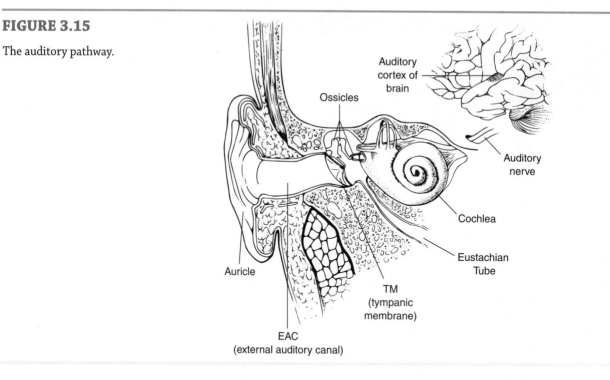

auricle include the earlobe, or lobule, which is the fleshy skin hanging from the bottom of the auricle; the tragus, which is the hard, cartilaginous triangle that protrudes over the entrance to the auditory canal; and the helix, which is the outer body of the auricle.

Opening from the auricle is the **external auditory canal,** or EAC. The role of the EAC is to conduct sound waves inward toward the brain. The EAC is a short tube, about 2.5 cm (1 in.) in length, that is shaped as a loose *S*. In children, the EAC curves downward, whereas in adults the EAC curves upward. The outermost portion of the EAC, nearest the auricle, passes through cartilage and is lined with skin, hair follicles, and glands that produce cerumen, or earwax. The hair follicles and cerumen serve as protective devices for trapping dust and other matter, preventing them from entering inner portions of the hearing apparatus. The innermost portion of the EAC passes through bone and is thus called the bony portion of the EAC. There are no cerumen-secreting glands or hair follicles in the bony portion.

Middle Ear

The EAC ends at the tympanic membrane, or eardrum. The **tympanic membrane** (TM) is a very thin, concave membrane that stretches across the bony portion of the EAC. The TM, when healthy, is pearly white and translucent. Although tiny—roughly 0.75 cm^2—the TM plays a large role in the hearing process, serving as a miniature loudspeaker (Zemlin, 1997). When sound waves travel through the EAC, they reach and strike the TM. The TM is highly sensitive to pressure, and its vibrations replicate the auditory information carried in the sound wave.

The TM serves as the boundary between the outer ear and the middle ear. The **middle ear** is an air-filled, bony cavity sometimes called the *tympanic*

DISCUSSION POINT:
Push your tragus in so that it lies over the external auditory canal. Have a conversation with someone nearby. Why does that person sound softer, but you sound louder?

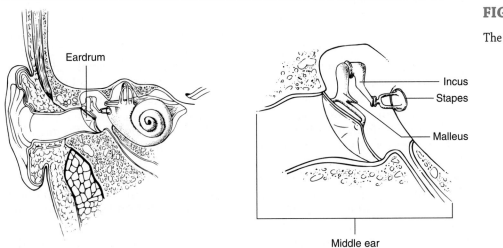

FIGURE 3.16

The middle ear.

cavity. The eustachian tube runs from the middle ear to the pharynx and serves as a pressure-equalizing tube (PET) for the middle-ear space. The middle-ear cavity is small, about 2 cm³, and holds the three smallest bones of the human body: the malleus, the incus, and the stapes. These three bones are called *ossicles* and form a linked chain, the **ossicular chain.**

The first of the three bones in the ossicular chain, the malleus, looks like a mallet, or hammer, with a long handle and head. The handle of the malleus is attached to the inside of the TM, and its head is attached to the second ossicle, the incus. In turn, the incus is attached to the stapes. When the TM is struck by sound waves traversing the EAC, it vibrates, transporting all the auditory information of those waves. The vibrations of the TM set in motion the conversion of the acoustical energy (sound waves) in the outer ear to mechanical energy in the middle ear. The vibrations are carried along the three ossicles as mechanical energy. The ossicular chain is shown in Figure 3.16.

> **DISCUSSION POINT:**
> One type of Valsalva maneuver involves holding your nose shut and pushing, as you might to relieve pressure in your ears when flying in an airplane. What is happening physiologically when you perform the Valsalva?

INNER EAR

Our look at the major structures and functions of the auditory pathway has so far included the auricle, the external auditory canal, the tympanic membrane, and the ossicles. In the outer ear, the auditory information is in the form of acoustical energy, or sound waves. In the middle ear, the auditory information is in the form of mechanical energy that travels along the ossicles. Next on the auditory pathway is the inner ear, which houses the cochlea. Here, the auditory information is converted from mechanical energy to hydraulic energy, as shown in Figure 3.17.

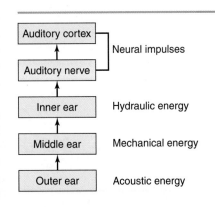

FIGURE 3.17

Energy transformations in the auditory pathway.

The **inner ear** is a fluid-filled cavity that resides deep inside the temporal bone behind the eye socket. It is sometimes called the bony labyrinth because it consists of a complex system of canals and cavities (Zemlin, 1997). The inner ear contains three major cavities: the vestibule, the semicircular canals, and the cochlea. The vestibule is the central portion, or entryway, of the inner ear that sits between the cochlea and the semicircular canals. The semicircular canals open off one side of the vestibule and consist of three canal systems that serve as the organs of balance. The **cochlea** opens off the other side of the vestibule and consists of a single, fluid-filled canal that serves as the organ of hearing. The cochlea is a relatively long (3.5 cm; about 1.4 in.) bony canal, coiled two and a half times into a snail shape. Along the inner length of the cochlea sits the important basilar membrane, which contains the **organ of Corti,** essentially a long row of hair cells that together form the hearing organ.

Auditory information is transported from the middle ear to the organ of Corti in a series of small but important gestures. The stapes, the third ossicle in the middle ear, is shaped like a stirrup. The footplate of the stirrup sits in a window of the inner ear's vestibule, called the *oval window.* When the ossicular chain vibrates, the footplate of the stapes vibrates in and out of the oval window. On the other side of the oval window is the fluid-filled vestibule. The in-and-out movement of the stapes's footplate sets the fluid of the vestibule in motion. The fluid waves carry the auditory information transmitted by the motion of the stapes, now transformed into hydraulic energy, into the cochlea. The fluid waves moving through the cochlea stimulate the basilar membrane. To understand the way the basilar membrane responds to sound, it's helpful to imagine unrolling the cochlea, depicted in Figure 3.15. The apex of the cochlea is relatively wide compared to the base at the other end, and the stiffness of the membrane varies as a result, with the basal end relatively stiffer than the apical end. As a result of this variation in thickness, different places on the membrane are put into vibration with different frequencies of sounds, with the apex vibrating mostly to lower frequency sounds and the base to higher frequency sounds. As an analogy, consider the xylophone, which is ordered tonotopically so that different regions correspond to different frequencies (see Figure 3.18). The basilar membrane also exhibits such tonotopic organization. This tonotopic representation of incoming sound frequency is maintained as the vibrations of the basilar membrane in turn stimulate the hair cells of the organ of Corti. These hair cells interpret the auditory information coming from the fluids of the cochlea and turn the information into neural energy that is transported from the cochlea along the auditory nerve of the brain.

DISCUSSION POINT:

Repeated exposure to loud noise can lessen the sensitivity of the organ of hearing. What are some professions in which repeated noise exposure is common? How can workers in these professions protect themselves?

FIGURE 3.18

Tonotopic organization of xylophone and basilar membrane.

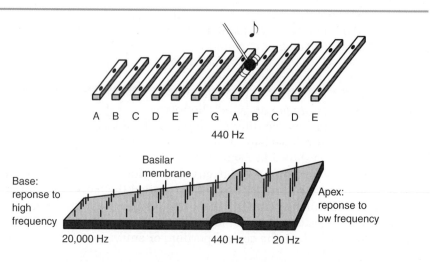

THE AUDITORY NERVE

The auditory information carried in the moving fluids of the cochlea is interpreted by the hairs of the organ of Corti. These hairs are connected to a bundle of nerve fibers that exits the cochlea and travels to the brain. This bundle is the auditory nerve, which is part of the VIIIth cranial nerve. It transports the auditory information, now in the form of neural energy, from the cochlea to the brain stem, the midbrain, and finally to the cerebrum. The temporal lobe of the cerebrum houses the auditory center of the brain.

AUDITORY BRAIN CENTER

Recall from our earlier discussion that the temporal lobe contains the auditory cortex (within both the right and left hemispheres). The auditory cortex processes incoming auditory information that includes both speech and nonspeech. It appears to be tonotopically organized, similar to the basilar membrane. Studies using functional MRI (see Spotlight on Technology: Functional Magnetic Resonance Imaging) have shown differential activation within the auditory cortex in response to auditory stimuli varying in different frequencies (Talavage et al., 2004). Recall also that the auditory cortex of the left hemisphere appears particularly specialized for speech and language processing within Heschl's gyrus; there are morphological differences between this region in the right and left hemispheres that may support the left-lateralization for language processing. Heschl's gyrus receives speech and language stimuli carried along the auditory pathway and analyzes it for frequency, loudness, timing, location, and so forth. A bundle of nerve fibers that runs between Heschl's gyrus and Wernicke's area enables the process of linguistic comprehension of auditory stimuli.

ANATOMY AND PHYSIOLOGY OF SWALLOWING ⬤

During the last few decades, disorders of swallowing have increasingly been considered within the scope of practice of speech-language pathologists. The act of swallowing—**deglutition**—involves many of the same neuroanatomical and anatomical structures involved in speech. When deglutition is inefficient or unsafe, a disorder of swallowing called *dysphagia* may be present.

It was previously noted that the evolution of speech by the human species did not require the creation of any new body structures. Rather, as speech evolved, it made use of many existing body structures, primarily those involved with deglutition. The chief articulators—including the maxilla and mandible, lips, teeth, hard and soft palates, and tongue—are all essential deglutition structures. When used for deglutition, these structures shift from producing speech to delivering food or drink for sustenance and survival.

The overlap in the anatomical functions and structures involved with speech and deglutition can have some grave repercussions. For instance, we all know we should not talk when we have food in our mouth. This is not simply an issue of manners. Rather, when we have food in our mouth, the body is focused on propelling that food from the pharynx to the stomach. When we eat and drink, the airway is closed to protect the respiratory system from penetration. When we talk, the body is focused on coordinating respiration and phonation to produce speech, which requires the airway to be open. If we try to talk and eat at the same time, food can enter the wrong tube—the larynx and trachea rather than the esophagus. When food or drink enters the laryngeal area, it is called *penetration.* If food or drink gets beyond the larynx and into the lungs, it is called *aspiration.* Coughing is a reflex that occurs with penetration to protect the larynx; a cough is often enough to propel foreign matter up and out of the laryngeal area. However, if the penetrating item is large enough, choking can occur, effectively shutting off the channel through which oxygen arrives to the lungs. Even if the item is not large enough to cause choking, or if drink is involved, penetration can result in small bits of food or drink entering the lungs, which can cause pneumonia and other serious respiratory problems. Thus, while the sharing of functions and structures for speech and deglutition keeps us from having to drag around extra body parts evolved just for talking, it also introduces some dangers of which we all need to be aware.

> **DISCUSSION POINT:**
> It is considered good manners not to eat and talk at the same time. From a physiological perspective, explain why this is an important lesson to learn as children.

THREE PHASES OF SWALLOWING

Deglutition is a carefully orchestrated three-phase process whose function is to move a bolus—the food or liquid matter that is being transported—from the lips to the stomach and to keep it from penetrating the larynx and respiratory system. Figure 3.19 depicts the three phases of deglutition.

Oral Phase

The foods humans eat come in many textures—mashed potatoes are soft, gumdrops are chewy, beef jerky is tough, pudding is creamy, pretzels are crunchy, and so on. Even liquids can vary, from the thin consistency of lemonade to the thick consistency of a milkshake. In the oral phase of deglutition, the bolus is manipulated and modified into a form that can be readily transported through the pharynx and esophagus to the stomach. Preparation of the bolus often requires mastication—chewing and grinding to break the bolus down. Some boluses require considerable mastication (e.g., popcorn), others require a moderate amount of mastication (e.g., rice), and others require little or no mastication (e.g., yogurt). The oral phase involves two stages: the oral preparatory stage and the oral transport stage. In all, the oral phase of swallowing takes about 1 second,

FIGURE 3.19

Three phases of deglutition.

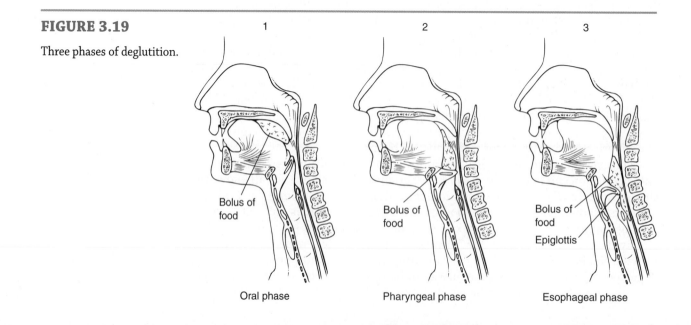

1   2   3

Bolus of food

Bolus of food

Bolus of food
Epiglottis

Oral phase   Pharyngeal phase   Esophageal phase

although age, disease, and various disorders can slow the swallowing process (Blonsky, Logemann, & Boshes, 1975).

Oral Preparatory Stage.   The oral preparatory stage consists of two activities: (1) bolus preparation and (2) bolus placement (Perlman & Christensen, 1997). Bolus preparation is needed for any food item that requires reduction to a more transportable and digestible form (e.g., popcorn, walnuts, rice). When the bolus enters the oral cavity, the tongue moves it to the middle of the cavity so that it sits on the blade of the tongue between the molars. Here the bolus is broken down through a chewing and grinding process using the molars. Saliva secreted by the salivary glands moistens the bolus to help reduce it. Saliva also has antifungal, antibacterial, and antiviral properties that protect the oral cavity from invading pathogens (National Institute of Dental and Craniofacial Research, 2003). After the bolus is appropriately masticated, it is again placed on the blade of the tongue between the molars, where it waits for transport via a swallow.

Key structures involved in the oral preparatory stage include the lips, the mandible and the maxilla, the teeth, the tongue, and the palate. When a bolus enters the oral cavity, the lips and jaws (mandible and maxilla) open and then close quickly. The lips are held tightly together, helping to create a pressure vacuum for easy movement and control of the bolus. The teeth and tongue are important

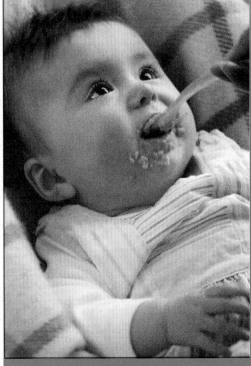

Swallowing involves the oral phase, the pharyngeal phase, and the esophageal phase.

for positioning the bolus so that it can be masticated. At the same time, the palate—particularly the soft palate—descends to make contact with the rear third of the tongue, or the tongue base. This action seals off the oral cavity from the nasal passage so that the person can breathe while masticating. The seal also keeps the bolus from exiting the oral cavity during its preparation.

Oral Transport Stage.   The oral transport stage begins once the bolus is fully prepared for propulsion. Note that for a swallow to be safely executed, breathing must stop. A swallow can be thought of as a "single pressure-driven event" (Perlman & Christensen, 1997, p. 18). To understand the process, try initiating a swallow using saliva as the bolus (or, if you have something nearby to drink or eat, take a sip or bite). Notice that in producing a swallow, the oral cavity is tightly sealed to create a pressure vacuum, and your tongue arches up to propel the bolus out of the oral cavity into the pharynx. There are four essential acts in the initiation of a swallow: (1) the soft palate elevates, effectively closing off the nasal cavity; (2) the lips contract, creating a tight oral seal; (3) the tongue blade drops, with the bolus descending slightly back into the oral cavity; and (4) the tongue tip rises to press against the hard palate (Perlman & Christensen, 1997). With all systems go, the muscular tongue arches to propel the bolus onward into the pharynx. In addition, during the execution of a swallow, the vocal folds close tightly within the larynx to protect the lungs from penetration by the bolus.

In both stages of the oral phase, the chief structure involved is the tongue. Normal tongue movement and sensation are needed to move a bolus to the appropriate place for preparation and then to transport the bolus from the oral cavity to the pharynx. The front two-thirds of the tongue help in preparation and then propulsion; the back one-third of the tongue makes contact with the velum (soft palate) to seal off the nasal cavity at the time of transport.

Pharyngeal Phase

The pharyngeal phase begins when the bolus reaches the tonsils. The tonsils are a ring of tissue around the entrance to the pharynx from the oral cavity. At about this time, the epiglottis drops to protect and seal the larynx from the bolus. From the tonsil ring in the rear of the oral cavity the bolus descends into the pharynx. The pharynx has been called "the gateway to the gut" (Sicher & DuBrul, 1975), although it is also the gateway to the lungs. The pharynx is lined with a series of constrictor muscles. The bottommost constrictor muscles blend into the muscles of the esophagus (Zemlin, 1997). The muscles lining the pharynx constrict during the pharyngeal phase to propel the bolus to the entrance of the esophagus. The entire pharyngeal phase lasts approximately 0.8 seconds (McConnel, Cerenko, Jackson, & Guffin, 1988).

Esophageal Phase

The esophagus is a long tube of muscle that runs from the bottom of the pharynx to the entrance of the stomach. The esophagus is about 25 cm (10 in.) long (Curtis & Barnes, 1989) and features two sphincter muscles, one at its upper end (the upper esophageal sphincter) and one at its lower end (the lower esophageal sphincter). The sphincters aid in propelling the bolus through the esophagus via a series of involuntary, wavelike contractions called *peristalsis*. Eventually, the bolus reaches the stomach and the intestines for digestion.

● CHAPTER SUMMARY

The human body consists of two major nervous systems: the central nervous system (CNS) and the peripheral nervous system (PNS). The CNS comprises the brain and spinal cord; the PNS comprises the cranial nerves and spinal nerves, which carry information to and from the CNS. The brain is the commander in chief of the entire human body; it consists of the cerebrum, the brain stem, and the cerebellum. The lobes of each hemisphere of the cerebrum include the frontal lobe, temporal lobe, parietal lobe, and occipital lobe; the frontal lobe controls the executive functions and is home to Broca's area; the parietal lobe controls sensory and perceptual processing; the temporal lobe contains the hearing and language centers; and the occipital lobe controls vision.

The production of spoken language involves respiration, phonation, and articulation. Respiration provides the power supply for speech through exhalation of air from the lungs. The power supply is sent from the lungs through the trachea to the larynx, which contains the vocal folds to create voice. The air supply further resonates in the pharynx and is articulated in the oral cavity to produce the variety of speech sounds.

The hearing process involves seven main areas: the outer ear, which serves as the entry point for sound; the external auditory canal, which channels sound inward; the tympanic membrane, which vibrates; the ossicular chain, which carries the sound as mechanical energy; the cochlea, which contains the organ of hearing and receives the sound as hydraulic energy; the auditory nerve, which transports neural energy from the cochlea to the brain; and the auditory center of the brain, which interprets the sound.

Deglutition refers to the three-phase act of swallowing. In the oral phase, the bolus is received and prepared through mastication for further transport. The bolus is then placed on the middle of the tongue and propelled posteriorly toward the pharynx with the initiation of a swallow. In the brief pharyngeal phase, the bolus moves from the oral cavity to the base of the pharynx. In the esophageal phase, the bolus traverses the esophageal tube to arrive at the stomach for digestion.

KEY TERMS

afferent, p. 83
anterior, p. 83
auricle, p. 103
axons, p. 84
brain stem, p. 85
Broca's area, p. 87
cerebellum, p. 86
cerebrum, p. 86
cochlea, p. 106
corpus callosum, p. 86
cranial nerves, p. 83
deglutition, p. 107
dendrites, p. 84
distal, p. 83
dorsal, p. 83
efferent, p. 83
executive functions, p. 87
external, p. 83
external auditory canal, p. 104

frontal lobe, p. 87
Heschl's gyrus, p. 88
hyoid bone, p. 96
inferior, p. 83
inner ear, p. 105
internal, p. 83
laryngopharynx, p. 96
larynx, p. 96
lateral, p. 83
medial, p. 83
meninges, p. 85
middle ear, p. 104
myelin, p. 84
nasopharynx, p. 96
neurons, p. 84
neurotransmitters, p. 84
occipital lobe, p. 89
organ of Corti, p. 106
oropharynx, p. 96

ossicular chain, p. 105
outer ear, p. 103
parietal lobe, p. 88
pharynx, p. 96
plasticity, p. 89
pleura, p. 94
posterior, p. 83
proximal, p. 83
spinal nerves, p. 83
superior, p. 83
synapse, p. 84
temporal lobe, p. 88
trachea, p. 100
tympanic membrane, p. 104
ventral, p. 83
vocal folds, p. 99
voice, p. 100
Wernicke's area, p. 89

ON THE WEB

Check out the Companion Website at www.pearsonhighered.com/justice2e! On it, you will find:

- suggested readings
- reflection questions

- a self-study quiz
- additional cases
- links to additional online resources, including information about current technologies in communication sciences and disorders

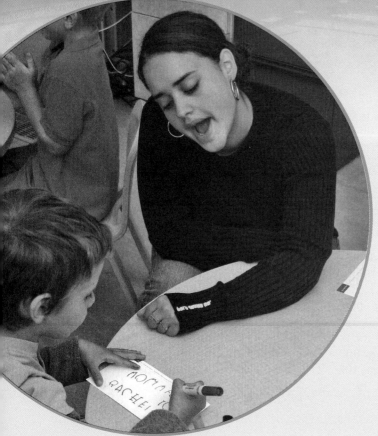

COMMUNICATION ASSESSMENT AND INTERVENTION
PRINCIPLES AND PRACTICES

FOCUS QUESTIONS

This chapter answers the following questions:

1. What is assessment?
2. How are assessment instruments categorized?
3. What is intervention?
4. How are interventions categorized?

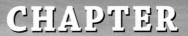

CHAPTER 4

INTRODUCTION

People are drawn to the discipline of communication sciences and disorders for diverse reasons. Students often come to an introductory course in communication disorders with some general impressions of the field derived from interaction with family members who have worked as speech-language pathologists, audiologists, or special educators. Some students have had direct exposure to the field because a family member or friend required evaluation or treatment for a communication disorder. Through direct exposure or indirect impression, many students are already aware of three benefits of a profession in communication sciences and disorders: (1) the opportunity to make a difference in the lives of others, (2) the potential to have a job that offers significant challenges and the promise of day-to-day variability, and (3) the excitement of working in a dynamic field in which new discoveries are constantly informing and enhancing practice. These features make the communication disorders disciplines highly desirable to many traditional university students who are looking toward their professional futures as well as to many nontraditional students who are considering reentry into the workforce or a change in their profession.

Although people in the communication disorders professions fill a variety of roles—from university faculty, to administrators, to consultants—the majority of them are direct service providers, working as therapists or educators. The key responsibilities of a direct service provider are assessment and intervention, or diagnosis and treatment. The daily responsibilities of assessment and intervention are what make it possible for these professionals to make a difference in the lives of others, to have a job that offers great challenges, and to ensure attention to new scientific discoveries that can inform and enhance our practice.

Because there are many varieties of communication disorders, there is great variability in the assessment and intervention techniques and tools used by professionals. This chapter provides an overview of terminology related to assessment and intervention, as well as key principles and practices associated with these two aspects of service delivery. The content of this chapter serves as a foundation for many of the concepts discussed in Chapters 6 through 15, which provide more detailed content on assessment and intervention as they relate to specific disorders of communication. ●●●

| CASE STUDY 4.1 | Communication Disorders Across the Life Span |

LILA is a 7-year-old who lives in St. Louis, Missouri. She entered first grade at a public elementary school this past fall. A routine developmental screening conducted at that time indicated that Lila might be showing some stuttering behaviors. Lila rarely speaks in class. During a recent round-robin reading activity in which the children took turns reading from their literature book, Lila got stuck on the first sound in a word four times in the first short paragraph she was asked to read. Her teacher, Mr. Kendall, stopped Lila in the middle of her turn because Lila seemed to be about to cry and the other children were giggling. Mr. Kendall referred Lila to the school speech-language pathologist, Ms. Tyler, for a comprehensive evaluation. Ms. Tyler, however, does not want to do an evaluation, because her caseload is too large; she currently serves 72 children in the elementary school.

Internet research

1. What is the typical caseload for a speech-language pathologist in an elementary school in St. Louis, Missouri? See what you can find out. Compare this to the caseload sizes recommended by the American Speech-Language-Hearing Association.

2. Mr. Kendall is using the Internet to find some suggestions for helping Lila in the classroom. What kind of materials will he find? How can he differentiate between good information and bad information?

Brainstorm and discussion

1. Ms. Tyler has agreed to interview Lila's mother to gather more information about Lila. What are some questions she will likely ask?

2. If Ms. Tyler decides to conduct an evaluation, what would be the goal of the evaluation?

● ● ●

MR. STEVENS is a morbidly obese man with diabetes who is unable to leave his home because of complications associated with these conditions. Mr. Stevens has vocal nodules, a voice disorder often characterized by hoarseness and breathiness. He is no longer able to use the telephone, because his voice quality is too poor for him to be understood. Mr. Stevens lives in a rural and remote area of Wyoming and does not have access to speech-language pathologists who might be able to work with him directly in his home. He has been referred to a telehealth model of voice therapy that is delivered using remote video teleconferencing from the Tripler Army Medical Center in Honolulu, Hawaii (Mashima et al., 2003).

Internet research

1. What is telehealth; and what kinds of medical conditions are currently treated using telehealth models?

2. For people who live in remote areas, what are options for treating communication disorders other than telehealth?

Brainstorm and discussion

1. In what ways does Mr. Stevens's communication disorder negatively impact his quality of life?

2. To participate in the Tripler Army Medical Center's telehealth program, a comprehensive interview will be conducted to judge the likelihood that Mr. Stevens will complete the voice therapy program. What kind of questions do you think will be included in this interview?

WHAT IS ASSESSMENT? ●

DEFINITION

Assessment is the systematic process of gathering information about an individual's background, history, skills, knowledge, perceptions, and feelings. In the field of communication disorders, assessment focuses on comprehensively gathering information in one or more of the following areas: language, speech, cognition, feeding, swallowing, voice, fluency, and hearing. Assessment is often a **multidisciplinary** process involving many professionals who bring their diverse knowledge, skills, and experiences to the assessment. It is also a systematic process that follows certain procedures so that its outcome will be comprehensive, nonbiased, and valid. Assessment is more than testing. A test is the administration of one task to examine a person's skills or knowledge in a particular area. A test might be part of an assessment, but a test alone is not assessment.

PURPOSES OF ASSESSMENT

Assessment has four purposes, as shown in Table 4.1. The first purpose is to identify skills that a person has and those that a person does not have in a particular area of communication. This information determines whether an individual's performance is consistent with a disorder. For instance, the assessment for 2-year-old Marcus, brought by his father to a speech-language pathologist (SLP) because he is not yet talking, focuses on identifying the language skills that Marcus does and does not have. The SLP carefully studies Marcus's skills to determine whether a disorder is present. The SLP may conclude that Marcus has a communication disorder and recommend treatment. Conversely, the SLP may conclude that Marcus's language skills are appropriate for his age and background, and thus not recommend therapy.

The second purpose of assessment is to guide the design of intervention for enhancing a person's skills in a particular area of communication. This purpose focuses on people who have an identified communication disorder, although it may also focus on people who do not have a disorder but would nonetheless benefit from some type of assistance, such as a prevention

TABLE 4.1 Four purposes of communication assessment	
Purpose	**Application**
1. To identify skills that a person does and does not have in a particular area of communication	To determine whether a person's performance indicates presence of a disorder
2. To guide the design of intervention for enhancing a person's skills in a particular area of communication	To identify specific short- and long-term goals and specific learning targets and to identify strategies and contexts for addressing these goals
3. To monitor a person's communicative growth and performance over time	To determine progress made in intervention and whether specific outcomes are reached and to monitor progress after discharge
4. To qualify a person for special services	To determine whether a person meets the eligibility requirements to receive coverage of educational and therapeutic services for a particular governing organization or institution

program designed to lower an individual's risk for developing a communication problem. In building a program of intervention for a particular individual, assessment enables the SLP to identify (1) specific short- and long-term goals and (2) strategies and contexts for addressing those goals. For Marcus, the assessment process identifies the language goals that are most appropriate for him at this time and how those goals should be addressed. Specifically, through the assessment, the SLP finds that Marcus is not yet using communication to meet his needs at home or at daycare and identifies (among others) the following short-term goal:

- Marcus will use gestures and single words to ask for objects and actions in interactions with his father and the daycare provider.

Marcus's SLP considers information gained from the assessment process in making decisions about where and when intervention will take place, identifying the people who will be involved in delivering the intervention and determining the types of techniques likely to be most effective for helping Marcus meet his communication goals.

The third purpose of assessment is to monitor a person's communicative growth and performance over time. Assessment measures progress made in intervention and reveals whether specific outcomes have been reached. Assessment is also used to periodically monitor people following their discharge from intervention or people for whom no intervention is provided but periodic assessment seems warranted. Assessment used for this purpose permits practitioners to be highly flexible in their intervention. Periodic assessments enable practitioners to change goals, modify treatment schedules, change treatment settings, and shift treatment approaches. For instance, after a 3-month period of implementation of techniques to facilitate Marcus's use of single words and gestures for requesting, the SLP used a reassessment to study Marcus's communication skills at home and at daycare. This assessment showed that Marcus was frequently using gestures and single words to meet his needs. The SLP used this information to revise Marcus's goals and strategies.

The fourth purpose of assessment is to qualify a person for special services. Treatments for communicative impairments are often expensive, although treatment benefits usually outweigh the costs. Whereas some people pay for communicative therapies out of their own pockets, often these services are paid for by public school divisions, Medicaid and Medicare, and private-pay health insurance. These organizations and institutions often have strict regulations governing what coverage they will provide. For instance, school districts are required by law to pay for a student's communicative therapies only if the communicative impairment has a measurable impact on educational achievement. School districts have considerable discretion both in how they determine whether a communicative impairment has a negative educational impact and in determining the level of impairment that must be exhibited for services to be provided. Nonetheless, the assessment process must document the adverse effects of a communication disorder on educational achievement for a child to qualify for special services. Federal health care coverage through Medicare and Medicaid, as well as private-pay insurance agencies, also set their own guidelines concerning eligibility for communication-related services. The purpose of assessment thus often includes determining whether an individual meets the eligibility requirements of a particular governing organization for speech, language, or hearing services.

DISCUSSION POINT:
Consider the case of Lila in Case Study 4.1 and these four purposes of assessment. Which of the four purposes are most relevant to her current needs?

FIGURE 4.1

Scope and sequence of communicative assessment.

1. Screening and referral
2. Designing and administering the assessment protocol
3. Interpreting assessment findings
4. Developing an intervention plan
5. Monitoring progress and outcomes

THE ASSESSMENT PROCESS

The assessment process is a systematic, comprehensive activity that includes a 5-stage scope and sequence (see Figure 4.1): screening and referral, designing and administering the assessment protocol, interpreting assessment findings, developing an intervention plan, and monitoring progress and outcomes.

Screening and Referral

Both screening and referral are used to identify people who may require a more comprehensive communicative assessment.

Screening. **Screening** is the delivery of a test or task that provides a quick check of an individual's performance in a particular area. Most readers have probably had an audiological screening at some point to check their hearing. This procedure provides a quick and relatively inexpensive probe of an individual's hearing at key levels, as shown in Figure 4.2. A pass on a screening such as this

FIGURE 4.2

Hearing screening protocol.

Name:	Date:
Date of Birth:	Age:
Screening Site:	Examiner:

Patient Background

___history of hearing loss	___ear infections
___earaches	___ringing in the ears
___head trauma	___medications
___noise exposure	___chronic disease
Comments:	

Screening Results

dB level (circle one)   25dB   30dB   35dB

Right	Left
___1000 hz	___1000 hz
___2000 hz	___2000 hz
___4000 hz	___4000 hz
___Pass ___Fail	
Notes:	
Referral:	

precludes the need for a lengthier, more expensive, and professionally administered audiological assessment.

Newborn hearing screening, formally referred to as Early Hearing Detection and Intervention (EHDI), is an increasingly common type of screening used in the field of communication sciences and disorders. In 1993, a panel convened by the National Institutes of Health (NIH, 1993) achieved consensus regarding the importance of conducting a hearing screening of all newborns within the first 3 months of life. This consensus statement emphasized that early identification of hearing loss is critical for providing early intervention services to promote the positive outcomes of children with hearing loss. The intent behind EHDI programs is to identify all children with hearing loss by 3 months of age so that early intervention services can be initiated by 6 months of age. Today, 42 states (as well as Washington, D.C., and Puerto Rico) have statutes regarding the importance of newborn hearing screening, although it is a universal practice applied to all newborns in only 26 states.

Screening differs in several important ways from assessment. First, screening probes an individual's skills broadly, whereas assessment examines an individual's skills in a focused, in-depth manner. Second, screening is conducted in just minutes, whereas assessment may take several hours. Third, screening typically costs just dollars per individual screened, whereas assessment may cost hundreds or even thousands of dollars per individual. Fourth, screening can be conducted by a person with relatively little training, whereas assessment is conducted only by highly qualified individuals.

Screening for communicative skills is typically done at key developmental junctures in a person's life; hence it is referred to as **developmental screening.** For many children, developmental screening starts at birth and continues with every visit to the pediatrician through their first 5 years. The newborn hearing screening described previously is an example of developmental screening.

Screening is also routinely used to identify the extent of an illness or injury; this is called **injury-related screening.** For example, a person who has had a

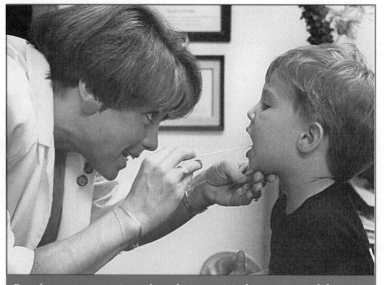

Development screening takes place at critical junctions in life.

stroke is screened for communication, because stroke is a leading cause of adult speech and language disorders. Likewise, a child who has a chronic history of middle-ear infections is routinely screened for hearing to establish the effects of the illness and the potential need for a more in-depth hearing evaluation.

Referral.   **Referral** often accompanies screening and describes the process by which the involvement of speech, language, and hearing professionals is formally requested. Referrals are typically made by parents or other caregivers and by educational and health care professionals. For example, young children routinely see their pediatricians at regular intervals over the first few years of life. At each visit, the pediatrician screens the child's communication skills, either by using a formal screening instrument or by informally questioning the parent and interacting with the child. If the pediatrician has concerns about any aspect of a child's communicative abilities, he or she is likely to refer the child to a speech, language, or hearing professional for a comprehensive assessment. As another example, nurses who provide care for people following stroke carefully observe their patients for signs of swallowing problems. If a patient shows evidence of a swallowing problem, the nurse will confer with the patient's physician to discuss the need for a referral to a speech-language pathologist. Once a referral is made, the speech-language pathologist will determine whether a more comprehensive swallowing assessment is warranted.

DISCUSSION POINT:
What factors might influence the likelihood of a physician referring a patient to a speech-language pathologist or audiologist?

Designing and Administering the Assessment Protocol

The screening and referral process typically identifies a specific area of concern for an individual. For instance, a speech-language pathologist may receive a referral from a physician that requests "diagnosis and treatment for hoarse vocal quality" or "assessment for possible stuttering." Professionals use their clinical skills and knowledge of current research to design a highly individualized assessment for each client that is sensitive, comprehensive, nonbiased, and family centered.

A sensitive protocol is one that accurately identifies whether a problem is present and characterizes the severity of the problem. A sensitive protocol is not affected by a false positive (the assessment reveals a problem when there is no problem) or a false negative (the assessment shows no problem when there is a problem).

A comprehensive protocol is one that accurately identifies all the dimensions of the problem. It characterizes the influences of the problem on diverse aspects of a person's life and skills, including how the problem affects daily living activities at home, school, and work.

A nonbiased protocol is one that accurately characterizes communicative performance regardless of a person's race, ethnicity, gender, socioeconomic background, culture, or native language.

A family-centered protocol is one in which family members are involved to share their understandings about strengths and needs of the individual being assessed, as well as their own priorities and values. Family members may be involved in many different ways in the assessment process. A family-centered assessment views family members as critical resources.

In designing the assessment protocol to meet these specifications, the professional uses many different techniques and materials to obtain information about areas of concern. Common techniques and materials include chart review, interviews, systematic observation, questionnaires and surveys, testing, and instrumentation.

DISCUSSION POINT: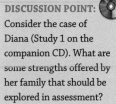
Consider the case of Diana (Study 1 on the companion CD). What are some strengths offered by her family that should be explored in assessment?

DISCUSSION POINT:
Consider the case of
Mr. Stevens in Case Study 4.1.
A chart review will be conducted in consideration of his
candidacy for the Telehealth
Voice Therapy Program. What
kind of information might
be useful in determining
whether he is an appropriate
candidate for this program?

Chart Review.   A **chart review** is the systematic examination of an individual's developmental, educational, and medical history that has been collected by other professionals. Chart review provides the professional with access to other practitioners' opinions and diagnoses, previous test results evaluating broad aspects of health and development, and descriptions of outcomes from other interventions. For professionals working with children who have received special services through state agencies, a chart review includes examining the family's Individualized Family Service Plan (IFSP) and the child's Individualized Education Plan (IEP). An IFSP is a document used to identify services and outcomes for infants and toddlers; an IEP is a document used to identify services and outcomes for children aged 3 and older. IFSPs and IEPs are federally required plans that identify specific goals for children and specific strategies for addressing these goals. The clinician's careful review of chart information, when available, provides an important vehicle for getting to know a client and his or her unique developmental, educational, and medical history.

DISCUSSION POINT: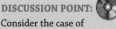
Consider the case of
Mr. Johnson (Study 4). If you
were to interview his wife,
Ms. Johnson, what are some
questions you would ask her?

Interview.   An interview is a unique vehicle for collecting information from individuals, their families and caregivers, and other professionals that can aid in understanding the nature, history, and extent of the problem. An interview provides indispensable information about the impact of a disorder on a person's life at home, at school, at work, and in the community. It may also reveal how the characteristics of a disorder have evolved and changed over time. Examples of interview questions used to collect information from people receiving a voice evaluation are presented in Figure 4.3. The interview is also an important tool in ensuring that assessment is family-centered (Rini & Hindenlang, 2007). It provides an opportunity for family members of those affected by a communication disability to share their perceptions about how communication is impacted in a range of daily activities and to share their priorities. It is very important that the interviewer develop a trusting relationship with family members before or during the interview process and that the information they provide be viewed as valuable. Additionally, the interviewer must be aware of his or her own biases and set these aside in order to allow family member input to become a valuable part of the assessment process (Rini & Hindenlang, 2007).

FIGURE 4.3

Sample interview questions for voice evaluation.

1. What specifically is bothering you about your voice?
2. Please describe the onset of your voice problem.
3. What do you think may be the cause of this problem?
4. Tell me how the voice problem progressed after you first noticed it.
5. How is your voice different now from before the onset of problems?
6. What terms would you use to describe your voice now?
7. Can you identify any environmental factors that may make your voice problems worse or improved?
8. In what ways does your voice problem affect your life at home and at work?
9. How important to you is it that your voice problem be resolved?

Sources: Stemple, Glaze, & Gerdeman (1995); Verdolini (2000).

FIGURE 4.4

Sample items from systematic observation to assess student performance in classroom discussion.

Classroom Discussion Behaviors	0 Never	1 Sometimes	2 Often or Always
1. Difficulty paying attention	0	1	2
2. Difficulty understanding abstract concepts	0	1	2
3. Difficulty answering questions from peers	0	1	2
4. Difficulty answering questions from teachers	0	1	2
5. Difficulty asking for help or clarification	0	1	2
6. Difficulty providing details	0	1	2
Notes:			

Systematic Observation. Systematic observation is the process of observing how an individual uses communication for functional purposes in real-life, authentic activities. It allows a professional to examine an individual's communicative performance at home, at school, at work, and in the community. The observational protocol presented in Figure 4.4 is used by speech-language pathologists to observe students' understanding of directions within the classroom. Figure 4.5 presents a sample instrument used to observe a caregiver-child interaction for a child with a language impairment. This same assessment strategy could be used to study how people with other types of communicative impairments, such as language disorder following stroke, interact with others in real-life contexts. Language sampling, or conversational sampling, refers to the process of collecting samples of language or conversation during functional activities. As described more fully in Chapter 6, the clinician transcribes the language an individual produces and then analyzes it carefully for content, form, and use to determine which skills are and are not present.

Questionnaire/Survey. Questionnaires and surveys are formal mechanisms for gathering information on particular topics. They are administered to individuals, their family members, and relevant professionals to gather input. For instance, a speech-language pathologist might ask a client to complete a self-rating scale to describe his voice quality (loudness, shakiness, hoarseness, monotone; Fox & Ramig, 1997). Or, a special educator might ask a pupil's parent to complete the Social Skills Rating System (Gresham & Elliott, 1990), on which parents rate their children's skills in cooperation, empathy, assertion, self-control, and responsibility. Questionnaires and surveys like these provide useful information about clients that might be difficult to collect through other avenues.

Testing. Professionals often use formal, commercial tests to evaluate a person's communicative skills in a standardized manner. A standardized test is given in a

FIGURE 4.5

Systematic observation of child communication initiations during caregiver-child conversation.

	Intervals									
	1	2	3	4	5	6	7	8	9	10
Communication Behavior Gesture (G) Eye Contact (E) Vocalization (Vo) Verbalization (Ve)										
Communication Intent Request Action (RA) Request Object (RO) Comment (C) Reject (R) Imitate (I) Other (O)										

Observations:

Directions: Complete this checklist in a 20-min. observation of child engaged in play-based interactions with primary caregiver. Watch continuously for a 1-min. period and then code for 1 min. all behaviors observed in child. Repeat this process for a total of 10 intervals (1-min. observation followed by 1 min. of coding).

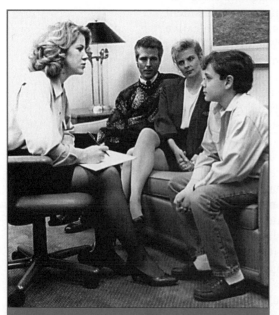

With language sampling, the clinician transcribes the language an individual produces for later analysis.

highly specific and uniform way so that its administration does not influence the individual's performance. With stringent rules governing administration, the results of a standardized test presumably can provide unbiased information about a person's achievements in a particular aspect of communication or can compare a person's achievement to that of a more general population. Principles associated with formal testing are discussed later in this chapter.

Instrumentation. Assessment for many types of communication disorders relies heavily on technological instrumentation. An individual's swallowing performance, for instance, can be evaluated using videofluoroscopic barium swallow studies, in which a person swallows food mixed with barium and the swallow is followed from the oral cavity through to the esophagus. An individual's vocal fold appearance and movement is evaluated using video stroboscopy, in which a long, flexible endoscopic tube is threaded through the nose into the pharynx to look down onto the vocal folds. The individual is instructed to make certain sounds, and the professional can watch the vocal fold movement either through an eyepiece or on a video monitor.

Technological innovations are useful for evaluating online performance in communication. **Online performance** refers to studying a communicative process as it happens (Shapiro, Swinney, & Borsky, 1998). Clinicians often use assessment tasks that study communicative processes after they happen; this is called *offline assessment.* For instance, if a clinician asks an adult patient to point to a picture of an umbrella from an array of four pictures, the pointing behavior (whether successful or not) occurs only after the client has comprehended the information. Many technological innovations now provide the means for clinicians to look at the process of communication, rather than the product. For instance, with technology we are able to examine a person's vocal folds while the person is talking and observe a person's brain while it is processing a command. Other technological innovations that influence communication assessments range from the use of computer software to evaluate language samples collected from children to the use of eye-gaze analyses to study comprehension in adults following stroke.

Interpreting Assessment Findings

When the assessment process is complete, the results must be interpreted. The first step, diagnosis, is to determine from the assessment findings whether a disorder is present and if one is, to identify it. Diagnosis is based on the preponderance of evidence from a variety of tools and techniques. Generally speaking, a disorder is diagnosed when the assessment shows that a particular aspect of communication is markedly discrepant from what is observed in the typical population or from what is expected in the individual being assessed. Also, there must be some adverse effect on the person's functional activities at home, at school, at work, or in the community.

Accurate diagnosis requires the clinician to engage in a process called **differential diagnosis,** or solving "diagnostic dilemmas" (Philips & Ruscello, 1998, p. 2). Sometimes it is difficult to differentiate disorders that share symptoms and causes. Differential diagnosis is the process of systematically differentiating a disorder from other possible alternatives to arrive at the most accurate diagnosis.

Once the presence of a disorder is confirmed, the clinician uses the available evidence to determine the severity of the disorder. Severity estimates typically range along a continuum of *very mild, mild, moderate, severe,* and *very severe* (e.g., Wingate, 1976). The American Speech-Language-Hearing Association (1998) provides guidelines for differentiating the severity of disorders on a 7-point scale, shown in Table 4.2, for adult language disorders.

Finally, the clinician characterizes the client's prognosis, or changes expected as a result of treatment. Prognosis statements are subjective predictions made by clinicians that are influenced by characteristics of the disorder (severity and cause) and of the client (age, family supports, motivation, general health, etc.).

Developing an Intervention Plan

The clinician uses the assessment process to develop an intervention plan based on the individual's strengths and needs in communication. Development of the plan involves identifying treatment goals, describing the possible length and frequency of treatment, and describing treatment contexts and activities. The goals that are identified vary with different types of communicative disorders. For instance, for a person with a swallowing disorder, goals are likely to focus first on ensuring safety while swallowing and second on improving

DISCUSSION POINT:
Some professionals might fear that technology will take over the assessment of communication disorders, making the clinician superfluous. How important, in your opinion, is the human factor in medical and educational assessments?

DISCUSSION POINT:
Consider the cases of Lila and Mr. Stevens in Case Study 4.1. What are some ways that stuttering and voice disorders can affect a person's functional activities at home, at school, at work, and in the community?

TABLE 4.2	Severity classifications for adult language disorders
Severity	**Description**
Level 1	Individual is alert, but unable to follow simple directions or respond to yes/no questions, even with cues.
Level 2	With consistent, maximal cues, individual is able to follow simple directions, respond to simple yes/no questions in context, and respond to simple words or phrases related to personal needs.
Level 3	Individual usually responds accurately to simple yes/no questions. Individual is able to follow simple directions out of context, although moderate cueing is consistently needed. Accurate comprehension of more complex directions/messages is infrequent.
Level 4	Individual consistently responds accurately to simple yes/no questions and occasionally follows simple directions without cues. Moderate contextual support is usually needed to understand complex sentences/messages. Individual is able to understand limited conversations about routine daily activities with familiar communication partners.
Level 5	Individual is able to understand communication in structured conversations with both familiar and unfamiliar partners. Individual occasionally requires minimal cueing to understand more complex sentences/messages. Individual occasionally initiates the use of compensatory strategies when encountering difficulty.
Level 6	Individual is able to understand communication in most activities but some limitations in comprehension are still apparent in vocational, avocational, and social activities. Individual rarely requires minimal cueing to understand complex sentences. Individual usually uses compensatory strategies when encountering difficulty.
Level 7	Individual's ability to independently participate in vocational, avocational, and social activities is not limited by spoken language comprehension. When difficulty with comprehension occurs, the individual consistently uses a compensatory strategy.

Source: *American Speech-Language-Hearing Association. (1998).* National outcomes measurement system. *Reprinted with permission.*

quality of life. For a child with a disorder of speech production, goals may focus first on developing other means of communication so the child's needs can be made known and second on improving speech intelligibility.

All goals identified through the assessment process should exhibit the following characteristics:

1. *Functional:* Goals should directly improve the client's life in some way.
2. *Measurable:* Goals should link directly to some aspect of measurement so that progress toward the goal can be documented.
3. *Attainable:* Goals should be realistic and achievable for the client so that progress, however incremental, is possible.

Monitoring Progress and Outcomes

Assessment is not a one-shot deal that stops when the diagnosis is made. Rather, assessment is an ongoing process that monitors progress and outcomes for the client. Assessment is used to monitor a client's progress during treatment, to modify the treatment plan as progress is made, and to determine when a client should be discharged from treatment. The use of assessment to guide intervention is a natural part of the treatment process for experienced clinicians. During every treatment session, the experienced clinician probes the client's skills and progress, making adjustments to the treatment process to enhance the effectiveness of the session and the overall treatment plan.

SPOTLIGHT ON LITERACY

Dolch Sight Words

The majority of words that we encounter in print are "high frequency"; representing somewhere between 50 and 75% of words on the typical page of text in a book, magazine, or newspaper, high-frequency words are those that occur most commonly in printed texts. Because these words occur so often in printed text, they are sometimes called *service words*. A number of these high-frequency words feature irregular sound-letter correspondences and therefore cannot be easily sounded out (e.g., *have, you, one*). Many experts contend that children should learn these high-frequency words early and well; if these words are committed to sight, they are processed so efficiently that cognitive resources can be devoted elsewhere (e.g., tackling unfamiliar words, comprehending main ideas).

In 1948, Dr. Edward William Dolch was the first to publish lists of high-frequency words organized by grade; his book was titled *Problems in Reading* and contained 220 words organized into five lists of increasing difficulty: preprimer (e.g., *a, and, big, can*), primer (e.g., *all, but, did, do*), first grade (e.g., *after, give, how, once*), second grade (e.g., *around, does, read, tell*), and third grade (e.g., *about, hold, kind, laugh*).

Dolch's lists were derived from analysis of children's books and did not include any nouns. His lists of words became known as *Dolch words* or *Dolch sight words,* and these are commonly used to both assess and teach early reading. For instance, children may be provided flash cards of the Dolch words during each of the early primary grades to commit these to memory. Many school districts publish these lists on their websites so that parents can access them to use at home (e.g., www.fcboe.org/schoolhp/shes/sight_words.htm at Spring Hill Elementary in Fayetteville, Georgia). In some schools, children may be tested on their knowledge of small sets of Dolch words at entry to kindergarten and first grade to determine whether they exhibit expected levels of reading ability (Invernizzi, Justice, Landrum, & Booker, 2004). Adults who are learning English as a second or foreign language may receive instruction in these Dolch words as a way to build their early English reading fluency, as will children who have significant developmental disabilities (Van der Bijl, Alant, & Lloyd, 2005). Parents, teachers, and therapists can use a variety of strategies to teach Dolch words to children and adults, including traditional modes of drill with flash cards or more inventive possibilities involving poems and puzzles. Attractive flash cards are available from the website of the children's author and illustrator Jan Brett, at www.janbrett.com/games/flash_card_dolch_word_list_main.htm. Clinical professionals can readily access the Dolch word lists at no cost on the Internet; consequently, assessment of one's knowledge of sight words can readily be incorporated into the speech-language assessment battery for individuals whose reading skills may be negatively affected by brain injury (e.g., aphasia) or developmental disability.

HOW ARE ASSESSMENT INSTRUMENTS CATEGORIZED?

Professionals use a variety of instruments to identify an individual's strengths and needs in communication and to develop an assessment protocol that is sensitive, comprehensive, and nonbiased. A variety of instruments is necessary because no one assessment instrument fulfills all these characteristics.

VALIDITY AND RELIABILITY

All assessment instruments should exhibit two critical qualities: validity and reliability. **Validity** is the extent to which a particular instrument measures what it says it measures. For instance, a test purporting to evaluate the oral language skills of Spanish-speaking children in the United States for the purpose of identifying children with a language disorder has questionable validity if it was designed based on English-language developmental data (Restrepo & Silverman, 2001). The validity of an instrument relates to the design and content of the instrument's tasks (Pankratz, Plante, Vance, & Insalaco, 2007). Three types of validity especially important to clinicians when selecting instruments include construct validity, face validity, and criterion-related validity (Pankratz et al., 2007).

Construct validity is the extent to which an instrument examines the underlying theoretical construct it was designed to examine. For instance, the items on a newly designed intelligence test should clearly reflect what experts know about intelligence and how it can be measured. For a test to have construct validity, it must measure a defined construct, or a definable aspect of knowledge or ability. In the field of communication sciences and disorders, important constructs include speech, language, cognition, communication, swallowing, and hearing. It is often hard to get experts to agree on the parameters and definitions of these and other important constructs. As expert opinion redefines or refines certain constructs, the tests used to measure these constructs change as well.

Face validity is the extent to which an instrument appears superficially to test what it purports to test. If you watch an experienced audiologist examine a client's auditory discrimination skills, it should be fairly obvious to you that the test is examining some aspect of auditory discrimination.

Criterion-related validity is the extent to which the outcomes of an instrument reflect the outcomes from other instruments measuring the same construct. There are two types of criterion-related validity. **Concurrent validity** describes how an instrument's outcomes relate to outcomes on other, similar measures. For instance, the results of a new test that examines adults' language comprehension after brain injury should be similar to those of prevailing tests. **Predictive validity** describes how performance on an instrument predicts future performance in the area examined. Many of you reading this text have taken the SAT. The SAT was designed to predict the likelihood that a particular student would be successful in the first year of university studies. If the SAT did not have adequate predictive validity, it would not make sense for so many high school students to take it. The same is true for all instruments used for evaluative purposes: Tests should be able to reasonably predict future performance.

Reliability is another important concept related to assessment and testing and is the extent to which a particular instrument is consistent in its measurement of a particular skill, behavior, area of knowledge, perception, or belief. For instance, if a person took a personality test on a Monday and was classified as outgoing and bold, and then took the same test the following Friday and was classified as shy and introverted, we would question the test's reliability, or consistency. Slight variation can be expected as a result of any number of factors (e.g., fatigue on one day); however, test outcomes should be fairly consistent. Two important types of reliability are test-retest reliability and inter-rater reliability (McCauley & Swisher, 1984).

Test-retest reliability describes the stability of an individual's test performance over time. A test has test-retest reliability when scores are similar over repeated administrations. In the example just cited, the personality test did not have good test-retest reliability. In the field of communication disorders, test-retest reliability is crucial because clinicians use tests to make important diagnostic decisions. For example, if a voice assessment shows that a person has a significant voice disorder, but the assessment instrument has inadequate test-retest reliability, the diagnosis may be in error.

DISCUSSION POINT:
What are some tests you have taken in the last few years? Think about a particular test and consider its validity. What was the purpose of the test? What did it purport to measure?

DISCUSSION POINT:
Consider video clip 5 of Diana (Study 1) as she is administered a norm-referenced test. What characteristics of the test situation might impact the reliability of the testing?

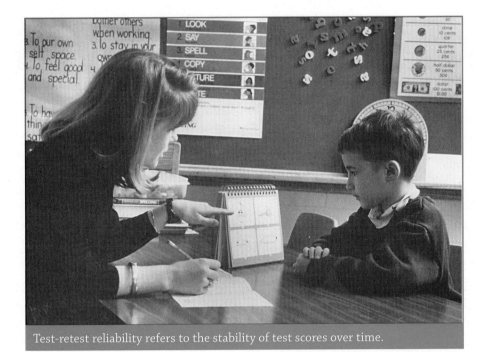

Test-retest reliability refers to the stability of test scores over time.

Inter-rater reliability describes the consistency of assessment outcomes over multiple observers. This type of reliability is particularly important for assessments that involve any level of subjective scoring. For instance, in administering a vocabulary comprehension test that involves pointing to pictures (as might be given to an elderly person who has had a stroke), will two observers reliably score the client's pointing behaviors as correct or incorrect? In using a stuttering observation to evaluate the stuttering behaviors of a young boy, will two observers reliably rate the stuttering as mild, moderate, or severe? If both observers consistently scored behaviors the same way, these tests would have inter-rater reliability. Assessment instruments need to be carefully designed to ensure that all observers of an individual's test performance will see the same thing.

TYPES OF ASSESSMENT

Five categories of assessments frequently are used by speech, language, and hearing professionals: norm-referenced, criterion-referenced, performance-based, dynamic, and progress-monitoring. These five types of instruments vary primarily on the basis of their outcome goals: What is the assessment task or tool designed to accomplish? Table 4.3 provides a description of these major assessment categories.

Norm-Referenced Instruments

The goal of **norm-referenced assessment** is to compare an individual's performance in a particular area of communication to that of his or her same-age peers. To achieve this goal, norm-referenced tests share three important qualities: (a) standardization, (b) normative sample, and (c) standard scores.

Standardization.   **Standardization** means that the test must be given in a uniform and scripted manner so that it is given in exactly the same way to everyone who

TABLE 4.3 Major types of assessment instruments	
Type of Instrument	**Purpose and Description**
Norm-referenced	Compares an individual's performance to that of same-age peers. Often required to establish an individual's eligibility for special services for organizations (e.g., school districts, insurance companies). Administered according to standardized guidelines; results interpreted against a normative sample to derive standard scores and percentile ranks.
Criterion-referenced	Determines an individual's level of achievement or skill in a particular area of communication. Individual's performance on a set of tasks is evaluated against a clear standard of performance. May use questionnaires, surveys, formal tests, informal tests, and observation.
Performance-based	Describes an individual's skills or behaviors within their actual contexts of use. Studies communicative performance across contexts that vary in the demands of the situation. May use questionnaires, surveys, observation, and collection of artifacts in portfolios for portfolio analysis.
Dynamic assessment	Identifies how much and what types of support are needed to bring an individual's communicative performance to a higher level. Uses graduated prompting after independent level of skill is identified to see how performance changes through interaction and assistance.
Progress-Monitoring	Identifies the rate of growth an individual exhibits during a course of intervention. Tracks rate using frequently administered brief probes of performance that come in multiple forms (to control for practice effects that would occur if the same form was given repeatedly). Performance results are typically plotted along a graph and compared against those of other individuals receiving the same intervention.

takes it. To accurately achieve the test's goal of comparing one person's performance to that of others, all test takers must be tested in the same way.

Normative Sample.   With norm-referenced testing, an individual's test performance can be compared to that of a **normative sample**—a group of individuals who were given the test to identify standards of performance at specific age levels. For instance, in developing an assessment of vocal quality to be used with adults aged 21 through 100, test developers would gather a normative sample of individuals representing the characteristics of the people who will ultimately be given the test. A normative sample ideally resembles those for whom the test is designed in terms of geographic residence, socioeconomic status, dialect, and disability status (McCauley & Swisher, 1984). In our example, the normative sample would be likely to comprise about 800 people, 100 from each major age band (21–30 years, 31–40 years, 41–50 years, etc.). When the test becomes commercially available, it will be able to compare a 45-year-old person's vocal quality to the vocal quality observed in the comparable age group of the normative sample.

When professionals use norm-referenced tests, they must ensure the appropriateness of comparing a client's performance to that of the normative sample. It may not be appropriate, for instance, to use a norm-referenced language test with adolescents with traumatic brain injuries if people with brain injuries were not included in the normative sample (Turkstra, 1999). Similarly, it may not be appropriate to use norm-referenced tests for members of particular ethnic or racial groups if their ethnic or racial peers were underrepresented in the test's normative sample (Laing & Kamhi, 2003).

Standard Scores.   The use of a standardized, norm-referenced test results in a **standard score,** the index that identifies how a person's test performance compares to that of their normative peers. Standard scores are frequently used by speech, language, and hearing professionals to determine whether a person has a disorder and whether a person qualifies for intervention services. Many public school special education programs depend on standard scores to determine whether a student qualifies for special education.

To understand standard scores, it is necessary to understand what happens when a person is administered a norm-referenced test. Let's take 8-year-old Garcia, who is given a norm-referenced test of speech intelligibility. On this test, Garcia is asked to say 20 words; the number of speech-sound errors is counted for each word. Garcia makes 32 speech-sound errors; this is his **raw score**—the number of items scored as incorrect or, on some tests, the number of items scored as correct. Because this is a norm-referenced test, we want to compare Garcia's performance to that of other 8-year-old children. The raw score is not helpful in this regard. Although we know that Garcia made 32 errors, we do not know how this compares to the number of errors made by other 8-year-old children. Thus, we must turn to the normative references gathered by testing a large number of children across the country. Normative references are available in the test manuals of standardized, norm-referenced tests. For Garcia, we look for the table describing performance of 8-year-old males, which indicates 71 as the standard score correlate of a raw score of 32.

Now that we have a standard score, we need to interpret it. It is easier to interpret a standard score than a raw score, because standard scores are derived from the same standard metric: the standard normal distribution. The **standard normal distribution** is derived from mathematical models of probability regarding how scores will range for a skill or aptitude that is assumed to be normally distributed within the population. The standard normal distribution assumes that certain percentages of the population will perform at particular levels; for instance, really poor scores on a test of speech intelligibility will be seen only for about 2% of 8-year-old children. Standard scores are mathematically arranged along a standard normal distribution, or **normal curve,** to approximate these probabilistic expectations.

The standard normal distribution is defined by two parameters: a mean of 100 and a standard deviation of 15. **Mean** refers to the average score, which in the standard normal distribution is a standard score of 100. **Standard deviation** (*SD*) refers to the spread of scores; on a normal curve, standard deviation units work their way outward from the mean, and scores are characterized in terms of how many standard deviation units they lie away from the mean. Figure 4.6 shows the parameters of the standard normal distribution: A score of 70, for instance, is 2 standard deviation units below the mean (−2 *SD*); a score of 110 is within 1 standard deviation unit of the mean; and a score of 149 is more than 3 standard deviation units above the mean (+3 *SD*). Standard deviation units are relative to the mean score expected for a person's age. On the basis of the normal distribution, we can expect that

- 68.3% of scores will be between 85 and 115, often referred to as "within normal limits";
- 13.6% of scores will be between 116 and 130, often referred to as "above average";
- 13.6% of scores will be between 70 and 84, often referred to as "below average";
- 2.3% of scores will be 131 or higher, often referred to as "significantly above average," with 0.13% of scores over 145 ("truly extraordinary");
- 2.3% of scores will be below 69, often referred to as "significantly below average," with 0.13% of scores under 55 ("severely/profoundly depressed").

FIGURE 4.6

Standard normal distribution.

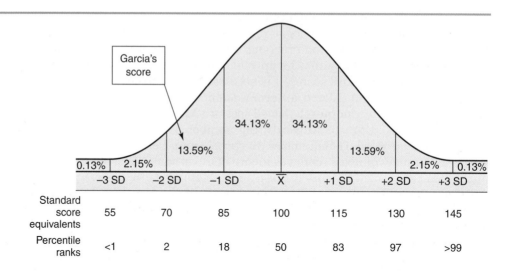

	−3 SD	−2 SD	−1 SD	X̄	+1 SD	+2 SD	+3 SD
Standard score equivalents	55	70	85	100	115	130	145
Percentile ranks	<1	2	18	50	83	97	>99

To return to our example, Garcia's standard score of 71 on the norm-referenced measure of speech intelligibility is significantly below average relative to the scores of his peers. His relative placement on the standard normal distribution is depicted in Figure 4.6.

In addition to standard scores, the outcome of a norm-referenced test provides several types of derived scores—scores that are derived from raw scores. A **percentile rank,** often used in conjunction with a standard score to interpret an individual's performance (see Figure 4.6), indicates the percentage of people in the normative reference group whose scores were at or below a given point. For instance, Garcia's percentile rank on the test of speech intelligibility was 6: only 6% of children within Garcia's age group received a score at or below Garcia's standard score of 71. Conversely, 94% of 8-year-old children in the normative sample had scores higher than 71.

Diagnostic Accuracy.   Norm-referenced tests are often used as diagnostic tools. When tests are used diagnostically, this means that their results are used to determine whether an individual has a disability or not. When tests are used for this purpose, it is important that they have strong diagnostic accuracy. For instance, a test used to identify whether children have language impairment should have evidence showing that it can reliably differentiate children with language impairment from those with typical language abilities. Unfortunately, many tests that are commonly used for the purpose of diagnosis do not have adequate diagnostic accuracy. For example, an analysis of four commonly used measures of vocabulary knowledge showed that all had relatively high rates of error in identifying children with language impairment, failing to identify about one out of four children tested (Gray, Plante, Vance, & Henrichson, 1999). An important point here is the need to ensure that the properties of specific tests be aligned to their intended use; a test that does not have good diagnostic accuracy should not be used for diagnoses. An additional point is that diagnoses should never rest on the results of a single test. Rather, diagnoses result from the careful integration of multiple forms of evidence.

DISCUSSION POINT:

Consider the case of Lila in Case Study 4.1. How useful would a norm-referenced test be in an assessment of her communicative abilities?

Criterion-Referenced Assessment

The goal of **criterion-referenced assessment** is to determine an individual's level of achievement or skill in a particular area of communication. The term *criterion* means that the individual's performance is judged against a particular standard (criterion). For example, audiologists often use criterion-referenced instruments to evaluate hearing acuity. These tests are designed to determine whether an individual can hear at a level considered adequate for daily living activities. If not, amplification, such as a hearing aid, may be indicated.

Criterion-referenced instruments are useful for probing intensively at what a person can do in a specific aspect of communication and are often used to document treatment progress. For instance, after fitting a client with a hearing aid, the audiologist uses several criterion-referenced instruments to determine whether the client's hearing has improved. These might include systematic observation of how the client performs in a conversation with his or her spouse, administration of several questionnaires and checklists, and evaluation with clinical instrumentation. All these methods of evaluation are considered criterion-referenced, because the goal is to evaluate the extent to which an individual has achieved established standards for hearing.

Criterion-referenced instruments are defined by three important qualities. First, criterion-referenced instruments require establishment of a clear standard of performance. The standard against which a person's performance is evaluated must be carefully defined. As an example, let's consider swallowing disorders and the use of criterion-referenced tasks to evaluate swallowing. In evaluating people with suspected swallowing disorders, it is of little relevance how they compare against normative references. What is important is whether their swallowing skills are consistent with a standard, which is based on knowing the standard level of skill needed to safely execute a swallow. Minimally, the standard requires a swallow to be coordinated and executed in a way that prevents any threat to nutrition or the airway.

Second, criterion-referenced instruments require design of specific tasks that reliably document an individual's performance against the standard. These instruments may include observation, questionnaires and surveys, formal tests, informal tests, and instrumentation. Continuing with the swallowing example, any one of these types of instruments may be used to document a person's performance against a standard. For instance, the professional might observe the client swallowing a variety of foods and liquids and watch for indicators that the standard of a safe swallow is not met.

Third, criterion-referenced instruments must provide clear guidelines for interpreting performance and determining whether an individual has achieved the standard. For instance, many toddlers and preschoolers go through a period in which they show stuttering behaviors, or dysfluencies. Criterion-referenced procedures for identifying a child's rate of stuttering must provide clear guidelines that enable professionals to determine whether the rate of dysfluencies observed is significantly higher than would be expected and thus whether some type of intervention is needed.

Performance-Based Assessment

Performance-based assessment (PBA), also called *authentic assessment,* describes an individual's skills or behaviors within authentic contexts of use, such as at home, in the workplace, in the classroom, or in the community (Secord & Wiig, 2003). One rationale for using PBA is that communicative skills are highly influenced by context and therefore vary across different situations (Klein & Moses, 1999). For communication assessment to be valid, it should document an individual's communicative performance in a variety of real contexts that have different performance demands. A second rationale for using PBA is that

DISCUSSION POINT:
View Clip 5 for Mr. Lamm (Study 2) on the companion CD and identify the type of assessment tool being used.

DISCUSSION POINT:
Describe a criterion-referenced task that would document a student's participation in your class. What does the task look like? How is it scored? How could you determine its validity and reliability?

traditional models of assessment, namely norm-referenced instruments, are of limited use in planning treatments. Whereas norm-referenced assessment is useful for making diagnoses, assessing severity, and recommending treatments, the outcomes from such assessment cannot be used directly to inform the design of treatments (Secord & Wiig, 2003). With PBA, by documenting the strengths and limitations of individuals' skills and behaviors within the contexts of their lives, professionals are better able to design interventions that promote functional, meaningful outcomes.

Several techniques are available for conducting PBA. These include many of the techniques already described, such as systematic observation, surveys, and questionnaires. For PBA, these techniques are employed within actual contexts. For instance, to study how well 10-year-old Adele is able to meet the communicative demands of the curriculum, a speech-language pathologist may use systematic observation to code and analyze her communication behaviors within the classroom. An important aspect of PBA is studying *how* an individual performs in relation to the context. In assessing Adele's communication in the classroom, PBA documents key features of the environment that relate to her performance, such as classroom organization and the teacher's instructional approaches.

An additional technique used in PBA is **artifact analysis,** or collection and analysis of communicative samples produced by an individual, such as a spelling test, a thank-you note, or a grocery list (Secord & Wiig, 2003). Often, artifacts are collected and maintained in portfolios for **portfolio analysis.** Professionals analyze the portfolio to identify patterns of communicative strengths and weaknesses across different contexts. This analysis is used to select communication targets and to identify contexts requiring intervention.

> **DISCUSSION POINT:**
> What kind of information does a portfolio provide about a person that might not be available through other types of assessment?

Dynamic Assessment

Dynamic assessment analyzes how much and what types of support or assistance are needed to bring an individual's communicative performance to a higher level. This approach is sometimes described as *interactive assessment* or *mediated learning* (Justice & Ezell, 1999), as it examines how interaction and mediation influence an individual's ability to complete a task (see Figure 4.7).

Dynamic assessment has its roots in the theories of Lev Vygotsky, a Russian psychologist who believed that the best indicator of a person's **learning potential** was how much he could achieve with the assistance of another (Vygotsky, 1978). As an example, consider two 20-month-old children—Danielle and Eli—who are at the single-word stage of language development. Neither child spontaneously produces two-word utterances (e.g., "doggie up"), but both can produce two-word utterances given some level of adult mediation. Danielle produces a two-word utterance following an adult model:

> ADULT: Doggie up
>
> DANIELLE: Doggie up

Eli produces a two-word utterance only when an adult breaks the two words into a succession of single words:

> ADULT: Doggie up
>
> ADULT: Tell me "doggie"
>
> ELI: Doggie
>
> ADULT: Up
>
> ELI: Up

FIGURE 4.7

Description of graduated prompting.

One common type of dynamic assessment is *graduated prompting,* in which the professional studies how an individual's performance changes as interactive supports are gradually introduced. Prompts are graduated in that they are arranged hierarchically in their intensity of support. For instance, the following hierarchical prompts might be used to examine how much support is needed to assist an adult to say his or her name:

Prompt 1: Ask client to say name ("Tell me your name.")
Prompt 2: Provide an auditory model ("Tell me, 'Will.'")
Prompt 3: Provide a visual model ("Look in this mirror. Try to say 'Will.'")
Prompt 4: Provide a starter ("Let's make the first sound: /w/.")

With this approach, the professional can determine how much and what type of assistance is needed to improve performance. For example, if Will can produce his name following prompt 3 (use of a mirror and a model), this type of support is most beneficial to Will and this response provides information that is useful to designing his treatment program.

Source: Gutiérrez-Clellen & Peña (2001).

Assessment techniques that focus on what a person can do *independently* would characterize both children similarly as being at the one-word utterance stage of language development. Dynamic techniques that focus on what a person can do *dependently* (within the context of assistance) differentiate the children by their learning potential. In our example, Danielle's language skills are more advanced than Eli's, as Danielle is able to perform at a higher level within the context of adult assistance. As this example suggests, we cannot document learning potential without considering how an individual performs with assistance. Dynamic assessment differs from other assessment approaches that withhold assistance to the individual to focus only on what the individual can do independently.

Dynamic assessment complements norm-referenced, criterion-referenced, and performance-based measures. Professionals may use dynamic assessment after other techniques have identified an individual's independent level of skill (the level achieved without any assistance) to identify the type of supports needed to bring performance to higher levels. Dynamic assessment is particularly valuable for use with people from culturally and linguistically diverse populations, as traditional methods of assessment may underrepresent their abilities and learning potential (Laing & Kamhi, 2003; Peña, Iglesias, & Lidz, 2001).

Progress-Monitoring Assessment

Progress-monitoring assessment analyzes an individual's progress during a course of intervention and is used to compare *actual* rates of growth to *expected* rates of growth, and adjust intervention techniques accordingly. Unlike the other measures discussed previously, progress-monitoring assessment is used specifically to look at rates of growth over time, or growth velocity (Carta et al., 2002). Typically, progress-monitoring measures are implemented frequently—perhaps as often as every week or every 2 weeks. An individual's rate of growth, also called *responsiveness to intervention,* is plotted on a graph, either by hand or by using specialized software. If he or she does not achieve the rate of growth expected from the intervention being utilized, then changes will be made to its intensity (e.g., shifting from one session per week to three

FIGURE 4.8

Results of progress-monitoring assessment for 18-month-old.

Adapted from: Carta et al. (2002).

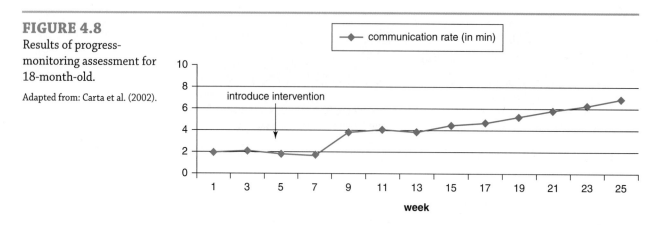

sessions per week) or the way it is being delivered (e.g., shifting from small-group sessions to one-on-one sessions).

Because progress-monitoring relies on frequent investigation of an individual's behaviors or skills, this type of assessment relies on a particular set of tools that are designed for frequent use—curriculum-based measures (CBMs, also called *individual growth and development indicators,* or IGDIs; Fuchs & Fuchs, 2007). Most CBMs are administered in a very short period of time. For instance, the Early Communication Indicator (ECI) is a type of CBM designed to study how frequently young children expressively communicate with others. It is administered in a 6-minute play-based interaction and can be repeated frequently to graph children's growth in expressive communication (Carta et al., 2002). Figure 4.8 provides an illustration of ECI used to monitor the growth of a child beginning at 18 months. As this graph shows, communication expression was low (averaging about two communicative acts per minute) during a 4-week period of observation; intervention was introduced at week 5, at which point steady increases in communication expression were observed.

WHAT IS INTERVENTION? ●

DEFINITION

The term **intervention** in the field of communication disorders refers to the implementation of a plan of action to improve one or more aspects of an individual's communicative abilities (Roth & Paul, 2007). Professionals may also use the terms *treatment, therapy,* and *remediation* to refer to this plan of action. Important considerations in designing and implementing interventions are effectiveness, efficiency, and adherence. Effectiveness is the likelihood that an intervention will have the expected outcome. An effective intervention has been shown by scientists to have value for a certain population. Efficiency is the time it takes for an intervention to result in change. An efficient intervention is one that effects change relatively quickly compared to other treatment options. Adherence is a person's implementation of an intervention following the professional's prescription; adherence is highly influential in treatment outcomes. When selecting interventions, professionals must consider the likelihood that an individual will show fidelity to a recommended course of treatment.

There is no "one size fits all" intervention that will meet the communicative needs and values of all people with communication disorders. In fact, for

> **DISCUSSION POINT:**
> In your opinion, what characteristics of an individual are most influential in determining whether that individual will adhere to a prescribed course of treatment?

one category of disorder, such as stuttering, there may be dozens of treatment variations from which to choose. Professionals must be knowledgeable about the many treatment options for different types of communication disorders and about related issues of effectiveness, efficiency, and adherence.

Making Treatment Decisions: The Knowledgeable Clinician

Some professionals work in a setting in which they treat only one type of communication disorder; for example, clinicians who work in a cleft palate clinic likely see only children with cleft palate. Many professionals, however, work in settings in which they serve a more diverse clientele. For instance, in any given week in a communication disorders outpatient clinic, a professional might treat children with communicative impairments associated with autism, apraxia, mental retardation, and vocal nodules, and may treat adults with communicative impairments associated with stroke, traumatic brain injury, dementia, and hearing loss. Being a competent clinician requires, more than anything else, a solid knowledge base that drives ongoing decision making with diverse clients. The knowledgeable clinician is one who can make sound treatment decisions for any client by integrating four areas of knowledge:

1. *Theoretical knowledge* about typical communication and how a particular disorder impacts communication

2. *Empirical knowledge* derived from the scientific literature on the disorder, including knowledge of the effectiveness and efficiency of different treatment options

3. *Practical knowledge* gained through clinical experience with other clients with this disorder

4. *Personal knowledge* of the values and needs of clients and their families.

Evidence-based practice is the process by which the clinician integrates these four areas of knowledge to arrive at the best plan of action for a particular client. This term emphasizes the use of empirical (scientific) literature for making treatment decisions but also recognizes the roles of theoretical knowledge, practical knowledge, and personal knowledge in designing interventions. Evidence-based practice provides a means for guarding against the use of fringe therapies—treatments for which there is no scientific evidence of validity. Fringe therapies are often inconsistent with theoretical models of communication and communication disorders. Many are touted as viable treatments for certain communication disorders despite these scientific and theoretical shortcomings. They may become popular through testimonials, which are easily disseminated through word-of-mouth and the Internet. Often, the authors of fringe therapies make statements that the therapy will "cure" a disorder and that "scientific evidence" has shown this to be so. Fringe therapies presented in this way frequently appeal to the families of people with communication disorders, particularly when the disorder has no known cure and treatment progress is slow.

Clinicians who engage in evidence-based practice take into account their personal knowledge of the values and needs of clients and their families. To do this, they must exhibit cultural competence as they gather information from clients and incorporate these understandings into intervention. Cultural competence is the "ability of service providers to recognize, honor, and respect the beliefs, interaction styles, and behaviors" of the individuals and families they serve (Coleman & McCabe-Smith, 2000, p. 3). The influences of one's cultural, ethnic, and linguistic background on beliefs, styles of interaction, and behaviors

DISCUSSION POINT:
Explore the Internet for available cures for autism. Which ones appear to be fringe therapies? Why?

are well established. For instance, Rodriguez and Olswang (2003) studied parents' beliefs about childrearing for 30 Mexican American and Anglo-American mothers. The Mexican American mothers in this study were either born in Mexico or were first-generation Mexican Americans. These researchers used surveys to study the mothers' beliefs about childrearing and parenting, and found that beliefs differed for the two cultural groups. For instance, Mexican American mothers held more traditional and authoritarian educational beliefs than did Anglo-American mothers—that is, Mexican American mothers viewed schools as having greater responsibility for the education of their children, with their own roles as subservient to those of the schools and teachers. Also, compared to Anglo-American mothers, Mexican American mothers placed relatively higher value on teaching their children characteristics of conformity, in terms of being polite to others, being a good student, and obeying elders; in contrast, the Anglo-American mothers placed relatively higher value on teaching their children to be self-directive. The details of this study are included to show how beliefs can vary across cultural groups and that speech, language, and hearing professionals cannot simply assume that their clients' beliefs and values are similar to their own. Cultural competence involves recognizing that culture shapes our values, beliefs, and experiences, and that in our clinical service to others, we must (1) learn about the cultural background of our clients and their families; (2) be aware of and work to eliminate our own judgments, biases, and preconceptions when working with clients and their families; and (3) build upon the unique strengths, values, and experiences of our clients and their families in the services we provide (Coleman & McCabe-Smith, 2000).

PURPOSES OF INTERVENTION

Intervention has three primary purposes: (1) prevention, (2) remediation, and (3) compensation. **Preventive interventions** attempt to prevent a disorder from emerging. They typically target all people who are considered at risk for developing a particular communicative disorder but who do not yet show signs of the disorder. Here are three examples:

Adelaide: At Adelaide's routine 12-month checkup, the pediatrician instructed Adelaide's mother to read storybooks to her daily. This is a preventive intervention designed to stimulate Adelaide's early language and literacy development and thereby reduce her risk for developing a language or literacy disorder.

Alfonso: Alfonso is a construction worker who builds office buildings in urban settings. Each worker in Alfonso's company is required to take an annual 2-hour hearing protection seminar designed by an audiologist and receives ear protectors to wear while working at sites with high levels of construction noise. This is a preventive intervention designed to reduce Alfonso's risk for developing hearing loss.

Matthew: Matthew is a professional opera singer who engages in vocal exercises daily. A speech-language pathologist designed these vocal exercises to strengthen Matthew's vocal cords and other muscles of the larynx. This is a preventive intervention designed to reduce Matthew's risk for developing a vocal disorder and experiencing vocal strain.

One challenge to delivering effective preventive interventions is outreach—the process of identifying people who are at risk of developing a particular disorder and ensuring that they have access to the preventive intervention.

Because these people do not have signs of the disorder, they may be hard to find, and they may not view themselves as in need of intervention. Also, outreach efforts can be expensive. To justify their implementation, the potential benefits must outweigh the possible costs.

Remediation interventions are clinical or educational interventions designed to slow the progress or reverse the course of a disorder once it has emerged. These are delivered to people who have been diagnosed with a communicative disorder. Here are three examples of remediation interventions:

Breah: For reasons unknown, 30-month-old Breah is producing very few words, although she seems to understand everything that is said to her. She has been diagnosed with an expressive language impairment. She sees a speech-language pathologist (SLP) twice weekly in individual sessions to promote expressive language skills; the SLP also provides Breah's mother with training in specific techniques to use at home. This is a remediation intervention designed to slow or reverse the course of Breah's expressive language impairment.

Maurice: Maurice is a second-grade teacher in a rural elementary school who has been diagnosed with vocal nodules resulting from overuse and misuse of the vocal cords. Maurice's voice is hoarse and breathy. He is seeing a speech-language pathologist for intervention for a voice disorder. The remediation intervention is designed to eliminate the cause and symptoms of the vocal disorder by retraining Maurice to use his voice properly.

Tenard: Tenard is a 4-year-old boy who has mild hearing loss and is experiencing a delay in language development. Tenard's audiologist helps his preschool teacher use sound-field amplification in large- and small-group activities in the classroom. This intervention is designed to speed up Tenard's learning and remediate early delays.

Remediation interventions, in contrast to preventive interventions, are delivered to people who show clear signs of having a disorder. These interventions are delivered with much greater intensity than are preventive interventions, and often at much greater cost.

Interventions designed for **compensation,** or compensatory interventions, are clinical interventions that help a person cope with a disorder whose symptoms are not likely to dissipate. Compensatory interventions are used when significant communicative difficulties remain after a course of remediation intervention, when a disorder is not amenable to remediation, and when it is unlikely that the progression of a disorder will be reversed. Here are three examples of compensatory interventions:

Riz: Sixty-year-old Riz had his larynx removed as a result of cancer. During the laryngectomy, Riz was fitted with a voice valve that allows him to speak by diverting air from the lungs to the back of the throat. Riz is working with a therapist to learn how to create voice using the valve. This is a compensatory intervention that will help Riz contend with a disorder that will not go away. Riz will learn a series of compensatory techniques that will allow him to be a functional communicator.

Quinton: Quinton is a 42-year-old surgeon. He has stuttered for as long as he can remember and has not received any intervention since middle school. Because his work increasingly requires him to speak publicly at conferences and training sessions, Quinton has sought the help of a speech-language pathologist to lessen the frequency of his stuttering during public speaking.

DISCUSSION POINT: Consider the case of Ashley (Study 3) and her use of hearing aids. Is this type of intervention prevention, remediation, or compensation?

This is a compensatory intervention: Quinton's stuttering is unlikely to go away, but he can be helped to manage his stuttering with specific compensatory techniques.

Leia: Leia is a high school student who has severe hearing loss resulting from use of a prescription drug during cancer treatment. Leia is working with the deaf-and-hard-of-hearing teacher at her school to learn how to use her residual hearing in the classroom in combination with her hearing aids. This is a compensatory treatment, as Leia's hearing loss is not going to go away. However, intervention will help her compensate for this loss and to participate more fully in educational activities.

Compensatory interventions help people who have disorders that significantly affect their communication and that are not likely to be resolved. Like remediation interventions, compensatory interventions often require a significant investment of time by both clinician and client.

DISCUSSION POINT:
Consider the three types of interventions and then study the cases in Case Study 4.1. Think about the purpose of the interventions discussed for Lila and Mr. Stevens.

INTERVENTION PLANNING

An array of professionals who are vested in preventing the emergence of communicative disorders, such as nurses, teachers, physicians, human resource managers, psychologists, and social workers, deliver preventive interventions, whereas speech-language pathologists, audiologists, and special educators are most intimately involved with the design and delivery of remediation and compensatory interventions. Preventive interventions often use a "one size fits all" approach, delivering the same intervention to everyone. In contrast, remediation and compensatory interventions are highly individualized to meet the unique needs and strengths of a particular client through the careful selection of goals and procedures (Klein & Moses, 1999).

An **intervention goal** is the targeted communication achievement of an individual, and an **intervention procedure** is the clinician's plan of action. The professional sets both short- and long-term goals and identifies specific procedures for achieving these goals. Intervention planning involves three decision-making phases, as described by Klein and Moses (1999).

In phase 1, the professional sets long-term goals for a client, the anticipated outcomes of therapy. The long-term goals identify the "best performance that can be expected of an individual in one or more targeted areas of communication within a projected period of time" (Klein & Moses, 1999, p. 98). Long-term goals specify broad changes expected to occur through treatment, and when these are achieved, treatment can be terminated (Roth & Paul, 2007). This phase involves specifying the general area of communication skill targeted, the time frame of the intervention, and the performance outcome anticipated. Examples include the following:

- Jason will achieve normal swallowing functions.
- Heather will be fully intelligible during conversations.
- LeShawn will use his voice appropriately in all speaking situations.
- Ava will exhibit expressive language skills that are consistent with her age.

In phase 2, the professional sets the short-term goals that will lead to the desired long-term goals. Typically, sequential short-term goals are identified that will lead to achievement of the long-term goal. These are also called *behavioral objectives.* For instance, a special educator sets the following sequence of short-term goals for Jequan, an eighth-grade student whose long-term goal stipulates that he "will produce complex fictional narratives linked to classroom literature" (Merritt, Culatta, & Trostle, 1998):

1. Retell a one-episode story while looking at a story map.
2. Retell a one-episode story following a peer model.
3. Answer questions about a two-episode story within class discussions.
4. Fill in character maps related to characters' motives and feelings from two-episode stories.

By achieving competence in each of these short-term goals, Jequan moves toward the long-term goal of producing complex fictional narratives.

In setting short-term goals, professionals use their knowledge of normal and disordered communication development to identify the steps needed to achieve desired long-term outcome. Professionals place priority on short-term goals that are achievable and linked to real-life communicative needs, as in the example of Jequan, for whom the short-term goals are directly linked to academic performance.

In phase 3, the professional sets session-level goals for a client that are written in measurable and observable terms (Klein & Moses, 1999). Session-level goals are addressed in a specific therapy session and over time lead to the attainment of the short-term and long-term communicative goals. Session goals are observable behaviors that represent "an act of learning" that presumably will lead to the acquisition of a communicative goal (Klein & Moses, 1999, p. 174). For example, consider the following three session goals for Gabby, a child with a feeding disorder. Gabby's long-term goal is to discontinue tube feeding, and a short-term goal is for her to "chew food on her own during each of three meals in a day":

1. Gabby will sit upright with her head and trunk remaining stable at the kitchen table for a continuous 10-minute meal.
2. Gabby will follow cues for tongue and lip movement with at least 90% accuracy prior to eating.
3. Gabby will swallow at least 5 ounces of rice cereal with jaw-support assistance.

These three session goals identify clearly observable behaviors that are linked to both short- and long-term goals for Gabby. The goals are functional, measurable, and presumably achievable. Importantly, these goals also reflect specific behaviors that the therapist believes represent acts of learning. Through participation in this session, Gabby will make incremental improvements in feeding skills, particularly those associated with positional stability, muscle tone, and sensory experiences (Kedesdy & Budd, 1998).

INTERVENTION MODELS

The design and delivery of effective interventions for people with communication disorders often requires the expertise and involvement of many professionals. Their involvement may be direct or indirect. Direct service is when the professional provides services directly to the individual who has the disorder; indirect service is when the professional serves as a consultant. Common models in the design and delivery of communication interventions include the following:

- *Pull-out/direct service:* A therapist or an educator provides an intervention to an individual or small group. This is one of the most common types of service delivery and is used in almost all clinical settings (e.g., schools, clinics, hospitals, nursing homes).

- *Co-teaching/parallel instruction:* Two or more therapists or educators work together to provide intervention to an individual or group. This collaborative model is becoming increasingly common in early intervention and school-based programs.
- *Intervention consultation:* The therapist or educator provides guidance to other professionals or to family members concerning assessment data and intervention approaches but does not work directly with the individual. This model is prevalent in many clinical settings (DiMeo, Merritt, & Culatta, 1998; Meyer, 1997).

HOW ARE INTERVENTIONS CATEGORIZED? ●

The intervention approach used with a client is uniquely designed to meet that client's needs and strengths in communication. Recall from earlier in this chapter that decisions involved in designing and delivering interventions are based on the clinician's combined theoretical, empirical, practical, and personal knowledge. Interventions are typically categorized on the basis of theoretical knowledge of how communication change is facilitated through intervention. Four prevalent models of intervention are behaviorist approaches, linguistic-cognitive approaches, social-interactionist approaches, and information-processing approaches. Combining two or more of these models is called a *hybrid approach* (Fey, 1986).

BEHAVIORIST APPROACHES

Behaviorist approaches are based on classic learning theory, which emphasizes the importance of the environment for shaping behavior and, in particular, the influence of consequences on behavioral change. Behaviorist approaches view communication as a behavior that is amenable to change through operant conditioning—the modification of behavior by environmental reinforcers, both positive and negative. Behavior that is positively reinforced improves, whereas behavior that is negatively reinforced is extinguished.

Inherent to behaviorist approaches is a focus on observable and measurable behaviors as the units of change and the use of systematic, hierarchical sequences of goals to structure and deliver intervention (Roth & Paul, 2007). In behaviorist approaches to intervention, a particular target behavior, or terminal behavior—the behavior that the clinician wants the client to achieve—is broken down into its smallest components. Examples of terminal behaviors in communication disorders include (1) saying one's own name fluently, (2) executing a swallow, (3) asking for help, (4) listening to conversational speech, and (5) understanding three-step directions.

Terminal behaviors are subjected to task analysis to identify all of their smaller components. Task analysis identifies the skills needed to perform a terminal behavior and determines the order of instruction for these component skills (Mercer, 1997). These components are then arranged into a systematic, hierarchical sequence of goals. In communication interventions, the client is gradually led to mastery in each of these components—a process called *shaping*—based on the assumption that mastery of each of the parts will lead to mastery of the whole. Figure 4.9 illustrates the behaviorist approach as applied to voice therapy; note the discrete, measurable objectives and the level of mastery required in each for an individual to progress to the next objective.

FIGURE 4.9

Behaviorist-oriented approach for training more appropriate voice volume.

Terminal Behavior: Use of appropriate volume in all situations with self-monitoring	
Specific Competency	Mastery Required
Appropriate volume in quiet room: monitor by clinician	Maintains for 30 minutes continuously
Appropriate volume in quiet room: monitor by client	Maintains for 30 minutes continuously
Appropriate volume in noisy setting: monitor by clinician	Maintains for 30 minutes continuously
Appropriate volume in noisy setting: monitor by client	Maintains for 30 minutes continuously
Appropriate volume with people talking: monitor by client	Maintains for 30 minutes continuously
Appropriate volume with people talking in noisy setting: monitor by client	Maintains for 30 minutes continuously

Source: Adapted from S. Goldberg, *Clinical intervention: A philosophy and methodology for clinical practice.* Published by Allyn & Bacon, Boston, MA. Copyright © 1993 by Pearson Education. Reprinted/adapted by permission of the publisher.

Behaviorist approaches to intervention tend to emphasize the role of the clinician over that of the learner or client in the intervention process, as it is the clinician who is responsible for organizing the environment and learning tasks to shape the learner's achievements toward mastery. Therefore, these approaches are referred to as clinician directed or trainer oriented, meaning that the clinician maintains a high degree of control in the implementation of the intervention. The clinician is responsible for (1) identifying observable and measurable goals arranged in a hierarchy, (2) specifying the level of mastery at each goal needed to move to the next level, (3) controlling each intervention session to focus systematically on the appropriate goal in the hierarchy, and (4) collecting data in each session to determine progress toward the targeted goal.

LINGUISTIC-COGNITIVE APPROACHES

Linguistic-cognitive approaches are based on theories of developmental psychology and cognitive science, which emphasize the developmental sequences and underlying rule-governed organization of communicative behavior (Klein & Moses, 1999). These approaches view communication development as the individual's achievement of a set of highly specific rules that inform different categories of communication. For instance, children learn the underlying rule for how to make requests (a category of communication) by combining the verb *want* with any number of actions or objects (e.g., want go, want car, want eat). The linguistic-cognitive perspective suggests that children do not need to be taught every possible way to produce a request; rather, they need only learn the general underlying rule governing this communicative category. This approach is influenced by the work of Noam Chomsky, a linguist who described the underlying grammatical rules of language acquisition, and Jean Piaget, a cognitive psychologist who described the developmental organization of early cognition.

Unlike behaviorist approaches, cognitive-linguistic interventions emphasize the role of the learner over that of the clinician in the intervention process. The learner's interaction with the environment is integral to the process of learning, as it is through interactions with the environment that an individual acquires new rules about effective communication. The extent to which these interactions enhance or accelerate learning is influenced by how the learner perceives, organizes, and interprets new information (Mercer, 1997). The role of the clinician is to study how learners interact with their environment in the learning process and to enhance the environment to promote rule-governed learning.

Linguistic-cognitive approaches to intervention are defined by three general parameters. First, the goals of communicative interventions are derived from knowledge of normal communication development, particularly *when, how,* and *why* individuals use communication. Professionals select and organize goals based on the normal process of communication acquisition and emphasize the interaction between an individual and the environment during communication.

Second, communicative goals focus on helping the individual learn the rules that underlie successful communication. By focusing on general rules rather than a smaller set of highly specific behaviors, linguistic-cognitive approaches attempt to induce an underlying change in communication that can then be applied to a wide variety of situations.

Third, the learner is engaged fully in the intervention process. Cognitive-linguistic approaches emphasize that learning takes place within an individual and that the clinician's role is to structure the environment to facilitate the individual's induction of rules that govern successful communication. The interventionist's role is to study how an individual perceives, organizes, and applies new information and to guide the learner to more efficient learning (Mercer, 1997).

The delivery of cognitive-linguistic interventions tends to be more client-directed than the delivery of interventions. In client-directed approaches, the client and clinician share control over the materials and the general structure of intervention. The emphasis on greater learner control is consistent with the cognitive-linguistic belief that learners themselves (rather than the clinician) are the critical agents in determining the effectiveness of communicative interventions.

SOCIAL-INTERACTIONIST APPROACHES

Social-interactionist approaches are based on theories of developmental psychology that emphasize the importance of social interactions among individuals as a critical means for development and learning. This approach is strongly influenced by the work of Lev Vygotsky, a Russian psychologist who believed that children's development and learning proceed from a social plane to a psychological plane (see Justice & Ezell, 1999). The **social plane** is the knowledge contained within the interaction between two individuals, whereas the **psychological plane** is the knowledge that one possesses internally and independently. According to Vygotskian theory, all knowledge exists initially on a social plane (in the interactions between two people), and then proceeds to the psychological plane. A concept must first be introduced to an individual on the social plane within the context of social interaction; only after this introduction can a concept move inward to the psychological plane.

Two additional important concepts of Vygotsky's theory that are relevant to communicative interventions are the zone of proximal development, depicted in Figure 4.10, and scaffolding. The **zone of proximal development** refers to the range between an individual's independent performance of a particular skill or behavior (what he or she can do by himself or herself) and the person's level of performance when aided by another person (what he or she can do with assistance). The zone of proximal development represents the skills and knowledge in the process of

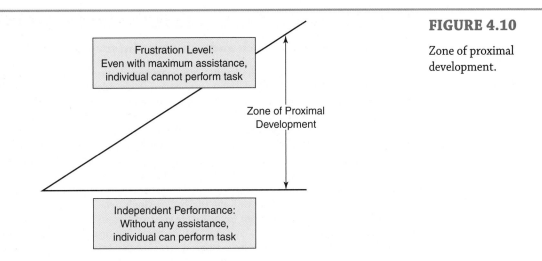

FIGURE 4.10

Zone of proximal
development.

maturation, or learning potential. **Scaffolding** is the assistance provided by another person to raise an individual's level of performance. Scaffolding provided within an individual's zone of proximal development is a primary vehicle of learning and is viewed as the essential mechanism for social-interactionist interventions.

Social-interactionist approaches to intervention are defined by three general parameters. First, the goals and methods of communicative interventions emphasize the function, purpose, and social nature of communication. Because communication skills are seen to advance from the social to the psychological plane, goals and methods used in intervention emphasize the social plane as a context for facilitating communication change. Goals are organized to emphasize an individual's engagement with others in socially relevant communication.

Second, communication interventions emphasize the importance of the zone of proximal development as the area in which learning is maximized and hence as the target for intervention. Goals at the lower end of the zone—the person's independent level—are too easy and will not result in much learning; goals at the upper end of the zone—the frustration level—are too hard and not achievable. The clinician must carefully identify an individual's zone of proximal development and ensure that therapy goals are within this zone, called the *instructional level* because it is where learning takes place.

Third, social-interactionist interventions emphasize the clinician's use of scaffolding as an essential ingredient to delivering effective interventions. Scaffolding allows a learner to perform skills that are within the zone of proximal development but beyond the level of independent skill. Scaffolds are the nonverbal and verbal support provided by professionals to help learners complete learning tasks they cannot achieve independently.

INFORMATION-PROCESSING MODELS

Information-processing approaches are derived from theories of cognitive science, which emphasize how the brain processes information and the interactions between brain processing and various aspects of communication, known as the *brain-behavior relationship* (Klein & Moses, 1999). The brain-behavior relationship suggests that communication problems are rooted in specific processing limitations. The processing of auditory and linguistic information during communication relies on many cognitive processes, including "encoding, organizing,

SPOTLIGHT ON TECHNOLOGY

Computer-Assisted Speech and Language Intervention

With the proliferation of personal computing, it is no wonder that computers are increasingly being incorporated into speech and language intervention for children, adolescents, and adults. Computer-assisted speech and language intervention involves use of computer software and hardware as supplemental tools in the delivery of intervention. In some cases, computer-assisted intervention may utilize general tools, such as word-processing software (Mander, Wilton, Townsend, & Thomson, 1995), but more often, it features software designed specifically to improve aspects of communication, speech, and language ability. One such example is the program AphasiaScripts, developed in collaboration between researchers at the Rehabilitation Institute of Chicago and the University of Colorado's Center for Spoken Language Research. This software is designed to promote the functional communication skills of individuals with aphasia. It allows individuals to create and then practice conversational scripts that are important to their daily life activities, such as ordering food in a restaurant. These scripts are entered into computer software that features a virtual therapist (see figure) with whom the individual practices the scripts and from whom different levels of support are provided (e.g., spoken models of sentences and words, highlights over certain words). Individuals who use this type of computer-assisted intervention can complete practice sessions in their homes with the virtual therapist. Pilot data collected for three adults with chronic aphasia indicated that use of AphasiaScripts improved their expressive communication at home and that they were greatly satisfied with this innovative treatment approach (Cherney, Halper, Holland, & Cole, 2008).

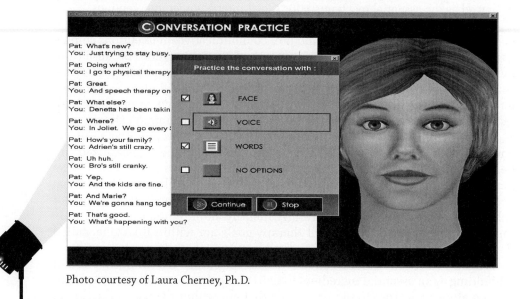

Photo courtesy of Laura Cherney, Ph.D.

storing, retrieving, comparing, and generating or reconstructing information" (Chermak & Musiek, 1997). Bottom-up processes are involuntary processes involved with moving perceptual information from the sensory systems toward the brain. Top-down processes are voluntary executive and self-regulatory strategies used to monitor information that has been received from the senses. A limitation in any of these basic processes can undermine effective communication.

During the last several decades, our understanding of how humans process information and how brain injuries or abnormalities affect this processing has advanced considerably. The literature on the processing of auditory information has been particularly influential in the design and delivery of speech, language,

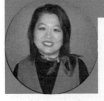

SPOTLIGHT ON RESEARCH AND PRACTICE

NAME: SHANNON WANG

PROFESSION/TITLE:
Research Director, Clinical Assessment Department
Pearson Assessment and Information

PROFESSIONAL RESPONSIBILITIES

As a research director, I am responsible for planning the research that goes into developing assessments. Depending on the research phase, I create test items, write administration and scoring directions, and specify the artwork to be rendered. I coordinate with the company's field research team to recruit clinicians across the United States to collect data for new tests. I provide scoring specifications to a scoring team so that the data are captured accurately. I consult with the psychometrics team to analyze the data and create norm-referenced and/or criterion-referenced scores. I also collaborate with editors to write examiners' manuals and production staff to create record forms and stimulus books.

A DAY AT WORK

One of the positives, as well as the negatives, of my job is that there are no "typical days at work." For example, within the same week, I spent Monday crawling around the floor with a 1-year-old, eating animal crackers with a 2-year-old, and drawing rainbows with a 4-year-old, all in the attempts to collect data for a new test in development. Tuesday, I sat at my desk pouring over data to decide on the final item order for another test that is soon to publish. Wednesday, I took a break from data analysis to shop at Costco and prepare "welcome bags" for the summer advisory board meeting. Finally, on Thursday, Friday, and Saturday, I had the privilege to sit around a table with 12 outstanding members of our profession to discuss current clinical practices, "hot" research topics, and future trends in areas such as Response to Intervention (RTI), bilingual assessment, and intervention for individuals who have suffered a traumatic brain injury. To repeat, there are no "typical days at work."

HOW INTERESTS IN COMMUNICATION SCIENCES AND DISORDERS BEGAN

I immigrated to the United States with my family in 1972. As my parents advanced in their careers, their respective employers compensated them for attending speech-language therapy for accent reduction. I frequently attended their therapy sessions and assisted with their "homework," such as correcting CVCV for CVC substitutions (e.g., "anda" for "and").

FUTURE TRENDS IN CSD

It seems that school SLPs are delivering services to students in the classroom rather than pulling them out for small group intervention. SLPs are requesting that assessment instruments provide the link of diagnosis to intervention planning rather than just providing a diagnostic standard score.

and hearing interventions. For instance, speech-language pathologists, audiologists, and special educators now have access to several computer programs designed specifically to help individuals learn to process auditory information in more efficient ways (e.g., Merzenich et al., 1996). However, these programs are not without controversy (Gillam, 1999) and are not more effective than clinician-directed treatment (Gillam et al., 2008). A major criticism is that our theoretical knowledge of how the brain processes certain types of information is incomplete and may even be erroneous in some cases (Nittrouer, 1999).

As our understanding of brain processing and neurological organization improves, information-processing approaches are likely to become more influential in the treatment of communication disorders. These approaches focus on identifying the processing limitations that result in communication limitations

(Torgesen, 1993) and then enhancing these processes. Remediation is directed to improving specific bottom-up processing abilities of the brain, such as the retrieval of words, discrimination of sounds, or auditory memory. Remediation is also directed to improving top-down processing, such as how to monitor one's own comprehension during communicative interactions. Improvement of bottom-up and top-down processing can be accomplished in several ways, including using technologies or programs designed to promote specific processing skills, heightening an individual's awareness of his or her own processing abilities (and disabilities), and manipulating the environment to improve processing.

FAMILY-CENTERED INTERVENTION

Regardless of the approach used, clinicians can adopt family-centered practices to improve the efficiency and effectiveness of treatment. Family-centered practices build upon the concept of family systems theory, which emphasizes that "the family as a whole is greater than the sum of its parts" (Rini & Hindenlang, 2007, p. 323). Treatment goals emphasize an individual's participation within and access to family activities and contexts, and may incorporate family members' perspectives regarding viable treatment approaches. Family members may also help to provide intervention, if this is a role with which they are comfortable. Parents of young children, for instance, may participate in parent programs that provide them information about communication development, disabilities, and therapeutic approaches they can use at home with their children. An example of such a parent program, developed in Canada, is It Takes Two to Talk, available from the Hanen Centre; this program provides parents with tangible techniques on how to foster their children's language skills during naturalistic activities at home. Spouses and children of adults with communication disorders may also serve as critical participants in intervention processes. For instance, the spouses and children of adults who have aphasia may benefit from training in Supported Conversation for Adults with Aphasia (CVA; see Kagan et al., 2001). Individuals learn a variety of strategies for communicating effectively with persons with aphasia, such as using gestures, writing, and pictures as communication aids. A family-centered approach, however, goes beyond enlisting the help of family members in providing intervention to those affected by communication disorders; it involves honoring the values, beliefs, perspectives, and contributions of families throughout all aspects of assessment and treatment.

● CHAPTER SUMMARY

Assessment is the methodological process of gathering information about an individual's background, history, skills, knowledge, perceptions, and feelings. It has four purposes: (1) to identify skills that a person does and does not have in a particular area of communication; (2) to inform a program of intervention designed to enhance a person's skills in a particular area of communication; (3) to monitor a person's communicative growth and performance over time; and (4) to establish eligibility for special services.

There are six stages of scope and sequence in the assessment process: screening and referral, design of the assessment protocol, administration of the assessment protocol, interpretation of assessment findings, development of an intervention plan, and monitoring of progress and outcomes. Tools for design and administration of the assessment protocol include chart review, interviews, systematic observation, questionnaires and surveys, testing, and instrumentation. The professional's responsibility is to use a variety of instruments so that the assessment protocol is sensitive, comprehensive, and nonbiased.

Intervention is the implementation of a plan of action to improve some aspect of an individual's communicative abilities and includes preventive, remediation, and compensatory approaches. Four categories of intervention, based primarily on theoretical perspectives of communicative development and disorders, include behaviorist, linguistic-cognitive, social-interactionist, and information-processing approaches. Behaviorist approaches, based on classic learning theory, emphasize environmental consequences for influencing change in observable be-havior. Linguistic-cognitive approaches are derived from an understanding of normal developmental sequences in communicative acquisition and the underlying rule-governed organization of communication. Social-interactionist approaches are based on the belief that all human communication moves from a social to a psychological plane and that skills emerge through socially meaningful interactions between two or more people. Information-processing approaches focus on the underlying processing mechanisms responsible for communication. Intervention that combines two or more approaches is considered a hybrid approach.

● KEY TERMS

artifact analysis, p. 132
assessment, p. 115
behaviorist approaches, p. 140
chart review, p. 120
compensation, p. 137
concurrent validity, p. 126
construct validity, p. 126
co-teaching/parallel instruction, p. 140
criterion-referenced assessment, p. 130
criterion-related validity, p. 126
developmental screening, p. 118
differential diagnosis, p. 123
dynamic assessment, p. 132
evidence-based practice, p. 135
face validity, p. 126
information-processing approaches, p. 143
injury-related screening, p. 118
inter-rater reliability, p. 127
intervention, p. 134

intervention consultation, p. 140
intervention goal, p. 138
intervention procedure, p. 138
learning potential, p. 132
linguistic-cognitive approaches, p. 141
mean, p. 129
multidisciplinary, p. 115
normal curve, p. 129
normative sample, p. 128
norm-referenced assessment, p. 127
online performance, p. 123
percentile rank, p. 130
performance-based assessment, p. 131
portfolio analysis, p. 132
predictive validity, p. 126
preventive intervention, p. 136
progress-monitoring assessment, p. 133

psychological plane, p. 142
pull-out/direct service, p. 139
raw score, p. 129
referral, p. 119
reliability, p. 126
remediation, p. 137
scaffolding, p. 143
screening, p. 117
social-interactionist approaches, p. 142
social plane, p. 142
standard deviation, p. 129
standardization, p. 127
standard normal distribution, p. 129
standard score, p. 128
test-retest reliability, p. 126
validity, p. 125
zone of proximal development, p. 142

● ON THE WEB

Check out the Companion Website at www.pearsonhighered.com/justice2e! On it, you will find:

- suggested readings
- reflection questions

- a self-study quiz
- additional cases
- links to additional online resources, including information about current technologies in communication sciences and disorders

AUGMENTATIVE AND ALTERNATIVE COMMUNICATION AND COMPLEX COMMUNICATION NEEDS

Julia M. King, Ph.D.

FOCUS QUESTIONS

This chapter answers the following questions:

1. What is AAC?

2. What is an AAC system?

3. What are complex communication needs?

4. What are some common causes of complex communication needs?

5. How are AAC systems and complex communication needs identified?

6. How can people with complex communication needs benefit from an AAC system?

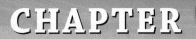
INTRODUCTION

Many people take the power of communication for granted. How many times have you thought about how you use your speech and language skills to greet a friend, order food, negotiate a transaction, or express your feelings? Imagine what it would be like if one day people did not understand your speech, you did not understand what people were saying to you, or you could use only eye blinks to express your thoughts. This is an everyday reality for many children and adults with communication disorders. Traditional approaches to treatment focus on eliminating or at least reducing the symptoms of an individual's communication disorder. This chapter will describe another approach to treatment, with a focus on understanding how the disorder affects individuals' daily lives and identifying ways to help them participate more fully in society. This approach is termed **augmentative and alternative communication** (AAC). The American Speech-Language-Hearing Association (2005c) refers to AAC as the area of research, clinical, and educational practice that "involves attempts to study and, when necessary, temporarily or permanently compensate for the impairments, activity limitations, and participation restrictions of individuals with severe disorders of speech-language production and/or comprehension."

An important point throughout this chapter is that communication is the essence of human life, and every person has the right to communicate to the fullest extent possible. No one should be denied this right because of a type or severity of a linguistic, social, cognitive, motor, sensory, perceptual, or other communication disability (ASHA, 2005c). To understand the way communication disorders affect an individual, we draw upon the model of disability from the World Health Organization (WHO). The WHO model provides a framework to investigate how a communication disorder can limit an individual's communication activities and restrict his or her participation in a variety of life situations (WHO, 2002). For example, a child who has a speech disorder may be limited in which activities he can engage in if people have difficulty understanding him; in turn, this may restrict the child's ability to participate in these activities. Table 5.1 provides an overview of the model of disability and examples of how communication disorders can impact activities and participation.

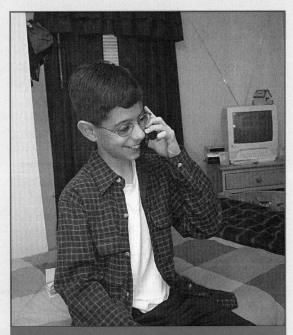

An unmet communication need is present if a young child is unable to call a friend on the telephone to invite him over to play.

TABLE 5.1	Examples of Disorders, Activity Limitations, and Participation Restrictions	
WHO Model of Disability	5-year-old kindergartener who has cerebral palsy	59-year-old car salesman who had a stroke
Disorder	Speech and language delay	Aphasia and apraxia
Activity Limitation (Example)	He has difficulty expressing himself during show & tell time and circle time in his class at school.	He has difficulty understanding questions from customers and explaining the features of cars he is trying to sell.
Participation Restriction (Example)	He is not fully participating in all aspects of kindergarten.	He cannot keep his job and will lose his societal roles as employee and financial provider for his family.

Adapted from: World Health Organization. (2002). Towards a common language for functioning, disability, and health: The international classification of functioning, disability, and health. Retrieved August 22, 2007, from www.who.int/classifications/icf/site/beginners/bg.pdf.

CASE STUDY 5.1   Complex Communication Needs and AAC

SARA is a 3-year-old twin who was born 6 weeks prematurely. She has a diagnosis of athetoid cerebral palsy, severe dysarthria, and a mild–moderate receptive and expressive language delay. Sara has significant gross and fine motor impairments because of her cerebral palsy. She communicates with gestures (eye gaze, reaching, pointing), vocalizations, and facial expressions but has no formal symbolic means of communicating at this time. At home she uses her voice to gain attention from and to protest to her parents, older brother, and twin sister, Susan, who has no documented disabilities. Sara also communicates with grandparents, aunts and uncles, and several older cousins at family gatherings. At school she communicates with her teacher and the teacher's aide but does not currently communicate with other children, because they do not know how to recognize and respond to her communication behaviors.

Recently, Sara's mother observed her looking out the window, watching neighborhood children pulling dolls in a wagon. When she asked Sara what she was doing, Sara gazed at the children, reached and pointed toward them, looked back at her mom, and then smiled. Sara's mother believes Sara comprehends much of what is said to her and has the potential to express much more than she is able to right now. Sara's mother wants to learn about what kind of help is available so she can better communicate with her daughter and help Sara participate in the activities her other daughter does.

Internet research

1. What is the rate of premature births in the United States? How often do children born prematurely exhibit developmental disabilities like Sara's?

2. What are Birth-to-Three programs? How might these programs assist children like Sara, who exhibit complex communication needs?

Brainstorm and discussion

1. What information could a speech-language pathologist learn from Sara's twin sister, Susan, during an assessment?

2. What are some possible AAC options for Sara that could be used at home and at preschool by her parents and teachers to facilitate communication now?

SCOTT is a 45-year-old male who has spastic cerebral palsy. He has dysarthria, which affects the intelligibility of his speech. Scott is a multimodal communicator; he uses speech, gestures, facial expressions, and a photo communication book when communicating with people. However, many people do not understand his communicative messages. Scott is interested in an AAC system to augment his speech and other modes of communication to help him communicate with unfamiliar **communication partners** (e.g., parent, friend, spouse, stranger) and in a variety of settings to enhance his independence and participation in desired life situations (e.g., work).

Internet research

1 What is cerebral palsy?

2 What barriers might exist that make it difficult for Scott to get a job?

Brainstorm and discussion

1 How might Scott's use of a photo communication book be helpful during a speech-language assessment?

2 What AAC features would be important for Scott in an AAC system?

WHAT IS AAC? ●

Traditionally, speech-language pathologists have designed treatment programs to remediate an individual's communication disorder or help an individual to compensate for the disorder. Another approach to treatment of communication disorders is called *augmentative and alternative communication (AAC)*. An AAC approach to treatment considers the manifestation of a disorder (e.g., the type of disorder and/or its severity) and how activities and participation are impacted. Both the people illustrated in Table 5.1 would benefit from an AAC approach to treatment to support their participation and engagement in desired activities while they work to improve their communication skills. An AAC approach also benefits people with temporary or degenerative causes of communication disorders.

This area of practice strives to improve the quality of life for individuals with severe disorders of speech-language production and/or comprehension by compensating, either temporarily or permanently, for impairments, activity limitations, and participation restrictions (ASHA, 2005c). The clinical practice of AAC involves a set of procedures and processes through which an individual's expressive and receptive communication skills are maximized for functional and effective communication (ASHA, 2002a).

Effective communication is **multimodal;** that is, people use a combination of communication modalities to meet their intended communication goals. Listening, reading, talking, writing, and sign language are all language-based modalities. Communicators also use modalities that are not language-based, including gestures, facial expressions, vocalizations, vocal inflection, speaker proximity, posture, and eye gaze. Many of us use gestures and facial expressions along with speech when communicating in face-to-face interactions. An AAC system is considered part of a multimodal approach to communication treatment. As the term *augmentative and alternative communication* suggests, meeting complex communication needs may involve augmenting (i.e., supplementing) current communication modes and/or providing an alternative mode or form of communication. An example of a communication augmentation is a speech-generating device with word-prediction software that helps to increase an individual's speed of typing and spelling of messages. An example of a communication alternative is a picture communication board that a person in an intensive care unit could use temporarily while on a ventilator and cannot speak. Some people with complex communication needs (CCNs) benefit from both augmentative and alternative forms of communication.

Severe communication disorders historically have been referred to as *severe communication impairments*. However, the International Society of Augmentative and Alternative Communication (ISAAC) and ASHA have adopted the term **complex communication needs** (CCNs) to replace previously used terms, such as *severe communication disorders* or *severe communication impairments* (ASHA, 2005c; Balandin, 2002). The term *complex communication needs* emphasizes the importance of speech, language, and/or cognitive abilities for a person's participation in society rather than focusing solely on the disorder. The term also emphasizes the complexity of communication—how it varies as a function of different contexts, participants, and modalities. The focus on needs emphasizes the individual's use of communication as a tool of personal expression.

Complex communication needs result from significant speech, language, motor, and/or cognitive impairments that prevent individuals from communicating in conventional ways. Successful communication is a challenge for many children and adults, but estimates vary on how many people with complex communication needs or challenges are meeting their daily communication needs. Beukelman and Ansel (1995) estimate that about 8 to 12 of every 1,000 Americans are unable to meet their daily communication needs, and the American Speech-Language-Hearing Association estimates that 2 million Americans currently have complex communication needs (ASHA, 2004b). Fortunately, numerous possibilities are now available to meet these persons' needs and help them participate more fully in society.

An AAC system utilizes symbols, aids, strategies, and techniques to supplement—or augment—an individual's current way of communicating; however, as we noted previously, in some cases, an AAC system provides an alternative way of communicating. For instance, an individual who loses hearing in late adolescence might learn to use sign language to augment other means for communication, such as gesturing and writing. A child with cerebral palsy who cannot coordinate the precise motor movements needed for speech might use a **speech generating device** (SGD) to produce words and phrases as an alternative to speaking in situations where he or she is not understood. Speech-language pathologists and other professionals determine whether people with communication disorders are meeting their daily communication needs and how the disorder is impacting communication activities and participation in life situations. Communication occurs in a variety of settings and with many different communication partners, so it is important to consider these factors in any intervention program.

DISCUSSION POINT:

Symbols are prevalent everywhere. What type of symbols do you use each day? What type of symbols does Scott use in Case Study 5.1?

WHAT IS AN AAC SYSTEM? ●

AAC intervention includes the design of an AAC system for an individual with CCNs. An **AAC system** consists of four different components that are used to enhance communication. The components include symbols, aids, strategies, and techniques, as presented in Figure 5.1. The selection set of an AAC system refers to the visual, auditory, and tactile presentation of messages, symbols, and codes available to the person (Beukelman & Mirenda, 2005).

FIGURE 5.1

AAC system components.

	Definition	Example
Symbol	Something used to represent an object, action, concept, or idea	A drawing of a DVD case used to represent the message "Let's watch a movie."
Aid	An assistive device used to augment communication modes or provide another method of communication	A talking photo album is an aid that can be used to assist a communicator in telling stories
Strategy	A method used to enhance communication performance	Word-prediction software enhances speed of communication by eliminating keystrokes and supporting spelling
Technique	A method used to select or access symbols and messages	Direct selection techniques include physically touching a symbol, using an instrument such as a head stick to select a symbol, or pointing without contact such as using an eye gaze system.

The AAC system becomes part of the AAC intervention plan to enhance communication via multiple modalities. Each AAC system is individualized to meet the person's unique communication needs.

SYMBOL

A **symbol** is something that stands for something else. For instance, a child might point to a line drawing of a glass to indicate "I want a glass of water." The line drawing is a symbol used to represent the communicative word *drink*. Each AAC system contains symbols that are typically classified as either aided or unaided (ASHA, 2004b). Regardless of type, symbols can be acoustic, graphic, manual, or tactile.

Aided and Unaided.   An **aided** symbol requires a device or accessory that is external to the body to transmit a message. Typing a message, drawing a picture, or pointing to photographs are all examples of aided symbols. **Unaided** symbols require only one's body—for example, speaking, gesturing, vocalizing, and signing to represent meaning (Fuller, Lloyd, & Stratton, 1997).

Acoustic Symbols.   Acoustic symbols are sounds or tones processed in the auditory system to interpret meaning. What meaning does the ring of a doorbell have? When you press the wrong key on your computer and it beeps, what does that mean? An example of an acoustic symbol set used in AAC systems is Morse code (see Figure 5.2). In Morse code, the different sounds represent letters, which can be used to access communicative messages and orthography in a computer-based AAC system.

Graphic Symbols.   Graphic symbols are printed symbols that are usually represented on paper, boards, or computer screens. Commonly used graphic symbols

FIGURE 5.2

Morse code symbols.

A	.—		N	—.
B	—...		O	———
C	—.—.		P	.——.
D	—..		Q	——.—
E	.		R	.—.
F	..—.		S	...
G	——.		T	—
H	....		U	..—
I	..		V	...—
J	.———		W	.——
K	—.—		X	—..—
L	.—..		Y	—.——
M	——		Z	——..

in AAC systems include photographs; black and white line drawings; colored line drawings; and orthographic characters, such as alphabet letters on a keyboard. Figure 5.3 shows one set of graphic symbols commonly used. These line drawings, coupled with written words, are known as picture communication symbols (PCS) and are available from a computer software package called Boardmaker that is distributed by the Mayer-Johnson Company.

Manual Symbols. Manual symbols are produced using the body; examples include gestures, sign language, and facial expressions. Figure 5.4 shows two manual symbols from American Sign Language (ASL).

Tactile Symbols. Tactile symbols can be physically manipulated. A well-known example is the braille alphabet, used by individuals with visual impairment to access written language for reading. Objects can also be used as tactile symbols by some people with complex communica-tion needs. For instance, an early childhood special educator might use a cracker or a yogurt container to symbolize or represent snack time in the classroom. A child understands the meaning of the symbol from the physical properties of the object.

Variations in the Use of Symbols

Symbols are used to represent objects, actions, concepts, and ideas. However, the way in which various AAC systems use symbols to promote communication varies. For instance, in some AAC systems, symbols are used alone, whereas in other systems symbols are combined with one another. As an example, a child might point to two pictorial symbols in succession to communicate "I don't want to go home" (i.e., *no* + *go home*). Many AAC systems permit use of symbols alone or in combination. For instance, in sign language, an individual can successfully communicate hunger using a single sign (*eat*) or can add additional signs to communicate hunger for a particular food (e.g., *eat* + *potato chips*). AAC symbol systems also vary in other ways.

Static and Dynamic Symbol Systems. **Static** symbols do not require movement or change to understand their meaning—for example, a photograph or an illustration. An AAC system using static symbols might be one in which a child points to photos in a book to request or talk about specific family members. In contrast, **dynamic** symbols require movement or change to understand their meaning (ASHA, 2002a). Gestures are one example of a dynamic symbol system—

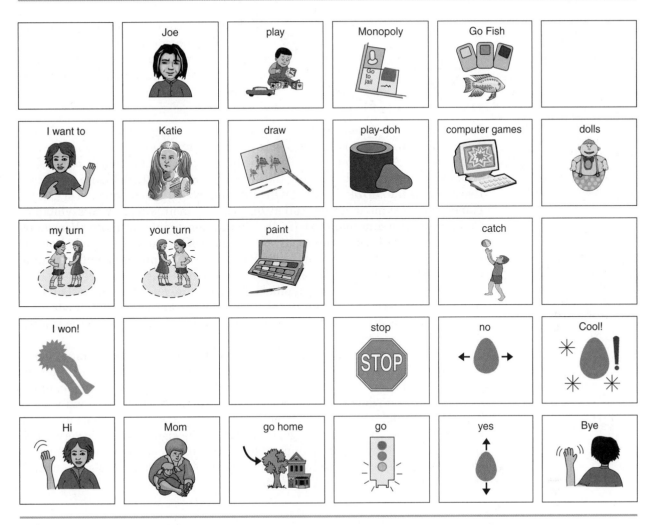

FIGURE 5.3   Graphic symbols in the form of line drawings on a communication board.

Source: Illustrations courtesy of Boardmaker™ (Mayer-Johnson, Inc.).

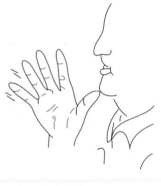

FIGURE 5.4

Signs for *mother* (left) and *father* (right) in American Sign Language.

FIGURE 5.5

An opaque (A) and an iconic (B) symbol for *carrot*.

Source: (A) From Online Blissword Dictionary (http://www.blisswords.co.uk). Reprinted with permission. (B) From *Picture Communication Symbols* by Mayer-Johnson, 1995, Solana Beach, CA: Mayer-Johnson. Reprinted with permission.

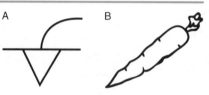

think of the gestures to signal *come here* or *go away*. Some speech generating devices (SGDs) feature an animated graphic system in which different symbols are expressed dynamically.

Iconic and Opaque Symbol Systems. Symbols also vary in their iconicity and opaqueness. **Iconicity** is the degree to which symbols visually resemble what they refer to. An **opaque** symbol has little resemblance to what it represents, whereas an iconic symbol is very transparent (ASHA, 2002a). Figure 5.5 shows two symbols for *carrot*; the one on the left—an example of an opaque symbol—comes from a symbol system called *Blissymbols* maintained by Blissymbolics Communication International (BCI). This system contains more than 3,000 symbols, many of which are relatively opaque (BCI, 2008). The symbol on the right is iconic and comes from a symbol system titled picture communication systems (PCS) in the Boardmaker software. Boardmaker is a set of more than 3,000 picture-communication symbols that are widely used in the design of individual AAC systems. Many of the PCS symbols are iconic, although more opaque symbols are needed for abstract or complex concepts, as in the symbol for "cool" in Figure 5.6.

> **DISCUSSION POINT:**
> Consider the pros and cons of AAC systems comprised entirely of iconic or opaque symbols.

Some AAC systems are built to use only iconic symbols—for example, a picture board with line drawings representing specific actions, such as an apple for *eat lunch* and a sun for *go outside.* Other AAC systems are very opaque, to the extent that those who do not know the system are unable to understand what is being communicated. However, even within one system, the symbols may vary in their iconicity. In sign language, for instance, the sign for *drink* is very transparent, produced by moving a cupped hand toward the mouth. And the sign for *think* uses the index finger tapped against the forehead. But other signs—such as those for *dream, cracker,* and *mother*—are relatively opaque.

AID

Many AAC systems include an aid. The term **aid** refers to a type of assistive device that is used to send or receive messages (ASHA, 2004). Aids often supplement natural speech or writing and can augment input of information. A visual display on an aid allows communication partners to see/read a communicative message if they have difficulty hearing because of a hearing loss or a noisy environment. Aids can also support language development by augmenting language comprehension. Goosens and Crain (1986 a, b) developed visual displays of graphic symbols that can be used as aids to augment input of language concepts during class activities or language therapy. Aids can be **electronic** and nonelectronic. Electronic AAC aids are usually referred to as *speech generating devices* (SGDs). Nonelectronic AAC aids are typically described as either *no technology* (no tech) or *low/light technology.* The term *assistive technology* (AT) is also sometimes used

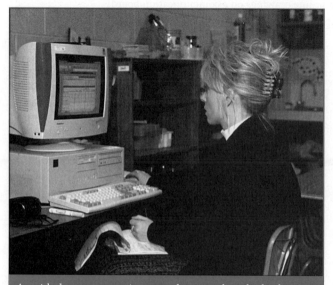

An aided system requires a tool external to the body, such as a computer.

to describe aids that promote communication and other aspects of well-being, such as physical or motor performance. Figure 5.7 presents examples of different commercially available electronic SGDs. For instance, a very young child might have a communication book with photographic symbols depicting a variety of activities (e.g., reading a book, playing blocks, using the computer, playing in the sand table) to request an activity during free time at school.

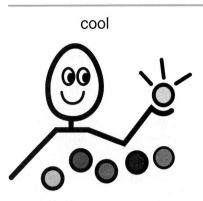

FIGURE 5.6

Symbol to represent the concept of "cool."

Source: From *Picture Communication Symbols* by Mayer-Johnson, 1995, Solana Beach, CA: Mayer-Johnson.

STRATEGY

Strategy is the third component of an AAC system and is the way symbols are effectively and efficiently conveyed (ASHA, 2004b). AAC strategies are intended

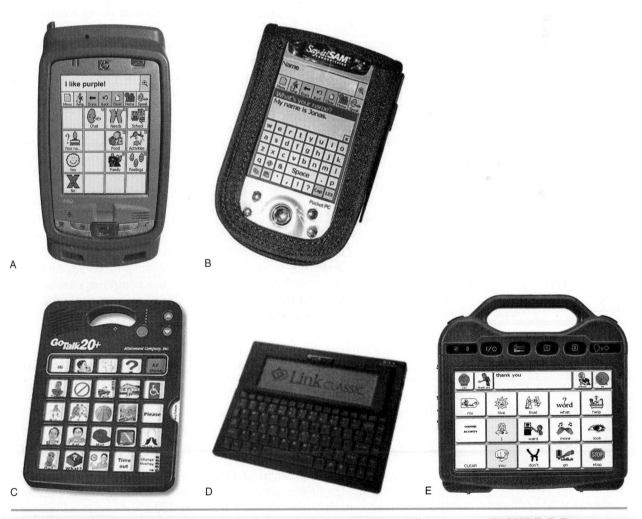

(A) Examples of SGDs. Dynavox V and Vmax. (B) Say-it! SAM by Words+. (C) Go Talk 20+ Attainment Company. (D) LINK. Assistive Technology Inc. (E) Springboard Lite. Prentke-Romich Company.

FIGURE 5.7

to improve message transmission time, support grammatical formulation of messages, and enhance communication rates (Beukelman & Mirenda, 2005). Examples of AAC system strategies include setting the topic before initiating a conversation, using software that predicts letters or words in order to eliminate keystrokes, and having an index card available for unfamiliar communication partners to explain how the individual communicates. A strategy is, in essence, how the AAC is used (the symbol and the aid). Much of AAC intervention involves supporting an individual's use of strategies to enhance his or her effectiveness and efficiency as a communicator.

TECHNIQUE

Technique refers to the way in which messages are transmitted—that is, how an individual selects or accesses symbols. There are two types of techniques: direct selection and indirect selection (Dowden & Cook, 2002).

Direct selection is a direct motor act that is not dependent on time (Dowden & Cook, 2002). There are four types (Beukelman & Mirenda, 2005): The first type is physical pressure, or depression; individuals select symbols using a controlled body movement to depress a key or apply sufficient pressure for activation to occur. This body movement can involve a body part, such as a finger, or an instrument attached to the body, such as a stick mounted to a headband. The second type of direct selection is physical contact. With this technique, the individual needs only to have physical contact with the AAC aid, such as touching a finger to a symbol on a communication board.

The third type of direct selection technique is pointing without contact, as shown in Figure 5.8. This example depicts eye pointing, in which an individual looks at an item long enough for a communication partner to assess the person's intent (Beukelman & Mirenda, 2005). After a severe spinal cord injury, an individual might use eye pointing to select a symbol (i.e., the words *TV* and *READ*) representing an activity on a communication board (e.g., watching television or reading a book). Eye pointing can also use a light beam attached to a headband to point to desired selections. Some computer systems allow eye pointing with an infrared light-emitting diode to type on keyboards or to activate certain images. For instance, a toddler who cannot speak because of severe muscular impairment might use eye pointing to activate songs on a computer screen.

The fourth direct selection technique is speech or voice input. Some AAC systems can be accessed by speech or voice input to activate messages and functions. Some cell phones come with voice activation for hands-free calling, an example of a system accessed by voice input. Some computers are also equipped with this technology; for example, saying "Computer turn on" accomplishes that feat. This same technology is used by some companies—for instance, when we're asked to "Say 1 for English or 2 for Spanish" when calling and navigating an automatic phone system.

Individuals with severe motor or sensory impairments can also access their AAC systems with one of three **indirect selection** techniques (Dowden & Cook, 2002). The first is **scanning** with single or dual switches. With scanning, a selection set of symbols is presented in a predetermined configuration by either a communication device or a communication partner (Beukelman & Mirenda, 2005). For instance, an electronic device might highlight pictures in a linear format following a preset, one-at-a-time order. The individual waits until the desired symbol is presented and then signals his or her choice using eye gaze, eye blinks, head nods, or switch activation. Because of the time needed for the

DISCUSSION POINT:
Motor and sensory skills often determine which technique is best for accessing communication symbols and messages. What AAC technique does Sara in Case Study 5.1 use? What about Scott?

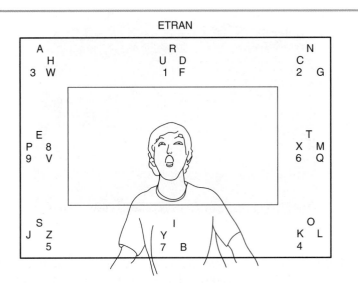

FIGURE 5.8

An eye gaze board.

Source: From *Augmentative Communication: An Introduction* by S. W. Blackstone, 1986, Rockville, MD: American Speech-Language-Hearing Association. Copyright 1986 by ASHA. Reprinted with permission.

device to scan through items, the number of possible symbols should be kept low. Figure 5.9 shows a switch attached to an SGD. As the SGD scans the letters, the individual depresses the attached switch when the desired symbol is lighted.

The second indirect technique is directed scanning, which is the use of multiple switches or a joystick interface to move a cursor to a specified target location (Dowden & Cook, 2002). This approach is considered a hybrid of typical scanning. An individual uses a joystick or other type of switch to select a scanning direction and then makes a selection. Directed scanning provides a more efficient approach to communication than regular scanning.

The third type of indirect selection is **coded access,** which requires an individual to use a sequence of movements to select a symbol from a set (Dowden & Cook, 2002). Morse code is an example of coded access that many individuals with complex communication needs have used successfully to access their SGD. Morse code can be inputted to an SGD with switches.

SELECTION SET

An AAC selection set is another important component of an AAC system. An AAC aid may display symbols on displays in different ways. Displays are usually

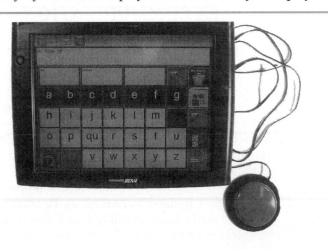

FIGURE 5.9

Scanning with a single switch.

Source: Photo courtesy of AbleNet, Inc., and DynaVox Systems, LLC.

FIGURE 5.10

Example of visual scene display.

Source: Photo provided courtesy of Tobii ATI.

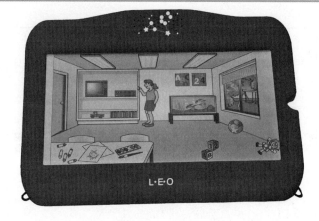

visual, auditory, or tactile, and can be described as fixed, dynamic, hybrid, or visual (Beukelman & Mirenda, 2005). A **fixed display** remains the same before and after a symbol is selected. For example, a picture of a TV on a picture communication board remains the same and does not change when you point to it. **Dynamic displays** are visual and change after a symbol is selected (ASHA, 2002a). A dynamic display usually involves a computer screen presenting a visual message, typically either letters or pictures. As symbols are selected, the screen changes automatically to another display (Beukelman & Mirenda, 2005). Dynamic displays are available in many commercially available AAC systems. This type of technology is also used on such common devices as cell phones and ATM mac-hines. For instance, the display of an ATM machine changes in response to input (e.g., "To continue in English, press 1; to continue in Spanish, press 2") to feature a new display with more options. **Hybrid displays** use a combination of display types on the AAC system. A new type of display is called **visual scene display** (VSD). VSDs are pictures, photographs, or depictions of virtual environments that represent situations, places, or experiences (Beukelman & Mirenda, 2005). VSDs can be static or dynamic; can be used in any AAC system; and can provide rich visual context to support communication about personally relevant people, topics, and places. Objects in the visual scene become the symbols or "hot spots" on the display rather than on a traditional grid layout. Figure 5.10 shows an example of a VSD.

WHAT ARE COMPLEX COMMUNICATION NEEDS? ●

DEFINITION

As we discussed earlier in this chapter, complex communication needs exist when individuals cannot meet their daily communication needs through their current method(s) of communication. Two important organizations, ISAAC and ASHA, endorse using the term *complex communication needs* over other terms that focus solely on impairment and disability. This shift in terminology allows an increased emphasis on the needs and purposes of communication and, as a result, the development of meaningful treatment goals. The presence of complex communication needs can restrict and limit children's and adults' ability to participate independently in society (Balandin, 2002, p. 2). To maximize participation in society, individuals benefit from alternative and augmentative ways to communicate. For example, if a 9-year-old girl has the desire to call her friend to come over to play but her speech is not intelligible over the telephone, she has an unmet communication need—that is, using the telephone to make a request. This unmet need is considered complex, because many factors must be considered in this situation. In order to make the communicative exchange happen successfully, several factors must be addressed—that is, the child's communication capabilities, the reasons she wants to communicate, and the capabilities and needs of the listener on the other end of the telephone.

Complex communication needs are as varied as individuals are unique and can occur in any modality of communication (i.e., listening, speaking, reading, writing, gesturing), in any environment (e.g., school, home, community), and with a variety of communication partners. Additionally, complex communication needs can occur when an individual is not able to use communication for all of its many purposes, which are described in Table 5.2. The purposes of communication presented in Table 5.2 vary in their focus, duration, and predictability.

Purposes of Communication

Needs and Wants.   One of the most basic purposes of communication is expressing our needs and wants. Within moments of birth, infants communicate for this very basic purpose. In communicating needs and wants, an individual is able to regulate the behavior of another person to obtain something—either a desired object or a desired action (Light, 1988). The content of the message is very important in relaying needs and wants. For example, a young boy pointing to the kitchen cupboard to indicate that he is hungry hopes that his communication partner, his father, will open the cupboard and remove some food for him. In this example, how the communication is conveyed (i.e., by pointing) is just as important as the message, which in this case is vaguely represented in the child's communicative

TABLE 5.2 The Purposes of Communication Interactions	
Purpose	**Description**
Needs and wants	Goal: regulate behaviors of others
	Focus: desired action or object
	Duration: limited
	Predictability: very predictable
Information transfer	Goal: share information with others
	Focus: shared information
	Duration: lengthy
	Predictability: not predictable
Social closeness	Goal: establish and maintain relationships with others
	Focus: interpersonal relationship
	Duration: lengthy
	Predictability: ranges from very predictable to not predictable
Social etiquette	Goal: engage in social conventions
	Focus: social conventions (e.g., being polite, greeting)
	Duration: limited
	Predictability: very predictable

Source: Based on Light (1988).

act. Communication for the purpose of expressing needs and wants is usually brief in duration and predictable.

Information Transfer.   We also communicate to give and to receive information—that is, **information transfer.** The information being conveyed may be novel and unknown to the recipient, posing special challenges for someone with complex communication needs. Communication for this purpose may be lengthy and unpredictable in its content. Consider an individual, for whom speech is unclear or unintelligible, being stopped by a stranger who asks for directions to a local restaurant. The individual with unintelligible speech may have a difficult time transferring this information with speech alone. Using more than one mode of communication may enhance the success of the information transfer. Giving directions, ordering food in a restaurant, giving medical personnel details of an illness, and telling about the day's activities are all examples of the need to communicate specific information in a message with varied communication partners.

Social Closeness.   **Social closeness** is another reason people interact and communicate with one another. Human beings are social creatures, and as such we strive to establish, develop, and maintain interpersonal relationships (Light, 1988). Individuals who have difficulty communicating may need intervention to assist them in finding ways to promote social closeness with their communication partners. One way people establish and maintain closeness is to share stories about their lives. Have you ever discovered that you had a similar experience to another person after hearing that person's story about childhood? Did you feel closer to the other person after learning about the common experience? Enabling persons with complex communication needs to tell their own stories of who they are and how their experiences have shaped their lives is an important focus of intervention. Communication for this purpose may be lengthy and unpredictable in its focus.

Social Etiquette.   Another purpose of communication is **social etiquette,** which has to do with being polite and conforming to the social conventions of one's culture. In mainstream North American society, examples include introducing oneself to someone new, saying hello and good-bye in phone conversations, and not interrupting others during conversations. Communication for this purpose is often brief in duration and highly predictable. Of course, what is considered a social nicety in one cultural community may not be so in another, and part of being an effective communicator is learning and using the communicative approaches that are appropriate in a given community. For individuals with complex communication needs, learning and using communication in a socially appropriate way can pose a special challenge. In social situations, the content of the message may not be as important as meeting the expectations of both familiar and unfamiliar communication partners.

MULTICULTURALISM AND CCNS

Children and adults who have complex communication needs belong to many different cultural groups, sometimes more than one culture at the same time. Culture is "a lens through which individuals see themselves in relation to others and to the world" (Soto, Blake Huer, & Taylor, 1997, p. 406). For AAC intervention to be successful, the members of an AAC team must understand the values, beliefs, behaviors, and communication styles of each identified culture of the person with complex communication needs. AAC service

SPOTLIGHT ON LITERACY

Literacy Development among Children with Complex Communication Needs

The development of literacy skills is as critical for children with CCNs who require AAC as it is for all children. Literacy skills provide access to opportunities in education and vocation, provide access to mainstream technology, and provide options for independent living (Light & Kent-Walsch, 2003). Literacy development—that is, learning to read and write—may proceed slowly for many children with CCNs. Risk factors that may affect literacy development include the limited use of speech, lack of opportunities to interact in conversations, and limited access to print (Hetzroni, 2004). Light, McNaughton, Jansen, Kristiansen, et al. (2005) have developed methods to teach literacy skills to young children who use AAC. The literacy instruction was developed from evidence in the literature on teaching literacy skills to children at risk as well as from evidence with individuals who use AAC. The instruction was adapted to accommodate the needs of children with CCNs by eliminating the need for spoken responses and providing alternative response modes, scaffolding support, and systematic data collection. The outcomes of this adapted literacy instruction are promising for children aged 3 to 5 years. Specific gains were seen in the areas of phonological awareness, letter-sound correspondences, independent reading, decoding novel words, and participating in story writing. Light and McNaughton (2007) highlighted the current evidence on literacy intervention for individuals who use AAC as well as indicators of effective evidence-based literacy instruction. These indicators include sufficient time allocated for instruction, appropriate instructional content, appropriate instructional procedures, and adaptations to allow active participation of individuals who require AAC. Light and McNaughton presented positive outcomes of literacy intervention for eight participants as young as 3 years old who had a variety of disabilities. Evidence-based literacy instruction is now available to help individuals who use AAC, so let's spread the word!

providers also need to be aware of their own cultural beliefs and practices and the ways those might influence their clinical practice (Soto et al., 1997).

People with complex communication needs, their families, and other communication partners from diverse cultural groups also exhibit heterogeneity in their linguistic backgrounds. Some may be monolingual, and others may be bilingual or multilingual. In addition, the language used at home may differ from that used at school or in the community, posing special challenges to the individual with complex communication needs:

> Individuals who use AAC who come from diverse cultural and linguistic backgrounds face additional demands in developing communicative competence; they must learn receptive and expressive skills in the language spoken by their family as well as receptive and expressive skills in the language of the broader social community (e.g., educational system, business community). (Light, 2003)

When designing an AAC intervention plan, service providers must respect culturally appropriate rules for social interaction and social participation (Soto et al., 1997). People with bilingual/bicultural communication needs may require different systems to meet the unique needs of each language and culture. A bicultural AAC system allows the individual to function and participate in both cultures. Many resources are available to assist professionals in providing appropriate AAC intervention plans for children from various ethnic and cultural backgrounds (Alant, 2007; Parette & Huer, 2002; Parette, Huer, & Wyatt, 2002; VanBiervliet & Parette, 2002).

WHAT ARE SOME COMMON CAUSES OF COMPLEX COMMUNICATION NEEDS?

Complex communication needs can result from developmental or acquired disorders that affect communication in the areas of speech, language, or cognition. Examples of disorders associated with childhood or development that may affect communication include intellectual disability, cerebral palsy, autism, and childhood apraxia of speech. Disorders affecting communication acquired later in life may result from traumas, illnesses, or degenerative diseases.

Intellectual Disability

The American Association on Mental Retardation (2002) defines an **intellectual disability** (also known as *mental retardation*) as having significant limitations in both intellectual functioning and adaptive behavior, as expressed in conceptual, social, and practical adaptive skills. Some children and adults with severe or profound intellectual disabilities may not be able to communicate effectively using only speech. An AAC system would expand modes of communication for these individuals. Consider Jane, a 42-year-old woman with a profound intellectual disability. She works 5 days a week (3 hours per day) placing caps on pens in a factory. She communicates with her job supervisor with an AAC system, an SGD with digitized speech output featuring a static display using photos as symbols. When Jane is finished with a set of pens, she selects a symbol (i.e., a photo of a set of pens on a static display) and communicates the message "I am done. I would like another set." When Jane is ready for a break, she selects a photo of the break room to tell her supervisor "I am ready for my break now." Just as in this example with Jane, AAC interventions can improve communication opportunities in natural environments for many individuals with intellectual disabilities (Beukelman & Mirenda, 2005).

Cerebral Palsy

Cerebral palsy is a neuromotor impairment resulting from trauma or damage to the developing child before, during, or soon after birth (McDonald, 1987). The impact of cerebral palsy on a child's ability to communicate ranges from little or no impact to a complete inability to use speech at all with accompanying changes in language development and sensory input. Children and adults with cerebral palsy may use AAC systems to meet the complex communication needs resulting from speech, language, cognitive, or sensory (i.e., vision, hearing) impairments. The type of AAC system selected is based on the individual's communication needs and on motor, language, sensory, and cognitive abilities.

Autism Spectrum Disorders

Autism spectrum disorders (ASDs) are a group of developmental disorders characterized by impaired social interaction; difficulty with verbal and nonverbal communication; and unusual, repetitive, or severely limited activities and interests (National Institute of Neurological Disorders and Stroke, 2006). Complex communication needs are commonly identified in children and adults who have an autism spectrum disorder. An AAC approach to intervention can facilitate the development of speech and language for children and adults with ASD, augment their current modes of communication, or provide alternative means of communication. All of these may help individuals with ASD to meet their communication needs and alleviate any activity limitations or participation restrictions in desired life activities. An example of a common AAC approach used with children with ASD is the picture exchange communication system (PECS; Frost & Bondy, 1994), in which individuals learn to exchange a symbol (usually a picture or a photo) for a desired object (e.g., a picture of a banana for a banana). Some reports on the use of PECS with children with autism indicate that it provides an important means for transitioning them to using spoken language to communicate, with the majority of children using PECS subsequently developing functional speech (Bondy & Frost, 1994, 1995).

Childhood Apraxia of Speech

Childhood apraxia of speech (CAS), also known as *developmental apraxia of speech*, is a speech disorder characterized by the inability to control the purposeful speech movements and sequences of speech movements (Hall, Jordan, & Robin, 2007). The impact of CAS on the intelligibility of speech can range from mild to severe, with some children unintelligible even to those with whom they are very familiar, including parents. Some children with severe CAS use AAC systems to help meet their communication needs as they work to improve their speech intelligibility or meet specific communication needs where speech alone is not successful. Although many parents and professionals may be concerned that using an AAC system may inhibit children's speech development, evidence in the literature has shown that such concerns are not warranted. This speech disorder is described in Chapter 12.

Traumatic Brain Injury

Traumatic brain injury (TBI) is an acquired injury to the brain caused by a traumatic event (e.g., head hitting the pavement at high speed after falling off a motorcycle or head hitting the windshield in a car accident). The brain damage from a TBI can result in motor speech disorders (dysarthria or acquired apraxia of speech) or cognitive-communication impairments, as described in Chapter 7. If the speech, language, or cognitive impairments affect communication to a point where communication needs are unmet, the person with a TBI may benefit from an AAC system. Most TBI survivors use an AAC system at some point in their recovery (Fager, Doyle, & Karantounis, 2007). AAC strategies and techniques can benefit TBI survivors at all phases of cognitive recovery. Early in recovery, AAC provides a means for consistent responses—for instance, pointing to a picture of a family member to ask "When are they coming to visit?" Some TBI survivors regain intelligible speech during their recovery; however, other survivors do not. An AAC system can be used as a temporary solution to an inability to communicate effectively or efficiently or as a long-term solution to meeting communication needs. In either case, an AAC system can improve the quality of life for a TBI survivor.

Stroke

A **stroke** occurs when the blood supply to part of the brain is interrupted or when a blood vessel in the brain ruptures (National Institute of Neurological Disorders and Stroke, 2008). Depending on where the brain damage occurs, a person may have motor, speech, language, sensory, or cognitive impairments. Language expression and comprehension are frequently impacted by left-hemisphere strokes (i.e., aphasia), although language use is also impacted by frontal-lobe and right-hemisphere strokes (i.e., cognitive-communication impairments). For people with communication impairments resulting in complex communication needs, an AAC system can improve functional and effective communication and increase their participation in society. Chapter 7 provides additional discussion of communication disorders that result from stroke.

Degenerative Diseases

Degenerative diseases can also result in the loss of motor, speech, language, cognitive, or sensory functioning. In many cases, this loss is progressive and becomes more severe over time. People with degenerative diseases often lose their ability to meet their communication needs independently and may become isolated from society. An AAC approach to intervention targets activities and participation in desired life situations to alleviate the potential negative consequences of illness and disease.

One degenerative disease that significantly affects communication is **amyotrophic lateral sclerosis** (ALS). Also known as Lou Gehrig's disease, ALS is a rapidly progressive disease (Yorkston, Miller, & Strand, 2004). People with ALS may experience a deterioration of speech skills, resulting in unintelligible speech (i.e., dysarthria), or may experience poor respiratory functioning, resulting in mechanical ventilation (e.g., causing aphonia). Dysarthric speech or dependence on a ventilator to breathe often present complex communication challenges for adults. AAC intervention can help individuals with ALS meet their complex communication needs at any stage of the disease. For example, consider the case of a 59-year-old farmer recently diagnosed with ALS. He has difficulty making his voice loud enough for the farm employees to hear him outside, and his speech is starting to sound imprecise. He needs a way to communicate in all environments without causing fatigue. The man met with a speech-language pathologist and discussed different voice amplification systems as well as how his voice and speech might be affected in the future. AAC systems are dynamic—that is, they are constantly changing to meet ongoing communication needs.

Parkinson's disease (PD) is a slowly progressive disease of the basal ganglia in the central nervous system. Complex communication needs usually stem from dysarthria, a motor speech disorder discussed in Chapter 12. A person with PD may have difficulty initiating voicing and will produce short rushes of poorly articulated speech (Yorkston et al., 2004). Thus, people with PD may benefit from AAC strategies and techniques to augment their speech and improve the success of communication exchanges.

Dementia is another degenerative disease that can affect communica-tion. Dementia can be caused by diseases such as Alzheimer's disease and Huntington's disease or from other disorders of the brain. Dementia results in significantly impaired intellectual functioning, resulting in disruptions to daily activities and relationships (National Institute of Neurological Disorders and Stroke, 2008). The change in intellect impacts communication. AAC strategies benefit many people with dementia at early, middle, and late stages by focusing on enhancing communication and by support-ing memory and participation and engagement in regular life activities (Bourgeois & Hickey, 2007).

HOW ARE AAC SYSTEMS AND COMPLEX COMMUNICATION NEEDS IDENTIFIED?

THE ASSESSMENT TEAM

DISCUSSION POINT:
AAC team members represent a diverse group of professionals. What important information do you think each of the team members brings to the assessment?

A **multidisciplinary team** of professionals conducts an AAC assessment. Possible team members include individuals with complex communication needs, parents, teachers, speech-language pathologists, physical therapists, occupational therapists, rehabilitation engineers, social workers, psychologists, vocational counselors, nurses, and doctors. Typically, one professional serves as the team leader; often the speech-language pathologist leads the team and coordinates the assessment process.

THE ASSESSMENT PROCESS

AAC teams work in many different locations. Assessments take place in schools, clinics, hospitals, and the natural environments in which people communicate (e.g., home, community, work site). The assessment process is described below.

Referral

A referral for an AAC assessment can be made by anyone who identifies unmet communication needs in a person or has concern related to a person's communication. Common referral sources include parents, speech-language pathologists, teachers, counselors, and nurses. After a referral is made, a member of the AAC team contacts the identified person and his or her communication partners to schedule a **comprehensive AAC assessment.**

Comprehensive Assessment

The purpose of a comprehensive AAC assessment is to identify, measure, and describe factors affecting communication, the effects of the communication impairment on the individual's activities and participation, what barriers exist to desired participation, what facilitates successful communication, and what AAC system (i.e., symbols, aids, strategies, techniques, selection set) would enhance communication and participation in life situations (ASHA, 2004b). Thus, the AAC team looks at the whole person from a functional perspective.

An authentic assessment considers individuals' communication skills and needs in relation to the communication skills of same-aged peers in natural environments and situations (ASHA, 2002a). This is accomplished by planning an AAC assessment that identifies participation patterns and communication needs of the individual, conducting an assessment of the individual's capabilities and understanding of symbols, and running trials with different AAC features. Each area is briefly described below (see Beukelman & Mirenda, 2005, for additional details).

> **DISCUSSION POINT:**
> Who do you think would be the best informant regarding the current communication abilities and needs of Sara and Scott in Case Study 5.1? Why?

Identification of Participation Patterns.   Beukelman and Mirenda (2005) describe a model of AAC assessment and intervention called the *Participation Model* (as shown in Figure 5.11). This model is helpful in identifying patterns and needs related to communication as well as possible barriers. The team looks specifically for the presence of opportunity and access barriers in the community. **Opportunity barriers** are imposed by other people and prevent an individual's participation in communication activities. There are five types of opportunity barriers (Beukelman & Mirenda, 2005): policy, practice, skill, knowledge, and attitude. Examples of opportunity barriers are when a school policy places children with complex communication needs in segregated classrooms so that they have little time to communicate with peers, or when a school practice does not allow students to take their AAC system home with them. Other opportunity barriers are caused by negative attitudes, lack of knowledge, or lack of skill, which impedes participation. **Access barriers** can also prevent participation in communication activities, but they stem from the capabilities, attitudes, and resources of the person using AAC (Beukelman & Mirenda, 2005). For instance, individuals with complex communication needs might resist participating in

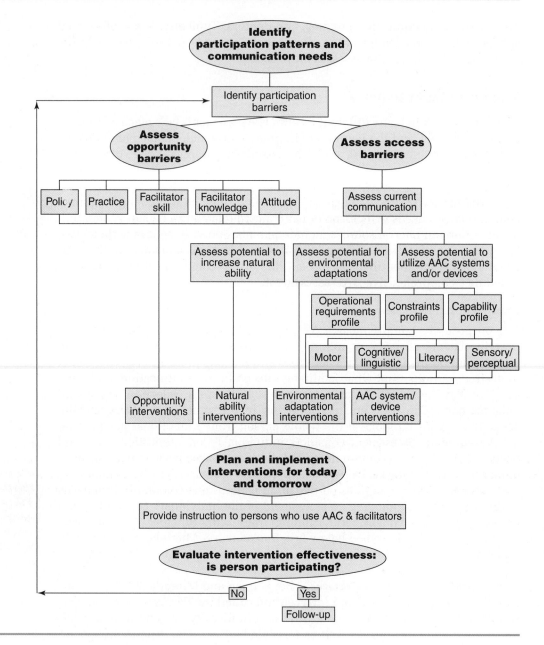

FIGURE 5.11   Participation Model.

Source: Beukelman, D. R., & Mirenda, P. (2005). *Augmentative and alternative communication: Supporting children and adults with complex communication needs* (3rd ed.). Baltimore, MD: Brookes.

community activities because they did not receive adequate training after receiving an AAC system and are not proficient in using the system in the community, or perhaps they do not have access to the vocabulary and communicative messages that would support their participation in that environment.

Social Networks: A Communication Inventory for Individuals with Complex Communication Needs and Their Communication Partners (Blackstone & Hunt-Berg, 2003) is an assessment tool available to help AAC teams identify

SPOTLIGHT ON TECHNOLOGY

AAC: More than Technology

An AAC system can be considered high-technology, but it also can be low or light technology, or no technology at all. An AAC system refers to any combination of devices, aids, techniques, symbols, or strategies that provide an additional mode of communication for a person with CCNs (ASHA, 2004b). For many people with CCNs, an AAC system that includes technology best meets their needs. Advances in mainstream technology have improved the features available on SGDs and other forms of assistive technology. Examples of recent advances that have improved communication options for people who use AAC include improved intelligibility of synthesized speech, more recording time for digitized speech, ability to import digitized photos into aids, access to e-mail and the Internet, and improved interfaces with environmental control units. Examples of technology that may be considered a part of an AAC system are Talking Photo Albums (Attainment Company), voice recognition software, eye gaze access (e.g., ERICA system, http://eyegazesystems.com/Disabilities/), vocal amplifiers, and speech generating devices (SGDs) (see Figure 5.7).

communication partners, modes of communication, AAC strategies and techniques, activities, environments, topics, and needed supports.

Identification of Communication Needs.   The AAC team must identify the individual's communication needs and determine which are not being met (Beukelman & Mirenda, 2005). Each AAC assessment begins with a case history to gather background information about the individual's communication development, current methods of communicating, medical history, the history of any treatment for a communication impairment, and pertinent family information. The team then interviews the individual and key communication partners and may also observe a range of natural environments, such as home, school, and work. The team focuses on how to support the individual to interact with family, friends, acquaintances, and others in order to improve the person's quality of life by enhancing communication in desired activities.

> **DISCUSSION POINT:**
> What communication activities might Sara and Scott (Case Study 5.1) be restricted from participating in, given their current methods of communicating?

In addition, the team must determine the extent to which the individual is participating in all of the communication activities of age-matched peers. To identify participation patterns and communication needs, the team initially conducts a Participation Inventory, which examines the range and type of everyday activities characteristic of same-age peers (Beukelman & Mirenda, 2005). AAC team members complete an inventory for each regularly occurring activity for each individual with complex communication needs in all the environments in which they interact. The team must then determine whether the individual is participating in the same activities. If there is a discrepancy, the team must determine what barriers are preventing participation.

Identification of Capabilities Related to Communication.   The assessment team identifies the individual's current level of communication skills using a variety of formal and informal assessment tools. It is imperative that the team assess capabilities in the areas of speech production, language (i.e., listening, speaking, reading, writing), cognition, perception (e.g., hearing, vision), and motor.

For the individual with complex communication needs, professionals must be prepared to adapt test materials to support motor, speech, cognitive, and language impairments. For instance, a child with cerebral palsy may not be able to point to pictures with her finger to show comprehension of vocabulary words;

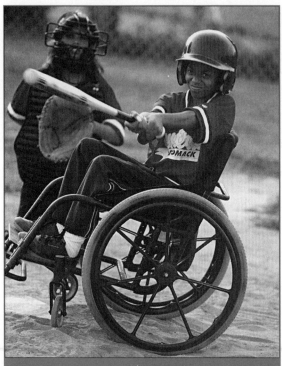

An activity inventory examines the range and types of activities engaged in by same-age peers.

DISCUSSION POINT:
Consider the case of Sara in Case Study 5.1. How do you think tests could be adapted to assess her language comprehension? How would that affect the standardization of the test?

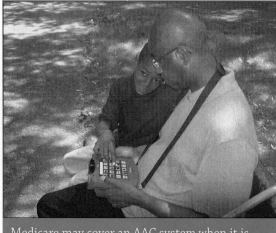

Medicare may cover an AAC system when it is needed to meet physical and medical needs.

thus, tests that require pointing need to be modified for this child. Of concern to the team is how to validly represent an individual's capabilities when motor or sensory challenges are present. AAC team members must be very knowledgeable about how to make accommodations in testing procedures and to validly interpret such findings (ASHA, 2002a).

Symbol Assessment. A symbol assessment is another component of a comprehensive AAC assessment. It is conducted to "select the types of symbols that will meet the individual's current communication needs and match his or her current abilities, as well as to identify symbol options that might be used in the future" (Beukelman & Mirenda, 2005, p. 191). Both unaided and aided symbols are presented and assessed.

Feature Match. During the assessment, different features of AAC systems are demonstrated and taught to the individual with CCNs, including display type, symbols type, voice output, size, and access options. Recommendations are made based on the match of features that the individual uses successfully and the features available in different AAC systems. Device Assistant (AAC Tech-Connect, 2008) is a database of high-technology AAC systems in which users can select features based on an assessment and then receive results of which AAC systems offer those features in a side-by-side comparison chart. This database saves AAC teams time by having up-to-date information about new AAC systems that are available as well as comparison data collected for them.

Recommendations. Once the comprehensive assessment is completed, the AAC team develops and implements "intervention plans that maximize effective and successful communication between individuals who use AAC and their conversational partners" (ASHA, 2002a, p. 9). Intervention plans include objectives to assist individuals with CCNs to understand and use their AAC system; to maximize communication activities and participation; and to train communication partners to provide opportunities for communication, facilitate communication interactions, and support the ongoing development and updating of the AAC system.

Funding. Funding for an AAC system and training can come from a variety of sources. School districts, insurance companies, and private organizations are examples of funding sources. The funding process can be complicated, but assistance is available. Many manufacturers of AAC technology have funding departments to help AAC teams with the funding process. Funding information is also available on the Internet at sites such as www.aacfundinghelp.com/ and http://aac-rerc.com/.

HOW CAN PEOPLE WITH COMPLEX COMMUNICATION NEEDS BENEFIT FROM AN AAC SYSTEM? ⬤

The long-term goal of treatment for people with complex communication needs is to maximize effective and successful communication between individuals who use AAC and their communication partners (ASHA, 2002). For anyone with CCNs, access to AAC treatment is a right, not a privilege; and for children in U.S. public schools, intervention for significant communication difficulties is legislated through the Individuals with Disabilities Education Act.

AAC intervention should be conducted in real-world, functional, and authentic contexts and organized to match the individual's needs and capabilities for today and for the future (Beukelman & Mirenda, 2005). The AAC team plans a treatment program that will achieve three purposes: (1) meet unmet communication needs, (2) increase communication competence, and (3) increase participation in society.

DISCUSSION POINT:

Researcher David Wilkins (2003) of the Max Planck Institute for Psycholinguistics has said, "There are no impaired communicators, only impaired conversations." To what extent do you agree or disagree with this statement, and why?

Meeting Unmet Communication Needs

Once the team identifies unmet communication needs, short-term treatment goals are developed to enable the individual to meet these needs. For example, an unmet communication need for a student in an elementary school might be greeting friends within the classroom, and a treatment goal might be to use this child's AAC system to greet friends independently. Specific activities are then designed to help the young student achieve the treatment goal—perhaps selecting vocabulary and identifying specific messages to convey, selecting symbols to represent vocabulary and messages, encoding messages, and developing approaches to increase the rate of communication delivery. It is important to consider age-appropriate vocabulary and symbols. It is unlikely that a young child would say, "Good morning, John. How are you today?" Conducting a Participation Inventory will assist AAC teams to identify age-appropriate vocabulary.

Improving Communication Competence

The process of working toward **communication competence** requires significant time and effort (Light, 2003). Many factors impact the attainment of communication competence—factors that are both intrinsic and extrinsic to an AAC user (Light, 2003). The intrinsic factors include the person's knowledge, judgment, skills, motivation to improve, attitude toward AAC, confidence, and resilience (Light, 2003). Extrinsic factors include the communication demands of interactions and the environment. Factors in the environment can support or hinder communicative competence.

In helping a person gain communication competence, the AAC team considers the level of support needed or the level of independence the person has when communicating. The level of support ranges along a continuum (Blackstone & Hunt-Berg, 2003; Dowden, 1999), from **emerging communication** to **context-dependent communication** to **independent communication.** These three descriptors describe what an individual is able to do communicatively at a given point in time but should never be used to define an individual's potential for communication (Dowden, 1999).

DISCUSSION POINT:

What level of support in communicating do you think Sara in Case Study 5.1 would need? What about Scott?

Emerging Communication.   Individuals at the point of emerging communication have no reliable method of symbolic expression and are limited to nonsymbolic methods of communicating, such as facial expressions, physical movements, or vocalizations (Blackstone & Hunt-Berg, 2003). The term *emerging communication* is often used to describe the presymbolic behaviors of infants, which others interpret as communicative, such as vocalizations and babbles, vegetative sounds like burps and coughs, and gross gestures. The term is also appropriate for the nonsymbolic behaviors of individuals with complex communication needs.

Context-Dependent Communication.   Individuals at the point of context-dependent communication have reliable symbolic communication but communicate in only a few contexts or with only a few partners. Thus, communication seems to be stuck to, or dependent on, a specific context. Such communication limits are usually due to strategies that require partner familiarity or a vocabulary that is limited to a highly specific context (Blackstone & Hunt-Berg, 2003).

Independent Communication.   Individuals at the point of independent communication are usually literate and interact with both familiar and unfamiliar communication partners in a variety of **communication environments** (Blackstone & Hunt-Berg, 2003).

Communication Partners.   The definition of *communication* emphasizes the importance of there being both a sender and a receiver—in other words, a communicative partnership. For AAC treatment to be successful, one or more communication partners must be involved with the person using an AAC system. Thus, an important part of treatment is helping communication partners develop positive and efficacious perspectives toward the use of AAC, understand how to provide opportunities for communication, and learn how to support communication and the AAC system. A good conversation partner shows patience and an interest in and comfort with many different methods or modes of communication. A good communication partner also makes an effort to understand impaired speech, interprets signs and gestures, is comfortable with silence, and admits any lack of understanding (Blackstone, 1999). Communication partners can benefit from explicit training to help them facilitate and support the use of a person with CCNs and the use of an AAC system.

INCREASING PARTICIPATION IN SOCIETY

Effective and successful communication is more than meeting communication needs and being competent. Communication is truly successful when an individual with complex communication needs can participate in any desired aspect of society. Any barrier to effective communication must be addressed in treatment to allow complete participation in all desired social and **communication roles**.

The AAC team specifically considers the social roles of the person with CCNs, seeking to increase the person's participation in society. **Social roles** are the roles each person has in society—the different hats people wear. Some roles may change over a lifetime; others remain constant. A current social role for you may be that of student, but this role will likely change in the future. Importantly, social roles determine communication demands (Light, 2003); each social role has corresponding communication roles that must be met. A student's communication roles include such things as communicating with teachers and classmates orally, corresponding with teachers and classmates using e-mail, preparing written papers and tests, and so forth.

DISCUSSION POINT:
Identify the social and communication roles of Scott in Case Study 5.1. What changes might occur if he develops a more effective way of communicating and can participate independently in more environments?

SPOTLIGHT ON RESEARCH AND PRACTICE

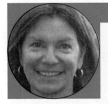

NAME: MARY HUNT-BERG, PH.D., CCC-SLP

PROFESSION/TITLE:
Education and Research Program Director
The Bridge School, Hillsborough, CA

A DAY AT THE BRIDGE SCHOOL

The Bridge School's education program serves 14 students with severe speech and physical impairment who participate in preschool, elementary, or middle-school educational experiences while concurrently learning to use AAC. Our program is designed to be short-term and intensive with the goal of transitioning students back to their respective local school programs. Our curriculum addresses communicative competence with AAC (Light, 2003), California state standards for general education (with emphasis on literacy), and specialized areas such as self-determination and adapted play.

My primary professional responsibilities include overseeing the innovative work of a highly skilled and talented team of professionals that includes special educators, speech-language pathologists, classroom instructional assistants, and an assistive technology specialist, as well as consultants for occupational therapy, visual impairment, and rehabilitation engineering. In doing so, I coordinate ongoing development and documentation of Bridge School's student curriculum and instruction. I have a lead role in guiding our staff as they tailor research findings to the Bridge School context. I lead our intake process for new students, recruit new staff, and design ongoing professional development for our staff and parents. I also explore how the knowledge gained through the work at the Bridge School can be disseminated in the larger AAC field.

Given that many people have a variety of social roles, the number of communication roles may be considerable. Consider a 14-year-old who is a student, a son, a brother, a friend, and a scorekeeper for his soccer team. Each of these social roles has expected communication roles: The student needs to be a listener, a responder, a reader, and a writer. At home, the brother needs to be an advisor to his younger siblings, and the son needs to be a listener and a negotiator with his parents. Figure 5.12 shows other examples of social roles and communication roles.

The individual with complex communication needs and other members of the AAC team must identify current and desired social and communication roles. Treatment should then focus explicitly on the skills necessary to meet the communication demands of each role so that the person can participate fully in society.

FIGURE 5.12

Examples of social roles and communication roles.

Social roles:	Communication roles:
Daughter/son	Listener
Mother/father	Director
Student	Advisor
Employee/employer	Reader
Friend	Storyteller
Consumer	Questioner

CHAPTER SUMMARY

Millions of Americans have complex communication needs—that is, they have difficulty meeting their daily communication needs with their current modes of communication. Children and adults with speech, language, sensory, or cognitive impairments are at risk of having complex communication needs that limit their activities and restrict their participation in society. The more common causes of these speech, language, sensory, or cognitive impairments include intellectual disability, cerebral palsy, autism, childhood apraxia of speech, traumatic brain injury, stroke, and degenerative diseases.

An AAC intervention approach addresses the complex communication needs and participation restrictions for individuals with communication disorders. No one should be denied the right to communicate. Implemented correctly, an AAC system and training can maximize effective communication and improve participation in society.

KEY TERMS

AAC system, p. 152
access barriers, p. 167
aid, p. 156
aided, p. 153
amyotrophic lateral sclerosis, p. 166
augmentative and alternative communication, p. 149
autism spectrum disorders, p. 164
cerebral palsy, p. 164
childhood apraxia of speech, p. 165
coded access, p. 159
communication competence, p. 171
communication environments, p. 172
communication partners, p. 151
communication roles, p. 172

complex communication needs, p. 152
comprehensive AAC assessment, p. 167
context-dependent communication, p. 171
dementia, p. 166
direct selection, p. 157
dynamic, p. 154
dynamic display, p. 160
electronic, p. 156
emerging communication, p. 171
fixed display, p. 160
hybrid display, p. 160
iconicity, p. 156
independent communication, p. 171
indirect selection, p. 158
information transfer, p. 162
intellectual disability, p. 164

multidisciplinary team, p. 166
multimodal, p. 151
opaque, p. 156
opportunity barriers, p. 167
Parkinson's disease, p. 166
scanning, p. 158
social closeness, p. 162
social etiquette, p. 162
social roles, p. 172
speech generating device p. 152
static, p. 154
strategy, p. 157
stroke, p. 165
symbol, p. 153
technique, p. 157
traumatic brain injury, p. 165
unaided, p. 153
visual scene display p. 160

ON THE WEB

Check out the Companion Website on www.pearsonhighered.com/justice2e. On it you will find:

• suggested readings

• reflection questions
• self-study quiz
• links to online resources

PART II

Communication Disorders Across the Lifespan

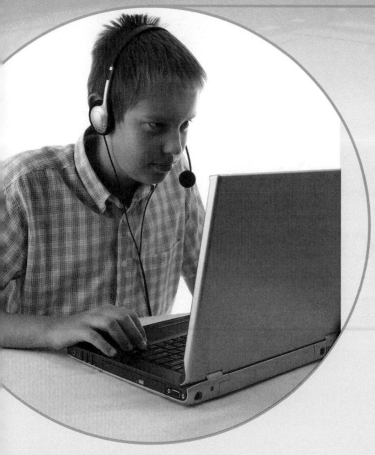

LANGUAGE DISORDERS IN EARLY AND LATER CHILDHOOD

FOCUS QUESTIONS

This chapter answers the following questions:

1. What is a language disorder?

2. How are language disorders classified?

3. What are the defining characteristics of prevalent types of language disorders?

4. How are language disorders identified?

5. How are language disorders treated?

CHAPTER 6

INTRODUCTION

For many children, the development of language follows a predictable pathway in both the rate and the type of accomplishments. Recall from Chapter 2 that most children say their first word at around 1 year, begin to combine words to form two-word sentences at about 18 months, are able to produce three-word sentences by 24 months, and so forth. In fact, one of the remarkable features of language is that it is *species uniform* (see Chapter 1), meaning that regardless of where a child is born and reared—whether in the Arctic, Laos, or Zimbabwe—critical language accomplishments adhere to a strikingly similar pathway.

However, for reasons that are sometimes never known, a small but consequential portion of young children have considerable problems with the development of language. These children have a **language disorder.** They typically show delays in obtaining critical language precursors, such as babbling and gesturing, in the first year of life. In the toddler and preschool years, they are slow to achieve important early language milestones, such as speaking the first word, combining words into sentences, and initiating conversation with adults or peers. During the school-age years, these children often struggle with academic skills that rely on language proficiency, including reading and writing. They also are likely to have problems with complex language tasks, such as using and understanding figurative (e.g., idioms, proverbs) and abstract language. As adults, persons with language disorders face ongoing challenges in living and working in a culture that places enormous value on language proficiency. ●●●

WHAT IS A LANGUAGE DISORDER? ●

DEFINITION

A language disorder refers to

> impaired comprehension and/or use of a spoken, written, and/or other symbol system. The disorder may involve (1) the *form* of language (phonology, morphology, and syntax), (2) the *content* of language (semantics), and/or (3) the *function* of language in communication (pragmatics) in any combination. (American Speech-Language-Hearing Association [ASHA], 1993, p. 40; emphasis added)

CASE STUDY 6.1   Language Disorders in Early and Later Childhood

ALEJANDRO is a 6-year-old student in Mr. Allen's kindergarten classroom in a small elementary school in rural Washington. Alejandro is the youngest child in a migrant Spanish-speaking family that travels annually from Texas to Washington state for the pear and apple harvest. Like many other migrant families, Alejandro's family is living in a small tent in a state-run temporary housing camp. Mr. Allen, a monolingual English speaker, has difficulty communicating with Alejandro, who speaks very little English. Mr. Allen recognizes that there is a language mismatch, which explains much of the difficulty in their communication with one another, but he is concerned that Alejandro may also have a communication disorder. Mr. Allen has noted that Alejandro does not interact well with his peers—for instance, he uses communication cues inappropriately (e.g., talks too loud, refuses eye contact) and is very clumsy and defensive in social interactions. Mr. Allen has asked the speech-language pathologist to come and observe Alejandro in the classroom and to consider the need for a comprehensive speech-language evaluation.

Internet research

1. Is Alejandro's circumstance common in the United States?
2. What educational resources are available for children like Alejandro?
3. What challenges face migrant families?

Brainstorm and discussion

1. What strategies can be used to identify whether Alejandro's suspected communicative difficulties are the result of a language difference or a language disorder?
2. What are some strategies Mr. Allen might use in the classroom to promote Alejandro's success when communicating with classmates?

• • •

NATASHA is a 28-month-old child adopted 4 months ago from Ukraine by Mr. and Mrs. Scarbrough. The adoption agency reported that Natasha had been abandoned by her parents at 3 months of age because of her severe lactose intolerance. From 3 months to 2 years of age, Natasha lived in an orphanage outside Kiev with 120 other children. Although the adoption agency indicated that Natasha had received a full developmental screening and showed no developmental delays or medical problems (aside from lactose intolerance), Mr. and Mrs. Scarbrough are very concerned about Natasha's communication development. When Natasha was adopted, she was not talking at all. Currently, she uses only about four English words (*mama, dada, wawa, car*) and understands several more. She rarely initiates communication with her parents, does not consistently respond to their initiations, and seems more content sitting and looking at storybooks than interacting with others. Mr. and Mrs. Scarbrough have heard friends talk about institutional delays in children adopted from foreign countries and are concerned that Natasha will have ongoing problems with speech and language, given her apparent late start. They have arranged for a comprehensive speech-language evaluation at the local foreign-birth adoption clinic and are eager for suggestions to help Natasha at home.

Internet research

1. Approximately how many children are adopted each year through international adoption agencies?
2. What community resources are available to families adopting children from overseas?
3. What is the developmental prognosis for children who have been institutionalized for long periods of time?

Brainstorm and discussion

1. What information concerning Natasha's first 2 years of life would be helpful for understanding her current communicative abilities?
2. To develop a comprehensive understanding of Natasha's current communicative patterns in the home environment, what questions would you ask her adoptive parents?

A disorder is present if a child's language skills in these areas—form, content, or use—are not consistent with what is typically seen in children of a similar age and a similar cultural and linguistic background (Paul, 2002). A language disorder may impact all three areas—whereby a child has difficulties with phonology, morphology, syntax, semantics, and pragmatics—or it may impact only one area. In addition, a language disorder can affect spoken or oral language as well as written language (e.g., reading, spelling) or another system of symbolic communication, such as sign language.

Additional Considerations in Defining Language Disorders

This definition of a language disorder is theoretical, and applying it to everyday clinical and educational work with children suspected of having language disorders can be quite challenging. Theoretical definitions must be refined for work with children by (1) considering the extent to which observed or suspected language problems have adverse social, psychological, and educational impact upon the children, (2) differentiating between language disorders and language differences, and (3) deciding when language problems are significant enough to be classified as disordered.

Social, Psychological, and Educational Impact.   If a child exhibits difficulty with language but the difficulty does not adversely affect the child socially, psychologically, or educationally, it could be argued that what appears to be a disorder is not a disorder at all (Fey, 1986). Emphasizing the social, psychological, and educational impact of language skills focuses attention on *functional consequences:* Does a child's language performance have a negative impact on the child's ability to function in society (Fey, 1986)? Some experts argue that a language disorder can exist only "when that person is at some risk

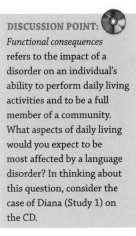

DISCUSSION POINT:
Functional consequences refers to the impact of a disorder on an individual's ability to perform daily living activities and to be a full member of a community. What aspects of daily living would you expect to be most affected by a language disorder? In thinking about this question, consider the case of Diana (Study 1) on the CD.

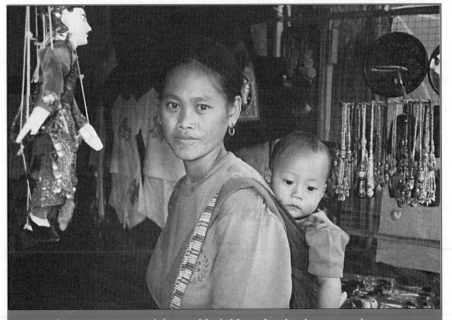

Across the communities of the world, children develop language along a predictable pathway.

FIGURE 6.1

Determining a language disorder.

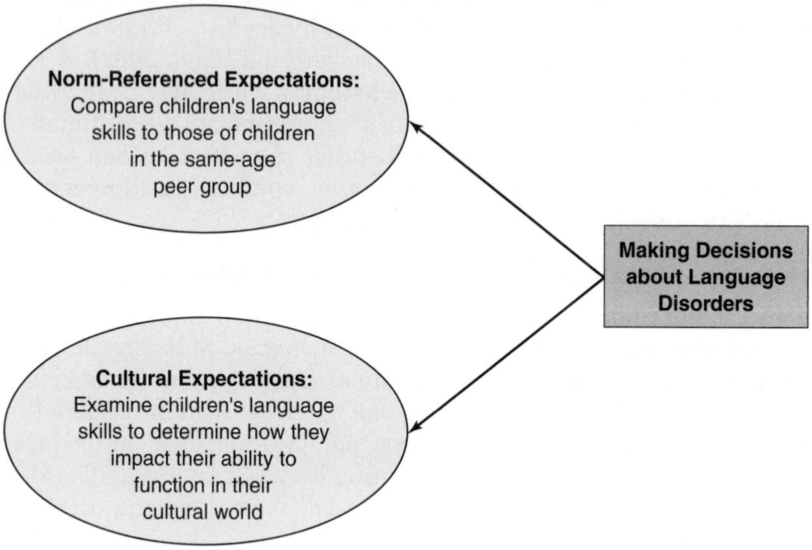

for disvalue in one or more domains of life function because of the person's current or projected language abilities" (Tomblin, 1983, as cited in Fey, 1986).

Language Disorder versus Language Difference. An accurate definition of *language disorder* must also take into consideration the cultural contexts in which a child is reared and is expected to perform. Consider, for instance, the case of Alejandro in Case Study 6.1. Alejandro's communication difficulties may be the result of a language disorder or a **language difference.** A language impairment should be evident when examining a child's language skills against both norm-referenced expectations and cultural expectations (see Figure 6.1; Paul, 2002).

Norm-referenced expectations are based on a child's peer group. For instance, to determine whether a boy who is 3 years, 6 months of age is experiencing impaired language development, his language skills would be compared to the language skills typically seen in boys of the same age. This is a normative reference. On the other hand, cultural expectations are based on the cultural contexts in which a particular child is raised. One would expect slightly different language patterns when comparing the oral language skills of a 3-year-6-month-old European American child reared in inner-city Boston and an African American child of the same age reared in an Appalachian region of southeast Ohio. Thus, definitions of language disorder should refer to language expectations based on normative references, as well as the expectations of a child's cultural group and the language-learning environment.

The Meaning of Significant. A definition of language disorder also must specify the difference between language difficulties that are not serious enough to be classified as disordered and those that are. By many accounts, a language disorder is present if *significant* problems are present (see Paul, 2002). However, it is difficult to determine when a child's language problems are serious enough to be called significant.

Because of the challenges in determining the presence or absence of signifi-cant difficulties, speech-language pathologists and other professionals who

DISCUSSION POINT:
What are some ways in which a child's culture may affect her language development? Consider its impacts on language content, form, and use.

DISCUSSION POINT:
In the case of Alejandro in Case Study 6.1, how would a professional charged with completing a speech-language evaluation find out about speech-language expectations of Alejandro's cultural group and language-learning environment?

diagnose language disorders tend to rely on the use of tests and their outcomes. However, even scores from norm-referenced tests are not always absolute when considering the meaning of *significant.* For instance, a child may receive a standard score of 81 on a standardized test of language development. (Recall from Chapter 4 that a standard score is a type of derived score from a norm-referenced test.) In many clinical or educational settings, this score of 81 would be interpreted as showing a significant problem with language development, because a score of 85 is used as a cutoff—that is, a score of 86 or over is not disordered, whereas a score of 85 or below is disordered. However, in other clinical settings, a score of 81 would not be considered disordered, or significantly different from normal. It is important to realize that these cutoff scores are arbitrary; there is currently no universally accepted test score that differentiates significant from nonsignificant problems with language (Aram, Morris, & Hall, 1993).

DISCUSSION POINT:
Consider Ashley's communication skills (Study 3 on the CD). Are her difficulties significant? Why or why not?

TERMINOLOGY

Many terms are used to describe language disorders in children, including *language delay, language impairment, language disability,* and *language-learning disability.* The terms *childhood aphasia* and *language deviance* are outdated and inaccurate classifications of this condition and are therefore no longer used. The term **language delay** carries the connotation that children exhibiting problems with language achievements are having a late start with language development and can be expected to catch up with their peers (Leonard, 2000). However, as can be seen in Figure 6.2, many children with language disorders do not catch up with their peers over time; rather, the gap in language skill between children with normal development and those with language disorders tends to widen. In addition, for some children with language disorders, their language skills plateau at a point of arrested development. Therefore, the term *language delay* is not really an accurate characterization. There are some children, termed **late talkers,** who do show delays in the earliest stages of language development; approximately half of these children will catch up with their peers by 3 or 4 years of age (Girolametto,

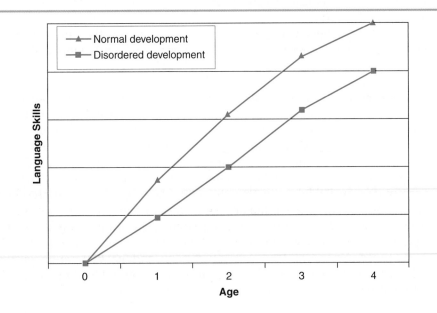

FIGURE 6.2

Normal and disordered language development over time.

Source: From *Children with Specific Language Impairment* by L. Leonard, 2000, Cambridge, MA: MIT Press. Copyright 2000 by MIT Press. Adapted with permission.

Wiigs, Smyth, Weitzman, & Pearce, 2001; Rescorla, Roberts, & Dahlsgaard, 1997), whereas the other half will continue to show ongoing difficulties with language development.

The terms *language disorder* and *language impairment* provide the most accurate representation and are currently preferred for describing children experiencing significant challenges in language development relative to other children (Paul, 2002). The term *language disability* may also be used to suggest that children's language difficulties are exerting a significant, negative impact on their daily-living activities or functions (Paul, 2002). The term *language-learning disability* often describes older children with language disorders who experience difficulties with academic achievement in areas associated with language, such as reading, writing, and spelling (Heward, 2003). Finally, federal legislation (Individuals with Disabilities Education Act, 2004) uses *specific learning disability* to describe children having substantial problems "in one or more of the basic psychological processes involved in understanding or in using language, spoken or written, which . . . may manifest itself in imperfect ability to listen, think, speak, read, write, spell, or do mathematical calculations" (p. 13).

PREVALENCE AND INCIDENCE

Language disorders are the most common type of communication impairment affecting children. They represent the most frequent cause for early intervention and special education services for children from toddlerhood through the elementary grades. About 15% of toddlers are late talkers (Rescorla & Achenbach, 2002), and some of these youngsters will go on to receive a diagnosis of primary language impairment in the later preschool years (Rescorla, 2002). **Primary language impairment** describes a significant impairment of language in the absence of any other developmental difficulty (e.g., mental retardation, brain injury); it affects about 7 to 10% of children over the age of 5 years (Beitchman et al., 1989; Tomblin et al., 1997). Many of these children will continue to experience significant problems with language skills into middle and later adolescence (Catts et al., 2001a; Catts, Fey, Tomblin, & Zhang, 2002; Johnson et al., 1999). Well over 1 million children receive special education services in American schools because of speech or language impairments (U.S. Department of Education, 2001).

A **secondary language impairment** is the result of other intellectual or developmental disorders or is acquired by a brain injury; it is more difficult to estimate in terms of prevalence. About 1 in 1,000 children exhibit mild to severe intellectual disability as a result of Down syndrome (a chromosomal anomaly; Lovering & Percy, 2007) and about 1 in 400 children exhibit autism or an autism spectrum disorder (Fombonne, 2003). In addition, approximately 2% of children experience significant head injuries each year (U.S. Department of Health and Human Services, 1999). Annually, these percentages translate into large numbers of pupils receiving services for speech, language, and communication challenges within the public school system. In the 2001–2002 school year (the most recent data available), more than 300,000 infants, toddlers, and preschoolers received services for speech-language impairments, and an additional 47,000 received services for intellectual, learning, and hearing impairments. In this same period, for school-age children (6 to 21 years), more than 1,000,000 pupils received services for speech-language impairments and 600,000 pupils received services for intellectual disability/mental retardation (U.S. Department of Education, 2003).

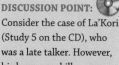

DISCUSSION POINT: Consider the case of La'Kori (Study 5 on the CD), who was a late talker. However, his language skills are now quite typical. Why might some children outgrow early language delays whereas others do not?

HOW ARE LANGUAGE DISORDERS CLASSIFIED? ●

Every child with a language disorder has an individual profile of language strengths and needs. To capture these differences among children, language disorders are usually classified according to etiology, manifestation, and severity.

ETIOLOGY

Primary and Secondary Disorders

Etiology refers to cause. Language disorders result from many diverse causes, although in some cases cause can never be determined. Language disorders are often differentiated as having primary versus secondary etiologies (Schuele & Hadley, 1999). As was mentioned earlier, a primary language impairment occurs in the absence of any other disability that can clearly be held accountable for the disordered pattern of language development. A secondary language impairment occurs as a consequence of another disorder. For instance, intellectual disability, hearing loss, and brain injury are primary conditions that often result in a secondary language disorder. Similarly, language disorders resulting from such conditions as prenatal or postnatal exposure to toxins (e.g., fetal alcohol syndrome, lead ingestion) or child abuse (e.g., shaken baby syndrome) may also be considered secondary language impairments.

> **DISCUSSION POINT:**
> Consider the case of Natasha in Case Study 6.1. Natasha clearly is showing some delays in acquiring the English language. If she is found to have a language impairment, would you consider it primary or secondary in etiology?

Developmental and Acquired Disorders

Language disorders also are often classified as developmental language disorders or acquired language disorders. A **developmental language disorder** is present from birth; it can describe a primary language impairment that has no obvious cause or an impairment that is secondary to another congenital disability, such as Down syndrome, which results in intellectual disability. An **acquired language disorder** is acquired sometime after birth, typically as the result of some type of insult or injury to the developing child (e.g., a car accident). For instance, lead exposure that occurs through ingestion of airborne lead particles (e.g., when lead dust is tracked inside the home) or lead-based paints can cause significant impairments to intellectual functioning (Centers for Disease Control and Prevention, 2005). Negative impacts on language abilities can also occur. A recent study of 42 adults who had significant lead exposure as children showed a relationship between higher levels of childhood lead exposure and diminished activity in regions of the brain associated with language processes (Yuan et al., 2006).

MANIFESTATION

Language disorders are also classified according to which aspects of language are affected or how the disorder is manifested. Does the disorder impact comprehension, expression, or both? Does the disorder affect form, content, and use, or just one or two of these domains?

Comprehension and Expression

Some children exhibit significant problems with comprehending language but have normal expressive language skills—this is a language comprehension disorder (Beitchman et al., 1989). Other children have problems only with expressive language—this is an expressive language disorder (Rescorla & Achenbach, 2002). This is also referred to as a **specific expressive language disorder** (SELD). Children who show impairments in both comprehension and expression have a **mixed receptive-expressive disorder** [American Psychiatric Association (APA), 1994]. Generally, children with only an expressive disorder during toddlerhood will have typical language performance by Kindergarten (Rescorla & Achenbach, 2002).

Form, Content, and Use

Children with language disorders differ in the area of language affected. Recall from Chapter 2 that *language form* refers to the structure of language (i.e., morphology, syntax, and phonology), *content* refers to the meaning expressed through language (i.e., semantics), and *use* describes how language is used in social contexts (i.e., pragmatics). Some children may have problems only with syntax and morphology—a language disorder of form. Children who have a disorder of phonology also have a form problem. Some children may have difficulties only with aspects of word meaning; word-finding problems, difficulties with abstract language, and slow vocabulary development would characterize a content problem. Some children have problems only with use, or pragmatics. These children may have problems initiating conversations with peers, engaging in extended discourse, or using a wide range of communicative behaviors (e.g., questions, requests, comments, greetings).

Although some children have a problem specific to one area or domain, a great number of children have difficulties in two or all three areas. A disorder affecting only one domain is a **focal disorder,** whereas a disorder affecting multiple domains is a **diffuse,** or widespread, **disorder.** Typically, a diffuse disorder is less likely to resolve and is viewed as more serious than a focal impairment (Beitchman et al., 1994).

However, even those children whose language difficulties are resolved by the time they enter school face a general vulnerability for ongoing challenges in the area of language. This is because some educational experiences make significant requirements of the underlying language system, as is the case when children begin to learn to read (Catts, Adlof, & Ellis Weismer, 2006; Scarborough, 2000); the process of learning to read may reveal an underlying language problem that seemed to be resolved. One way of describing this phenomenon, whereby children manifest different language problems at different points in time, is presented in Figure 6.3. This figure shows how a child's language symptoms may vary across time; a language disorder may be a lasting condition that persists across the life span (Botting, Faragher, Simkin, Knox, et al., 2001; Girolametto et al., 2001; Johnson et al., 1999).

SEVERITY

The severity of language disorders ranges from mild to profound, as shown in Figure 6.4. Mild impairments may be perceptible only to a child, parent,

---

FIGURE 6.3

Symptom variations of language disorders over time.

Source: Based on Scarborough, H. S. (2000).

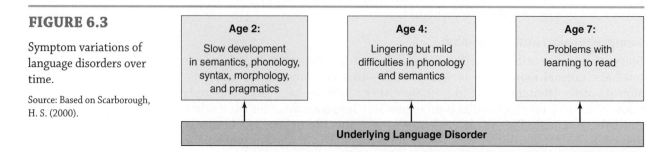

Age 2:	Age 4:	Age 7:
Slow development in semantics, phonology, syntax, morphology, and pragmatics	Lingering but mild difficulties in phonology and semantics	Problems with learning to read

Underlying Language Disorder

> ## FIGURE 6.4
>
> **Variations in severity of language disorders.**
>
> | Mild | Has some impact on child's ability to perform in social or academic situations but does not preclude participation in normal, age-appropriate activities in school or community |
> |---|---|
> | Moderate | Involves a significant degree of impairment that necessitates some special accommodations for the child to participate in mainstream community and academic settings |
> | Severe | Usually makes it very difficult for a child to function in community and educational activities without extensive supports |
> | Profound | Implies that the child has little or no ability to use language to communicate and is unable to function in community and educational activities |

Source: From *Language Disorders from Infancy Through Adolescence* by R. Paul. Copyright 2002. Reprinted with permission from Elsevier.

or professional and may have little impact on a child's ability to function at home or at school. In contrast, children with a profound impairment may have no language skill at all and therefore may be severely limited in their ability to participate in many home, school, or community functions (Paul, 2002).

DUAL LANGUAGE LEARNERS

Children who are under 5 years of age and are acquiring two languages simultaneously (e.g., English and Spanish) are described as *simultaneous bilinguals;* children who are over 5 years of age and who have a native (home) language but are learning a second language, such as English, are described as *sequential bilinguals* (August & Hakuta, 1997). Children who are simultaneous and sequential bilinguals develop language differently than children who are acquiring English only and are native English speakers. Some children with limited English proficiency (LEP, also referred to as *English language learners,* or ELLs) may appear to have a language disability but, in fact, are simply going through the normal stages of learning a new language. These differences must not be mistaken for a language disorder; federal law legislates that children who are struggling academically should not be identified as having a disability when their difficulties are associated with LEP.

Learning two or more languages—either simultaneously or sequentially—should have no negative impact on a child's ability to acquire language. Fears that learning multiple languages can confuse children are derived from flawed research in the early 1900s in which bilingual immigrant children in the United States were given intelligence tests and found to have lower test scores than monolingual children had. These early studies were flawed for many reasons, including the fact that many more of the immigrant children studied were from low socioeconomic households, whereas the monolingual children were from more advantaged homes. More recent and well-conducted studies have shown bilingualism to have an overwhelmingly positive impact on children's cognitive and linguistic development, once the effects of socioeconomic status are accounted for (August & Hakuta, 1997).

Large numbers of children who are learning English as a second or foreign language are being educated in American schools. Today, ELL students represent more than 7% of public school students, corresponding to more than 3 million students. In some regions of the United States, the ELL student population is particularly concentrated, such as the West, which educates more than half of all ELL students (National Center for Education Statistics, 2004). About 10% of these children can be expected to exhibit a primary or secondary language disorder on the basis of epidemiological estimates of the prevalence of language impairment in young children. For some groups of children within the broader population of LEP students, the incidence may be slightly higher, particularly among children who are being reared in poverty conditions or whose families have had limited access to health care. In such cases, however, language disorders are not arising from limited English proficiency or second/foreign language acquisition, but rather from socioeconomic and broader cultural influences that have impacted the children's language-learning conditions.

WHAT ARE THE DEFINING CHARACTERISTICS OF PREVALENT TYPES OF LANGUAGE DISORDERS? ●

Four types of language disorders are particularly prevalent among young children. **Specific language impairment** is a primary, developmental language impairment with no known cause. **Autism spectrum disorder** and intellectual disability (mental retardation) are two types of developmental disabilities that often result in secondary language impairments. Traumatic brain injury is an acquired disorder that also often results in a secondary language impairment.

SPECIFIC LANGUAGE IMPAIRMENT

Defining Characteristics

Specific language impairment (SLI) describes preschool and school-age children who show a significant impairment of expressive or receptive language that cannot be attributed to any other causal condition. Children with SLI have typical hearing skills (although they may have a history of middle-ear infections), normal intelligence, and no obvious neurological, motor, or sensory disturbances, such as seizures or brain injury.

Children are typically diagnosed with SLI after their third birthday (Rescorla, 2002). Although signs of language difficulty may be present as early as the first and second years of life, toddlers who are slow to talk are typically classified as late talkers rather than language impaired. Because at least 35% and as many as 60% of late talkers outgrow their language problems by 3 years of age (Rescorla, Roberts, & Dahlsgaard, 1997; Thal & Tobias, 1992), the diagnosis of SLI is usually not made until age 3 or later, when it is clear that a child is exhibiting a true disorder of language rather than a late start.

The language profile of children with SLI is difficult to capture, because these children are a very diverse group. Some children with SLI have problems in only one area of language, whereas others have problems that transcend all areas of language performance. Some children have difficulties with expressive

DISCUSSION POINT:
What are some benefits of early diagnosis of SLI? Can you think of any drawbacks of early diagnosis?

language only (SELD), while others have problems with both expression and comprehension (a mixed disorder).

An overview of language challenges for children with SLI from toddlerhood through adolescence is presented in Table 6.1. Hallmark characteristics include the following:

1. Inconsistent skills across different domains; for instance, a child might have a strength in phonology and a weakness in syntax and morphology.

2. A history of slow vocabulary development: on average children with SLI produce their first words at about 2 years of age and continue to struggle with learning new words through the elementary years (see Leonard, 2000).

3. A tendency toward **word-finding problems**—that is, difficulties in coming up with the right words at the right time (Oetting, Rice, & Swank, 1995). Word-finding problems are usually accompanied by frequent pauses, filler words (e.g., *um, uh*), a reliance on nonspecific and general words (e.g., *thing, stuff*), and naming errors (e.g., calling a plate a glass; McGregor, 1997).

4. Considerable difficulty with grammatical production and comprehension that begins during toddlerhood and continues through school age (Conti-Ramsden & Jones, 1997). This problem is particularly evident with verbs. Children with SLI use verbs less frequently than do their same-age peers, use fewer types of verbs, and show delayed development of verb morphology (Conti-Ramsden & Jones, 1997; Rice, 1996; Watkins & Rice, 1994). Leonard (2000) has written that verb use is an "extraordinary problem" for children with SLI (p. 61).

TABLE 6.1 Language difficulties associated with SLI	
Age	**Language Difficulties**
Infancy and toddlerhood	Late appearance of first word (average age of 23 months); delayed use of present progressive (-*ing*), plural (*s*), and possessive (*'s*); late use of two-word combinations (average age of 37 months); less frequent use of verbs and less variety in verbs; slow development of pronouns; longer reliance on gestures for getting needs met; difficulty initiating with peers; difficulty sustaining turns in conversation
Preschool	Use of grammar that resembles that of younger children (e.g., pronoun errors, as in *me want dolly*); late use of verb markers (e.g., third-person singular *is* as an auxiliary); frequent errors of omission (e.g., leaving out key elements of syntax); shorter sentence length; problems forming questions with inverted auxiliaries; difficulty with accurate use of *be* as an auxiliary or copular verb form; slow development of pronouns; requests similar to those of younger children; difficulty with group conversations (i.e., conversing with more than one child); difficulty with verbal resolution of conflict
Early and later elementary	Word-finding problems accompanied by circumlocutions and pauses; naming errors (e.g., *shoes* for *pants*); slower processing speed; use of earlier developing pronoun forms; low sensitivity to the speech of others (e.g., difficulty responding to indirect requests); difficulty maintaining topics; difficulty recognizing need for conversational repair
Adolescence	Difficulty expressing ideas about language; inappropriate responses to questions and comments; poor social language; insufficient information for listeners; redundancy; inadequate sense of limits or boundaries; difficulty expressing needs and ideas; difficulty initiating conversations with peers; immature conversational participation

Sources: Based on Conti-Ramsden and Jones (1997); Leonard (2000); McGregor and Leonard (1995); Ratner and Harris (1994); Watkins, Rice, and Molz (1993).

5. Problems in social skills and behaviors (Fujiki, Brinton, Morgan, & Hart, 1999; Fujiki, Brinton, & Todd, 1996; Stanton-Chapman, Justice, Skibbe, & Grant, 2007). This includes difficulties making friends, initiating conversations with others, and being relatively withdrawn in social settings. Children with SLI have difficulty inferring (or reading) the emotions of others during conversations (Ford & Milosky, 2008).

6. The likelihood of language difficulties persisting over time. Well over 50% of children who exhibit SLI at kindergarten age continue to show language weaknesses in adolescence and adulthood (Johnson et al., 1999; Stothard, Snowling, Bishop, Chipchase, et al., 1998).

Causes and Risk Factors

There is currently no known cause for SLI, a fact that is frustrating for both parents and professionals. Recent advances in brain imaging, epidemiological investigations, and molecular genetics suggest a strong biological and genetic component to this disorder (Flax et al., 2003). Linkages of SLI to specific chromosomes is progressing to a point where specific susceptible genetic loci have been identified (Bartlett et al., 2002). The current theoretical view is that biological or genetic factors predispose a child to SLI. For instance, children who have immediate family members with language impairment are more likely than other children to develop SLI (Ellis Weismer, Murray-Branch, & Miller, 1994; Rice, Haney, & Wexler, 1998; Tomblin, 1989; Van Der Lely & Stollwerck, 1996). About 20 to 40% of children with SLI have a sibling or a parent with a language disorder (Flax et al., 2003).

Whether a biological or genetic predisposition to SLI is eventually manifested as a disorder is linked to a child's exposure to additional risk factors. Not all children who are genetically or biologically predisposed to SLI will experience it. Specifically, it appears that sensory deprivation due to environmental factors (e.g., limited language input) or biological factors (e.g., chronic middle-ear infections) contributes to a developmental fragility that increases the risk for SLI, as can physical health challenges resulting from adverse perinatal influences (e.g., low birth weight, prematurity) and postnatal influences (e.g., exposure to toxins, undernutrition).

DISCUSSION POINT:
Survey your classmates to find out how many had chronic middle-ear infections as children. These infections can increase a child's risk for language difficulties, although the connection has been difficult for researchers to establish. Why would it be difficult to study ear infections in young children?

AUTISM SPECTRUM DISORDER

Defining Characteristics

Autism spectrum disorder (ASD) is an umbrella term describing a variety of developmental conditions that are characterized by significant difficulties in social relationships, communication, repetitive behaviors, and overly restricted interests (Lord & Risi, 2000). While the prognosis for autism has historically been poor (Heflin & Simpson, 1998) and few individuals with autism have been able to live and work independently, recent advances in early identification and intervention provide increasing promise for individuals with autism and their families.

Autism spectrum disorder includes four types of disabilities: autism, childhood disintegrative disorder, Asperger's syndrome, and pervasive developmental disorder–not otherwise specified (PDD). These four conditions are childhood disabilities that together impact about 1 in 400 children (Fombonne, 2003). There is a higher rate of these disorders in children with family members who are also affected, indicating a strong genetic component. The prevalence of autism across the genders is markedly uneven: With the exception of childhood

FIGURE 6.5

Language characteristics of children with ASD.

Infancy/ Toddlerhood	• Limited engagement in joint attention • Few signals to others to draw attention to self or objects, such as showing or pointing • Communication focused exclusively to regulate behaviors of others (rejecting and protesting) • Low responsiveness to caregivers' smiles • Low responsiveness to caregivers' bids for shared attention • Low levels of positive affect during interactions with caregivers • Low use of vocalizations to communicate • Low use of conventional symbolic gestures to communicate (waving, pointing, nodding) and overreliance on presymbolic gestures (leading and pulling)
Preschool and Primary Years	• Low use of nonverbal behaviors during communication (e.g., eye-to-eye gaze, facial expression, gestures) • Difficulty in initiating conversations with others • Difficulty participating in multiturn conversations • Limited interest in participating in communicative exchanges with others • Restricted vocabulary • Echolalia, or repetitive use of language (often phrases or sentences heard elsewhere) • Lack of use of language for imaginative purposes or make-believe play • Limited or inconsistent response to spoken communication or other auditory stimuli • Limited engagement in play with others • Use of challenging behaviors to communicate and procure attention (e.g., tantrum, self-injury)
Adolescence	• Difficulty understanding nonliteral uses of language (e.g., jokes, idioms) • Difficulty understanding abstract language concepts • Dysprosody (use of unusual pitch, rhythm, and pace) • Difficulty with nonverbal behaviors during communication (e.g., eye-to-eye gaze, facial expression, gestures, proximity to others) • Difficulty comprehending written text (although word recognition may be strong) • Difficulty entering peer conversations and initiating conversation with others • Limited range of communicative functions or purposes

Sources: American Psychiatric Association (1994); Nelson (1998); Wetherby, Prizant, & Schuler (2000).

disintegrative disorder, boys are about four times as likely as girls to be affected (Fombonne, 2003). However, when girls are affected, they tend to have more severe symptoms than boys.

Children with any one of the autism spectrum disorders usually will exhibit a mild to severe or profound secondary language impairment. The language characteristics of children with ASD are presented in Figure 6.5.

Autism. Autism is a severe developmental disability with symptoms that are present before a child's third birthday. Diagnostic criteria from the most recent *Diagnostic and Statistical Manual of Mental Disorders* (*DSM;* APA, 1994) are presented in Table 6.2. The three hallmark characteristics of autism are

TABLE 6.2	Diagnostic criteria for ASD	
Disorder	**Onset**	**Hallmark Characteristics**

Autism	Prior to 3 years	Abnormal functioning in social interaction, communication, and behavior, with at least six specific areas of deficit from the following (at least two must be in social interaction, and at least one in the other two categories):
		
		 1. Social interaction
		    a. Marked impairment in using multiple nonverbal behaviors (eye-to-eye gaze, facial expression, body posture, gestures)
		    b. Failure to develop peer relationships appropriately
		    c. Lack of spontaneous seeking to share enjoyment, interests, or achievements with others
		    d. Lack of social or emotional reciprocity
		
		 2. Communication
		    a. Delay in or total lack of development of spoken language
		    b. Marked impairment in ability to sustain conversation with others
		    c. Stereotyped and repetitive use of language or idiosyncratic language
		    d. Lack of varied, spontaneous, or make-believe play or social imitative play
		
		 3. Behavior
		    a. Preoccupation with one or more stereotyped patterns of interest that are abnormal in intensity or focus
		    b. Inflexible adherence to specific nonfunctional routines or rituals
		    c. Repetitive motor movements
		    d. Persistent preoccupation with parts of objects

Childhood disintegrative disorder	Between 2 and 10 years	Normal development for at least first 2 years, significant loss of skills in two or more of the following: language, social skills, or adaptive behavior; bowel or bladder control; play; and motor skills. Significant impairment must also be observed in at least two of the following: 1. Social interaction, including impaired nonverbal behaviors, failure to develop peer relationships, and lack of emotional reciprocity 2. Communication, including lack of spoken language, inability to sustain or initiate conversation, and repetitive use of language 3. Behavior, including restrictive, repetitive, or stereotyped patterns of behavior and interests

Asperger's syndrome	Onset before or after 3 years	No clinically significant delay in language, cognitive, self-help, and adaptive behavioral skills, but significant impairment in two or more areas of the following:
		
		 1. Social interaction
		    a. Impairment in use of nonverbal behaviors
		    b. Failure to develop peer relationships
		    c. Lack of spontaneous seeking to share enjoyment, interests, or achievements with others
		    d. Lack of social or emotional reciprocity
		
		 2. Behavior
		    a. Preoccupation with one or more stereotyped patterns of interest that are abnormal in intensity or focus
		    b. Inflexible adherence to specific nonfunctional routines or rituals
		    c. Repetitive motor movements
		    d. Persistent preoccupation with parts of objects

Pervasive developmental disorder	Onset before or after 3 years	A severe and pervasive impairment in social interaction, communication, and/or behavior without meeting criteria for diagnosis of autistic disorder, childhood disintegrative disorder, or Asperger's syndrome

Source: From Diagnostic and Statistical Manual of Mental Disorders *(4th ed.) by American Psychiatric Association, 1994, Washington, DC: APA. Copyright 1994 by APA. Adapted with permission.*

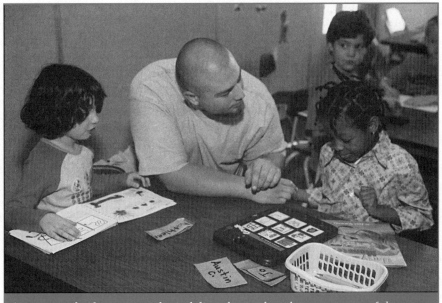

Autism results from a neurological disturbance, but the exact cause of the disorder remains unknown.

difficulties with social interactions with others, severe impairment of communication skill, and restricted and stereotypical behaviors and interests.

Children with autism show significant difficulties in interacting and relating with others. This includes impaired nonverbal behaviors (e.g., eye contact, posture, facial expressions), an inability or lack of interest in developing relationships with peers and participating in social games or routines, and little awareness of the feelings or needs of others (APA, 1994). Children with autism also have severely impaired communication skills, and some never develop any functional oral language skills; the language of those who do develop it is often characterized by idiosyncratic, repetitive language (e.g., **echolalia,** stereotypical repetitions of specific words or phrases) and an inability to initiate or reciprocate in communicative interactions with others.

In addition, children with autism also show "restricted, repetitive, and stereotyped patterns of behaviors, interests, and activities" (APA, 1994, p. 67). These children may have very few interests and are overly preoccupied with certain objects or activities. For instance, a child may be preoccupied with a set of plastic dinosaurs and may spend hours each day lining up the dinosaurs along the edge of a table in a particular order. **Stereotypical behaviors** are also common, such as rocking back and forth, humming, or flapping the arms.

Childhood Disintegrative Disorder. **Childhood disintegrative disorder** describes children under 10 years of age who appear to be developing normally until at least their second birthday but then display a significant loss or regression of skills in two or more of the following areas: language, social skills, bowel control, play, or motor skills (APA, 1994). Like children with autism, children with disintegrative disorder display significant problems in their social interactions and communication skills and show restricted and repetitive behaviors and interests.

Asperger's Syndrome. Children with **Asperger's syndrome** are often referred to as "higher functioning" children with autism. Like children with other autism

DISCUSSION POINT:
Even though children with Asperger's syndrome tend to have well-developed language skills, they still benefit from language intervention to enhance their pragmatic skills, such as conversational participation and initiating with peers. Can you think of some ways these skills might be targeted in a therapy session?

spectrum disorders, children with Asperger's have substantial problems with social interaction and show restricted and idiosyncratic behavioral patterns and interests. The language skills of children with Asperger's tend to be relatively well developed and are not viewed as clinically disordered. However, because of their challenges with social relationships, children with Asperger's often have considerable difficulty using language as a social tool and a means of developing and maintaining social relationships. They may, for instance, have difficulty initiating conversations with peers and may use language that is situationally inappropriate.

Pervasive Developmental Disorder (PDD). PDD describes children who have severe problems with social interactions and communication and who display repetitive behaviors and overly restricted interests but do not otherwise meet the criteria for autism, childhood disintegrative disorder, or Asperger's syndrome.

Causes and Risk Factors

Autism spectrum disorders are currently viewed as neurobiological disorders resulting from an organic brain abnormality (Lord & Risi, 2000). These disorders likely result from multiple causes that result in similar patterns or appearance of disability (Perry, Dunlap, & Black, 2007). Several risk factors may contribute to the likelihood of a child's developing an autism spectrum disorder. Prenatal and perinatal complications, particularly maternal rubella and **anoxia** (i.e., lack of oxygen to the brain), have been associated with increased risk for autism (APA, 1994). The presence of other developmental or physical disabilities, such as encephalitis (an inflammation of the brain) and fragile X syndrome (a genetic disorder that results in mental retardation), also can contribute to the occurrence of autism. Seizure disorder is seen in 25% of children with autism (APA, 1994). Severe sensory deprivation, as seen in severe cases of neglect and child abuse, can have a profound impact on communication and social development and in extreme cases may result in patterns of development similar to that of autism spectrum disorders (Kenneally, Bruck, Frank, & Nalty, 1998).

Some professionals and parents believe there is a link between childhood vaccinations and autism, particularly the MMR (measles, mumps, rubella) vaccine. However, the most extensive study to date examining the evidence for the autism-vaccination connection found no link between this vaccine and the risk for developing autism. Published in 2002 in the *New England Journal of Medicine* (Madsen et al., 2002), this study examined the incidence of autism in 537,303 children in Denmark, of whom 440,655 had received the MMR vaccine. The study showed the rate of autism to be no higher for children who had received the vaccine than for children who had not. Research focused on determining the cause of autism, including further study of the vaccine-autism link, is currently under way in the United States.

INTELLECTUAL DISABILITY

Defining Characteristics

Intellectual disability, also described as *mental retardation,* is a "condition of arrested or incomplete development of the mind, which is especially characterized by impairment of skills manifested during the developmental period." (American Association on Mental Retardation [AAMR], 2002, p. 103). The term *intellectual disability* is used internationally to describe this condition;

in the United States, the term *mental retardation* is often used (Brown, 2007). Generally, the terms may be used synonymously, although some view the term *intellectual disability* to be less pejorative (Acharya & Msall, 2008). The term *developmental delay* is also often used to describe children with intellectual disability; this term carries the connotation that development is still progressing and that the disability may not persist (Brown, 2007). About 1% of children in American schools have a diagnosis of mental retardation, reflecting about 10% of children receiving special education services (U.S. Department of Education, 2002). The diagnosis of mental retardation is made in children under the age of 18 years who experience "significant limitations both in intellectual functioning and in adaptive behavior as expressed in conceptual, social, and practical adaptive skills" (AAMR, 2002, p. 1).

In accordance with this definition, an accurate diagnosis of intellectual disability/mental retardation is made on the basis of two key considerations (AAMR, 2002):

1. Limitations in intelligence, to include difficulties with reasoning, planning, problem solving, abstract thinking, comprehending abstract and complex concepts, and learning skills

2. Limitations in **adaptive behavior** and the activities of daily living, including difficulties in conceptual skills (communication, functional academics, self-direction, health and safety), social skills (social relationships, leisure), or practical skills (self-care, home living, community participation, work)

By this definition, we can view intellectual disability as a "cognitive-adaptive" disorder (Acharya & Msall, 2008). Consideration of limitations in both intelligence and adaptive behavior is made in reference to the broader context of an individual's peers and community and must include the impact of linguistic and cultural diversity (AAMR, 2002). In other words, the unique contexts in which an individual is reared—referring to the "conditions within which people live their everyday lives"—must be closely examined for any determination of mental retardation to occur (AAMR, 2002, p. 15). Examination of context should include an individual's *microsystem* (close family), *mesosystem* (neighborhood and community), and *macrosystem* (society).

Intellectual disability can affect an individual only minimally, with the person exhibiting mild learning difficulties but able to participate fully in society and develop strong social relationships, or it can affect an individual profoundly. People with profound intellectual disability may be unable to care for themselves, communicate, or participate in any community or employment activities. Four levels of intellectual disability/mental retardation, ranging from mild to profound, are presented in Table 6.3 and can be determined by considering both intellectual limitations and adaptive behavior limitations. Of the four levels presented in Table 6.3, mild and moderate levels are much more prevalent (about 95% of persons with mental retardation) than severe and profound levels of disability (only about 5% of cases; AAMR, 2002).

The language skills of a person with intellectual disability usually approximate the degree of cognitive impairment. In general, children with intellectual disability show delays in early communicative behaviors (e.g., pointing in order to request, commenting vocally) and are slow to use their first words and to produce multiword combinations (Rosenberg & Abbeduto, 1993). The path of language acquisition tends to be the same as that of children who are developing typically, albeit at a slower rate.

TABLE 6.3   Classification of intellectual disability/mental retardation

Classification	IQ Range	Adaptive Skills
Mild (85% of MR)	50–69	Mild learning difficulties; able to work, maintain good social relationships, and make contributions to society. Can acquire academic skills up to about a sixth-grade level. By adulthood usually achieve social and vocabulary skills adequate for minimum self-support; apt to need supervision and assistance. Usually live successfully in community, either independently or in supervised settings.
Moderate (10% of MR)	35–49	Marked developmental delays in childhood; able to develop some degree of independence in self-care and acquire adequate communication and academic skills. As adolescents may have problems with peer relationships because of difficulties with social conventions. Can benefit from vocational training. Need varying degrees of support to live and work in community but are able to perform unskilled or semiskilled work with supervision. Adapt well to community life, usually in supervised settings.
Severe (3–4% of MR)	20–34	Significant developmental delays; acquire little or no speech and language skill in preschool years but may later develop minimal communication skills. Can master some preacademic skills (sight reading of important words). Need continuous levels of support to care for self and participate in community activities but can adapt well to community life with close supervision.
Profound (1–2% of MR)	<20	Severe limitations in self-care, continence, communication, and mobility; usually identified with a neurological condition that accounts for mental retardation. Need constant aid and supervision; may perform simple tasks with much support.

Source: From Diagnostic and Statistical Manual of Mental Disorders *(4th ed.) by American Psychiatric Association, 1994, Washington, DC: APA. Copyright 1994 by APA. Adapted with permission.*

Children with mild forms of intellectual disability may have well-developed oral language skills, particularly in vocabulary, with minor difficulties with abstract concepts, figurative language, complex syntax, conversational participation, and communicative repairs (Ezell & Goldstein, 1991; Kuder, 1997). For instance, children with mild intellectual disability often have difficulty understanding abstract notions such as *liberty* or *cooperation,* understanding and using idiomatic expressions (e.g., *hit the books*), using conjunctions to temporally and causally sequence their thoughts, and recognizing when communication breakdowns have occurred. Despite these difficulties, many children with mild levels of intellectual disability exhibit oral language skills that allow them to fully participate in the academic curriculum, communicate competently with peers and adults, and relay their needs and interests to others.

Comparatively, children with more severe forms of intellectual disability display severe to profound levels of language disorder. Some individuals with intellectual disability never learn to express themselves through verbal means. They may produce only a few words or sounds and few gestures. For some individuals, an augmentative and alternative communicative (AAC) device can facilitate their ability to express themselves. AAC devices and other means of enhancing the communicative abilities of individuals with severe communicative disabilities are described in Chapter 5.

Historically, it was thought that individuals with intellectual disability reached an early plateau in language development. Research has shown, however, that new language skills can continue to emerge well into adolescence for persons with intellectual disability. Chapman and colleagues' research on persons with Down syndrome, which is a fairly prevalent cause of intellectual disability, show significant gains in syntax and vocabulary development through later childhood and adolescence (Chapman, Seung, Schwartz, & Kay-Raining

Bird, 1998). For instance, children who are 5 to 8 years of age produce utterances that average about two words in length, compared to utterances of about 4.5 words in length for older adolescents. Although continuing to develop over time, the language skills of children and adolescents with Down syndrome tend to be characterized by short sentences (about three words in length), a fairly small expressive vocabulary, a slowed rate of speech, and often compromised intelligibility. Function words, such as copular and auxiliary verbs (e.g., *is, were, does*), may be frequently omitted, as are pronouns, conjunctions, and articles. Language comprehension tends to be better than language expression.

When considering the language achievements of individuals with intellectual disability, it is important to consider whether one's disability is *static* or *progressive*. An individual whose intellectual disability is static will typically show a steady but slow rate of language development over time. For children and adolescents with Down syndrome, language growth approximates this description. An individual whose disability is progressive, however, likely will show regression and loss of skills over time. Children with certain metabolic disorders, such as untreated hypothyroidism and Rett syndrome, can experience a halt in language progress followed by a regression (Acharya & Msall, 2008). Sometimes these distinctions are blurred in individuals with intellectual disability. For instance, Down syndrome (typically a static disability) can co-occur with progressive disabilities, such as hypothyroidism, which can contribute to intellectual dysfunction if left untreated (Acharya & Msall, 2008).

Causes and Risk Factors

Intellectual disability can occur for many reasons, although in about 30 to 40% of cases, the cause cannot be identified (APA, 1994). For the other 60 to 70% of cases, causes stem from both biomedical and psychosocial factors (Acharya & Msall, 2008). Prenatal damage to the developing fetus due to chromosomal abnormalities or maternal ingestion of toxins accounts for the majority of cases (about 30% overall). Environmental influences and other mental conditions, such as sensory deprivation (e.g., neglect), abuse, or the presence of autism, account for about 15 to 20% of all cases. Pregnancy and perinatal problems— such as fetal malnutrition, prematurity, anoxia (lack of oxygen to the child's brain before, during, or following birth), and viral infections—account for an additional 10% of cases. Medical conditions such as trauma, infection, and poisoning cause about 5% of cases of mental retardation, and heredity alone accounts for 5% of cases.

BRAIN INJURY

Defining Characteristics

Brain injury refers to damage or insult to an individual's brain. Although brain injuries can occur in utero (before birth) and perinatally (during the birthing process), this chapter focuses on *acquired* brain injuries. Brain injuries sustained before or near the time of birth that result in significant intellectual challenges are usually viewed as cases of intellectual disability. Acquired brain injuries are a leading cause of death and disability among young children, and many of these injuries result from transportation-related accidents, falls, and recreational accidents (Christensen et al., 2008). Serious brain injuries can result from infection (e.g., meningitis), disease (e.g., brain tumor), and physical trauma. Brain damage resulting from physical trauma, particularly blunt trauma to the head, is referred to as *traumatic brain injury*, or TBI. Causes of TBI in children include abuse (e.g., shaken baby syndrome), intentional harm (e.g., being hit or shot in the head), accidental poisoning through ingestion of toxic substances (e.g., prescription medications, pesticides), car accidents, and falling.

Acquired injuries occur sometime after birth as a result of an incident that inflicts damage on the brain matter. Brain injuries affect approximately 1.5 million persons each year, the majority of whom do survive but often with significant, lasting neurological damage. Young children, adolescent males, and the elderly are at greatest risk, and males are affected twice as often as females. By age 15, 4 out of 100 males will experience a brain injury, as will 2.3 girls (Christensen et al., 2008). The impact of a brain injury on children and their families can be enormous; more than half of those affected by moderate to severe brain injury have lifelong serious impairments that negatively impact daily living activities (Christensen et al., 2008). The financial costs of brain injuries are substantial. Many families directly impacted by a brain injury deplete all or most of their financial resources to care for the injured person, and the annual economic burden to the United States is billions of dollars (U.S. Department of Health and Human Services, 1999).

The severity of a brain injury is typically defined based on the level of consciousness the injured individual experiences after the injury as well as during subsequent monitoring. The Glasgow Coma Scale (GCS; Jennett & Teasdale, 1981) is the most commonly used metric for quantifying consciousness. Up to 4 points are given to describe an individual's eye responses (1 = does not open eyes, 4 = opens eyes spontaneously), up to 6 points are given to describe motor responses (1 = makes no movements, 6 = obeys commands), and up to 5 points are given to describe verbal responses (1 = makes no sounds, 5 = converses normally). Points are summed, and the lowest score (3 points) indicates a serious coma state. Typically, a severe brain injury equates to a score of 3 to 8 (when coma lasts for 6 hours or longer), a moderate brain injury equates to a score of 9 to 12, and a mild Traumatic Brain Injury (TBI) equates to a score of 13 to 15. Mild TBI, typically accompanied by a concussion and loss of consciousness for 30 minutes or less, are the most common type of brain injury and have the least serious repercussions. Children with mild brain injury show little residual difficulties in intellect and language, although they may experience an elevated risk for hyperactivity and other psychiatric illnesses (Massagli et al., 2004). For moderate and severe cases of brain injury, persistent difficulties in intellect, language, and behavior are common; typically, the more severe the injury, the more likely it is for severe impairments to persist (Christensen et al., 2008).

The most common type of TBI is a closed-head injury (CHI), in which brain matter is not exposed or penetrated. CHI is frequently associated with rapid acceleration and deceleration, as in a car, in which people may hit their heads on the dashboard or steering wheel. Among children, CHI may result from child abuse, sports injuries, falls, and pedestrian-vehicle accidents (National Institute on Deafness and Other Communication Disorders [NIDCD], 2003a). In contrast, in open-head injuries (OHI), brain matter is exposed through penetration.

Injuries may be diffuse, affecting large areas of the brain, or they may be focal, affecting only one specific brain region. The frontal and temporal lobes of the brain, which house the centers for much of our executive functions (e.g., reasoning, planning, hypothesizing) and our language functions, are often damaged in head injuries, as they sit more anterior in the brain where damage is most likely to occur (e.g., during a car accident; NIDCD, 2003). CHI tends to be associated with diffuse damage to the brain, whereas OHI, such as injury from a gunshot wound, usually results in a focal injury.

Most children with an acquired brain injury have a history of normal language skills. Language disorders resulting from brain injury are influenced by the severity of the injury, the *site* of the damage, and the characteristics of the child before the injury occurred (Christensen et al., 2008). Children with more severe injuries have less of a chance for full language recovery. Contrary to popular thought, the brains of young children are not better able to withstand and heal from injury than those of older children. Infants, toddlers, and preschoolers can show long-lasting cognitive and language impairments following moderate or severe TBI (Aram, 1988). However, some young children may have a delayed onset of impairment; that is, problems sustained during a brain injury may not be evident until later years when damaged areas of the brain are used for certain skills and activities (Goodman & Yude, 1996).

In many cases of CHI, the brain injury affects the frontal lobe of the brain, resulting in difficulties associated with language use and cognitive, executive, and self-regulatory functions. About 75% of children with severe CHI have language use problems in the area of discourse (Chapman, 1997). Major language difficulties commonly associated with brain injury are presented in Figure 6.6 and include giving less information in discourse, producing language that is fragmented and difficult to follow, and having difficulties with word retrieval (Chapman, 1997; Russell, 1993).

Brain injury can also impact a child's cognitive, executive, and behavioral skills (Massagli et al., 2004; Taylor, 2001). These include difficulties with sustained and selective attention (e.g., maintaining attention during an ongoing activity, when distractions might be present), storing new information, retrieving known information, planning and goal setting, organizational skills, reasoning and problem solving, self-awareness, and behavioral monitoring (Taylor, 2001). Children and adolescents with brain injury may be more likely to exhibit aggression, irritability, depression, and anxiety. Because the prevalent long-term repercussions of brain injury are more subtle than obvious physical manifestations, brain injury is often referred to as an invisible epidemic (U.S. Department of Health and Human Services, 1999).

Causes and Risk Factors

The most common causes of brain injuries are automobile accidents, falls, and sports injuries (Christensen et al., 2008). For children, recreational and sports injuries—such as bicycling, football, and horseback riding—are

> **DISCUSSION POINT:**
> Contrary to historical belief, infants, toddlers, and preschoolers show long-lasting cognitive and language impairments following a moderate or severe TBI. A prevalent cause of TBI in children is shaken baby syndrome. What are other causes of TBI in children? What are some ways to decrease the occurrence of TBI in children?

FIGURE 6.6

Language problems associated with brain injury.

- Language comprehension difficulties, affected by decreased attention and decreased speed in processing information
- Difficulty with abstract information, such as identifying a main idea and understanding abstract concepts
- Disruption of newly learned language information (e.g., new vocabulary) due to long-term memory deficits
- Problems organizing complex or main ideas and information in verbal and written language
- Difficulties in word retrieval and rapid naming
- Ineffective, tangential, or socially inappropriate discourse
- Impaired coherence in discourse: fragmented, irrelevant, and lengthy utterances

Source: Based on Russell (1993).

common causes of brain injury. Risk factors include participating in contact sports or other recreational activities that may result in a fall or a collision and using drugs or alcohol during these activities or when driving or riding in vehicles. Adolescents who are new drivers are at increased risk for brain injury as well.

The potential for experiencing a brain injury has no social or economic boundaries. For example, skiing, which is a sport associated with affluence, places an individual at an increased risk for brain injury. Brain injuries occurred at a rate of about 0.77 per 100,000 ski visits to Colorado resorts from 1994 through 1997 (Diamond, Gale, & Denkhaus, 2001). Males were more likely to be injured than females, and children and older adults were also at increased risk. Of injured skiers, 24% experienced a skull fracture, and 79% experienced amnesia; their average hospital stay was 4.3 days. However, it is important to note that risks for brain injury are not evenly distributed within the population (Christensen et al., 2008). In fact, risks for brain injury are inversely related to income level, and we see higher rates of injury among those children who reside in low socioeconomic communities and homes. Some potential reasons for this include (1) increased exposure to faster moving traffic, (2) increased exposure to violence in the surroundings, (3) decreased supervision, and (4) less caregiver knowledge regarding preventive strategies (Rivara, 1994). Additionally, some research findings show that children who have certain learning and behavioral disabilities, including attention-deficit/hyperactivity disorder, have increased rates of brain injury (Gerring et al., 1998).

HOW ARE LANGUAGE DISORDERS IDENTIFIED? ●

THE ASSESSMENT PROCESS

DISCUSSION POINT:

Referral is a critical first step in beginning the assessment process. What are some barriers to referral? Consider the case of Alejandro in Case Study 6.1 in answering this question.

Identifying children who exhibit language disorders is a multistage process that often involves many team members working together at each stage of the process; team members often include speech-language pathologists, special and general educators, audiologists, pediatricians, psychologists, and parents. Referral and screening are the first steps in the process, followed by a comprehensive language evaluation to gather evidence concerning the extent of linguistic strengths and weaknesses. On the basis of this evidence, a diagnosis is made.

Referral

For children under 5 years of age, referral for language assessment is usually made by pediatricians in consultation with the children's parents. Generally, referrals are made because children exhibit a developmental or acquired disorder, such as Down syndrome or traumatic brain injury, that places them at increased risk for language problems or because warning signs signal the presence of a language disorder. By the time children enter their second year of life, they should be babbling often with a variety of consonants, using some gestures (e.g., pointing and showing), showing pleasure and excitement toward others, comprehending several common words (e.g., *daddy, mommy, bye-bye, up*), engaging in periods of joint sustained attention with others, and participating in vocal routines. For children between 1 and 5 years of age, delayed attainment of key language milestones is usually viewed as a warning sign of a possible language disorder and the need for referral.

Table 6.4 provides a checklist that can be used to determine whether infants, toddlers, and preschoolers are meeting milestones according to expectations. Children who are not displaying particular behaviors should be seen by their pediatricians to determine whether a referral for a comprehensive speech-language evaluation is needed. Although some pediatricians prefer to take a wait-and-see approach, children who show delays in attaining early communication milestones should always be referred for further evaluation by a speech-language specialist, particularly children who have a history of abuse or neglect, medical problems, developmental disability, trauma, hearing loss, exposure to drugs or

TABLE 6.4 Key milestones in early language development: A parent checklist	
Age	**Does Your Child . . . ?**
0–3 months	____ startle to loud sounds? ____ smile when spoken to? ____ seem to recognize your voice and quiet if crying? ____ increase or decrease sucking behavior in response to sound? ____ make pleasure sounds (cooing, booing)? ____ cry differently for different needs? ____ smile when seeing you?
4–6 months	____ move eyes in direction of sounds? ____ respond to changes in tone of your voice? ____ notice toys that make sounds? ____ pay attention to music? ____ produce babble that sounds more speechlike with many different sounds, including *p*, *b*, and *m*? ____ vocalize excitement and displeasure? ____ make gurgling sounds when left alone and when playing with you?
6 months–1 year	____ enjoy games like peekaboo and pat-a-cake? ____ turn and look in direction of sounds? ____ listen when spoken to? ____ recognize words for common items like *cup, shoe, juice*? ____ respond to some requests? ____ produce babble that has both long and short groups of sounds such as "tata upup bibibibi"? ____ use speech or noncrying sounds to get and keep attention? ____ imitate different speech sounds? ____ have 1 or 2 words (*bye-bye, dada, mama, no*) although they may not be clear?
1–2 years	____ point to pictures in a book when named? ____ point to a few body parts when asked? ____ follow simple commands and understand simple questions ("Roll the ball," "Kiss the baby," "Where's your shoe?")? ____ listen to simple stories, songs, and rhymes? ____ say more words every month? ____ use some 1–2-word questions ("Where kitty?" "Go bye-bye?" "What's that?")? ____ put 2 words together ("more cookie," "no juice," "mommy book")? ____ use many different consonant sounds at the beginning of words?
2–3 years	____ understand differences in meaning (*go/stop, in/on, big/little, up/down*)? ____ follow two requests ("Get the book and put it on the table")? ____ have a word for almost everything? ____ use 2–3-word sentences to talk about and ask for things? ____ produce speech that is understood by familiar listeners most of the time? ____ often ask for or direct attention to objects by naming them?

(*continued*)

TABLE 6.4	(continued)
Age	**Does Your Child . . . ?**
3–4 years	_____ hear you when you call from another room? _____ hear television or radio at the same loudness level as other family members? _____ understand simple who, what, where questions? _____ talk about activities at school or at friends' homes? _____ usually talk easily without repeating syllables or words? _____ produce speech that people outside the family are able to understand? _____ use a lot of sentences that have 4 or more words?
4–5 years	_____ pay attention to a short story and answer simple questions about it? _____ hear and understand most of what is said at home and in school? _____ use sentences that give lots of details (e.g., "I like to read my books.")? _____ tell stories that stick to a topic? _____ communicate easily with other children and adults? _____ say most sounds correctly except a few like *I, s, r, z, j, ch, sh, th*? _____ use adultlike grammar?

Source: From "How Does Your Child Hear and Talk?" Retrieved October 1, 2004, from www.asha.org/. Copyright 2004 by American Speech-Language-Hearing Association. Reprinted with permission.

DISCUSSION POINT:

Infants can be screened for early indicators of language disorder (e.g., slow start in babbling, few gestures, and limited periods of joint attention). What are some other possible indicators? If you were interviewing La'Kori's mother (Case 5) about his early communication development, what questions would you ask?

other poisons, or any other significant risk factor (Paul, 1996). There is no good reason to wait and see when the topic is a young child's health and development.

Once children enter school, referrals for language evaluation are usually made by classroom teachers or by other school personnel. Language disorders are not always readily recognizable, however. Speech-language pathologists and other knowledgeable specialists can provide in-service workshops and develop referral checklists (see Figure 6.7) to help teachers recognize signs of possible language difficulties (Paul, 2002). There are a range of Kindergarten readiness screening tools available that include examination of language as well, such as the Early Development Instrument, portions of which are presented in Table 6.5.

Screening

Screening should follow referral to determine the need for a comprehensive language assessment. After the referral, a speech-language pathologist, a special educator, or another trained professional may administer a screening tool that is specially designed to efficiently and effectively determine whether a child has difficulties using or understanding language (Paul, 2002). Some formal tests, such as the Early Screening Profiles (Harrison et al., 1990) and the Denver II (Frankenburg et al., 1990) are available for this purpose and can be administered in about 10 or 15 minutes.

If a child does not achieve a benchmark score on such screening tests, then a full evaluation is conducted to determine whether a language disorder is present and, if so, what the nature and type of language difficulty is. If the child passes the screening test, a full evaluation is not conducted. Obviously, then, the quality of a screening test is important. Children who pass a screening test but show minor communication difficulties or exhibit significant developmental risk factors should be continually monitored, with screening repeated every 3 to 6 months for children under 3 years and every 6 to 12 months for children between 3 and 5 years (Paul, 1996).

Many preschools and kindergarten programs regularly conduct language screening when children enter these programs. In such cases, all children in a particular program are administered a brief language screening; children who

FIGURE 6.7

Example of a referral checklist for teachers of older students.

Does the student's language or communication exhibit:

_____ 1. Insufficient information: Student does not provide the amount or type of information needed by listener.

_____ 2. Nonspecific vocabulary: Student uses pronouns, proper nouns, and possessives without supplying appropriate referents. Student overuses generic terms like _thing_ and _stuff._

_____ 3. Informational redundancy: Student continues to stress a point or relate a fact even when the listener has acknowledged its reception.

_____ 4. Need for repetition: Student requires repetition of material for accurate comprehension even though material is not difficult.

_____ 5. Poor topic maintenance: Student makes rapid and inappropriate changes in topic without providing transitional cues to listener.

_____ 6. Inappropriate response: Student makes responses that are radically unpredictable interpretations of meaning.

_____ 7. Failure to ask relevant questions: Student does not seek clarification of material that is unclear.

_____ 8. Situational inappropriateness: Student produces utterances that are irrelevant to the discourse and the situation.

_____ 9. Linguistic nonfluency: Student's language use is disrupted by frequent repetitions, pauses, and hesitations.

_____ 10. Frequent revision: Student speaks with many false starts and self-interruptions.

_____ 11. Delay in responding: Student responds to utterances following pauses of inordinate length.

_____ 12. Turn-taking difficulty: Student does not attend to cues indicating the appropriate exchange of conversational turns.

_____ 13. Failure to structure discourse: Student's speech lacks forethought and organizational planning.

_____ 14. Inappropriate intonation: Student uses inappropriate vocal intensity, pitch levels, and inflectional contours.

Source: From "Clinical Discourse Analysis: A Functional Approach to Language Assessment" by J. S. Damico, 1991, in C. S. Simon, _Communication Skills and Classroom Success,_ Eau Claire, WI: Thinking Publications. Copyright 1991 by Thinking Publications. Reprinted with permission.

do not pass the screening are referred for a more comprehensive language evaluation. However, because language screening programs are uncommon after kindergarten, it is important that classroom teachers are well aware of warning signs for possible language difficulties.

Comprehensive Language Evaluation

A comprehensive assessment determines whether a language disorder is indeed present. The language evaluation develops a profile of linguistic strengths and weaknesses and identifies needed supports for improving language form, content, and use. A comprehensive language evaluation includes a case history, an interview, a comprehensive analysis of language skills and communicative behaviors, and an evaluation of collateral areas of performance.

Case History. The case history involves a questionnaire administered to parents by an examiner or completed on their own. Older children can also provide information, but parents are always important to document children's

TABLE 6.5	Kindergarten readiness screen: Early Development Instrument, sample language items			
How would you rate this child's . . .	Very Good/ Good	Average	Poor/Very Poor	Don't Know
1. Ability to use language effectively in English				
2. Ability to listen in English				
3. Ability to tell a story				
4. Ability to take part in imaginative play				
5. Ability to communicate own needs in a way understandable to adults and peers				
6. Ability to understand on first try what is being said to him/her				
7. Ability to articulate clearly, without sound substitutions				

Source: From Early Development Instrument, Offord Centre for Child Studies, McMaster University, Hamilton Health Sciences Corporation. ©2007. Reprinted with permission.

DISCUSSION POINT:
When interviewing older students, it is important that students are fully informed of the reason for the interview. Students should be guided through a self-assessment that allows them to identify areas in which they excel, areas in which they do fine, and areas in which they need help. Why is this important?

history of early and later language skills. The questionnaire examines a child's developmental history and gathers information about general health; medical conditions and allergies; family size and resources; the child's language and communicative history; current skills, interests, and behaviors; and the parents' and the child's perceptions of suspected problems.

Interview.   Personal interviews are an important part of the evaluation process. For infants, toddlers, and preschoolers, a parent interview follows the case history to focus on particular issues identified in the case history, to further explore parental perceptions of the child's language difficulties, and to determine parental goals for the evaluation. For older children, interviews with teachers and the child are critical for developing an accurate profile of the child's language abilities.

Comprehensive Language Analysis.   To be comprehensive, a language evaluation must be broad-based and functional and use multiple methods of inquiry.

A **broad-based assessment** examines all domains of language (form, content, use) in both comprehension and production. For younger children who are not yet talking, a broad-based evaluation can examine the development of critical language precursors, including babbling, gesturing, affect and expression, participation in early communicative routines, and periods of joint attention. For older children, a broad-based assessment examines both oral and written language skills—including reading, writing, and spelling—and performance on classroom and curriculum-based tasks.

A **functional assessment** characterizes the extent to which children's language skills impact their ability to function in home, school, and community environments. For young children, the assessment must examine their ability to use language skills to get their needs met through various communicative functions, including requesting objects and actions; expressing feelings of interest, pleasure, and excitement; responding to the questions, requests, and comments of others; and using social behaviors, such as greeting (Halliday, 1975). For older children, the language assessment must examine the extent to which their language skills impact their ability to participate in the school curriculum and to interact effectively with friends, teachers, and parents.

An assessment that uses multiple methods of inquiry involves a variety of assessment tools, including criterion-referenced and norm-referenced tests, dynamic assessment, and observational measures. Criterion-referenced tasks examine the level of performance on a particular type of language task against a standard, or criterion, such as the percentage of one-step directions the child can correctly follow. Norm-referenced tasks examine the level of language performance against a national sample of same-age peers. Dynamic assessment examines children's performance with different types of assistance, providing valuable information about what kinds of supports are needed to optimize children's language performance. Observational measures examine children's language form, content, and use in naturalistic activities with peers or parents. Particularly important is an examination of children's conversational skills—the ability to initiate conversation, to take turns, to maintain topics, to identify breakdowns in conversation, and to attend to listener needs.

For older children, language assessment must also include curriculum-based assessment, which examines their strengths and weaknesses in participating in the academic curriculum. Methods of curriculum-based assessment include classroom observations of children's ability to work independently, work collaboratively with peers, complete assignments, and gain information from lectures and other assignments. Curriculum-based assessment also involves close examination of curriculum artifacts, including assignments and tests.

Evaluation of Collateral Areas.   To determine whether other difficulties may be present that impact a child's development of language, the language evaluation should screen cognitive skills, oral-motor structure and function, and hearing. If any of these areas are not developing appropriately, a more comprehensive evaluation by a specialist or other team member may be warranted.

Cognitive abilities can be estimated by examining play development for younger children; play and cognitive achievements are highly interrelated. Table 6.6 provides an overview of the major milestones in early play development that may guide the screening process. For older children, a formal cognitive screening may be administered, such as the Kaufman Brief Intelligence Test (Kaufman & Kaufman, 1990). Oral-motor structures are screened by examining the structures of the lips, teeth, and oral cavity (e.g., hard and soft palate), whereas oral-motor function involves children's ability to use the oral structures for different purposes. Screening of function might involve asking children to purse their lips, blow a bubble, lick a lollipop, and repeat the sound sequence "puh-puh-puh," among other tasks. A hearing screening is a quick check of hearing acuity.

Diagnosis

How does one determine whether a language disorder is indeed present? The answer to this million-dollar question comes through careful consideration of the evidence gained through the case history, interviews, comprehensive evaluation of all areas of language performance, and screening of collateral areas. An evaluation of the evidence indicates whether observed problems are serious

> **DISCUSSION POINT:**
> Curriculum-based assessment examines students' linguistic strengths and weaknesses when performing authentic academic tasks in the classroom. What are some examples of authentic academic tasks?

TABLE 6.6	Milestones in early play development
6–12 months	Handles objects with simple motor schemes (banging, mouthing) Drops objects (e.g., spoon after eating) Bangs two objects together Acquires objects on own (e.g., desired toy) Gives object to another Pushes a ball
By 12 months	Is aware objects exist when not seen Uses some toys appropriately (without mouthing or banging) Explores moving parts of toys Finds a hidden toy
By 18 months	Dumps objects out of containers Places objects into containers Hands toy to adult for assistance Attends to operating components of toys (buttons, knobs) Discovers how to use toys through exploration Uses toys appropriately (e.g., pushes car) Engages in symbolic play with self (e.g., pretends to eat pretend food)
By 24 months	Engages in symbolic play with toys (e.g., brushes doll's hair, feeds doll) Combines two toys in sequenced actions (e.g., pours from pot to cup) Imitates familiar routines (e.g., sweeps, irons, reads) Refers to toys not present Uses books and other literacy props in play (e.g., pretends to write)
By 30 months	Represents personally experienced events, including those that occur infrequently (e.g., going to the doctor, going to grandparents' house) Re-creates sequences during play (e.g., take baby's clothes off, put baby in bath, dry baby, dress baby) Uses considerable language during play, including questions (e.g., what, why, when)
By 36 months	Engages in role play with toys (stuffed animals, dolls) and other children Uses toys to act out scenarios or plays Acts out scenarios in which child was not directly involved (e.g., a firefighter fighting a fire) Engages in highly imaginative play (e.g., exploring planets on a spaceship)

Sources: Westby (1980); Widerstrom (2005).

DISCUSSION POINT:

A prognosis statement might differ for children who make quick progress versus those who progress more slowly. What other factors might influence prognosis? Consider the case of Natasha in Case Study 6.1 in answering this question.

enough to be considered significantly different from normal and ensures that observed problems are not the result of cultural or linguistic factors. Once the decision is made that a language disorder is present, the diagnosis usually designates the type of impairment (primary, secondary), impacted domains (form, content, or use; comprehension or production), and the severity (mild, moderate, severe, profound). Additionally, diagnosis may include a prognosis statement; a good prognosis states that a disorder is likely to resolve, whereas a poor prognosis states that a disorder is unlikely to resolve. In some cases, professionals withhold a statement of prognosis, pending further information from other specialists or a period of observing how children respond to treatment.

THE IMPORTANCE OF ACCURATE DIAGNOSIS

The importance of accurately determining whether a child has a language disorder cannot be overemphasized. Of two possible scenarios for inaccurate diagnosis, one is that of a **false-positive,** meaning that a child who does not have a language disorder is diagnosed as having one. The other scenario is a **false-negative,** whereby a child who has a language disorder is not accurately identified as having one.

Misdiagnoses happen for a variety of reasons. False-positives can occur because of poorly constructed tests or tests that are biased in cultural or linguistic factors. In addition, children may perform poorly during a language evaluation because of illness, fatigue, or shyness or because they have another condition (e.g., behavioral problem, attention deficit disorder) that shares characteristics with language disorders (e.g., difficulty following directions). There is also the alarming tendency of professionals to misdiagnose language differences as language disorders. Children who speak a nonstandard dialect of English or who are learning English as a second language may be diagnosed as language disordered when, in fact, their underlying language capabilities are culturally, linguistically, and age appropriate. This problem is at least partly to blame for the overrepresentation of children from diverse linguistic, racial, or ethnic backgrounds in special education (Rueda & Windmueller, 2006).

What are the implications of a false-positive? First, children receive a label that is inappropriate and that may have serious and practical consequences, including the possibility that the children will be stigmatized by their peers or that educators may hold low expectations for them (Heward, 2003). Second, children inaccurately diagnosed with a language impairment are likely to receive speech-language services to remediate their perceived language problems. Treatment for a language disorder is an expensive and time-consuming process on the part of the health and educational professionals involved, as well as the children and their families. And providing services to children who do not need them may keep those services away from children and families who really do need the help.

False-negatives happen for many of the same reasons that false-positives occur, including the use of poorly constructed tests or tests that are inappropriate for children of a particular cultural, ethnic, or language group. In addition, for children who have other disorders (e.g., mental retardation, attention deficit disorder), a clinician may mistakenly view poor language performance as a result of that disorder rather than as evidence of a language disorder.

The implications of a false-negative are also of serious consequence to the child and family affected. Children with a language disorder that is not identified do not receive the services to which they are entitled by federal law. Thus, these children are denied the services that might help them overcome or at least better cope with their disorders.

When assessing the language skills of children and adolescents who are culturally and linguistically diverse (CLD), including English language learners, it is particularly important that professionals look very closely at language performance within the classroom. Some children's observed challenges with language may stem not from a language disability per se, but rather from their lack of understanding of how to perform pragmatically within classrooms designed for a mainstream culture. They may not know, for instance, "what to say to whom, how it is to be said, why it is said, when, and in what situations" (Brice, 2002, p. 107). Observations of CLD students in mainstream American classrooms using the Adolescent Pragmatics Screening Scale (APS; Brice, 2002) have shown that they exhibit language behaviors that can look similar to those of children with language impairment, including difficulties with making requests to others and listening to speakers (Brice, 1992). Sample items of the APS examine students' abilities to

1. ask for a favor of a friend/classmate;
2. ask for help;

> **DISCUSSION POINT:**
> A false-negative occurs when a child with a language disorder is identified as developing typically in language. What are some reasons this might occur?

3. ask for teachers' or adults' permission;
4. describe personal feelings in acceptable manner; and
5. stay on topic for an appropriate amount of time.

If a student who is from a nonmainstream cultural or linguistic group is going through the assessment process, the SLP can directly observe these types of classroom behaviors and then provide instruction in them. Students who make rapid progress in the context of such direct instruction may be more likely to have a language difference than a language impairment.

HOW ARE LANGUAGE DISORDERS TREATED? ●

The nature of a child's language impairment drives the treatment. In other words, difficulty with language form requires a treatment approach focused on developing form; if problems are severe, the treatment approach will be more intensive than it will be if problems are mild. A child whose language disorder is secondary to autism will receive a treatment approach distinct from that of a child whose language disorder is secondary to traumatic brain injury. Treatment approaches are tailored to the unique needs of individual children in terms of targets, strategies, and contexts.

TARGETS, STRATEGIES, AND CONTEXTS

Treatment Targets

Treatment targets are the elements of language that are addressed during intervention. For instance, a treatment target for a 2-year-old child might be to produce two-word utterances to communicate needs, whereas a treatment target for an adolescent might be to comprehend figurative language (e.g., jokes heard on the playground). A treatment target for a young child with autism might be to communicate nonverbally for a variety of purposes (e.g., to request, reject, comment), whereas a treatment target for a first grader with traumatic brain injury might be to answer questions with appropriate, on-topic responses. Some professionals may emphasize only one or two targets at a time, whereas others may target many goals at once.

Treatment Strategies

Treatment strategies describe the manner in which treatment targets are addressed. **Child-centered approaches** are those in which the child is "in the driver's seat" (Paul, 1995, p. 68). The child sets the pace and chooses the materials, and the professional seeks ways to facilitate language form, content, or use in the context of child-selected activities. One example of a child-centered treatment approach is *focused stimulation* (Cleave & Fey, 1997; Ellis Weismer & Robertson, 2006; Girolametto, Pearce, & Weitzman, 1996). With focused stimulation, the adult provides multiple and highly salient models of language targets that are goals for the child. For instance, if a child is not able to request using the word *want,* the clinician would set up communication temptations in the context of play-based interactions to entice the child to use the word *want.* The clinician would also model use of this word repeatedly ("I want the cookie," "The boy wants candy," "The dog wants the bone"). To make the word stand out, the clinician might say it loudly, slowly, or with dramatic pitch changes (Fey, Long, & Finestack, 2003). During focused stimulation, the child is not required to

SPOTLIGHT ON LITERACY

Reading Development among Children and Adolescents with Down Syndrome

Historical perspectives of reading development took a "reading readiness" approach, which views strong oral language skills as a necessary precursor to reading instruction. Consequently, for many children with significant disorders of language, including those with Down syndrome, this meant that reading instruction was delayed if not absent completely from their academic curriculum. Current perspectives of reading development recognize that reading—or at least its important precursors— begins to develop at birth and can be supported in children simultaneous to their achievement of a strong language foundation.

With appropriate supports, ideally to begin soon after birth, many children with Down syndrome can become proficient readers. Typically, the reading skills of persons with Down syndrome will be similar to those of children of the same "mental age" (i.e., similar in nonverbal intelligence; Boudreau, 2002). Therefore, a 15-year-old adolescent with Down syndrome and a 7-year-old typically developing child would exhibit similar patterns of reading skill if they are matched on nonverbal intelligence. Given that the typical 7-year-old reads at a second- or third-grade reading level and is certainly able to use reading skills for a variety of functional purposes, this means that many individuals with Down syndrome can become proficient readers. In fact, survey data suggest that the majority of adults with Down syndrome have reading skills at a fourth- to sixth-grade level (Trenholm & Mirenda, 2006).

Professionals who work with parents of young children with disabilities, including Down syndrome, must support parents' understanding of the importance of encouraging reading development from birth forward. Even during infancy and toddlerhood, children can begin to develop an awareness of the organization and use of storybooks and the many purposes of print in the environment. Some survey data have suggested that parents of children with significant disabilities may provide fewer opportunities for their children to engage in home literacy activities, including reading storybooks to them (Skibbe, Justice, Zucker, & McGinty, 2008). Although children with disabilities may have exposure to many reading and writing materials in the home environment, it is possible that parents may be unsure of how to use these materials to support their children's early reading development (Trenhold & Mirenda, 2006). Professionals can work closely with parents to provide them with materials to support their children's reading development in the home environment as well as information about their role in promoting the likelihood that their children will become lifelong readers.

respond at all; however, the parent or professional arranges the environment and uses verbal techniques to *entice* the child's verbal participation and use of language targets. Focused stimulation and other child-centered strategies are often used with young children (infants and preschoolers) and can be implemented by parents in the home following training by a professional (Ellis Weismer & Robertson, 2006).

Clinician-directed approaches are those in which the adult (i.e., therapist, teacher, parent) is in the driver's seat. The adult selects the activities and materials and sets the pace of instruction. Rather than waiting for opportunities to occur that address a particular treatment target, the clinician deliberately structures a therapy session for frequent, ongoing opportunities for the child to experience and practice a form, content, or use target. Clinician-directed approaches are useful for older children in particular and can be used to target skills that arise infrequently in naturalistic communications. These approaches are also used to teach children with language disorders how to apply strategies to compensate for underlying challenges with language comprehension and production.

A strategy is the way an individual approaches a task; it includes both cognitive and behavioral components—that is, how one thinks and acts when doing something. Strategy training can be an effective way to improve children's abilities with diverse language tasks, such as understanding jokes, initiating conversation with friends or adults, or deciphering unknown words when reading. Strategy instruction focuses on teaching students specific ways to approach a linguistic task. Figure 6.8 shows the typical sequence of strategy instruction and ways to maximize its success.

Treatment Contexts

Treatment contexts describe the settings in which treatment targets and strategies are used. Treatment contexts should include as many settings as possible to promote generalization of skills learned in treatment—that is, the application of skills to many diverse settings. For instance, children may experience treatment targets and strategies at home with their parents, in the classroom with their teachers,

DISCUSSION POINT:
Home-based interventions are also useful for observing the quality of parent-child interactions, including maternal and child affect, mood, proximity, and initiations and responses to one another. What would this information tell us? If you were conducting a home visit to document Diana's (Study 1) interaction with her parents, what would you look for?

FIGURE 6.8

Stages in strategy instruction.

Stage 1: Pretest and make commitments

- Give rationale and overview, administer pretest, describe the strategy, discuss results others have achieved, ask for a commitment to learn the new strategy

Stage 2: Describe the strategy

- Describe situations in which the strategy can be used, describe the overall strategic process, set goals for learning the strategy, discuss self-instruction

Stage 3: Model the strategy

- Review previous learning, state expectations, present the strategy using think-aloud and self-monitoring, perform task while student observes, check student understanding

Stage 4: Verbal elaboration and rehearsal

- Have student describe intent of strategy and the process involved, have student describe each step and what it is designed to do, work until student is automatic in describing each step

Stage 5: Controlled practice and feedback

- Review the strategy steps, prompt reports of strategy use and errors, prompt student completion of steps as teacher models, prompt increasing student responsibility, provide peer-mediated practice opportunities

Stage 6: Advanced practice and feedback

- Repeat last stage with grade-appropriate materials, fade prompts and cues for use and evaluation

Stage 7: Confirmation of acquisition and generalization commitments

- Congratulate student on meeting mastery, discuss achievements, explain goals of generalization, prompt commitment to generalize

Stage 8: Generalization

- Identify settings for strategy use, discuss how to remember to use strategy, prompt and monitor application to other settings, help other teachers cue use of strategy, help student set goals for long-term use

Source: From *Students with Learning Disabilities* (5th ed.) by Cecil D. Mercer, © 1997. Adapted by permission of Pearson Education, Inc., Upper Saddle River, NJ.

and in the clinic with their speech-language pathologists. Clearly, collaboration among parents, teachers, speech-language pathologists, and other professionals is critical for ensuring that treatment occurs in many contexts.

For many young children receiving language intervention, treatment is provided in the home environment, allowing parents to directly observe and even implement treatment targets and strategies. Home-based interventions are particularly prevalent for children under the age of 3 years who receive language therapy. The professional providing intervention comes to the child's house and collaborates with the child's parent(s) and possibly other professionals (e.g., a physical therapist). For older children, treatment is usually provided in the school setting—preschool, elementary, middle, or high school—although parental involvement remains important and should be pursued at all opportunities. Some children also receive language treatment in outpatient hospital clinics or private centers.

In the school setting, treatment contexts can vary. Although historically children have received language intervention in a pull-out model, in which language therapy was provided in a speech room, this model is less common today. Frequently, children receive language intervention through collaborative classroom-based models, with teachers and speech-language pathologists working together to target language goals within the classroom environment (Throneburg, Calvert, Sturm, Paramboukas, et al., 2000). Speech-language pathologists may work individually with children during small-group or center times, may team-teach particular lessons with teachers, or may train teachers to integrate special language enhancement techniques into their classroom instruction (DiMeo et al., 1998). Several research teams have attempted to identify the most effective venue for delivery of language intervention to children by comparing language gains for children who receive treatment in collaborative classroom-based settings versus the more traditional pull-out setting (Throneberg et al., 2000; Wilcox, Couri, & Caswell, 1991). These studies suggest that collaborative classroom-based settings may have larger impacts on children's language growth, although clearly more research is needed to understand how best to align treatment contexts to the individual needs of children.

THE TREATMENT PLAN

A treatment plan is the guide to a particular child's treatment targets, strategies, and contexts. A treatment plan is established following a comprehensive language evaluation and is updated periodically as children progress. For children who are served through public agencies governed by federal law—such as early intervention programs, public preschools, and elementary schools—the treatment plan can appear in two forms. An individualized family service plan (IFSP) is required to provide any early intervention services to infants and toddlers with disabilities. The IFSP states the frequency, intensity, method, location, and expected duration of services; it must be reviewed every 6 months and updated annually. An individualized education program (IEP) is used to provide special services to preschoolers and school-age children with disabilities. The IEP includes a series of measurable annual goals and short-term objectives and describes the services, programs, and aids the child will be provided to meet those objectives and goals. An annual goal for language might state that "by the end of the academic year, Juan will improve his receptive and expressive vocabulary skills to levels consistent with his chronological age."

INTERVENTION PRINCIPLES

Researchers are continually seeking more effective and efficient strategies for reducing or ameliorating the consequences of language disorders. This chapter presents 10 key research-based principles for providing effective treatments to children with language disorders: five principles focus on working with younger children (infants, toddlers, and preschoolers), and five focus on working with older children.

SPOTLIGHT ON TECHNOLOGY

Speech Recognition and Dictation Software

Professionals who serve children and adolescents with language disorders do a great deal of collecting, transcribing, and analyzing language samples. Language samples are a critical part of every diagnostic battery (used to identify presence of a language disorder) and are used to monitor a child or adolescent's progress over time toward specific language goals. With all this sampling, it is no wonder that speech-language professionals are exploring technologies that can decrease the time it takes to transcribe a sample, such as speech recognition and dictation software. This software, such as Dragon NaturallySpeaking, has been used in the medical profession as a way to increase the accuracy and efficiency of medical transcription (Zick & Olsen, 2002). To use this software, an individual spends about 30 minutes in a training session during which the software learns the individual's voice pattern. Subsequently, the software will prepare a written transcript of the individual's spoken input. The benefits are primarily time, in that people typically speak much faster than they type (about 140 versus 40 words per minute, on average); it is also quite accurate, achieving similar levels of accuracy as compared to professional transcriptionists (Zick & Olsen, 2002). For the purpose of language sampling, a professional would collect a language sample on audio or video. Then, he or she would listen to the sample and pause periodically at junctures (e.g., after a phrase or sentence) and repeat the content into the speech recognition software, as shown in the photo below. The resulting transcript would be about 99% accurate and potentially would have saved the professional a considerable amount of time.

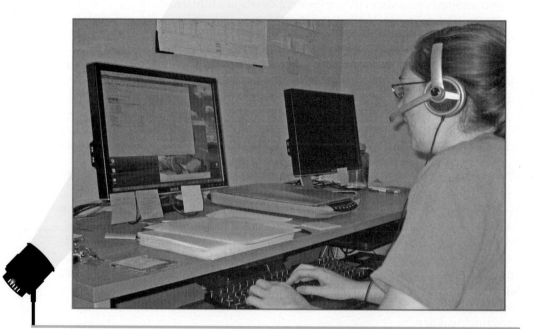

Intervention Principles for Infants, Toddlers, and Preschoolers

Key principles for providing language intervention to infants, toddlers, and preschoolers include early intervention, parental involvement, naturalistic environments, social interaction, and functional outcomes.

Early Intervention.   *Early intervention* refers to therapeutic interventions for children 3 years of age and under. Children receiving early intervention may have a developmental disorder, such as Down syndrome; an acquired disorder, such as a brain injury; or may be vulnerable for developing a disorder because of various risk factors. Early intervention is a primary prevention strategy aimed at keeping a disorder from developing at all or at least reducing its severity. Early intervention services, when applied in a timely and rigorous manner, can be very effective in both regards (Guralnick, 1997).

Critical to such efforts is identifying children with established disorders and those at risk for developing disorders as early as possible and enabling them to access needed therapeutic interventions. For some types of language disorders, such as SLI and autism, there may be a tendency to ignore early warning signs that can signal a possible problem with language development. Professionals and parents may be overly optimistic about the likelihood of problem resolution (Schuele & Hadley, 1999), or there may be a lack of information concerning early indicators of possible problems. Regardless, scientific evidence shows that early intervention is an effective route for reducing the negative outcomes associated with early language difficulties (Maclean & Cripe, 1997; Reynolds, Temple, Robertson, & Mann, 2001).

Parental Involvement.   Parental involvement is important for a variety of reasons when working with young children. First, the interactions between children and their primary caretakers are critical to developing firm language foundations (Tamis-LeMonda, Bornstein, & Baumwell, 2001). For instance, the number of words children experience in their interactions with family members contributes to how fast those children learn new words and what types of words they learn (Hart & Risley, 1995).

Second, parental involvement respects the role of parents in their children's lives. Involving parents in interventions helps professionals understand the values and beliefs of the families with whom they work. Third, parents can play key roles in language intervention programs (e.g., Kashinath, Woods, & Goldstein, 2006). Parents can be trained to use certain techniques when they interact with their children to stimulate development of important language skills. This is a cost-effective and family-centered way to provide early intervention treatments.

Naturalistic Environments.   The provision of services in children's most natural environments is an important part of working with young children. For many children receiving early intervention, therapists and special educators come to the home to provide treatment, and parents are hands-on partners. Working in the child's most natural environment promotes the child's sense of control and comfort and allows treatment to involve familiar activities and objects, thereby increasing the generalization of intervention to other situations of use. Working in the child's home also helps parents to learn specific language stimulation strategies. For example, a home-based interventionist might observe a mother and child eating lunch together and afterward suggest ways the mother can structure the mealtime routine to encourage the child's use of requesting behaviors. For medically fragile children, providing services in the home can also offer protection for their health (Rossetti, 2001).

DISCUSSION POINT:
Hart and Risley's book *Meaningful Differences* (1995) shows that the differences in language experienced by children can be large; for instance, in a given year, some children will hear about 11 million words, whereas others will hear only 3 million words. How important are these differences? Consider the case of Natasha in Case Study 6.1. What do you think the first 2 years of her life were like?

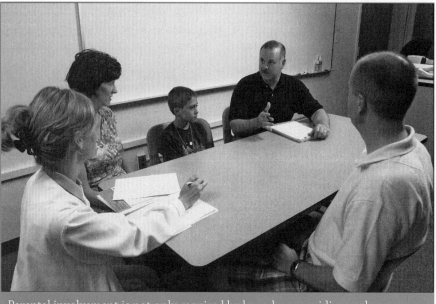

Parental involvement is not only required by law when providing early intervention services, but also respects the roles of parents as their children's first teachers.

Social Interaction.   A social interactionist account of language acquisition argues that language is learned through children's meaningful interactions with others. Social interaction creates opportunities for children to apply new language forms, content, and use. An important part of social interactionist perspectives is that therapies should embrace the communicative value of language; children need to be engaged in meaningful social interactions during which their use of emerging forms and functions is recognized as having communicative value. Social interactionist approaches would not value a speech-language pathologist or early childhood educator showing a young child a series of pictures and having the child repeat the name of each picture. Rather, engaging children in meaningful, authentic opportunities to communicate (e.g., asking for a real toy) is an integral part of therapies that embrace social interactionist accounts of language development (Kaderavek & Justice, 2002).

Functional Outcomes.   Language interventions for young children must target language outcomes that have real value—outcomes that improve children's ability to be valued members of home, school, and community. All language goals should apply directly to improving children's ability to communicate with others. For example, for a child struggling with grammatical development, a language goal that targets repetition of 10 noun phrases (*the* + *noun*) per therapy session has little direct functional value. The goal must have a functional aim that adds value to the contexts in which the child lives. For this child, the goal might be to use noun phrases to accurately specify the child's wants during mealtime routines (e.g., *the* + *milk, my* + *cup, big* + *bite*).

Intervention Principles for School-Age Children

The goals and techniques of language intervention with older children differ somewhat from those used with younger children. First of all, enlisting the support and commitment of older children is critical to the intervention process;

children who are unmotivated or who do not want to participate in therapeutic activities make it hard to achieve positive outcomes. Second, intervention goals shift for older children from primary prevention (i.e., keeping a disorder from manifesting) to secondary and tertiary prevention (i.e., helping children compensate for a disorder that is already present). Third, intervention for older children must be linked directly to the academic curriculum. Because children with language impairment are likely to struggle academically, improved academic performance should be a principal goal of intervention. And fourth, intervention with older children tends to move at a much slower pace than intervention with younger children. The rate of language acquisition slows as children age, and the types of skills that are targeted in later intervention are usually quite complex, requiring considerable time for learning to take place.

Five key principles for providing language intervention to older children include functional flexibility, curriculum access, career development, discourse-level skills, literacy achievement, and least restrictive environment.

Curriculum Access.   When working with adolescents with language impairment, it is critical that attention be paid to strengthening those aspects of language that will facilitate access to the academic curriculum. Once children enter the primary grades, they utilize their language skills to access the curriculum of science, social studies, literature, mathematics, and so forth. Language disorders can compromise learning across the curriculum; consequently, careful investigation of pupils' access to and participation in the general curriculum is necessary. As an example, learning experiences within a pupil's social studies curriculum may regularly feature higher-order language concepts, such as solving cause-and-effect problems in an economics unit (Coyne, Kame'enui, & Carnine, 2007). The student with a language disorder may have difficulty acquiring the economics concepts due to difficulty with the vocabulary that specifies causal relationships. Speech-language pathologists must work closely with content area educators, such as social studies teachers, to identify ways to mitigate the effects of language disorders upon curricular access.

Career Development.   Many occupations rely on effective communication skills for success. For adolescents with communication disorders, achieving gainful employment can be a particular challenge. Today, far too many students with disabilities do not complete high school, which lowers one's likelihood of successful employment and long-term earning potential (National High School Center, 2007). Currently, the federal regulations that govern the education of pupils with disabilities (Individuals with Disabilities Education Act, 2004) specifies the need to develop and monitor postsecondary/employment transition plans for students with disabilities, to begin at age 14. At this point, students begin to participate in career counseling and vocational assessments to help develop their transition plans. Speech-language professionals can play key roles in developing and monitoring these plans. They can, for instance, help students learn interviewing techniques, develop résumés, and participate in employment-setting role plays, among many other possibilities.

Discourse-Level Skills.   Language intervention for school-age children requires an intensive focus on discourse-level skills. *Discourse* refers to the stream of language that occurs when a person produces a series of sentences, as in relating a personal event or a fictional story (narrative) or participating in a conversation. Too often, language intervention focuses on smaller units of language—such as the word, the sound, or a part of speech—rather than on the child's ability to use language for narrative and conversational purposes.

Discourse is the unit of language used in the curriculum; *instructional discourse* refers to the exchanges that occur in the classroom between teachers and students. The goal of instructional discourse is to teach—to give new information and to teach new skills (Merritt, Barton, & Culatta, 1998). However, instructional discourse can be very challenging to children with language disorders, because it requires the integration of form, content, and use—all of which may be areas of weakness. Typically, classroom discourse is decontextualized, meaning that it is not accompanied by cues to help with meaning interpretation. Children must rely solely on their linguistic skills to interpret what is being relayed through the discourse.

Rather than focusing on discrete subcomponents of language, language intervention for school-age children needs to engage children at the level of instructional discourse (Brice, 2002). Indeed, intervention should provide them with ample opportunities to participate in discourse at various levels of complexity—conversation, narrative, and instructional discourse—with the interventionist providing supports to maximize the children's ability to participate and learn (Merritt et al., 1998).

Literacy Achievement.   Children with language disorders are more likely to struggle with reading and spelling. Language intervention should therefore help children develop skills that are critically linked to success in these areas. One area of particular difficulty for children with language impairment is phonological awareness (PA; Justice & Schuele, 2004). *Phonological awareness* is the ability to attend to the units of sound that make up running speech. A sentence, for instance, can be broken into a series of smaller sound units, including words, syllables, and phonemes. The phoneme is the smallest unit of sound, and in the English alphabetic system, the mapping between phonemes and graphemes (i.e., sounds and letters) is the key to unlocking the alphabetic system.

Children with language impairment tend to have problems with phonological awareness; during the preschool years, they are slower than other children to begin to play phonological awareness games (e.g., making rhymes; Magnusson & Naucler, 1993), and in the early elementary grades, they have difficulty identifying the number of phonemes in words. Figure 6.9 provides an overview of key developments in phonological awareness. Timely attainment of these skills helps children become successful readers.

Problems with phonological awareness contribute to the problems with reading and spelling that are prevalent among children with language disorders (Catts et al., 2001a, 2002). Integrating literacy goals into language intervention is becoming increasingly important for school-age children with language disorders. For instance, when working on specific speech targets, children can be prompted to think about the phonological composition of words (e.g., the word *wasp* has four sounds, and the word *wasps* has five sounds).

Another aspect of literacy to be addressed in language intervention is metalinguistic awareness. *Metalinguistic awareness* refers to the ability to focus on language as an object of scrutiny. When a teacher asks a child, "Is the word *caterpillar* a long word or a short word?" or tells the child to "circle all the nouns in this passage," these are metalinguistic tasks that require conscious reflection on language as an object of thought (Chaney,

FIGURE 6.9

Development of phonological awareness.

Stage I: Recognition that running speech can be broken into words (word awareness)

- Child can identify how many words are in a sentence.
- Child can clap with each word in a sentence.

Stage II: Recognition that multisyllabic words are made up of syllables (syllable awareness)

- Child can identify how many syllables are in a word.
- Child can delete the first or last syllable in a multisyllabic word.

Stage III: Recognition that syllables and one-syllable words can be divided into onset and rime* units

- Child can identify the first sound in a word.
- Child can match or produce words that rhyme.
- Child can segment the first sound from the rest of a syllable.

Stage IV: Recognition that syllables and words can be divided into a series of phonemes

- Child can identify how many sounds are in a word.
- Child can segment a word into all of its phonemes.
- Child can blend a series of phonemes into a syllable.

Sources: Based on Justice and Kaderavek (2004); Justice and Schuele (2004).

*Rime is a linguistic term. It is the part of a syllable that remains when the initial consonant(s) are removed (e.g., the rime of *dog* is "og," and the rime of *pay* is "ay").

1998; Justice & Ezell, 2001). Being able to scrutinize language is a highly abstract activity, one that does not come easily for children with language impairment. Providing frequent opportunities for children with language disorders to engage in metalinguistic tasks—with support and guidance—is an important aspect of language intervention for school-age children.

Least Restrictive Environment. Providing language intervention to children in the least restrictive environment (LRE) is federal law (IDEA 94-142). The law stipulates that children with disabilities are to be educated with their peers "to the maximum extent possible" (20 U.S.C 1412 [a][5]). Many children with language disorders receive their general education within regular classrooms but receive language intervention through pull-out therapies provided in a speech-language laboratory or resource room. This model has garnered a lot of criticism in recent years, because pull-out therapies remove children from the very context in which they need to learn to perform (Bashir, Conte, & Heerde, 1998).

The premise behind LRE, in contrast, is that children need to "learn, practice, and apply skills with their classmates in the communicative context of the classroom" (DiMeo et al., 1998, p. 39). Alternative models of language intervention are therefore receiving increased attention. These include providing therapy to children directly in their classrooms and using a consultant or collaborative model in which speech-language pathologists and teachers address children's language goals together.

DISCUSSION POINT:
Just the act of thinking about the meaning of the term *metalinguistic awareness* is itself a metalinguistic activity. Think of a metalinguistic activity that might take place in a preschool classroom, a first-grade classroom, and a third-grade classroom. Which children in the classroom would struggle with these activities?

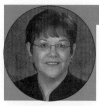

SPOTLIGHT ON RESEARCH AND PRACTICE

NAME: MARIA DIANA GONZALES, PH.D., CCC-SLP

PROFESSION/TITLE
*Chair and Associate Professor of the Department of Communication
Disorders at Texas State University–San Marcos*

PROFESSIONAL RESPONSIBILITIES
My responsibilities include managing and leading a department that offers undergraduate and graduate degrees in communication disorders. As department chair, additional duties include teaching, maintaining a research agenda, and engaging in departmental, college, university, and professional service.

A DAY AT WORK
I engage in numerous and varied activities to ensure that the department is in compliance with federal, state, and university standards. On any given day, I will need to meet with various constituents such as faculty, students, administrators, or community members. Even though I have scheduled appointments, I still need to be prepared for new and unplanned challenges each day.

HOW INTERESTS IN COMMUNICATION SCIENCES AND DISORDERS BEGAN
I first became interested in speech-language pathology when I completed an Introduction to Communication Disorders course that I took as an elective as a sophomore in college.

CURRENT RESEARCH AND PRACTICE INTERESTS
My research interests include the developmental outcomes of infants discharged from neonatal intensive care units. Additional research interests include the parent-child interaction skills exhibited by bilingual parents with typically developing and language disordered infants as well as the emergent literacy skills of typically developing and language disordered bilingual preschoolers.

MOST EXCITING/INTERESTING PROFESSIONAL ACCOMPLISHMENT IN CSD
My most exciting professional accomplishment has been the development and implementation of a bilingual/multicultural cognate in speech-language pathology at Texas State University–San Marcos in 2004. I was able to develop and implement this specialty track without external funding. Students who are bilingual (Spanish/English speakers) now have the opportunity to gain the necessary academic and clinical coursework to provide assessment and intervention services to bilingual clients who happen to have communication disorders.

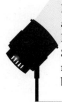

CASE ANALYSIS

Review the diagnostic report for Evan (Case Study 2) on the companion website at www.pearsonhighered.com/justice2e. Reflect on the possible long-term consequences of a childhood language disorder.

● CHAPTER SUMMARY

A language disorder refers to significant difficulties in the content, form, or use of spoken, written, or other symbol systems used for the purpose of communication. For a language disorder to be present, it must adversely impact an individual socially, psychologically, or educationally.

Language disorders are classified by etiology, manifestation, and severity. A primary language disorder describes an impairment attributable to no other cause, whereas a secondary impairment is caused by another primary source, such as hearing loss. Developmental disorders of language are present from birth; acquired disorders result from an insult or injury sometime after birth. Language disorders can affect comprehension, expression, or both. Disorders can affect all three domains of language (form, content, and use) or only one. These are described as diffuse and focal disorders, respectively.

Four of the most prevalent language disorders are specific language impairment (SLI), autism spectrum disorder (ASD), intellectual disability, and traumatic brain injury (TBI). SLI is a primary language impairment in which children show significant challenges with language development in the absence of any other known developmental difficulty. ASD is an umbrella term that encompasses four neurologically based developmental disorders characterized by disordered communication, repetitive behaviors, difficulties with social relationships, and restricted interests. Intellectual disability is a developmental disability associated with language disorders ranging from mild to profound. Language disorders resulting from TBI are typically characterized by discourse problems and additional executive difficulties.

A multistep assessment process includes referral, screening, comprehensive language evaluation, and diagnosis. Treatment principles for infants, toddlers, and preschoolers include early intervention, parental involvement, naturalistic environments, social interaction, and functional outcomes. Treatment principles for older children include career development, curriculum access, discourse-level skills, literacy achievement, and least restrictive environment.

● KEY TERMS

acquired language disorder, p. 183
adaptive behavior, p. 193
anoxia, p. 192
Asperger's syndrome, p. 191
autism spectrum disorder, p. 186
broad-based assessment, p. 202
child-centered approaches, p. 206
childhood disintegrative disorder, p. 191
clinician-directed approaches, p. 207

developmental language disorder, p. 183
diffuse disorder, p. 184
echolalia, p. 191
false-negative, p. 205
false-positive, p. 204
focal disorder, p. 184
functional assessment, p. 202
language delay, p. 181
language difference, p. 180
language disorder, p. 177
late talkers, p. 181
mixed receptive-expressive disorder, p. 184

primary language impairment, p. 182
screening, p. 200
secondary language impairment, p. 182
specific expressive language disorder (SELD), p. 183
specific language impairment, p. 186
stereotypical behaviors, p. 191
word-finding problems, p. 187

● ON THE WEB

Check out the Companion Website, www.pearsonhighered.com/justice2e. On it you will find:

- suggested readings
- reflection questions

- a self-study quiz
- links to additional online resources, including current technologies in communication sciences and disorders

ADULT LANGUAGE DISORDERS AND COGNITIVE-BASED DYSFUNCTION

Cynthia R. O'Donoghue
Carol C. Dudding

FOCUS QUESTIONS

This chapter answers the following questions:

1. What is aphasia?

2. How is aphasia classified?

3. What are the defining characteristics of aphasia syndromes?

4. How is aphasia identified and treated?

5. What are right-hemisphere dysfunction, traumatic brain injury, and dementia?

CHAPTER 7

INTRODUCTION

When stroke, progressive neurological disease, or tumors damage the tissues of the brain, one's ability to effectively accomplish everyday tasks—like watching a movie, reading the newspaper, and conversing with friends—is often compromised. This chapter describes language and cognitive disorders associated with acquired neurological injury, specifically aphasia, right-hemisphere damage, traumatic brain injury, and dementia.

Aphasia is an acquired language disorder that typically results from injury to the left cerebral hemisphere, most often due to a stroke. Difficulties in expressing, understanding, reading, or writing oral and written language are some characteristics of aphasia. *Right-hemisphere dysfunction* (RHD) is an acquired cognitive disorder associated with damage to the right cerebral hemisphere. Like aphasia, RHD can result from stroke, and typical symptoms include memory impairment, attention and impulsivity problems, and visual dysfunction. These symptoms are often accompanied by a lack of insight into or awareness of these problems. *Traumatic brain injury* (TBI) is another type of acquired neurological injury, which can result from car accidents, severe falls, and acts of violence. A variety of cognitive and linguistic difficulties can arise from TBI, with the symptoms varying based on the site and severity of the injury. *Dementia* describes a loss of linguistic and cognitive ability due to a progressive brain disease, such as Alzheimer's disease (AD). The linguistic and cognitive abilities of persons with dementia become increasingly affected as the disease progresses.

The language and cognitive-based problems associated with acquired neurological injury can have far-reaching consequences on a person's ability to live life in a full and meaningful way. This chapter provides an overview of adult communication problems following neurological injury that causes impairment of language or cognitive-based processes. The chapter first focuses on aphasia, which is primarily a disorder of language resulting from damage to the left hemisphere. The chapter then focuses on disorders of cognitive-based functions that affect communication, including RHD, TBI, and dementia. ●●●

| CASE STUDY 7.1 | **Adult Language and Cognitive-Based Dysfunction** |

RONNIE LAMM is a 68-year-old insurance agent retired from a successful career. He resides with his wife and has many family members living nearby. Ronnie experienced a left-hemisphere stroke approximately 10 years ago. At the time of his stroke, his medical evaluation revealed coronary artery disease, arteriosclerosis, hypertension, and three previous "ministrokes" from which he recovered fully. His communication profile immediately following his stroke fit a Broca's aphasia classification. He actively participated in speech-language therapy. He now communicates effectively but does experience hesitations when talking and difficulty recalling words. You can view his case on the companion CD-ROM (Study 2).

Internet research

1 Could Ronnie's word-retrieval errors be the result of the normal aging process?

2 What percentage of the current U.S. population is considered geriatric (over 65 years)?

3 What are some common warning signs of stroke?

Brainstorm and discussion

1 What are some reasons that survivors of stroke are at greater risk for depression?

2 How might the family dynamics in this scenario influence Ronnie's outcome?

3 Why do you think Ronnie did not recover fully from this stroke the way he did from the previous strokes?

● ● ●

THOMAS DRIVER is a 61-year-old, right-handed Caucasian male who recently suffered a left middle cerebral artery stroke. After Mr. Driver was initially stabilized at St. Patrick's Hospital's neurological intensive care unit, he was transferred to the rehabilitation unit. His current problems include right hemiparesis of the face, arm, and leg; visual field deficits; and communication difficulties. His past medical history reveals hypertension, elevated cholesterol, and noninsulin-dependent diabetes (adult onset, type 2), and tobacco use.

Mr. Driver is an architect who resides with his wife, Alice, of 40 years. They have four adult children, two of whom reside in the area. When time permits, Mr. Driver has enjoyed golfing and building model airplanes as hobbies. His goal is to return to his previous lifestyle at work and at home.

Internet research

1 What age group of the population is most at risk for experiencing a stroke?

2 How often do persons with strokes return to their jobs?

3 What information is available about leave of absence from gainful employment following a stroke?

Brainstorm and discussion

1 What psychological and social issues need to be considered by the rehabilitation team working with Thomas?

2 What factors in Thomas's life support his recovery and ultimate return to work?

WHAT IS APHASIA? ●

DEFINITION

Aphasia is a language disorder that is acquired sometime after an individual has developed language competence. Aphasia results from injury to the language functions of the brain. For most people, these language functions are contained in the left hemisphere, although for a small percentage of the population, the right hemisphere is language-dominant. The more common causes of neurological injury to the language-dominant hemisphere include stroke, infectious diseases such as meningitis or encephalitis, tumors, exposure to toxins or poisons, hydrocephalus, and nutritional or metabolic disorders. Of these, stroke is the neurological disorder that produces most aphasias. Stroke, also called a *cerebrovascular accident* (CVA), occurs when the blood supply providing nutrients and oxygen to the brain is interrupted by a blood clot or other clogging material in an artery serving the brain. Aphasia results when this interruption damages the tissue of the language areas of the brain (see Figure 7.1).

Aphasia literally means "the absence of language," or "without language." Although this suggests that the individual with aphasia has no language abilities, people with aphasia exhibit a broad range of language difficulties, from mild deficits to the most severe, in which an individual has few or no language functions. A classic definition of aphasia follows:

> A disturbance of one or more aspects of the complex process of comprehending and formulating verbal messages that results from newly acquired disease of the central nervous system. (A. Damasio, 1981, p. 51)

This early definition by Damasio is used frequently in the aphasia literature (Rao, 1994; Rosenbek, LaPointe, & Wertz, 1989). However, it does not clearly address two very important facts about aphasia. First, aphasia is not limited solely to problems of spoken language; it also encompasses disturbances in written language skills, including reading and writing. Second, the damage to the central nervous system can be more specifically defined; it interrupts the language-dominant hemisphere of the brain (Brookshire, 2003).

Therefore, a more comprehensive definition of aphasia includes these points:

1. Aphasia is a disturbance in the language system *after* language has been established or learned.

2. Aphasia results from neurological injury to the language-dominant hemisphere of the brain.

3. Aphasia includes disturbances of receptive or expressive abilities for spoken and written language.

It is important that aphasia be differentiated from other types of communication disorders, such as developmental disorders of language, psychiatric problems, and motor speech disorders. First, aphasia is not a developmental disorder. Rather, it is an acquired disruption in the language system following neurological injury. It most often affects adults who have experienced a stroke and thus is often considered an adult language disorder, although it can also affect children and adolescents who experience a stroke. Because aphasia is acquired later in life for most people, its symptoms vary widely across those affected as a function of premorbid factors, which are characteristics of a person before an illness, in this case the neurological injury. The way aphasia affects a person is influenced by such factors as health, emotional well-being, occupational and educational attainment, and language abilities.

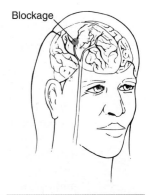

Blockage

FIGURE 7.1

Damage to the brain due to stroke.

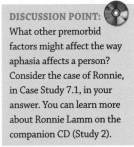

DISCUSSION POINT:
What other premorbid factors might affect the way aphasia affects a person? Consider the case of Ronnie, in Case Study 7.1, in your answer. You can learn more about Ronnie Lamm on the companion CD (Study 2).

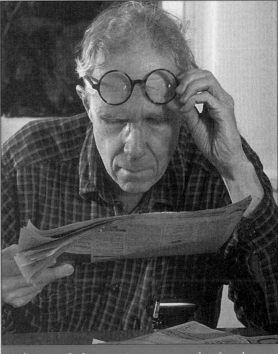

Aphasia includes impairment not only of spoken language but also of writing and reading.

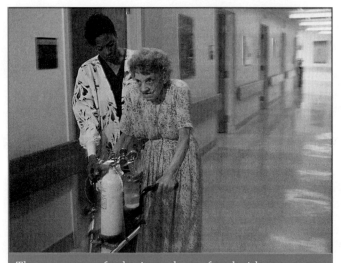

The symptoms of aphasia can be confused with symptoms of psychological disturbance.

DISCUSSION POINT:
Motor speech disorders often coexist with aphasia. Considering Thomas's case in Case Study 7.1, what information suggests that a motor speech disorder may be present as well as aphasia?

Second, aphasia is not a psychiatric problem, even though it has sometimes been misdiagnosed as such (Palmer, 1979; Sambunaris & Hyde, 1994). Some psychological disorders—such as psychosis, schizophrenia, or delirium—may yield bizarreness in language (H. Damasio, 2001) that can also occur with aphasia. For example, some language oddities, such as difficulty coming up with the names of objects, may be the residual effects of a stroke after other functions have returned but might be confused with signs of a psychological disturbance. A language deficit is not the same as a psychological disturbance, even though the symptoms of both may, at times, appear similar. Thus, it is important that the language weaknesses of persons with aphasia are not mistaken for a more general psychological disturbance.

Third, aphasia is not a motor speech disorder. *Motor speech disorders,* as discussed in this text, refer to an inability to plan, program, or execute the motor movements required for efficient, intelligible speech production as a result of neurological deficits. **Dysarthria** is a motor speech disorder characterized by disruption in the range, speed, direction, timing, and strength of movements in the respiratory, phonatory, articulatory, or resonatory components of speech. **Apraxia,** another motor speech disturbance, is a difficulty in planning and executing the volitional movements of speech. Aphasia is a language-based, not a motor-based, dysfunction, but the symptoms of dysarthria, apraxia, and aphasia can similarly impact a person's ability to communicate effectively. Additionally, motor speech disturbances often coexist with aphasia, thus challenging professionals to identify which aspects of an individual's communication are undermined by motor speech problems and which by aphasia.

PREVALENCE AND INCIDENCE

Stroke, or CVA, is the cause of most aphasias. The National Stroke Association reports that a stroke occurs every 45 seconds in the United States, with approximately 750,000 citizens suffering strokes each year. The estimate of the total number of surviving stroke victims is 4 million in the United States alone. The associated health care costs are staggering, consuming about $60 billion annually.

TYPES OF STROKES

Strokes occur when the blood circulating to the brain is disrupted, thereby robbing the brain tissue of the oxygen it needs to function properly. There are two major types of CVAs. **Ischemic strokes** happen when the blood supply to the brain is inhibited because of an occlusion (blockage) somewhere in an artery. An ischemic stroke can occur because of a thrombosis or an embolism. A stationary ischemic blockage, or **thrombosis,** occurs when plaque builds up in an artery and eventually closes it off, prohibiting the flow of blood. A traveling ischemic blockage, or **embolism,** occurs when a piece of accumulated plaque breaks off of an artery and then migrates from larger arteries into smaller arteries where it ultimately will lodge, blocking the flow of blood. In contrast to the ischemic strokes,

hemorrhagic strokes result when a blood vessel or artery ruptures and excessive amounts of blood enter the brain. These occur less often than ischemic strokes. Both ischemic and hemorrhagic strokes have similar underlying risk factors.

RISK FACTORS

Risk factors for stroke, and subsequent aphasia, include both uncontrollable factors (those beyond an individual's control) and modifiable factors (those that can be controlled). Uncontrollable risk factors include age, gender, racial or ethnic background, and family history. Risk for stroke increases with age. In fact, for each decade over 55 years, the risk for stroke doubles. African Americans are twice as likely to suffer a stroke as are European Americans, and males are at greater risk than females. These are not factors a person can change.

> **DISCUSSION POINT:**
> Consider Thomas's case in Case Study 7.1. What are his controllable and uncontrollable risk factors?

Controllable, or modifiable, risk factors include hypertension (i.e., high blood pressure), diabetes, tobacco smoking, and alcohol use. With behavioral changes, these factors can decrease the likelihood of a stroke occurring. For example, lifestyle changes, such as improving eating habits and exercise, as well as pharmaceutical intervention, can often improve symptoms of hypertension. And diabetes, although incurable, can be managed so that blood sugar levels remain within more normal ranges. Alleviating or reducing tobacco and alcohol use also decreases the risk of stroke. The National Stroke Association (NSA), the National Aphasia Association (NAA), and the National Institute on Neurological Disorders and Stroke (NINDS) are just a few of the many organizations working diligently on issues of stroke prevention, assessment, and treatment.

HOW IS APHASIA CLASSIFIED? ●

Aphasia is a global term used to describe language disorders following neurological injury. The way in which language is affected varies widely based on the location of the damage to the brain. Thus, aphasia is differentiated into different types according to the location of the damage and the language-disorder symptoms that occur. This classification system for the aphasias is known as **taxonomy;** it draws upon those characteristics of aphasia that most differentiate disorders from one another and is similar to the way we might classify automobiles. Although automobiles might be grouped by year and color, the most useful taxonomy would use the factors that best differentiate one car from another. For example, saying, "I have a red car made in 1965" tells us much less than "I have a 1965 red Mustang convertible." Similarly, to differentiate aphasias, we need to describe each profile by using the most important factors.

Historically, there has been great debate over the best taxonomy by which to characterize aphasia. Some experts have advocated using the "locus of the lesion and the set of behavioral characteristics" (Rosenbek et al., 1989, p. 40) to differentiate aphasias. In this approach, aphasia would be categorized by the cause and location of the brain damage, also called the *site of the lesion.* Based on this taxonomy, we would describe Ronnie in Case Study 7.1 as having an aphasia resulting from an infarct (i.e., damage) affecting the superior portion of the frontal lobe. The illustration in Figure 7.2 contrasts the effects of anterior and posterior sites of injury, which result in different kinds of aphasia symptoms.

Other experts prefer taxonomies based on the language skills, both strengths and weaknesses, that characterize the aphasia (Goodglass & Kaplan,

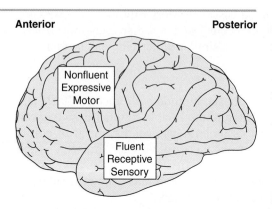

Anterior   **Posterior**

Nonfluent
Expressive
Motor

Fluent
Receptive
Sensory

1983). Such taxonomy categorizes the aphasia by the most prominent language characteristics. For instance, this system might differentiate aphasias into those that result in nonfluent speech (i.e., short, choppy utterances) and those that result in fluent speech (i.e., long, flowing utterances that are devoid of content).

Both of these approaches carry advantages and disadvantages. The most discriminating taxonomy differentiates aphasias by both the behavioral symptoms and the site of the lesion, and knowledgeable clinicians use all relevant factors when assessing and treating those patients with aphasia.

BEHAVIORAL SYMPTOMS

A person with aphasia has an impairment of language. With this noted, it might be the only thing that two people with aphasia have in common. Indeed, the way acquired impairments of language are expressed varies widely across individuals. Some persons with aphasia are unable to initiate speech at all; others can initiate speech well but produce extended, flowery monologues that seem void of content and contain odd names for things. Still others with aphasia show relatively few symptoms of language impairment but cannot seem to retrieve the names of common objects in the environment.

In general, the language deficits seen in aphasia are differentiated by their impact on fluency, motor output, comprehension, repetition, naming, and reading and writing. Problems in these areas, and the terminology used to identify them, are listed and described in Table 7.1.

Fluency

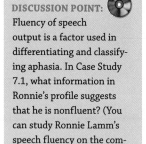

Fluency is a qualitative aspect of communication and speech that is used to describe its forward flow, including its phrasing, intonation, and rate. Fluent speech is easy, smooth, and well paced. Some people with aphasia exhibit a significant lack of fluency due to impairments in formulating and producing verbal output. This type of aphasia is called *nonfluent* and has these features:

- Short, choppy phrases
- Slow, labored production of speech
- Grammatical errors
- Telegraphic quality

However, some aphasias are considered fluent, also called *sensory aphasia.* With these, the individual's speech flows well with adequate phrase length, although often the content of the language is affected. To the extent to which a person with aphasia has fluent versus nonfluent speech gives insight into the location of the neurological injury. Generally, nonfluent aphasia correlates to injury anterior in the brain (i.e., the frontal lobe), whereas fluent aphasia correlates with posterior brain damage (i.e., the temporal-parietal regions).

TABLE 7.1 Common speech-language problems seen in aphasia syndromes

Problem	Definition	Syndrome
Agrammatism	Leaving out grammatical markers in sentences and phrases, including verb inflections, articles, and prepositions (e.g., "He go store")	Broca's aphasia, transcortical motor aphasia
Word-finding problems (anomia)	Inability to come up with words or names of items in spontaneous conversation or in structured naming tasks	Broca's aphasia, transcortical motor aphasia, global aphasia, Wernicke's aphasia, conduction aphasia, transcortical sensory aphasia, anomic aphasia
Telegraphic speech	Phrases and sentences made up of mostly content words (nouns and verbs) with function words omitted (e.g., "Tom go store")	Broca's aphasia, transcortical motor aphasia
Paraphasias	Substitution of one word for another (e.g., *table* for *desk*)	Transcortical motor aphasia, Wernicke's aphasia, transcortical sensory aphasia
Jargon	Production of language that is meaningless and may run on and on	Wernicke's aphasia
Neologisms	Making up a new word (e.g., "The *bramble-thingie* is over there")	Wernicke's aphasia
Effortful articulation	Production of speech that seems physically laborious, often accompanied by reduced phrases or sentence length; may grope with the articulators for positioning	Broca's aphasia, global aphasia
Initiation difficulties (adynamia)	Great difficulty or inability to initiate speech	Transcortical motor aphasia, global aphasia
Comprehension deficits	Compromised understanding or an inability to understand language	Wernicke's aphasia, transcortical sensory aphasia
Impaired repetition	Inability to repeat sounds, words, or phrases	Global aphasia, Wernicke's aphasia, conduction aphasia

Sources: Based on Rao (1994); Shipley and McAfee (1998).

Motor Output

For some people with aphasia, particularly those whose speech is nonfluent, motor systems involved with speech are compromised, resulting in a motor speech disorder. This occurs when the areas of the brain controlling motor planning and programming for speech are injured. These individuals may show slow and labored articulation of sounds, with some groping of the articulators as they seek accurate placement.

Language Comprehension

Language comprehension, also called *auditory comprehension,* is the ability to understand spoken language; this is not acuity or the ability to hear the message but rather the interpretation of what is heard. Most individuals with aphasia experience some degree of auditory comprehension deficit; some types of aphasia are characterized by significant problems with auditory comprehension, whereas other types correlate with more mild difficulties. The extent of comprehension difficulties is useful for classifying the aphasias.

Aphasia characterized by comprehension problems is often referred to as *receptive aphasia,* to emphasize its impact on language reception. More posterior aphasias, particularly those affecting the left temporal lobe, where language resides, tend to be coupled with more severe comprehension deficits. This contrasts with expressive aphasia, in which comprehension is relatively spared but expression is compromised. With anterior aphasias, which affect the left frontal lobe, comprehension is relatively intact or only mildly to moderately affected.

Repetition

Repetition is the ability to accurately reproduce verbal stimuli on demand, as in the following tasks:

- Say "eeee"
- Say "sofa"
- Say "no ifs, ands, or buts"

DISCUSSION POINT:
Repetition ability is informative for classifying aphasia when compared to spontaneous speech and auditory comprehension skills. Why would an individual with aphasia be able to repeat better than he or she might speak spontaneously?

The ability to repeat verbal stimuli is a major factor in differentiating among the aphasias, and for many people with aphasia, it is an ability that is seriously compromised. In a repetition task, a person must receive and process the incoming stimulus, convey that information to regions of the brain that formulate and plan motor acts for speech, and then articulate to reproduce the initial stimulus. Repetition ability is most informative when considered in conjunction with performance in spontaneous speaking and in comprehending language; there are certain aphasia profiles in which repetition skills are preserved even though spontaneous expression or comprehension is severely impaired. Repetition abilities alone cannot differentiate between fluent and nonfluent or between receptive and expressive aphasia profiles. However, after these general groupings are established, an individual's repetition skills provide further details about the exact nature of the person's language impairment.

Naming

Naming, or word retrieval, is the ability to retrieve and produce a targeted word during conversation or more structured tasks. **Anomia,** which literally means "no name," is the term used to describe word-finding problems or the inability to retrieve a word. We have all experienced anomia at one time or another, perhaps when we were tired, ill, or simply stressed. Thus, it is a language difficulty with which we are all familiar. However, more serious deficits in word-finding are a typical symptom of aphasia, with nearly all persons with aphasia exhibiting some degree of difficulty with naming tasks (Best, Herbert, Hickin, Osborne, et al., 2002). Anomia is also one of the most persistent deficits in aphasia, meaning that problems with word retrieval are most likely to remain even after recovery from aphasia (Basso, Marangolo, Piras, & Galluzzi, 2001; Cao, Vikingstad, George, Johnson, & Welsh, 1999).

Anomia patterns, or the type of word production errors seen in a person with aphasia, give insight into the type of aphasia. These patterns are called **paraphasias,** and they come in two varieties. A *phonemic paraphasia,* or literal paraphasia, occurs when there is a substitution or transposition of a sound. For example, looking at a picture of a sofa but producing "tofa" or "fosa" is a phonemic paraphasia. In "tofa" the /t/ is substituted for /s/. With "fosa," the /f/ and /s/ are transposed. In a *semantic paraphasia,* or verbal paraphasia, a word is substituted, often one that is in the same category as the targeted word. Looking at a picture of a sofa but producing "chair" or

DISCUSSION POINT: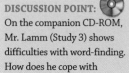
On the companion CD-ROM, Mr. Lamm (Study 3) shows difficulties with word-finding. How does he cope with anomia during normal conversations with others?

"furniture" is a semantic paraphasia. Typically, phonemic paraphasias are more prevalent in nonfluent, expressive aphasias, whereas semantic paraphasias are associated with the fluent and receptive classifications.

Reading and Writing

The language deficits of people with aphasia may extend to the domains of reading and writing, which involve the comprehension and expression of written language. Often, reading and writing deficits parallel the verbal language deficits. For example, persons who are nonfluent in spoken language frequently exhibit nonfluent oral reading. Likewise, persons who cannot understand sentence-length verbal messages often cannot comprehend sentence-level written information. It is unlikely that a person with mild to severe aphasia is unimpaired in reading and writing ability.

> **DISCUSSION POINT:**
> Paraphasias are typically viewed as either phonemic or semantic. How would you characterize these paraphasic errors: "chair" for *bed,* "apple" for *orange,* and "food" for *kitchen?*

SPOTLIGHT ON LITERACY

In rare instances, individuals with aphasia may experience "mirrored" reading and writing. When this unusual disturbance in literacy occurs, the individual will typically write with letter reversals and with script running from the right to the left side of the paper. Often the individual is aware that something is wrong but cannot self-correct the behaviors. When this mirror writing happens, the text is legible when reading the image reflected into a mirror. Test it out for yourself in the mirrored writing samples provided in the figure below. Individuals with mirrored reading and writing also demonstrate left-right confusion for pictured images. For example, when asked to identify the right side of a pictured object/person, they point to the left side. In creating a clock face, the affected individual will write the numbers counterclockwise. Interestingly, many of these individuals easily read mirrored writing without the use of a mirror. For example, the word *saw* would be read "was." Mirrored writing has been linked to dyslexia in individuals without a history of brain injury. One famous individual who reportedly wrote often in a mirrored format was Leonardo da Vinci. When this phenomenon presents itself in the stroke patient, the underlying cause is suspected to be from a disruption in the motor, visual, or spatial orientation systems. The clinician works to remediate the mirrored errors by increasing self-awareness of the behavior, training left to right reading/writing patterns, and encouraging spell checks. Most affected individuals do show a rapid recovery from this writing deficit (O'Donoghue & Dudding, 2004).

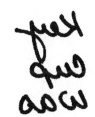

Note: Mirrored writing sample of name, address, and words written to dictation (key, cup, was).

WHAT ARE THE DEFINING CHARACTERISTICS OF APHASIA SYNDROMES?

Studying the language difficulties of people with aphasia provides information for classifying the types of aphasia into syndromes. We use the term *syndrome* to discuss aphasia, because certain language difficulties tend to cluster for different aphasias.

The following discussion describes the seven major aphasia syndromes, based on the most prevalent clinical system (Rao, 1994): Broca's, transcortical motor, global, Wernicke's, transcortical sensory, conduction, and anomic (Goodglass & Kaplan, 1983; Kertesz, 1982). Five of these categories are depicted in Figure 7.3 according to the most common site of the lesion.

The discussion includes the most salient traits of all seven syndromes. Table 7.2 summarizes the description of each: the site of the lesion, the impact on speech fluency and expression, and the impact on language and auditory comprehension.

Broca's Aphasia

Broca's aphasia results from damage to the frontal lobe of the brain, specifically Broca's area. This region, situated at the inferior portion of the premotor planning strip, plans and orchestrates the intricate motor movements for speech. In general, damage in Broca's area produces a nonfluent, expressive, motor aphasia profile.

Fluency and Motor Output

The individual with Broca's aphasia typically produces slowed, halting, and labored speech, yielding what some describe as a telegraphic or robotlike quality. Additional characteristics include a decreased phrase length, typically no more than four to five words in an utterance. Because of the short phrasing, the melody of speech is affected. An additional characteristic is agrammatical speech, in which function words are omitted, such as articles, prepositions, and conjunctions. Missing or inaccurate tense markers (e.g., *-ed, -ing*) are also frequent. Yet despite these significant difficulties with expression, the individual with Broca's aphasia is likely to have intact self-monitoring abilities and an awareness of these spoken language difficulties, resulting in extreme frustration.

Language Comprehension

The person with Broca's aphasia exhibits mild to moderate auditory comprehension problems, particularly when messages increase in length and complexity or

---

FIGURE 7.3

Aphasia syndromes and their lesion locations.

Source: From H. Damasio. (1981). Cerebral localization of the aphasia. In M. T. Sarno (Ed.), *Acquired aphasia* (p. 29). New York: Academic Press. Copyright 1981, with permission from Elsevier.

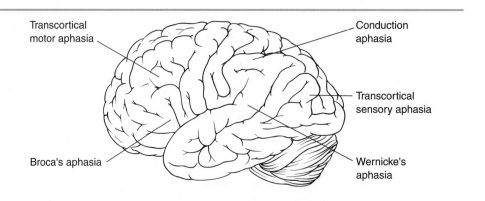

TABLE 7.2	Defining characteristics of the aphasia syndromes		
Aphasia Syndrome	Site of Lesion	Speech Fluency and Expression	Language and Auditory Comprehension
Broca's	Frontal lobe (posterior inferior region of left hemisphere)	Nonfluent, effortful articulation, telegraphic speech (mostly nouns and verbs), short phrases, impaired prosody, apraxia of speech	Fair to good
Transcortical motor	Prefrontal cortex (medial frontal region of left hemisphere)	Nonfluent, difficulty initiating speech, paraphasias, short utterances, good repetition	Good
Global	Multiple lobes and diffuse lesions	Nonfluent, delayed, or no speech initiation and output, naming and word-finding problems	Poor
Wernicke's	Temporal lobe (posterior portion of left hemisphere)	Fluent, meaningless speech and jargon, paraphasias, naming difficulties	Poor
Transcortical sensory	Parieto-occipital region	Fluent, meaningless speech and jargon, paraphasias, naming difficulties	Poor
Conduction	Arcuate fasciculus	Fluent, imitation problems, naming difficulties, normal prosody and articulation	Fair to good
Anomic	Angular gyrus	Fluent, word-finding problems (loss of words)	Fair to good

Sources: Based on Brookshire (2003); Rao (1994).

when contextual cues are removed. For instance, an individual may be able to follow simple directions, like "Point to the chair," but not more complicated directions with more complex language structures, such as "Point to the cat that is not white" or "Point to the chair and then to the table."

Repetition

Individuals with Broca's aphasia are highly variable in their repetition abilities, ranging from mildly to severely impaired. In large part, these abilities reflect the extent of difficulty in verbal expression.

Naming

The individual with Broca's aphasia is likely to have mild to severe anomia, characterized typically by phonemic paraphasias.

Reading and Writing

Reading and writing are unlikely to be spared in Broca's aphasia. Typically, the impact of the neurological injury on reading and writing parallels its impact on verbal performance. Reading aloud is slow and laborious with misarticulations or distortions, and writing is effortful, characterized by oversized printing called **macrographia.** Misspellings are also common, with incorrect letter choices and letter transpositions.

TRANSCORTICAL MOTOR APHASIA

Transcortical motor aphasia results from damage to the frontal lobe, typically the superior and anterior portions. Like Broca's aphasia, this syndrome is characterized as nonfluent, expressive, and motor in its typology. The symptoms of transcortical motor aphasia are also similar to those of Broca's aphasia *except*

DISCUSSION POINT: Consider Ronnie in Case Study 7.1. What aphasia syndrome might he have, based on the information supplied? What other information is needed to make this decision? (also see Mr. Lamm on the companion CD, Study 2).

that these individuals have repetition skills that are far better than their spontaneous speech. Thus, these individuals may have slow and labored expressive output on their own but are able to perform reasonably well on a repetition task. The relatively well-preserved repetition ability, in conjunction with the previously described language behaviors of Broca's aphasia, is the hallmark of transcortical motor aphasia. Most clients with this syndrome also demonstrate strong performance in oral reading.

GLOBAL APHASIA

Global aphasia occurs as a result of a large region of brain damage or multiple sites of brain injury in the language-dominant hemisphere. Because this aphasia syndrome results in deficits across all language modalities, a person is likely to be nonfluent *and* have poor language comprehension. Such individuals experience severe problems communicating, since they have difficulties receiving and sending messages. They are often nonverbal with limited gestures (e.g., head nods for yes or no, pointing to indicate a want). Likewise, understanding messages, even at the short-phrase or the single-word level, is usually impaired. And reading and writing abilities are similarly affected.

WERNICKE'S APHASIA

Wernicke's aphasia results from brain injury to the superior and posterior regions of the temporal lobe, possibly reaching to the parietal lobe of the language-dominant hemisphere. This area corresponds with auditory comprehension abilities. Wernicke's syndrome is a fluent, receptive, and sensory aphasia.

Fluency and Motor Output

The person with Wernicke's aphasia produces spontaneous speech that flows well with normal prosody. **Prosody** refers to the melody, intonation, and rhythm of speech. In addition, the length of utterances is not affected; utterances are typically at least five or more words in length. In fact, people with Wernicke's aphasia may appear verbose or may talk excessively, which is called **logorrhea.** However, the meaningful content of their utterances is limited, and they use frequent semantic paraphasias. These individuals are also prone to **neologisms,** the use of made-up words (e.g., *polyo* for *chair*), and **jargon,** the use of real words put together without any meaning (e.g., "days bone they could arms four kite"). Thus, although the spontaneous speech is quite fluent, the message is often empty or lost.

Unlike persons with Broca's aphasia, those with Wernicke's aphasia may have difficulty monitoring their own language production. Some people with Wernicke's aphasia may lack the insight that what they are attempting to say is not what they are actually saying. For this reason, it can be difficult to treat these clients; they may think that the therapist is the one with the communication problem, not them!

Language Comprehension

Comprehension problems are the key disturbance in Wernicke's syndrome. Unfortunately, persons with this syndrome have great difficulty interpreting verbal and written messages. Even simple language can be difficult to comprehend, such as sentences like "Put your finger on the button." And when language becomes decontextualized to describe events away from the here and now or becomes more grammatically complex, such as "Put your finger on the button and then stand up and smile," the comprehension deficits become even more profound.

Repetition

Most persons with Wernicke's aphasia have difficulty with repetition. As discussed previously, repeating something spoken by another involves both comprehension and production of that message. For someone with this type of aphasia, the comprehension system is usually significantly impaired, which impacts the ability to repeat.

Naming

Moderate to severe naming difficulties are associated with the Wernicke's profile, along with frequent paraphasias of both the phonemic and the semantic variety. In trying to describe a picture of a sailboat, for instance, an individual might say, "Yep, that's a, uh, booty-dock, a nooty-dock, yep a nooty-boat, soap, it's a, uh, saily-boaty, taily-boaty."

The difficulties in coming up with the word *sailboat* result in paraphasias and a behavior called **circumlocution,** which is, essentially, talking around a word that cannot be retrieved. A client trying to produce *refrigerator* might circumlocute and say, "That big box in the kitchen, it keeps food fresh, not spoiled, it is cold." These naming traits, coupled with the auditory comprehension deficits, contribute to the empty speech typical of Wernicke's aphasia.

Reading and Writing

With Wernicke's aphasia, reading may be intact, although comprehension of the text is likely to be degraded to the level of comprehension of spoken communication. Writing also parallels verbal expression. Although the writing is usually fluent and is in legible cursive with normal letter size, the message is unclear.

TRANSCORTICAL SENSORY APHASIA

Transcortical sensory aphasia results from injuries to the language-dominant hemisphere at the border of the temporal and occipital lobes (more inferior) or the superior region of the parietal lobe. Transcortical sensory aphasia is to Wernicke's aphasia as transcortical motor aphasia is to Broca's aphasia. These clients have the classic symptoms of a Wernicke's profile *except* they have stellar repetition skills. Further, they may also frequently repeat auditory stimuli, a phenomenon called **echolalia.**

CONDUCTION APHASIA

Conduction aphasia results from injury to the temporal-parietal region of the brain, typically to a connecting pathway called the *arcuate fasciculus.* This pathway provides communication between the speech production areas and the speech reception areas in the language-dominant hemisphere.

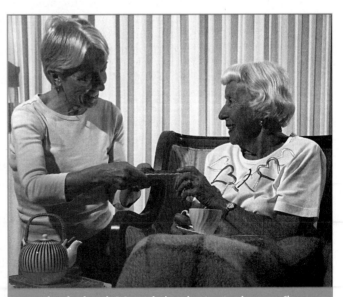

An individual with Wernicke's aphasia may be very fluent and talkative, but the speech lacks meaning and coherence.

Fluency and Motor Output

The conduction profile is fluent, with only mild to moderate deficits in expressive output. Prosody and articulation tend to be normal.

Language Comprehension

Language comprehension in conduction aphasia also tends to be fair to good with relatively little impairment.

Repetition

Difficulties with repetition and reading aloud are the hallmark of conduction aphasia. These individuals receive and process the verbal or written stimuli to repeat or read aloud, respectively, but cannot transfer this input to the verbal output area (i.e., Broca's region) because of the impaired pathway between these processing centers. Therefore, they are unable to produce the target response despite intact comprehension. However, they are aware of their repetition and reading errors and will attempt to revise and improve their production, possibly numerous times and with considerable frustration.

Naming

Conduction aphasia, like all the other syndromes, causes mild to moderate difficulties in naming and word retrieval.

Reading and Writing

An inability to read aloud is a hallmark characteristic of this disorder. Reading comprehension abilities are similar to those of auditory comprehension.

ANOMIC APHASIA

Anomic aphasia is not identified with a specific area of the brain or a site of lesion (i.e., injury). Anomic aphasia is fluent and expressive with relatively few deficits in language expression and comprehension with the exception of naming. Persons with anomic aphasia, as its name suggests, show significant impairment in word-retrieval skills in both spoken and written language. This form of aphasia is the most pervasive type of chronic condition, even after treatment (Raymer, 2001), and it is the most common of aphasia profiles.

HOW IS APHASIA IDENTIFIED AND TREATED? ●

THE ASSESSMENT PROCESS

For the individual who has sustained neurological damage, the interdisciplinary rehabilitation team includes physicians, nurses, physical therapists, occupational therapists, recreational therapists, social workers, respiratory therapists, registered dietitians, neuropsychologists, and, of course, speech-language pathologists. These specialists work cooperatively to treat the client using a holistic approach that attends to all problem areas, as opposed to focusing solely on isolated deficits. They may consult with still other disciplines, based on the client's individualized needs.

The speech-language pathologist's assessment of speech and language functioning provides insight for the entire rehabilitation team, as they determine appropriate goals and treatment strategies. For example, if the client's aphasia impairs the ability to understand long phrases, it is important for the other team members to incorporate this finding into their treatment approaches. In this case, the physical therapist should be using short phrases for instructions in treatment activities since multiple-step directions are beyond the client's ability (e.g., "Stand up straight" rather than "Lift up your head, straighten your back, and tuck your bottom in").

When evaluating an individual with suspected aphasia, the speech-language pathologist seeks to answer a series of questions:

1. Is aphasia present?
2. If so, what type or syndrome of aphasia is indicated by the symptoms and the site of injury?
3. What treatment plan will be most beneficial?
4. What is the prognosis for recovery?
5. Are any referrals to other professionals needed?

Immediately after a neurological injury, the affected individual may be too ill to participate in extensive testing. If so, screening is recommended in the client's hospital room, often at the bedside.

A screening typically examines orientation and responsiveness, speaking ability, listening skills, and possibly reading and writing in an abbreviated manner. The Aphasia Language Performance Scales (ALPS; Keenan and Brassell, 1975), a standardized aphasia assessment tool, is a relatively brief aphasia battery that is often appropriate for clients at this stage. The Bedside Evaluation Screening Test (BEST; Fitch-West & Sands, 1987) is also well suited for this purpose. Both of these instruments survey speech and language performance using a limited, yet informative, number of items; the testing takes about 30 minutes. Such informal bedside screening provides the starting point (i.e., baseline performance) for ongoing assessment and the start of a treatment plan.

As the client becomes more medically stable, improved endurance will permit more extensive, comprehensive assessment. Most individuals will exhibit at least some level of recovery on their own as part of the healing process. This **spontaneous recovery** is the natural healing of the brain without therapeutic interventions.

When the client is able to participate for longer periods of time, standardized comprehensive aphasia batteries can be administered to evaluate levels of functioning and to develop a detailed treatment plan. Numerous aphasia batteries are available from which the speech-language pathologist can choose. Often the choice of test is influenced by clinician preference, test availability, guidelines of an organization, or unique client needs (e.g., a bilingual client or a client who speaks only Spanish). The areas assessed include language expression and motor output, language comprehension, repetition, naming, reading, and writing. Generally, test items have a hierarchical arrangement, moving from easier to more difficult tasks. Table 7.3 provides a sample of typical items included in an aphasia battery.

The speech-language pathologist studies other variables that may affect communication. For example, a thorough examination of the oral structures and functions might reveal a coexisting dysarthria or apraxia. A hearing screening would indicate whether an audiologist should be consulted for further auditory and hearing assessment. A psychological screening could determine how any communication problems might be impacting the individual's psychological well-being, possibly warranting mental health counseling.

DISCUSSION POINT: Consider the areas of testing presented in Table 7.3. For a person with conduction aphasia, which tasks would be more difficult? What about a person with Wernicke's aphasia?

TABLE 7.3 Typical items included in aphasia batteries	
Area of Testing	**Typical Items**
Spontaneous speech	• Answering questions • Describing a picture • Participating in informal or structured conversations
Auditory comprehension	• Answering yes/no questions • Pointing to objects or pictures as they are named • Following directions (single-step, multistep, and complex commands)
Repetition	• Repeating real words, phrases, and sentences • Repeating nonsense words and phrases
Naming	• Naming objects and pictures • Completing phrases • Naming items in a category • Providing names of general categories
Reading	• Reading words, phrases, sentences, and paragraphs
Writing	• Copying letters, words, and sentences • Writing from dictation • Writing about fictional or real experiences

Prognostic Indicators

Determining treatment approaches and making prognostic judgments requires knowledge of those factors that predict which clients will benefit from what kind of therapy. **Prognostic indicators** are those variables that assist in predicting recovery: the site of the brain injury, the type and the size of the injury, the type and the severity of aphasia, handedness, age, preinjury health, and motivation for treatment (Robey, 1998a; Yamamoto & Magalong, 2003). Often, prognostic indicators are used to specify treatment approaches, including the amount and the type of treatment. However, some clients do not respond as predicted. For this reason, a trial period of intervention is often worthwhile to evaluate an individual's responsiveness to the intensity and the approach.

Designing Treatment Plans

The goal of aphasia treatment is to correct or compensate for speech and language deficits so that individuals can communicate functionally in their daily routines. Therapy should improve a client's communication skills beyond the level attributed to spontaneous recovery alone (Helm-Estabrooks & Albert, 1991). Since the time spent in treatment is positively associated with language improvements, a greater magnitude of change can be expected with a longer duration of treatment (Robey, 1998a). However, in the current health care climate of cost monitoring for services provided, there are often strict limits on the number of sessions allowed for aphasia treatment.

Treatment approaches focus on specific deficit areas identified in the evaluation and the underlying processes that produce these impairments. For example, consider a client with poor naming performance who consistently demonstrates phonemic paraphasias—a pictured flower is "tower." Rather than working specifically on improving the production of the word *flower,* the clinician wants to improve the underlying process that is impaired. Here, a

FOCUS ON TECHNOLOGY

Persons with neurological disorders may experience a loss of the ability to communicate verbally with others. These persons may seek an augmentative and/or alternative communication device (AAC) to meet their communication needs, as discussed in Chapter 5. Researchers are currently investigating the use of **visual scene displays** for people with chronic severe aphasia. These will allow users to communicate a wide variety of topics and messages in a visually contextualized manner that is highly individualized to the user. A visual scene is created around a single or related group of pictures that are meaningful to the individual (e.g., a wedding photo), and a series of communicative elements (e.g., questions, messages) are tied to that key picture(s), as shown below. Early research suggests that the use of visual scene displays may improve communication (Seale, 2007) and aid in transitions across themes (McKelvey, Dietz, Hux, Weissling, & Beukelman, 2007). A number of resources are available on the Internet to facilitate use of this low-tech AAC approach for individuals with aphasia, including a manual with step-by-step directions on how to build visual scene displays (http://aac.unl.edu/).

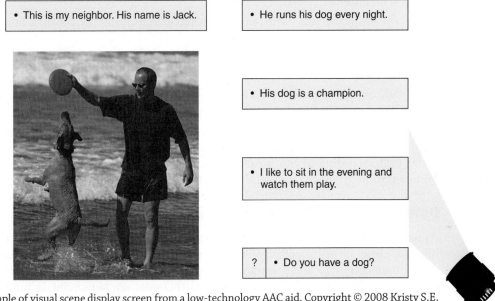

Example of visual scene display screen from a low-technology AAC aid. Copyright © 2008 Kristy S.E. Weissling. Used with permission.

motor planning or execution process is likely the cause of the naming error, because it appears that the client knows the correct label. The challenge is to produce gains in the therapy session that carry over or generalize into functional communication improvements. Designing a treatment regimen requires knowledge of **evidence-based practice,** which includes giving special consideration to those interventions that have been studied in a controlled manner and demonstrate improvement for a particular disorder.

Working with Culturally and Linguistically Diverse Clients

A relatively new frontier of adult language rehabilitation is the evaluation and treatment of bilingual individuals. Intervention with bilingual speakers requires the clinician to have knowledge of the languages spoken as well as the cultural backgrounds that influence language use. For individuals who speak multiple languages, optimal testing procedures will evaluate them in all spoken languages.

Although there are now tests that are standardized in multiple languages, therapists who are competent in multiple languages are scarce. Translators can be used to assist with this process, but they may miss subtle deficits in language or cognition. Further complicating matters are the multiple levels of bilingualism. For example, the individual who acquired both Spanish and English as a young child may have a different level of bilingual competency from that of the Spanish speaker who acquired English as a second language after moving to the United States at age 18.

Although there is still much to learn in this area of aphasia research, studies of bilingual persons with aphasia show several possible impacts (Roberts, 2001):

1. *Parallel impairment,* with both languages demonstrating similar strengths and weaknesses
2. *Differential impairment,* with one language showing greater impairment than another
3. *Differential aphasia,* with varying aphasia symptoms or profiles between languages
4. *Blended impairment,* with the individual appearing to mix features of the languages
5. *Selective aphasia,* with only one language revealing deficits and the other being preserved

These variations in aphasia profiles require much research. The rapidly expanding diversity in languages, dialects, and cultures in the United States necessitates better understanding of the most effective methods for evaluating and treating bilingual individuals (Niemeier, Burnett, & Whitaker, 2003).

DETERMINING THE TREATMENT SETTING

Aphasia therapy is not limited to the speech-language pathologist and client working in a clinic or office setting. Therapy should encompass other environments to facilitate carryover and generalization of progress to different settings. For example, cotreatments with the occupational therapist are beneficial as the client works on activities of daily living (ADLs), such as grooming or dressing. This provides an opportunity for the speech-language pathologist to assess generalization of skills as the client interacts with the occupational therapist to sequence, follow directions, and communicate. Community reentry programs are also excellent simulations for carryover, with the client venturing out, accompanied by therapists, to practice therapy skills in real-world settings such as banks, restaurants, and grocery stores.

A group approach is another consideration for treating aphasia. Group therapy provides a functional setting for clients to practice communicating and provides an avenue for cooperative learning (Avent, 1997, 2004). At present, group treatment appears to be most beneficial for clients who have chronic or persistent aphasia (Bollinger, Musson, & Holland, 1993) and who participate in individual treatment (Robey, 1998b). The group setting provides socialization and support for clients and their families.

DISCUSSION POINT:
What are some additional specific ways that group therapy could benefit clients and their families? Consider the cases in Case Study 7.1.

MEASURING OUTCOMES

Effective language treatment for persons with aphasia should be measured based on their ability to communicate in real-world situations (Elman & Bernstein-Ellis, 1995). *Real-world communication* refers to communication used in functional and authentic communication acts, and many third-party payers of communication therapy services emphasize the need for treatment to address real-world needs. For instance, Medicare guidelines focus on communicative interventions that enable individuals to "communicate basic physical needs and emotional states, and carry out communicative interactions in the community" (as cited in Busch, 1994). Thus, speech-language pathologists must consider how to measure treatment outcomes to document improvements such as these.

Tools that measure **functional outcomes,** or functional communication improvements, are considered an essential part of the speech-language pathologist's practice. The Communication Abilities of Daily Living (2nd ed.; Holland, Frattali, & Fromm, 1999), a standardized aphasia battery, is one example of a way to measure functional outcomes, as is the ASHA Functional Assessment of Communication Skills (Frattali, Thompson, Holland, Wohl, et al., 1995). These measures examine what individuals are able to do with independent and authentic communication tasks. Using such assessments to measure clinical effectiveness reminds speech-language pathologists of the importance of targeting real communication within therapeutic activities.

Most jobs require the ability to communicate, problem-solve, and reason. Some estimates suggest that only about 10% of stroke survivors return to work without impaired performance (Rosenbek et al., 1989). With federal regulations such as the Family Medical Leave Act and the Americans with Disabilities Act, individuals now have greater potential to maintain their previous employment. These acts provide some degree of job protection and encourage reasonable accommodation for employees with disabilities.

However, even with these guidelines, gainful productive employment following a stroke can be challenging. Individuals may remain employed but may need to function in an altered capacity. Such changes may represent a change in status within the organization (i.e., a loss of responsibility); reduced wages because, for example, a 10-hour workday is now physically impossible; or job reconfiguration. Such modifications can result in work that is no longer professionally satisfying. Such factors likely contribute to the elevated incidence of depression following neurological injury (Bays, 2001).

WHAT ARE RIGHT-HEMISPHERE DYSFUNCTION, TRAUMATIC BRAIN INJURY, AND DEMENTIA? ●

Thus far, this chapter has focused on aphasia, one of the most common acquired communication disorders. However, there are other adult language disorders and cognitive-based dysfunctions that merit discussion. The rest of this chapter focuses on three additional acquired disorders of communication— right-hemisphere dysfunction, traumatic brain injury, and dementia. Table 7.4 provides a summary of these disorders and their major impacts.

Right-Hemisphere Dysfunction

Right-hemisphere dysfunction (RHD) results from neurological damage to the right cerebral hemisphere. When an individual experiences a stroke, the injury to the brain tissue can occur anywhere. For about 90% of the adult population, the left hemisphere is dominant for language. Aphasia can result with left-hemisphere damage; when damage affects the right hemisphere, language and cognition may be impacted, but the symptoms are quite different from those

TABLE 7.4	Acquired disorders of language and cognition other than aphasia		
Disorder	**Description**	**Common Causes**	**Major Impacts**
Right-hemisphere dysfunction	Neurological damage to brain tissue in the right hemisphere due to loss of nutrients and oxygen to the brain	Stroke, illness, disease	Lack of attention to the left side of the body, including visual field Difficulty recognizing faces Compromised pragmatics (e.g., taking turns, reading others' cues) Wordy expression, including tangents Lack of awareness of communicative and cognitive impairments Problems with higher-level abstract thinking and language use Possible dysarthria and dysphagia
Traumatic brain injury	Neurological damage to brain tissue due to closed- or open-head injury	Motor vehicle accident, fall, recreational sports accident, act of violence	Possible significant personality changes Widespread language expression and comprehension problems, including expressing ideas, comprehending what others say, using and expressing humor, displaying and understanding emotions, and engaging in higher-level abstract uses of language and cognition, particularly memory
Dementia	Gradual onset of declines in cognitive, language, and daily living functions due to progressive central nervous system dysfunction	Neurological disease (Huntington's disease, Parkinson's disease, Pick's disease, Creutzfeldt-Jakob disease), multiple strokes	Memory impairment (both short- and long-term memory) Impairment in cognitive skills (abstract thought, judgment, and executive functions) Presence of aphasia, apraxia, or agnosia

seen with aphasia. The right hemisphere is responsible for many nonlanguage functions, including comprehension of visual-spatial information and emotional expression. Because the two hemispheres do communicate, RHD may include a language disturbance, but cognitive, perceptual, and behavioral disruptions are the more consistent findings with this disorder. For this reason, RHD is commonly referred to as a *cognitive-linguistic disorder.*

Characteristics of RHD

DISCUSSION POINT:
Treatment for RHD focuses on higher-level cognitive-linguistic tasks, such as making inferences. What are some tasks that require inferencing?

There is currently no universally recognized taxonomy for RHD. However, there are behavioral symptoms that appear with relative consistency:

1. Lack of awareness of cognitive-linguistic deficits and possible denial of problem areas (Hartman-Maeir, Soroker, Oman, & Katz, 2003)
2. Lack of awareness, or complete neglect, of the left side of the body and external stimuli to the left side, including physical limitations, such as paralysis of the left leg or arm (*left hemiparesis*), and visual-spatial neglect, in which the individual does not process information in the left visual field and which can negatively impact reading and writing (Heilman, 2004)
3. Difficulty recognizing faces (*prosopagnosia*)
4. Compromised pragmatics, such as ability to "read" other people's cues, recognize others' communication interests, and use physical space and affect appropriately during communication

5. A tendency toward using wordy expression and providing tangential information

6. Difficulty understanding or using higher-level cognitive-linguistic skills, such as problem solving or abstract thought

7. Dysarthria or dysphagia when neuromuscular systems are compromised

These characteristics vary in severity based on the size and the location of the injury; however, even mild cognitive-linguistic deficits can hinder functional abilities. This may include writing or even copying tasks, as seen in Figures 7.4 and 7.5.

Identification of RHD

Like left-hemisphere injury, right-hemisphere damage requires a comprehensive speech-language assessment as part of an interdisciplinary team assessment. The speech-language pathologist should assess all aspects of communication, speech, and language performance, including those abilities examined in the aphasia battery (e.g., expression, motor control, auditory comprehension, naming, repetition, reading, and writing). When right-hemisphere dysfunction is suspected, testing must assess higher-level language skills including predicting, reasoning, understanding humor and figurative language, and problem solving. Assessment should also study visual-perceptual performance and pragmatic appropriateness. And most individuals with RHD also benefit from comprehensive neuropsychological testing.

Specialized batteries are available specifically for the RHD population, such as the Mini Inventory of Right Brain Injury (MIRBI; Pimental & Kinsbury, 1989), the Right Hemisphere Language Battery (Bryan, 1989), and the Clinical Management of Right Hemisphere Dysfunction—Revised (Halper, Cherney, & Burn, 1996). Because evaluation of RHD is complex, it is best accomplished through an interdisciplinary team, whose collective findings can identify the strengths and weaknesses of cognitive, linguistic, and neuropsychological functioning that are pertinent to an individualized rehabilitation plan.

Treatment of RHD

Knowledge of treatments for RHD is more limited than that for left-hemisphere damage and aphasia. Initial therapy for RHD targets the management of attention and visual disruptions, since these impact productive treatment activities. For instance, if the individual does not attend to visual stimuli in the left visual field, treatment materials in that space are not processed. Thus, improved attention to stimuli across both visual fields is a key factor in resolving reading and writing disturbances. A therapist can improve attention to the left visual field by placing a heavy, bright red marking, such as a line, on the left side of reading materials to direct the individual's attention to the left.

Therapy also targets higher-level cognitive-linguistic tasks,

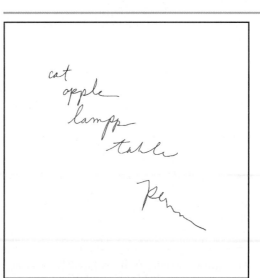

FIGURE 7.4

Writing sample of RHD patient with left visual field neglect.

FIGURE 7.5

Clock drawing by RHD patient.

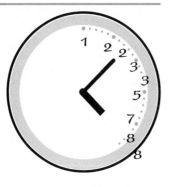

such as thinking through functional problems (What would you do if you locked yourself out of the house? What are the steps to changing a flat tire?) and making inferences (If the alarm doesn't go off, what might happen?). Further, the pragmatics of communication interactions require careful attention; improvements in facial expression, voice variation, turn-taking, topic maintenance, and eye contact are frequent goals with RHD. Again, there is benefit to both individual and group settings for delivering intervention. Given the frequency of pragmatic issues, group treatment is especially helpful for building competence in functional interactions with others.

TRAUMATIC BRAIN INJURY

Traumatic brain injury (TBI) refers to neurological damage to the brain resulting from the impact of external forces. TBI most frequently occurs as a result of motor vehicle accidents (both cars and motorcycles), falls, or acts of violence. Incidence and prevalence statistics tend to vary because of difficulties in defining a TBI. For example, the mild concussion of a football player who briefly loses consciousness and memory of the incident may or may not be included in TBI numbers (Kaut, DePompei, Kerr, & Congeni, 2003). Chapter 6 described TBI as it affects children and adolescents; however, TBI also affects adults.

Epidemiology studies show that TBI is a leading cause of death and disability in the United States. The yearly incidence of TBI in Americans is approximately 1.5 million, with 50,000 deaths (Bruns & Hauser, 2003). Of those surviving TBI, 85,000 suffer long-term disabilities (Thurman, Alverson, Dunn, Guerrero et al., 1999). Males are twice as likely to experience TBI as females, particularly males of lower socioeconomic backgrounds (Hanks et al., 2003). Certain age groups are also more prone to TBI, such as infants, adolescents, and senior citizens over 65 years of age.

Given the frequent long-term medical, vocational, and social needs of affected individuals, TBI represents a substantial health care issue in the United States. Recently, attention has focused on those who have suffered mild head injuries yet go undetected. These include people who experience "blackouts," dizziness, or disorientation after a blow to the head. Surprisingly, many of these injuries occur in high school sports; however, the true numbers are difficult to track. Of high school football players sustaining head injuries, only 47% reported the incident. Common reasons for a concussion going unreported included players' underestimation of the severity of their injury, fear of being withheld from competition, and lack of awareness of the significance of a concussion (McCrea, Hammeke, Olsen, Leo et al., 2004). The cumulative effects of these injuries can be devastating. Athletes with repeated concussions are eight times more likely to have a decline in memory than athletes with no concussion (Iverson, Gaetz, Lovell, & Collins, 2004; McClincy, Lovell, Pardini, Collins et al., 2006).

Characteristics of TBI

Head injuries are grouped by the nature of the injury, whether open-head or closed-head. **Open-head injuries** occur when the skull and the meninges (i.e., the layers of tissue that encase the brain) have been penetrated. These injuries often stem from violent acts using guns, ice picks, and other sharp instruments. The injuries tend to be relatively localized (i.e., focal) with regard to the size and the extent of neurological damage.

One of the most famous cases of TBI was an open-head injury sustained by Phineas Gage and described by Damasio (1995) in *Descartes' Error*. A railroad worker, Gage's brain was seriously damaged and his personality significantly changed when a metal rod went through his frontal lobe. The study of Gage's personality changes was important in advancing the field of psychology and explaining how traumatic brain injuries affect personality.

Closed-head injuries, by contrast, typically result from motor vehicle accidents, falls, sports injuries, physical assault, or abuse such as shaken baby syndrome. Although the outer protection of the brain remains intact, the brain is jostled within the skull, yielding diffuse (i.e., nonfocal) neurological injury. The *open* or *closed* labeling is common in the clinical setting for diagnostic purposes.

An unfortunate result of recent wars is that traumatic brain injury has become the signature injury of military personnel. The use of improvised explosive devices (IED) has created a new category of traumatic brain injury known as **polytrauma** (Roth, 2008). Polytrauma injuries refer to a mixture of open- and closed-head injuries, multiple medical concerns (e.g., fractures, lacerations, internal organ injuries, etc.), and posttraumatic stress disorder (Okie, 2005).

Regardless of the mechanism of injury, the cognitive and linguistic impacts of TBI vary considerably across individuals and are often not the only aspects of well-being that are affected. As shown in Figure 7.6, TBI affects the psychosocial realm as well, including emotions, temperament, motivation, and self-awareness. In fact, following a TBI, an individual's personality may seem totally changed. The combined impairments of cognition, language, and psychosocial functioning create significant difficulties with communication—expressing ideas, comprehending what others say, using and understanding humor, and displaying and comprehending emotions. As with other neurological injuries, there is often a correlation between the size, the location, and the overall severity of the injury and the impact on the individual's functioning. In short, there are numerous areas of impairment for most people following TBI. Consequently, comprehensive interdisciplinary testing by a team of professionals is imperative to determine baseline skills and target areas for rehabilitation.

Identification of TBI

The speech-language pathologist works as a member of an interdisciplinary rehabilitation team to plan for treatment following a TBI. Initially, many individuals who have sustained TBI are comatose and require advanced medical support to survive. At this stage, testing for communication ability and potential for communication recovery relies on subjective, behavioral observations. Two instruments commonly used in the early phases of TBI recovery include the Glasgow Coma Scale (Teasdale & Jennett, 1974) and the Rancho Los Amigos Levels of Cognitive Function (Hagen, 1998). These are presented in Tables 7.5 and 7.6, respectively.

The Glasgow Coma Scale (GCS) rates the best-observed response for eye opening, verbal response, and motor

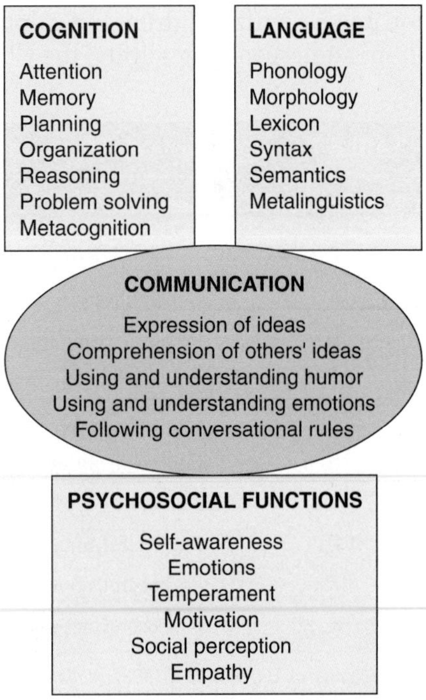

FIGURE 7.6

Impact of TBI on communication, cognitive, linguistic, and psychosocial realms.

Source: From *Traumatic brain injury: Rehabilitation for speech-language pathologists* by R. J. Gillis, 1996, Boston: Elsevier. Copyright 1996 by Elsevier, Inc. Adapted with permission.

COGNITION	LANGUAGE
Attention	Phonology
Memory	Morphology
Planning	Lexicon
Organization	Syntax
Reasoning	Semantics
Problem solving	Metalinguistics
Metacognition	

COMMUNICATION

Expression of ideas
Comprehension of others' ideas
Using and understanding humor
Using and understanding emotions
Following conversational rules

PSYCHOSOCIAL FUNCTIONS

Self-awareness
Emotions
Temperament
Motivation
Social perception
Empathy

TABLE 7.5 Glascow Coma Scale	
Behavior Observed	**Score**
Best Eye Response	
Spontaneous eye opening	4 points
Eye opening to speech	3 points
Eye movement/opening to painful stimulus	2 points
No observed eye response	1 point
Best Verbal Response	
Oriented	5 points
Confused, Disoriented	4 points
Inappropriate, incoherent speech	3 points
Unrecognizable, understandable speech	2 points
No verbal response	1 point
Best Motor Response	
Follows commands	6 points
Localized movement to pain	5 points
Withdrawal from pain	4 points
Decorticate posturing (flexion)	3 points
Decerebrate posturing (extension)	2 points
No motor response	1 point

Adapted from Teasdale & Jennett (1974).

response to characterize an individual's functioning, from severe TBI (score of 3) to mild TBI (score of 15). Recall from Chapter 6 that the GCS was described for its use with children and adolescents with TBI. Whether used with children, adolescents, or adults, the GCS is a predictor of eventual recovery. As an

TABLE 7.6 Rancho levels of cognitive functioning	
Rancho Level	**Behavior**
I	No response to stimuli, total assistance
II	Generalized response to stimuli, total assistance
III	Localized response to stimuli, total assistance
IV	Confused and agitated, maximal assistance
V	Confused, not agitated, inappropriate, maximal assistance
VI	Confused, not agitated, appropriate, moderate assistance
VII	Automatic, appropriate, minimal assistance
VIII	Purposeful, appropriate, stand-by assistance
IX	Purposeful, appropriate, stand-by assistance as requested
X	Purposeful, appropriate, modified independence

Sources: Based on Hagen (1981, 1998); Malkus, Booth, & Kodimer (1980).

alternative estimate, the Rancho levels of the Rancho Los Amigos Levels of Cognitive Function (Hagen, 1998) use a subjective rating that outlines ten levels of cognitive functioning. These range from nonresponsiveness, total assistance (Level I) to purposeful/appropriate behavior, modified independence (Level X), as shown in Table 7.6. Since this scale reflects the entire continuum of TBI recovery, it applies throughout the rehabilitation process.

As the client with TBI improves medically and stabilizes in functioning, the speech-language pathologist completes more extensive testing to evaluate the impact of the brain injury on communication performance. Several specialized tests are available, such as the Brief Test of Head Injury (Helm-Estabrooks & Hotz, 1991) and the Ross Information Processing Assessment (2nd ed.; Ross, 1996). These tests complement the additional testing that will examine oral motor performance to determine whether dysarthria or apraxia is present and will examine swallowing ability to ensure that dysphagia is not present. The speech-language pathologist then completes and shares a cumulative report with other rehabilitation team members. Because persons with TBI have many needs, the appropriate professionals collaboratively generate an interdisciplinary rehabilitation plan of care for the client.

Treatment of TBI

Treatment interventions will vary according to an individual's level of impairment as reflected by the Rancho scale. In the early stages of recovery, which correspond to severe impairment (Rancho levels I through III), stimulation treatment is common. Activities focus on arousing the individual's responses, such as being alert to the environment, and attending to incoming stimuli, particularly visual and auditory. For example, the therapist might use an irritating noise like an alarm clock or a bell to attract attention. Tracking the consistency of responses and the modes of stimuli yielding these responses is critical. At this early stage, responses will be inconsistent even for basic commands, such as "Blink your eyes" or "Make a fist."

Rancho levels IV to VI correspond to the middle phase of recovery. At this stage of moderate impairments, tasks focus on establishing basic communication systems—whether verbal, gestural, or augmentative (i.e., alternative)—and enhancing the reliability of communication efforts. Initial communication systems may use a picture board, to which the client can point to indicate *bathroom, water,* or *food.* These clients need much structure and assistance from the therapist, as they are still highly distractible and are frequently agitated or aggressive. Compensatory strategies, such as notebooks or schedule cards, can support orientation and memory and can improve goal-directed behavior. More structured therapy tasks are appropriate to improve memory, word retrieval, simple problem solving, and following directions as the client progresses.

Persons at Rancho levels VII through X are in the later phases of recovery and exhibit mild impairments. The focus at this stage is facilitating independence. Treatment stresses insight or judgment to solve problems encountered in daily activities. For example, a client might be helped to problem-solve the following scenario:

> You need to catch the bus and be at work by 9:00 AM. Look at the bus schedule and tell me which bus you should catch to get there on time.

Although much recovery has occurred prior to this stage, new or stressful situations are often difficult for the individual with TBI. Applying new communication and cognitive-linguistic skills to novel situations can cause anxiety and stress. Independence and safety issues should be addressed, using progressive community-based reintegration (e.g., planning a meal, making a grocery list, shopping at the store). Community outings can provide opportunities to apply treatment gains to real-world situations.

Treating clients with TBI requires great flexibility on the part of the therapist to meet their individualized needs as they progress through the Rancho stages. Many clients achieve an independent return to home, work, and society. Unfortunately, some clients do not and remain in early or middle Rancho stages. These individuals will require a structured, supervised, and supportive environment, such as a group home.

DEMENTIA

Dementia is a chronic and progressive decline in memory, cognition, language, and personality resulting from central nervous system dysfunction (Bayles & Tomoeda, 1995). Illnesses such as Alzheimer's disease, Huntington's disease, Parkinson's disease, Pick's disease, Creutzfeldt-Jakob disease, acquired immune deficiency syndrome (AIDS), and multiple cerebral infarcts (i.e., strokes) can cause dementia. Alzheimer's is the most common cause, representing about 70% of all diagnosed cases (Brookshire, 2003). Dementia is most prevalent in the elderly, with as many as 35% of those 85 years or older exhibiting signs of dementia (Kart & Kinney, 2001). Because the geriatric population (i.e., those over age 65) represents the most rapidly growing demographic segment in the United States, dementia will continue to be a major health concern for this country.

The diagnostic criteria of the American Psychiatric Association (1994) identify three defining traits of dementia:

1. Memory impairment (both short- and long-term memory)
2. Impairment in cognitive skills (abstract thought, judgment, and executive functions)
3. Presence of aphasia, apraxia, or agnosia (i.e., inability to recognize objects, words, or sounds)

In addition, dementia must have a gradual onset with progressive functional decline over time. Dementia does not result from psychological disturbances such as psychosis, schizophrenia, or delirium, although these conditions may coexist in some cases. It is important to determine the cause of dementia, since there are medical conditions that produce dementia-like profiles but are reversible, such as metabolic disturbances, infections, drug toxicity, vitamin deficiency, and thyroid disease.

Characteristics of Dementia

Since dementia is a progressive decline of skills, its characteristics are relative to how far the disease has progressed. People with dementia often progress from mild to moderate to severe deficits, with that progress ranging from a slow to a rapid decline.

Characteristics of Mild Dementia.   Individuals with mild dementia exhibit forgetfulness, even of basic information or common routines. These memory problems include frequently losing or misplacing items, missing appointments, or forgetting a familiar phone number. Language skills at the mild dementia level show decreased vocabulary, reduced or verbose conversation, or anomia, in

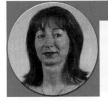

SPOTLIGHT ON RESEARCH AND PRACTICE

NAME: CATHERINE M. REYNOLDS, M.A., CCC-ACE-SLP/VAL

PROFESSION/TITLE
Senior Speech-Language Pathologist for Adult Acute Care, University of Virginia Medical Center, Charlottesville, Virginia

MOST MEMORABLE PATIENT
The very first patient with TBI of my career was particularly memorable. He was a man in his thirties who had been in a fight in the prison dining hall. A rival had rammed a table leg through his skull just above the left ear. His left facial nerve was severed, so his face was permanently paralyzed on that side. He had enough attention and comprehension to participate in therapy, but reading and writing were challenging. We played cards, and used the daily newspaper photographs and photographs of his young children to stimulate interaction using gestures. As he progressed, he became very aware of his word-finding problems and the errors he made when speaking, but he had no memory. Often my therapy plan was halted to repeatedly explain his injury and the consequences. He was always surprised: "Oh, is da ih? I taw I wuz goin' crazy!" (Oh, is that it? I thought I was going crazy!") I was fascinated by the multitude of deficits he displayed with, what seemed to me at the time, a very discreet injury. I continue to be intrigued by the workings of the brain, still not fully understood by scientists but revealing its interconnected complex functions as impairments occur.

which the name of something cannot be retrieved. Typically, language comprehension is preserved even though information may not be remembered. Pragmatics and social skills are well preserved at this stage, and motor function is intact, so that the individual is walking, eating, and toileting without difficulty.

Characteristics of Moderate Dementia. The moderate dementia profile is the phase of most dramatic functional change. Here, the individual becomes increasingly disoriented in time and place, and exhibits poor attention, memory, and marked language difficulties. Deficits of language include significant anomia, difficulty repeating, problems understanding humor, and often empty conversations. At this stage, motor skills are still adequate for walking and eating, although restlessness and roaming are likely.

Characteristics of Severe Dementia. Extreme disorientation and minimal, if any, cognitive ability are defining characteristics of severe dementia. At this stage, language skills are profoundly compromised, with limited meaningful communication and frequent repetitions (i.e., parroting) and jargon. Comprehension skills are also severely impaired. Motor skills at this stage vary, although many individuals are wheelchair dependent and unable to control bladder and bowel functions.

Identification of Dementia

A team of professionals evaluates suspected dementia to verify its presence, cause, and course of intervention. Medical testing will rule out other treatable illnesses that may appear like dementia (e.g., vitamin deficiency, drug toxicity). Imaging studies such as MRI or CT may reveal neurological changes suggestive of dementia such as loss of gray and white matter (i.e., atrophy), brain lesions, enlarged ventricles, or neurofibrillary plaques and tangles.

After the physician renders a diagnosis of dementia, referrals are requested to assess the patient's functional abilities. The speech-language pathologist assesses cognitive and linguistic skills in comparison to normal behaviors. Instruments commonly used to screen mental status include the Mini Mental State Examination (Folstein, Folstein, & McHugh, 1975) and the mental status subtest of the Arizona Battery for Communication Disorders of Dementia (Bayles & Tomoeda, 1993).

More comprehensive testing by the speech-language pathologist typically involves the complete Arizona Battery for Communication Disorders of Dementia (ABCD; Bayles & Tomoeda, 1993). This standardized battery assesses and evaluates key areas of performance, including linguistic comprehension, linguistic expression, verbal memory, visuospatial skills, and mental status. Scores of the ABCD guide clinical judgments on the presence and severity of dementia. Individualized intervention plans are then developed based on these findings.

Treatment of Dementia

Researchers continue to develop more effective pharmocological treatments to combat degenerative changes associated with dementia (Birks, 2006). The majority of medications currently approved by the Food and Drug Administration (FDA) for dementia target those individuals in the mild to moderate stages. These drugs are not cures but appear to improve the symptoms or slow the disease progression (Schmidt-Luggen, 2005). Even with medications, therapy to improve functional communication skills is typical.

Speech-language treatment is determined largely by the severity of the dementia. In mild to even moderate cases, treatment can help to compensate for deficits (Bayles & Kim, 2003). Environmental changes to promote safety are imperative, and education for family members or caregivers is emphasized to provide specific training. Family members might be trained, for instance, to give verbal cueing for dressing or eating (e.g., "First you pick up the spoon"). Strategies to manage potential behavioral issues are important, as well as measures to minimize frustration for the client and the caregiver. Active support groups for care providers are encouraged. In cases of severe dementia, the speech-language pathologist and other professionals serve as consultants, providing management strategies. Unfortunately, the resources to provide care in many of these cases are beyond the physical, emotional, and financial capabilities of some families. At this point, long-term placement is necessary in a nursing home or supportive group environment where the client has professional caregivers.

CASE ANALYSIS

Study the case of Mr. Driver, Case Study 3 on the Companion Website at www .pearsonhighered.com/justice2e. Reflect on the importance of treatment to remediating aphasia.

CHAPTER SUMMARY

Adult aphasia and other cognitive-based dysfunctions result from neurological injuries such as stroke, traumatic brain injury, or progressive diseases. These disorders occur after language and cognition are mature or established.

Aphasia occurs when the language-dominant hemisphere, typically the left hemisphere, is damaged. Stroke is the most common cause of aphasia. Aphasia is differentiated into several different syndromes based on analysis of fluency and motor output, language comprehension, repetition, and naming. The predominant aphasia syndromes include Broca's, Wernicke's, global, anomic, conduction, transcortical motor, and transcortical sensory.

Other acquired communication problems include right-hemisphere dysfunction, traumatic brain injury, and dementia. Right-hemisphere dysfunction (RHD) most often results from stroke, which damages regions of the right hemisphere. Characteristics of RHD may include difficulties with receptive and expressive language as well as significant problems in perception, behavior, and cognition. Traumatic brain injury (TBI) occurs with both open- and closed-head injuries. TBI is most frequently a result of motor vehicle accidents, falls, or acts of violence. Deficits following TBI are highly diverse but may include alterations in consciousness, cognition, language, and behavior. *Dementia* describes a progressive decline in functional skills, most notably cognitive abilities. There is variability across performance profiles of individuals with dementia, largely based on the disease progression or stage.

The adult communication disorders of aphasia, RHD, TBI, and dementia hinder an individual's ability to function in daily routines and responsibilities. Affected adults often face disruptions in their social, vocational, and psychological well-being. Family roles are also affected. An interdisciplinary team approach to prevention, evaluation, treatment, and education for these adults and their families is necessary. The speech-language pathologist plays a key role in the rehabilitation of aphasia and other cognitive-based disorders through comprehensive evaluation, efficacy-based and personalized treatments, and education.

KEY TERMS

anomia, p. 226
aphasia, p. 220
apraxia, p. 222
circumlocution, p. 231
closed-head injuries, p. 241
dementia, p. 244
dysarthria, p. 222
echolalia, p. 231
embolism, p. 222
evidence-based practice, p. 235

functional outcomes, p. 237
hemorrhagic strokes, p. 223
ischemic strokes, p. 222
jargon, p. 230
logorrhea, p. 230
macrographia, p. 229
neologisms, p. 230
open-head injuries, p. 240
paraphasias, p. 226
polytrauma, p. 241

prognostic indicators, p. 234
prosody, p. 230
right-hemisphere dysfunction, p. 237
spontaneous recovery, p. 233
taxonomy, p. 223
thrombosis, p. 222
traumatic brain injury, p. 240

ON THE WEB

Check out the Companion Website at www .pearsonhighered.com/justice2e! On it you will find:

- suggested readings
- reflection questions

- a self-study quiz
- hot topics
- current technological innovations
- links to online resources

READING DISABILITIES

Laura M. Justice
Sonia Cabell

FOCUS QUESTIONS

This chapter answers the following questions:

1. What are the key components involved in skilled reading?

2. What is a reading disability, and how are reading disabilities classified?

3. What are the defining characteristics of prevalent types of reading disabilities?

4. How are reading disabilities identified?

5. How are reading disabilities treated?

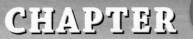

CHAPTER 8

INTRODUCTION

Many adolescents and adults in the United States do not exhibit the level of basic reading skills needed to succeed in school and work settings. By some estimates, about one-third of fourth-grade students in the United States are not proficient readers (National Assessment of Reading Progress, 2006). In 2003, national data showed that 14% of adult Americans (30 million) exhibited no more than the very basic literacy skills (National Assessment of Adult Literacy, 2003). This means that many students and adults currently do not have the reading abilities necessary to engage in such literacy-based tasks as using a map, ordering from a menu, completing a job application, following a recipe, or reading instructions on a prescription.

Not all of these students and adults who struggle with reading exhibit a reading disability, per se, although they certainly face significant handicaps when trying to achieve their basic needs in school, work, and society. In fact, the U.S. prison population is largely made up of persons with limited literacy skills, perhaps implying that being unable to read so greatly compromises a person's ability to succeed in society that crime presents the only alternative (National Assessment of Adult Literacy, 2003). Certain circumstances that many individuals face in life—particularly intergenerational poverty at home, limited home support for literacy, and enrollment in chronically underperforming schools—make achieving proficient reading skills out of reach. These circumstances are largely environmental in nature; such cases of reading difficulties may be attributable to experiential deficits, including poverty or poor instruction (e.g., Scanlon & Vellutino, 1997; Vellutino et al., 1996).

Reading difficulties or disabilities may also be attributed to intrinsic or neurobiological factors. For example, **dyslexia,** often used synonymously with the term *reading disability,* is defined as poor reading that is unexpected and constitutional in origin, with a core difficulty in phonological processes (Piasta & Wagner, 2008). Research has shown that dyslexia may be a heritable condition; the child of a parent with dyslexia has about a 50% chance of acquiring it (e.g., Hawke, Wadsworth, & DeFries, 2006). It is often difficult to separate children with experiential deficits and those with neurobiological deficits. Speech-language pathologists, audiologists, and their allied school and health professionals are troubled by these conditions, and many are involved with systematic efforts to prevent reading difficulties among at-risk children and remediate difficulties among adolescents and adults who exhibit reading disability. After providing a framework for understanding the key processes involved in skilled reading, this chapter defines and classifies reading disabilities and provides information on appropriate identification and treatment. ●●●

CASE STUDY 8.1	**Reading Disabilities**

BARCLEY is a 22-year-old single mother in St. Louis, Missouri. She is attending the local Adult Education Literacy Center (AELC) as part of a social services program in which she participates. Barcley goes to AELC three nights a week for 2 hours and works on developing basic reading skills. She has always considered herself dyslexic and has always had problems with even basic skills, like remembering the letters of the alphabet. When she was a child, she also had lots of problems talking and recalls seeing a speech therapist to work on making different sounds. A new teacher in the center, Ms. Shan, was formerly a reading specialist in the city school system. Ms. Shan has been working for the last 2 weeks with Barcley on learning the alphabet letters and practicing the sounds that go with them. Ms. Shan believes that Barcley might have a serious problem with phonological awareness, and she gave Barcley a few tasks to test her hypothesis, like making rhymes (*cat, hat*) and identifying when two words share the same first sound (*hat, hope*). Barcley could not do any of these activities and told Ms. Shan that she has "never been able to rhyme." Ms. Shan has a program she used to use with first graders that helped them develop phonological awareness, and she wants Barcley to go through the 36 lessons of this program. Barcley is definitely game and hopes to start next week.

Internet research

1. What proportion of adult Americans are unable to read at a basic level?

2. What types of community resources are commonly available for adults who cannot read?

Brainstorm and discussion

1. What might the connection be between Barcley's early problems with speech production and her current problems with reading?

2. What kinds of activities might be included in Barcley's phonological awareness training program? What is the goal of such a program?

3. In your opinion, how likely is it that Barcley will become a reader at age 22? What factors will most affect the likelihood of her success?

● ● ●

SAVANNAH WASSERSTROM is a 9-year-old student in a suburban elementary school in Ohio. She lives with her mother and is an only child. Savannah struggled with speech and language development when she was little. She did not start talking until she was nearly 3, and even then she was very hard to understand. Savannah received speech-language therapy at Head Start for 2 years, until she entered kindergarten. In kindergarten and first grade, Savannah had a lot of difficulty learning the letters of the alphabet and understanding the relationships between letters and sounds; she was consistently in the "low" reading group in her classroom and occasionally was paired with a tutor. Savannah, now a fourth-grade student, continues to have difficulty with some aspects of language (e.g., understanding jokes), problems following classroom directions, challenges in participating in conversations with other children, and serious struggles in comprehending what she reads. She refuses to participate in any oral-reading activities (e.g., reading aloud to her reading group) in her classroom.

Savannah's teachers view her as a "late bloomer" whose problems with communicating with others are due to shyness and embarrassment that stem from early speech difficulties. They see her struggle with reading as a result of "not trying hard enough." Savannah's mother, Mrs. Wasserstrom, is not assuaged by these perspectives and is growing more concerned about Savannah's communication and reading difficulties. Savannah struggles with reading at home and at school, and she never wants to look at books or talk about her reading problems. Mrs. Wasserstrom is wondering if Savannah's reading problems are related to her communication problems and is concerned that she will not be able to pass the state reading tests scheduled for the end of the year. If Savannah does not pass, she will probably be held back, and Mrs. Wasserstrom has concerns about Savannah having to repeat a grade. Mrs. Wasserstrom has requested that the school provide a speech-language and reading evaluation for Savannah, but the school personnel has rejected her request, noting that

Savannah's problems are too mild for an evaluation to be necessary.

Internet research

1 How many states have mandated fourth-grade reading tests? Do children with disabilities have to take these tests?

2 What does the 2001 No Child Left Behind Act say about mandated testing in reading for children?

Brainstorm and discussion

1 Is it legal for a school district to reject a request for a speech-language and reading evaluation if a parent requests it?

2 A comprehensive language evaluation involves investigation of classroom curriculum-based performance. What types of classroom artifacts of Savannah's should be examined?

3 Savannah does not like to read. How common is it for children who struggle with reading development to express resistance or dislike toward reading?

WHAT ARE THE KEY COMPONENTS INVOLVED IN SKILLED READING?

This section presents the key components involved in skilled and fluent reading. The first section describes the Simple View of Reading, which is a useful model for understanding the multidimensional nature of reading skill. The second section describes specific cognitive processes associated with reading. As a conclusion, we discuss how speech, language, and hearing professionals are involved with the identification and treatment of reading disabilities.

SIMPLE VIEW OF READING

The **Simple View of Reading** presents an equation for understanding what reading is: $D \times C = R$ (Gough & Tunmer, 1986; Hoover & Gough, 1990). In this equation, R is reading (or reading comprehension), in which a person draws meaning from written text and is the end goal of reading; D is decoding (or word recognition); and C is language comprehension. The multiplication sign in this equation is important, as it shows that reading is the multiplicative product of decoding and language comprehension. If performance on each component ranges from 0 to 1, it becomes clear that at least some skill in each is necessary. In short, skilled reading requires both decoding and language comprehension.

Decoding

Decoding as applied to reading an alphabetic language, as in English, Spanish, and French, involves applying the alphabetic principle to identify the spoken word that corresponds with a written word. The **alphabetic principle** is the understanding that speech and print correspond in a predictable, systematic fashion (Snow, Burns, & Griffin, 1998). Alphabetic languages are based on the systematic correspondences between each sound in the language and a unique symbolic representation of that sound (e.g., S = /s/). Consequently, every sound used in spoken English—of which there are 44—is represented by one or more written letters or, in some cases, a group of letters (e.g., "gh" for the final sound in *rough*).

Although it might seem that children need only to learn the letter or letter sequences corresponding to the 44 sounds of English to successfully acquire the alphabetic principle in English, this is hardly the case; rather, there are 251 different spellings corresponding to the 44 phonemes of English (Catts & Kamhi, 2005)! This makes learning the alphabetic principle a time-consuming process that, for many children with reading disabilities, can be extremely difficult.

As children learn to read an alphabetic language, they must learn these systematic correspondences between letters and sounds and then apply these correspondences to decode the many unfamiliar words they encounter as they read. Because of your knowledge of English orthography, you can decode virtually any word containing the English graphemes, even if you have never seen the word before, as in these:

drup, pram, doil, toud, wrin, dwin

These are called _pseudowords_ (or _nonsense words_), and are used to test students' ability to apply the alphabetic principle to unfamiliar words (Ekwall & Shanker, 1985; Gough & Tunmer, 1986).

DISCUSSION POINT:

Read the phrase _Drago mi je_. Likely, you had no trouble decoding it, but unless you know Croatian, you could not comprehend it. Before reading further, discuss the difference between the meaning of decoding and comprehension in the act of reading.

Educators must rely on pseudowords to test decoding skills, because once a child has decoded an unfamiliar word on one or several occasions, it will then be processed automatically on sight, in essence becoming a sight word for that child. Indeed, facility in decoding leads to automatic recognition of words (Ehri, 2005; Juel, 1988). Skilled readers, likely anyone who is reading this text, do not decode the words they encounter, per se; rather, they recognize these words effortlessly and automatically on sight. Therefore, for mature readers, the term **word recognition** is perhaps a better term than _decoding_ to describe the process of reading individual words, although _decoding_ and _word recognition_ are often used interchangeably (Catts & Kahmi, 2005).

Language Comprehension

Obviously, decoding or word recognition is not all that is involved with reading. If that were the case, everyone who successfully decodes the following question should be able to readily answer it:

Wie ist es Ihnen denn so ergangen?

However, since this question is posed in German, only those readers who know how to comprehend German reasonably well will be able to answer it. This is a reasonable illustration of the difference between decoding/word recognition and **language comprehension.**

When an individual reads, cognitive resources must be shared across word recognition and language comprehension. Consequently, comprehension is enhanced for the individual who recognizes words fluently and automatically, but it is compromised for the individual who struggles to decode what is read (Francis, Fletcher, Catts, & Tomblin, 2005). However, reading comprehension entails more than the ability to adequately translate print to speech (Kintsch, 2004). When the reader fluently decodes, text is immediately processed with little effort at the literal level, but reading is also a problem-solving process in which inferences must be made (Kintsch, 2004;

Skilled readers recognize words automatically and effortlessly on sight.

van Kleeck, Vander Woude, & Hammett, 2006). In fact, reading comprehension involves the interaction between the reader, the text, and the purposes of reading (National Reading Panel [NRP], 2000; RAND Reading Study Group, 2002). Readers are simultaneously drawing meaning from the text and constructing meaning based on their prior knowledge and experiences. In short, word recognition and language comprehension are related and, as represented by the Simple View model, dependent upon one another in the reading equation.

Spelling and Writing

This chapter focuses largely on reading, but the important constructs of spelling and writing require comment. **Spelling** represents the output of one's knowledge of the sound and symbol correspondences represented in the alphabetic principle; it is the encoding correlate of decoding. Spelling involves the encoding of sophisticated linguistic knowledge of the many rules that govern the correspondences between letters and sounds, such as those rules governing the spelling of various vowel patterns (e.g., "ea" vs. "ee" for *beat* and *beet,* respectively) and changes in spelling that occur when suffixes are appended (e.g., *healthy/healthier*). However, it does not involve rote memorization of rules; rather, spelling develops in conjunction with decoding ability and increases in sophistication as children grow in their knowledge of the alphabetic principle. Spelling is often studied by examining the patterns an individual uses to spell various words, such as whether all the sounds in a word are represented and how these sounds are represented (Ganske, 2000). For instance, analysis of a 6-year-old child's spelling of *bride* as *bid* shows that she has not yet mastered the spelling patterns of the vowel sound /aɪ/ and is not representing both sounds in the initial consonant cluster ("br.") Children's spelling typically develops in synchrony with their decoding ability (Bear, Invernizzi, Templeton, & Johnston, 2008). However, persons with reading disabilities typically will have problems with both decoding (word recognition) and encoding (spelling), and the latter can be quite pervasive (Cassar & Treiman, 2004).

Writing is a multidimensional process involving not only spelling but also mechanics and composition (Berninger et al., 2006). *Mechanics* (or handwriting) refers to the physical or manual act of producing writing, and it is often associated with fine motor development and visual-motor/eye-hand coordination. Writing mechanics is often studied by looking at the rate of writing speed as well as legibility. *Composition* refers to the meaning expressed by writing, associated with oral language skill, including grammar, vocabulary, and pragmatics. Writing composition is often studied by looking at the form of writing (the specific words and grammar used), the organization of the content, the genres produced (e.g., letters, stories, essays), and the way in which meaning is expressed, or creativity. Figure 8.1 provides an example of a 5-year-old's writing for examination of its mechanics, composition, and spelling.

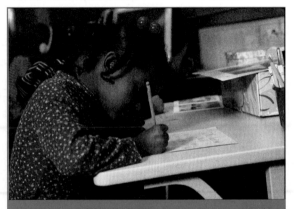

Writing is a multi-dimensional process that involves spelling, mechanics, and composition.

READING PROCESSES

Reading is a highly complex act that involves a number of core cognitive processes that interact to result in skilled word recognition and comprehension (Vellutino, Fletcher, Snowling, & Scanlon, 2004). Some

FIGURE 8.1

Writing sample of 5-year-old child.

Writing sample courtesy of Adelaide J. Mykel.

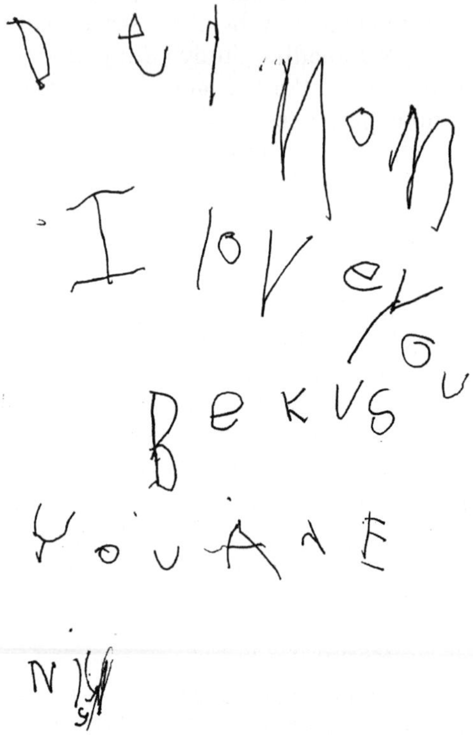

of these processes are specific to language, such as phonological processing, whereas others are more general, such as working memory. Some of these processes appear to be encapsulated, in that they act independently to process a highly specific type of input (e.g., visual information, phonological information), and many current perspectives of reading disability focus on problems specific to a single type of encapsulated processing ability. For instance, many experts view deficits in phonological processing (described shortly) as a key culprit in many cases of reading disability (Shaywitz & Shaywitz, 2005). While this perspective holds considerable merit, for skilled reading to occur, these basic perceptual processes become highly interactive at some stage of processing, presumably in the language-processing centers of the left hemisphere. Recent models of skilled reading emphasize the interactive nature of the many basic processes involved with skilled reading and suggest that this interactivity is an important source of compensation when one or several processing capabilities is weak (Stanovich, 2000). Thus, it is important to recognize that many individuals who become skilled readers do so not because they are strong in all basic processes associated with reading, but because the interactive nature of these processors serves to compensate for areas of limitation.

DISCUSSION POINT:
Describe this writing sample in terms of the child's spelling (representation of letters and sounds), mechanics (eye-hand coordination), and composition (expression of meaning).

Generally, several of the more critical processes involved with reading are differentiated into those that are code-related and those that are comprehension-related. *Code-related processes,* sometimes called *bottom-up processes,* directly support the act of decoding and word recognition, whereas *comprehension-related processes,* sometimes called *top-down or meaning-related processes,* directly support the act of language comprehension. Figure 8.2 provides a graphic illustration of several of the important processes involved with skilled reading.

Code-Related Processes

Two sets of processes are particularly important to word recognition and decoding: phonological processing and orthographic processing. To understand the importance of these processes, recall from earlier in this chapter that successful decoding requires application of the alphabetic principle. For developing readers to learn to apply the alphabetic principle and ultimately become automatic in its application, they must be able to process the two sets of symbols upon which alphabetic correspondences are based: phonemes and graphemes.

Phonological processing is the brain's processing of the phonological information contained within speech stimuli, to include the highly specific features of each phoneme. For instance, the phonemes /b/ and /p/ are quite similar, differing only on the characteristic of voicing (/b/ is voiced, while /p/

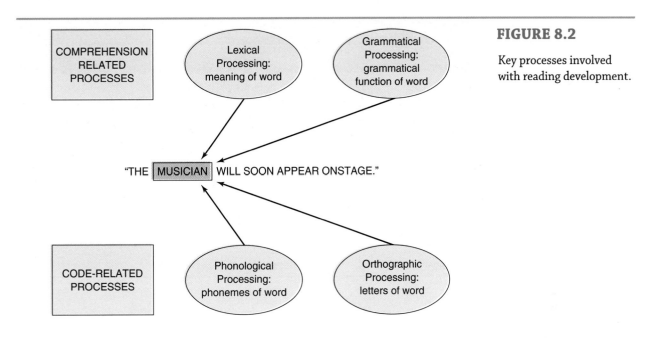

FIGURE 8.2

Key processes involved
with reading development.

is voiceless), and the brain must process these very fine distinctions between phonemes. Many people may have difficulties with such fine distinctions, yet for most everyday life activities that involve communication, such difficulties do not cause much concern. However, with respect to reading development, persons with phonological processing difficulties may find it extraordinarily difficult to learn to read, as phonological processing is a core element in successfully attaining the alphabetic principle and developing as a reader. When persons learn the alphabetic principle, they must have strong representations of the individual phonemes if they are to successfully learn the many phoneme-grapheme correspondences needed to be a good decoder.

Phonological processing difficulties appear to undermine an individual's ability to conduct three activities involved in the process of learning to read or the ability to read fluently: phonological awareness, phonological memory, and phonological retrieval. **Phonological awareness,** also called *phonological sensitivity,* is the ability to analyze and manipulate the phonological units of which words and syllables are composed (Gillon, 2004). This includes, for instance, being able to identify whether two words rhyme and to count the number of syllables in a word. *Phonemic awareness,* the most complex form of phonological awareness, refers to the sensitivity to individual phonemes and is critical for success in decoding. Indeed, phonemic awareness is one of the best predictors of reading ability (NRP, 2000). Tasks that involve phonological awareness appear in Table 8.1. The child who has poor phonological awareness will likely have difficulties learning to associate phonemes and graphemes and, as a result, may have significant delays in reading development (Gillon, 2004).

Phonological memory, also called *phonological coding,* is the ability to hold phonologically encoded information, such as words and sentences, in memory (Catts & Kamhi, 2005). When one wants to hold verbal information in memory, such as a telephone number, one will typically recite it from memory, a task that involves phonological processing. An example of a simple exercise requiring phonological memory is the digit-span task, in which an individual must repeat back to an examiner longer and longer spans of numbers, as in

TABLE 8.1	Types of phonological awareness tasks
Task	**Sample**
Rhyme production	*Tell me a word that rhymes with **map.***
Rhyme detection	*Which of these words rhymes with **map**: hip, hap, top?*
Syllable counting	*Clap with me for each syllable in the word **umbrella.***
Word counting	*Clap for each word in this sentence: **The butterfly is red.***
Syllable elision	*Say butterfly without the **fly.***
Sound elision	*Say hat without the **h.***
Beginning sound identification	*What is the first sound in the word **fire?***
Final sound identification	*What is the last sound in the word **frog?***
Sound blending	*Blend these sounds to make a word: / f /. . . /ɪ /. . . /s/. . . /t/*
Sound analysis	*Tell me each sound in the word **psych.***

7-5-1-4-6

8-6-3-6-8-5

9-1-4-2-5-7-3-1

Persons who have reading difficulties often perform poorly on such tasks, as compared to persons who read typically; these problems are confined to memory tasks that involve phonological or verbal stimuli, rather than nonverbal or visual stimuli, such as listening to strings of nonverbal tones (Nittrouer, 1999; Rvachew, 2007).

Phonological retrieval is the ability to retrieve phonological information about words. When one wants to produce a word, the word must be accessed within the lexicon, and at least two types of information must be retrieved: lexical information (the meaning of the word or concept) and phonological information (the sounds sequenced in the word; Levelt, 1999). This phonological information is then encoded into a string of phonemes to be produced by the articulators. We have all had moments when we cannot come up with the word to describe something; sometimes the word may be on the tip of our tongue, whereby we know the meaning of the word we want to express but cannot encode it phonologically. Some persons have significant problems with naming, referred to as *word-finding* or *naming difficulties,* whereas others are relatively slow in producing names of objects; both are generally attributable to difficulties with phonological processing, specifically imprecise phonological representations within the lexicon. To assess one's rate and accuracy of naming, researchers and clinicians use rapid naming tasks, in which individuals must identify as many pictured objects as they can within 1 minute (e.g., comb, dart, globe). Persons who are poor readers tend to name items more slowly and with more errors than good readers (Fowler & Swainson, 2004).

Orthographic processing is distinct from phonological processing and refers to the brain's ability to process the printed stimuli involved with reading words and letters. Orthographic processing relies on visual processing; the visual processes involved with reading are differentiated into *low-level visual processes* and *high-level visual processes* (Badian, 2005). Low-level visual processes include, for instance, tracking visual stimuli and recognizing different visual patterns, whereas high-level visual processes involve attending to and analyzing

DISCUSSION POINT:
Do you sometimes have difficulty coming up with the names of things? If so, try to discern some reasons for these naming difficulties—for instance, does it happen when you are tired or for certain types of words?

orthographic patterns (e.g., identifying differences between visually similar letters), holding orthographic patterns in memory, and accessing orthographic codes associated within a specific word (e.g., its spelling). A mental orthographic image (MOI) refers to the stored orthographic code for a given word. Some research evidence shows that orthographic information about words is stored separately from phonological information (Miceli, Benvegnù, Capasso, & Caramazza, 1997). Whereas lower-level visual processes do not appear to be causally related to reading disability (Vellutino et al., 2004), higher-level visual processes, referred to as *visual-orthographic processing,* may account for some types of reading difficulties, as children with reading difficulties perform relatively poorly on orthographic measures, such as identifying letters printed backward (Badian, 2005).

Comprehension-Related Processes

When people read, they must decode printed words and sentences and must understand what is read. Comprehension-related processes are those processing abilities that directly and indirectly facilitate reading comprehension, and these include lexical processing and grammatical processing. **Lexical processing** refers to accessing the meaning of words encountered in reading, called *lexical retrieval.* The end goal of decoding a word is, in fact, to access its meaning, which is stored in one's lexicon for words that are already known. Consequently, word recognition is largely a task of lexical retrieval, although it relies on code-level processing of letter-sound relationships (unlike listening, which involves processing only of sounds). Obviously, we do not have lexical entries for all words we encounter in text, as in the following (Taft, 1991):

> Even with hard yacka, you've got Buckley's of understanding this dinkum English sentence. (p. 1)

As Taft (1991) points out, the average Australian will have no problem comprehending this sentence, as the words *yacka, Buckley's,* and *dinkum* are likely to be entries in their mental lexicon; for others, this sentence may be incomprehensible. Lexical processing involves matching sensory information (phonological and visual-orthographic features of words) to semantic information contained about a word that is stored within the mental lexicon. This matching of sensory and semantic information involves accessing the lexicon—termed *lexical access*—from which we retrieve words. Some experts suggest that when individuals read, "bins" are accessed that represent sets of potential word matches constrained by the nature of the input received (Taft, 1991). For instance, when reading the word *spleen,* only bins containing words that start with the orthographic form "spl" and are nouns would be accessed (this bin would be activated based on features of the word being processed). Potential matches are sorted through until the best fit is represented. This obviously makes lexical access much more efficient than having to sort through all words contained in one's lexicon; in fact, lexical processing typically occurs so rapidly and automatically that we are unaware of it except in those relatively rare instances when we literally cannot find a word.

Some individuals have difficulty with lexical processing that transcends both oral and written language (Montgomery, 2002). Children with specific language impairment, described in Chapter 6, are much slower on lexical processing tasks involving listening and reading compared to other children, and it is unclear why (Montgomery, 2002). Lexical processing difficulties can contribute to delayed progress in establishing a strong vocabulary base, and smaller vocabularies are associated with poorer reading comprehension (Storch & Whitehurst, 2002).

Grammatical processing refers to the processing of grammatical functions of words in relation to other words in a sentence when reading. It also involves processing morphological components of words, including suffixes and prefixes. As individuals read, they appear to immediately assign grammatical categories to words, which then facilitates efficient comprehension of larger chunks of words, termed *phrases* (Perfetti, 1999). In English, knowledge of morphemes is particularly important in such tasks; for instance, one's knowledge of the past tense *-ed* marker facilitates the grammatical assignment of verbs (e.g., *chased, danced*). This automatic processing—and immediate assignment of words to syntactic categories—is illustrated through this example:

The horse raced past the barn fell.

If you felt momentarily confused and had to reread the sentence, this is because you automatically assigned the word *raced* to the category of main verb in this sentence, which created a problem when you reached the "real" main verb, *fell*. As this example suggests, two main syntactic elements of sentences— the subject (the horse raced past the barn) and the predicate (fell)—are particularly important to processing and comprehending a sentence (Leikin, 2002). Persons with reading difficulties may exhibit poor grammatical comprehension compared to those with typical reading skills, indicating that grammatical processing may be impaired (Catts, Fey, Zhang, & Tomblin, 2001b). However, given that persons who have reading difficulties may read much less often than those who read well and consequently get less exposure to written grammar, it is also possible that reading difficulties themselves may, over time, lead to difficulties in grammatical comprehension.

SPEECH, LANGUAGE, AND HEARING PROFESSIONALS' ROLES

To this point, this chapter has discussed key abilities related to reading, including word recognition and language comprehension, and described the importance of phonological processing, among other abilities, to achieving skills in word recognition. Because speech, language, and hearing are critical processes that underlie each of these abilities, individuals who identify and treat communication disorders have, in recent years, become more directly involved with providing services to persons with reading disability. The SLP, for instance, has a scope of practice related to reading that defines four sets of relevant activities (ASHA, 2001):

- Prevention of reading problems
- Identification of reading problems
- Assessment of reading problems
- Treatment of reading problems

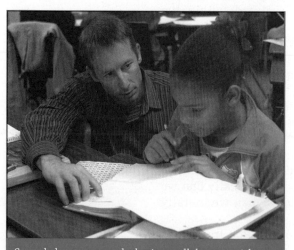

Speech-language pathologists collaborate with other professionals to prevent, identify, assess, and treat reading problems.

Largely, the SLP's involvement in these activities is one of consultant and collaborator, particularly regarding treatment of reading problems for which they may not

SPOTLIGHT ON LITERACY

Collaborating for Reading Success

Within America's schools, far too many children struggle to achieve skilled and fluent reading. Estimates from the U.S. Department of Education show that at least one-third of fourth-graders are not reading beyond very basic levels (National Center for Education Statistics, 2005). If the professionals who work within public schooling are to produce solutions to this pressing but complex issue, they must actively and effectively collaborate with one another.

Those specialists involved with ensuring the success of a pupil who is struggling with reading, whether a reading disability is present or the struggles are attributable to another cause, include the general educator, the learning disabilities specialist, the reading specialist, the speech-language pathologist, and possibly the school psychologist. An educational audiologist may be involved if processing problems are present. Each of these learning specialists has a scope of practice that pays some attention to reading development and reading difficulty, and all have specific types of expertise to share in the process of remediating the pupil's struggles. Yet, the ability for these diverse professionals to work together in schools can be difficult and oftentimes is not as seamless or effective as it ought to be. In part, this may reflect the insulated preprofessional training of these specialists, in which too little time is afforded to helping them develop an understanding of what other professionals may know and contribute to treatment of reading disabilities. Likewise, preprofessional training often provides little attention to what effective collaboration looks like and the processes involved with working with others on teams. Unfortunately, specialists who are not explicitly trained in the process of collaboration may find little time to develop these skills once they become busy professionals who face pressing issues each day.

have specialized training. Many other professions share these roles with the SLP and have expertise to offer. For instance, reading specialists have training in how to prevent, identify, assess, and treat reading problems, as do educators who specialize in this area. Adult literacy specialists may fulfill these roles with the adult population. For this reason, it is critically important that professionals who serve children, adolescents, and adults are knowledgeable of specific types of expertise various professionals have regarding reading disability and that they are able to work collaboratively, as discussed in the box Spotlight on Literacy: Collaborating for Reading Success.

WHAT IS A READING DISABILITY, AND HOW ARE READING DISABILITIES CLASSIFIED? ⬤

The first published paper on reading disability, prepared by British doctor W. Pringle Morgan in 1896, described an adolescent boy who, despite being apparently intelligent, had never been able to learn to read. Morgan labeled this condition as *congenital word blindness,* building upon the term *word blindness* used in the medical literature of the time to describe adults with acquired reading problems (Rawson, 1986). Although the term *word blindness* is no longer used today, Morgan's initial description largely holds, with dyslexia generally defined as unexpected difficulties with accurate or fluent recognition of words, often accompanied by spelling problems (Lyon, Shaywitz, & Shaywitz, 2003). In recent years, the umbrella of reading disabilities has widened to include children who have extreme difficulty with reading comprehension; indeed, there are cases of children whose reading

DISCUSSION POINT:
What comes to mind when you hear the word *dyslexia?* Explore your perceptions of dyslexia and consider which of your perceptions are valid versus those that are myths.

comprehension is compromised despite adequate word-recognition abilities (Catts, Hogan, & Fey, 2003; Catts & Kamhi, 2005).

HOW ARE READING DISABILITIES CLASSIFIED? ⬤

READING DISABILITIES: DYSLEXIA, SPECIFIC COMPREHENSION DEFICIT, AND MIXED READING DEFICIT

One way to classify reading disabilities is to identify whether an individual's difficulties with reading are primarily attributable to problems with decoding or with language comprehension (Catts et al., 2006; Catts & Kamhi, 2005). The Simple View of Reading, as discussed previously in this chapter, emphasizes the dual importance of decoding/word recognition and language comprehension to succeeding at reading. Corresponding to this premise, the individual who does not read well will have difficulties in decoding, comprehension, or, in some cases, both. Consequently, we may classify reading disabilities as to the extent of impacts in these two areas.

Doing so is a relatively recent advance in the field of reading disabilities (Catts et al., 2006; Catts & Kamhi, 2005). For some years, emphasis in the field of reading difficulties has focused nearly exclusively on identifying and understanding problems with word recognition, as this is the area in which problems with reading development usually first become apparent in children. Specifically, one of the most well-documented causes of reading disability is a core deficit in phonological processing; this deficit will manifest itself in the earliest stages of reading as children learn the alphabetic principle and begin to apply it to decoding tasks. The astute kindergarten or first-grade teacher is likely to recognize when a child is having difficulty learning this. Thus, the term *reading disability* has been used synonymously with *dyslexia* (Piasta & Wagner, 2008). More recently, researchers have recognized that there is a group of children who develop word-recognition skills relatively seamlessly but who then have unexpected difficulties with reading comprehension; these comprehension problems are attributable to core deficits in language ability, such as grammar and vocabulary, whereas phonological processing abilities are relatively intact (Catts et al., 2003, 2005, 2006).

Individuals with reading difficulties may be classified into three subgroups on the basis of whether they have difficulties in word recognition, language comprehension, or both, as presented in Figure 8.3 (Catts & Kamhi, 2005; Gough & Tunmer, 1986; Hoover & Gough, 1990). Individuals with poor word recognition and good comprehension are classified as having dyslexia; individuals with good word recognition and poor comprehension have a **specific comprehension disability;** and individuals with poor word recognition and poor comprehension have a **mixed reading disability** (Aaron, Joshi, & Williams, 1999; Catts, Adlof, & Ellis Weismer, 2006; Catts et al., 2003, 2005; Leach, Scarborough, & Rescorla, 2003).

FIGURE 8.3

Catts and Kamhi classification scheme for differentiating types of reading disabilities.

Source: From Catts et al., 2006.

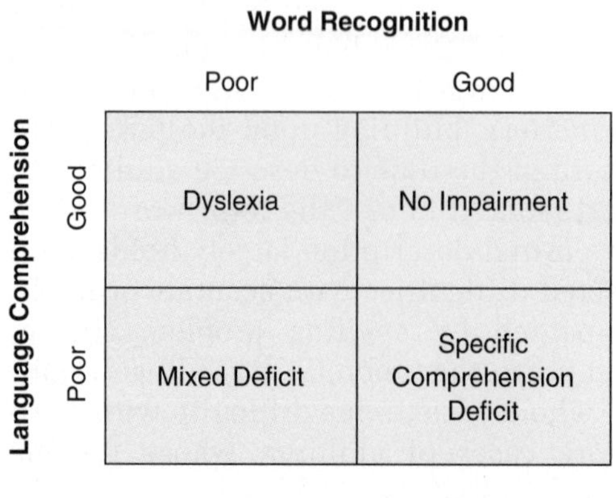

	Word Recognition	
	Poor	Good
Language Comprehension Good	Dyslexia	No Impairment
Language Comprehension Poor	Mixed Deficit	Specific Comprehension Deficit

WHAT ARE THE DEFINING CHARACTERISTICS OF PREVALENT TYPES OF READING DISABILITIES? ◉

In this section, we discuss defining characteristics for three types of general reading disabilities using the classification scheme presented in Figure 8.3: dyslexia, specific comprehension disability, and mixed reading disability.

DYSLEXIA

Defining Characteristics

Dyslexia, also known as *specific reading disability,* is a term that has a long and somewhat confusing history. First used more than a century ago to describe reading disability attributable to brain injury (i.e., acquired dyslexia), the term eventually came to identify (for many people) a reading disability characterized by letter and word reversals (see Catts & Kamhi, 2005). The term itself, as used by many researchers and clinicians, has no such connotation and generally refers to reading disabilities attributable to a core deficit in word recognition with at least adequate listening comprehension (Bruck, 1990; Vellutino et al., 2004). Sometimes the terms *learning disability, language-learning disability,* or *specific learning disability* are used within public schooling to describe reading difficulties to qualify children for special education services. In this context, reading disabilities are viewed as a specific type of learning disability.

Dyslexia (or developmental dyslexia), as the term is used in this text, describes a reading disability characterized by significant difficulty in achieving skilled word recognition and decoding abilities. This is the most common type of reading disability and is the most studied (for review, see Vellutino et al., 2004). We present four defining characteristics:

1. *Slow development of emergent literacy and early language skills.* In the years prior to formal reading instruction (from toddlerhood to kindergarten), children with dyslexia show relatively slow development of such important emergent literacy skills as **alphabet knowledge** and phonological awareness (Heath & Hogben, 2004). For instance, children who later are identified as dyslexic tend to know fewer alphabet letters at 4 years of age than children without dyslexia, and they have more difficulty identifying rhyming patterns. Also, relatively slow development of oral language in the areas of grammar, vocabulary, and phonology during the toddler and preschool years is characteristic of children later identified as dyslexic (Scarborough, 1990). At 30 months of age, children later identified as having dyslexia speak in shorter sentences (average of 2.4 morphemes in length) than children without dyslexia (average of 3 morphemes in length), and they make more errors in speech production (average of 43 consonant errors per 100 words) than children without dyslexia (average of 26 errors per 100 words; Scarborough, 1990). For some children with dyslexia, these early language difficulties signal the presence of a specific language impairment, which is present in about 15 to 20% of children with dyslexia (Catts et al., 2005).

2. *Specific disability in phonological processing.* A hallmark characteristic of dyslexia is a core deficit in phonological processing (Stanovich, 2000). Indeed, phonological processing seems to be the core "trouble spot" for children who fail to develop as readers despite being seemingly typical in all other areas of development (Nittrouer, 1999; Vellutino et al., 2004). Persons with dyslexia appear to have difficulty processing the phonological structure of spoken language, and

this difficulty seems specific to language rather than a general processing limitation that affects all auditory stimuli (Nittrouer, 1999). For most persons with dyslexia, these phonological processing limitations are not sufficiently serious enough to produce problems with comprehending or producing spoken language in everyday conversations, but they do present a specific handicap when one must carefully attend to phonemes for the purpose of mastering and applying the alphabetic principle. Difficulties with phonological processing are present early in life for the child with dyslexia and typically will persist over time, making learning to read much more difficult than it is for children who have no difficulties with phonological processing.

Perhaps as a result of core phonological processing limitations, the phonological representations of words within the lexicon of the person with dyslexia are underdeveloped, imprecise, or "fuzzy" (Fowler & Swainson, 2004). Because we use phonological information about a word we hear or read to access its meaning within the lexicon, the person with dyslexia typically has difficulty with lexical access. This difficulty is seen in rapid naming tasks, in which persons are asked to produce the names of items presented in pictures as quickly as possible. As described earlier in this chapter, persons with reading disabilities name items more slowly and make more naming errors than children without reading disabilities (Fowler & Swainson, 2004; Semrud-Clikeman, Guy, Griffin, & Hynd, 2000). These problems with naming are believed to reflect inadequacies in storage of phonological information about words within the lexicon and therefore seem symptomatic of deficits in phonological processing. However, some researchers believe that the naming problems seen in many persons with dyslexia do not reflect phonological processing deficits, but rather represent a separate and unique dimension of reading disability (Wolf & Bowers, 1999). Individuals who have deficits in both phonological processing and rapid naming are believed to have more severe dyslexia—termed a *double deficit*—compared to those with only phonological processing or naming difficulties.

3. *Slow development of decoding/word-recognition abilities.* With a core deficit in phonological processing seen as the primary cause of many reading disability cases, the primary result of this processing glitch is extreme difficulty in learning to read words (Piasta & Wagner, 2008). As discussed early in this chapter, learning to read relies on one's ability to represent sound-symbol correspondences. When one's representations of sound are faulty, this undermines one's learning of the alphabetic principle and the numerous correspondences that represent the relations between print and sound; in turn, the development of word-recognition skills occurs much more slowly in children with dyslexia relative to those who are not dyslexic, as shown in Figure 8.4. Note that children with dyslexia begin first grade with comparatively low scores in word recognition and that the gap separating them from typical readers becomes larger over time. For many children with dyslexia, this slow growth in decoding skills during the early years of reading instruction—typically first through third grade—is the first signal to parents and teachers that something is wrong.

4. *Less fluent reading.* Fluent reading occurs at a rapid pace and with little error, and involves the successful integration of the phonological, orthographic, and linguistic processes (i.e., grammatical, lexical) involved with reading (Wolf & Katzir-Cohen, 2001). Fluent reading is important for achieving practice in reading (fluent readers are able to read more words than nonfluent readers and thus get more practice reading) and for comprehending what is read. When one reads slowly or with error, reading comprehension can be compromised. Fluent reading involves rapid and accurate processing of letters, words, and connected

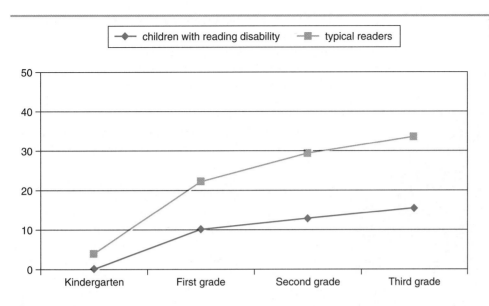

FIGURE 8.4

Growth in decoding skills over time for children with specific reading disability (dyslexia) compared to typical readers.

Source: Adapted from Vellutino, Scanlon, Small, and Fanuele (2006). Reprinted with permission.

text, and a breakdown at any level can impede reading fluency (Katzir, Kim, Wolf, O'Brien, et al., 2006). Perhaps because of core deficits in processing letters and words, persons with dyslexia tend to read much more slowly and make more errors when reading than persons without dyslexia; this can negatively impact the overall accuracy and rate of reading connected text.

Causes and Risk Factors

The causes of dyslexia are not well understood, although it affects slightly more boys than girls and tends to run in families, indicating that the disability is genetic (Hawke et al., 2006; Rutter et al., 2004). Having an immediate family member with specific decoding disability is one of the predominant risk factors for dyslexia. Recent neuroimaging studies show the presence of a specific brain difference among persons with dyslexia, in that language-processing regions of the left temporal and parietal lobes, including Broca's and Wernicke's areas, are underactivated during phonological processing and word-recognition tasks (Paulesu, Démonet, Fazio, McCrory, et al., 2001).

Epidemiological studies that examine a large group representative of the population have been used to determine the prevalence of children with dyslexia. One such effort (Rutter et al., 2004) involved examining the reading abilities of nearly 10,000 school-age students in Wales, England, and in New Zealand; the researchers identified the percentage of children who performed below the 15th percentile on standardized measures of reading. About 19% of boys and 11% of girls were identified with a reading disability according to these methods. This approach provides an objective and robust indication of how many children performed relatively poorly on standardized tests of reading in these countries; however, with no knowledge of these children's instructional experiences in reading, we cannot differentiate whether they had a legitimate reading disability or simply had poor instruction. Perhaps one of the most innovative approaches to determining the prevalence of reading disability involves determining the percentage of children who show profound difficulty learning to read in the context of intensive, high-quality instruction provided for a given time period. This method of identifying reading disabilities, termed *response to intervention,* seeks to differentiate children who have experientially based difficulties (who should be

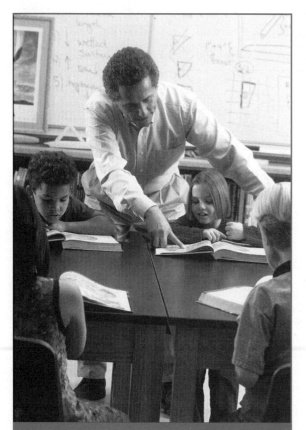

Response to intervention involves identifying children who show profound difficulties learning to read even with intensive reading interventions.

readily remediated given that their processing abilities are intact) from those with disabilities (who will be difficult to remediate given inherent processing difficulties). When intervention responsiveness is used to identify children with reading disabilities, studies find that about 2 to 6% of children show extreme difficulty in learning to read (Torgesen, 2004).

The prevalence of dyslexia is known to differ across cultures; for instance, it affects about half as many Italians as it does Americans (Lindgren, De Renzi, & Richman, 1985). This variability in prevalence rates seems attributable to differences in the orthographies being learned by members of a culture rather than differences in the actual base rate of the condition. Some orthographies are transparent, in that sound-letter mappings are consistent and unique (e.g., featuring one sound to one letter correspondence, as in Italian), whereas other orthographies are opaque, in that sound-letter mappings are more variable and oftentimes ambiguous (as in English; Paulesu et al., 2001). A person with dyslexia learning to read a transparent orthography is less likely to have difficulties than one who is learning to read an opaque orthography, although the level of impairment exhibited on processing tasks would be quite similar (Paulesu et al., 2001).

SPECIFIC COMPREHENSION DISABILITIES

Defining Characteristics

Compared to dyslexia, relatively little is known about reading disabilities that affect only reading comprehension. However, the condition clearly exists, with prevalence estimates indicating that about 5 to 10% of school-aged children experience this pattern of reading disability (Nation & Snowling, 1999). The three key characteristics of this disability are the following:

1. *Significant impairment in reading comprehension.* The primary characteristic of a specific comprehension disability is having significant deficits in the ability to comprehend what is read but having normal abilities in decoding and word recognition. In essence, these individuals have difficulty deriving meaning from what they read. This is particularly apparent when individuals with specific comprehension disabilities are asked questions about what they have read. Even when these questions focus on content explicitly presented in a text (e.g., where a story took place), these persons will have difficulty answering, as shown in Figure 8.5. These data depict the percentage of questions (out of 20) answered correctly by eighth graders after reading a grade-level passage and compare performance for pupils with specific comprehension disability, specific decoding disability (dyslexia), and typical reading skills. Those in the former group (pupils with specific comprehension disability) answered an average of 4 out of 20 questions correctly, about half as many as those in the other two groups.

2. *Comprehension difficulties attributable to core impairments in language ability.* Persons with specific comprehension disability have problems comprehending what they read, and these difficulties appear to be largely attributable to core impairments in language ability. In the early primary grades through the later

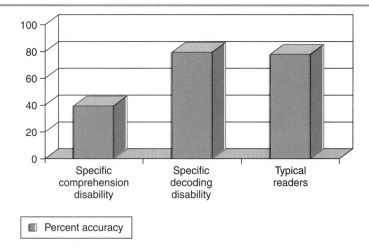

FIGURE 8.5

Performance of eighth graders with specific comprehension disability on reading comprehension questions.

Source: Adapted from Catts, Adlof, and Ellis Weismer (2006).

years of schooling, pupils with primary comprehension problems exhibit poor performance on measures of vocabulary knowledge, grammatical comprehension, and inferential language (the ability to infer meaning when it is not explicitly stated; Cain, Oakhill, Barnes, & Bryant, 2001; Catts et al., 2006). At eighth grade, for instance, children who are poor comprehenders score about 20 standard score points lower than children who read typically on measures of receptive vocabulary knowledge and score about 10 points lower than children with specific decoding abilities (Catts et al., 2006). Although these core difficulties with language ability may not be severe enough to signify the presence of language impairment in many children who are poor comprehenders, they are severe enough to compromise the process of reading comprehension.

　　3. *Unimpaired phonological processing and word recognition.* Individuals who have specific comprehension disabilities progress relatively normally in their reading development during the early primary grades, when the emphasis in reading instruction is largely focused on development of decoding skills. This is because children who are poor comprehenders have intact phonological processing capabilities, and as a result, typically exhibit no difficulties in learning the alphabetic principle and developing skilled word recognition. It is when reading instruction turns to focus on comprehension, typically in the later primary grades, that these youngsters' reading growth will explicitly begin to falter.

Causes and Risk Factors

The cause of specific comprehension disabilities appears largely attributable to language-based deficits, including developmental difficulties in vocabulary knowledge and grammatical performance. Some children with specific comprehension disabilities may meet criteria for a clinical impairment of language, such as specific language impairment (discussed in Chapter 6), although this is certainly not the case for all. Rather, many children with specific comprehension disabilities likely exhibit subclinical language problems, meaning that the signs and symptoms are not severe enough to surface as a clinical impairment. The cause of language difficulties, whether clinical or subclinical, is not well understood, but like dyslexia, it appears to be genetic, affects more boys than girls, and has been linked to specific structural brain differences (Flax et al., 2003; Watkins et al., 2002).

　　A particular challenge regarding persons with a specific comprehension deficit is that their reading difficulties are not likely to be apparent until the later grades of schooling. Figure 8.6 displays the lag in reading performance for this

FIGURE 8.6

Reading comprehension lag after grade 4 for children with specific comprehension deficit (poor comprehenders).

Source: From Catts, Adlof, and Ellis Weismer (2006). Reprinted with permission. GORT-3 = Gray Oral Reading Test-3 (Wiederholt & Bryant, 1992), a standardized and norm-referenced measure of reading comprehension.

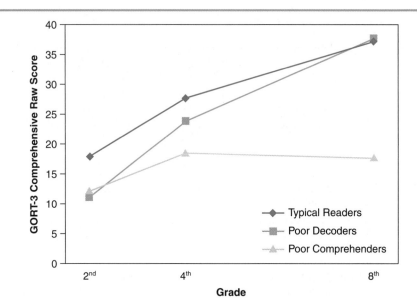

DISCUSSION POINT:
Many children, not only those with specific comprehension deficits, show a slump in reading performance at about fourth grade. Why do you think this happens?

group of children relative to those who are reading typically and those who have a reading disability specific to decoding. Developing approaches that can effectively identify this group of children well prior to their reading "slump" is an important area of future clinical practice and research.

MIXED READING DISABILITIES

Persons with mixed reading disabilities exhibit significant difficulties in both word recognition and language comprehension. Other terms used for mixed reading disabilities include *garden-variety poor readers* and *low achievers* (Gough & Tunmer, 1986; Fletcher et al., 1994). These individuals exhibit characteristics of dyslexia *and* specific comprehension disability simultaneously (Stanovich & Siegel, 1994), and as a result have long-standing challenges in both learning to read in the primary grades and reading to learn in the later years of schooling. About one-third of second graders in one study were found to have a mixed reading disability (Catts et al., 2003), indicating that this form of disability occurs about as commonly as the specific decoding and specific comprehension variants. The causes underlying mixed reading disabilities are not well understood. Ongoing research is exploring genetic linkages between reading disabilities and specific language impairment (Flax et al., 2003); it may be that persons with a mixed reading disability inherit vulnerabilities for both reading disability and language impairment.

HOW ARE READING DISABILITIES IDENTIFIED? ●

Too often, children with reading disabilities are not identified until they have exhibited problems with reading development for several years. Savannah's case, presented in Case Study 8.1, is all too familiar to many professionals who treat reading disabilities. In this case, Savannah showed many warning signs of a reading disability, including problems with early language acquisition followed by difficulties in kindergarten with learning the letters of the alphabet. If Savannah is identified as having a reading disability now, at fourth grade, it will be quite difficult for her to "make up" the loss in reading experience of the last several years. As a relatively challenged reader, Savannah has now missed out on literally hundreds of hours of exposure to new words, sentence types, prefixes and suffixes, and subject-matter knowledge to which she could have been exposed if she had been reading. In addition, Savannah is now reluctant to read. It is important to ask whether her reading disability, if in fact she does have one, could have been identified at a much earlier time—perhaps at kindergarten or even earlier. Likewise, we must also ask whether early intervention offered in response to earlier identification could have prevented the current problems Savannah is experiencing.

The approach to assessment of reading disabilities is currently changing dramatically, with an increasing emphasis on early identification of reading disabilities before children begin to read or in the earliest stages of reading development. Rather than waiting until children show obvious and persistent difficulties with reading in the later primary grades, which has long been the prevailing approach to identifying a reading disability, experts are now focusing on ways to identify reading disabilities much earlier in children's lives, sometimes even before they start reading, through use of **screening assessments.**

Screening Assessments

Chapter 4 described the importance of screening for the early identification of difficulties within any communication domain. In the area of reading, screening is particularly important for identifying children who show early indicators of difficulty, as these early difficulties can be readily remediated for many children, particularly for those whose reading difficulties are attributable to experiential issues (e.g., limited home literacy experiences).

Screening for Prereaders

Screening for children's reading disabilities typically employs a systematic approach involving administration of a small set of reading-related tasks. While reading disabilities are not generally diagnosed during preschool and kindergarten, common screening tasks examine children's development of precursory reading skills that are associated with later reading performance. Such skills include phonological awareness, alphabet knowledge, **print-concepts knowledge,** and early writing skill (Justice, Invernizzi, & Meier, 2002). Children's performance in each of these dimensions of early reading development, as measured during preschool and kindergarten, is predictive of future reading performance; children who perform poorly on such tasks may be at risk for future reading difficulties. A screening tool may include several different subtests to examine children's performance in each of these areas—for example the Phonological Awareness Literacy Screening-PreKindergarten (Invernizzi, Meier, & Sullivan, 2004) contains six subtests and a total of 67 items, as shown in Table 8.2. This tool was designed for professionals, including teachers, to use as a way to identify children who may need extra support developing important early reading skills. A child who performs poorly on one or more subtests would be a candidate for early intervention that addresses the areas of identified need (Invernizzi, Justice, Landrum, & Booker, 2004).

A potentially more efficient way to screen for early indicators of reading disability, albeit one that is potentially less informative, is to sample only a few items illustrative of each dimension of early reading development, including phonological

TABLE 8.2   Subtests of the Phonological Awareness and Literacy Screening—PreKindergarten (Invernizzi, Meier, & Sullivan, 2004)

Subtest (Number of Items)	Description
Rhyme awareness (10)	Examines ability to identify words that rhyme (e.g., *hen/pen*)
Beginning sound awareness (10)	Examines ability to identify words that share a common initial sound (e.g., *sink/sad*)
Name writing (1)	Examines ability to produce own written name
Alphabet knowledge (26)	Examines ability to name the 26 uppercase alphabet letters
Print and word awareness (10)	Examines knowledge of 10 concepts about print (e.g., location of book title, difference between letters and words)
Nursery rhyme awareness (10)	Examines knowledge of common nursery rhymes

awareness, alphabet knowledge, print-concepts knowledge, and early writing skill. The Get Ready to Read! (GRTR) screening instrument developed by the National Center for Learning Disabilities (NCLD) features a total of 20 items to sample 4-year-old children's skills across these different dimensions of development (available at the NCLD website for free at www.getreadytoread.org).

Screening for Readers

Once children are able to read some written material, typically toward the end of kindergarten, most screening tasks feature word-reading exercises in addition to exercises that examine underlying processes involved with reading skill, including phonological processing. Some tasks may also examine reading comprehension, particularly for older readers. The Dynamic Indicators of Basic Early Literacy Skills (DIBELS) provides one illustration of what typical screening tasks look like for readers. This is available free of charge at http://dibels.uoregon.edu (note that costs are involved to use the DIBELS online data entry and reporting system). DIBELS screening tools are designed to detect difficulties in reading development for kindergarten through sixth-grade pupils. Sample tasks used with readers include the following:

1. *Nonsense Word Fluency (middle of kindergarten to beginning of second grade):* This task identifies the number of nonsense words (e.g., *sig, rav, ov*) a child can decode in 1 minute. At the end of kindergarten, children who decode fewer than 25 words per minute are considered at risk for reading difficulties, as are first graders who decode fewer than 30 words per minute at the end of the year.

2. *Oral Reading Fluency (middle of first grade to end of sixth grade):* This task identifies the number of words a child can read correctly within a grade-level passage in 1 minute. Words produced in error (e.g., substitutions, omissions) are not counted. At the end of first grade, children who read fewer than 40 words per minute are considered at risk for reading difficulties, as are second graders who read fewer than 90 words per minute at the end of the year and third graders who read fewer than 110 words per minute at the end of the year. Guidelines for interpreting performance of fourth through sixth graders are also available.

DIAGNOSES AND DESCRIPTION

Screening tasks are not sufficient for identifying the presence of a reading disability; rather, they are used to signify a child's risk for reading disabilities and to identify candidates for supplemental or specialized reading interventions. Within U.S. schools, all children in kindergarten through third grade receive reading instruction as part of the general education curriculum, and many preschool programs include a prereading focus in response to state standards specifying the importance of attending to prereading development in early childhood programs. Screening tasks are typically used to identify children whose development of fundamental prereading or reading skills seems delayed relative to expectations or normative comparisons, and who require reading interventions above and beyond that available in the general education curriculum. Children who exhibit low response to intervention—that is, who fail to make sufficient prereading or reading gains even within the context of high-quality intervention delivered for a reasonable period of time—are candidates for a comprehensive reading assessment designed to (1) diagnose a reading disability and (2) describe one's reading ability and disability.

Diagnosing a Reading Disability

Traditionally, the diagnosis of a reading disability was based on a person exhibiting significantly lower reading achievement than is expected based on age, intelligence, or educational experiences (American Psychiatric Association, 1994). The disability could be present in reading accuracy (decoding/word recognition) or reading comprehension, and for a diagnosis to be made, difficulties with reading must be sufficiently severe so as to interfere with one's academic achievement or daily living experiences. Diagnosis of a reading disability per this definition involves administration of a comprehensive standardized normreferenced test of reading achievement, such as the Woodcock Reading Mastery Test—Revised (WRMT-R; Woodcock, 1987), suitable for kindergarteners through adults. A reading disability may be diagnosed if an individual exhibits poor performance on the WRMT-R (e.g., at the 10th percentile) in the presence of average to above-average nonverbal intelligence, also as measured by a standardized norm-referenced test.

This definition, used within many school and clinical settings today, is problematic to many experts because of its emphasis on diagnosis requiring a discrepancy between one's reading achievement and intelligence, and the implicit assumption that an individual who exhibits a reading disability must have normal or near-normal intelligence. As reading researcher Keith Stanovich (1991) pointed out some time ago, the use of intelligence scores as benchmarks for diagnosing reading disability has seriously "led us astray," given that a discrepancy between one's intelligence and reading achievement appears to have no real relevance—theoretically or scientifically—to confirming the presence of a reading disability. Increasingly, alternative approaches to the discrepancy approach to diagnosis of reading disability are being explored, including (1) an intraindividual differences approach, (2) a low achievement approach, and (3) the **response to intervention (RTI) approach** (Fletcher, 2003). Professionals today use any one of these approaches, and there is little consensus regarding which one, if any, is the most effective way to identify persons who have a reading disability.

Intraindividual Approach. The **intraindividual differences approach** is based on the premise that individuals with a reading disability have a core deficit in one or more underlying processes involved with reading achievement, such as lexical access or rapid naming (Fletcher, 2003). As a result, a comprehensive examination of reading and reading-related skills should show uneven performance across various skills, with uncharacteristically low performance in one or more basic processes. Diagnosis based on this approach examines an individual's test performance to look at patterns of strengths in relation to unexpected weaknesses or limitations that may contribute to difficulties in reading growth.

Low achievement approach.   The **low achievement approach** bases diagnosis of reading disability solely on the presence of low achievement in reading, relative to a specific cutoff point (Fletcher, 2003). For instance, persons who receive standardized reading scores below the 25th percentile may be diagnosed as having a reading disability. The problem with this approach is that it does not take into consideration the role of experience and instruction in learning to read; consequently, a child who failed to learn to read because of poor attendance at school would be diagnosed with a reading disability, thereby conflating experientially based reading problems with a neurobiologically based disability.

Response to Intervention.   In the last decade, a novel approach has emerged by which to identify cases of reading disability. This approach is termed **response to intervention,** or RTI (Fuchs & Fuchs, 2005). RTI is based on the premise that identification of reading disability requires assurance that children have high-quality opportunities to learn to read and that those who fail to "respond" to these opportunities exhibit a reading disability (Vellutino et al., 1996). RTI approaches are important for differentiating between children who have experientially based difficulties with reading achievement and those who have a neurobiological impairment that makes learning to read extremely difficult (Justice, 2006). Children in the former group, if provided high-quality opportunities to learn to read, should respond to these interventions by progressing well in reading development; by comparison, those in the latter group should exhibit low response to intervention (sometimes called **treatment resistance**), because they have a reading disability.

Frank Vellutino, a pioneer in early studies of RTI, used this approach to identify reading disabilities. Vellutino and colleagues (2006) implemented high-quality kindergarten and first-grade reading programs with more than 1,000 kindergarteners and first graders in upstate New York. Many of the children came to school with experiential risks to their reading development, as indicated by low performance on school-entry screenings. The researchers implemented multi-tier interventions for the students, focusing specifically on those who appeared at risk on the basis of periodic reading screening tasks. A multi-tier intervention involves the coupling of high-quality classroom-based reading programs with supplemental tiers of support—typically in the form of small-group and one-on-one tutorial sessions delivered several times per week. These tutorials focused on important reading skills with which children seemed to have difficulty (e.g., phonological awareness, vocabulary). By the end of third grade, the research team showed that most of the students, even those identified as at-risk, had responded to the reading interventions provided. Some children were no longer at risk by the end of kindergarten, whereas other children were more difficult to remediate and needed extra tiers of support in first grade. Only about 2% of children did not respond to intervention and exhibited poor word-reading skills at third grade; their lack of responsiveness to intervention likely signifies the presence of a reading disability (Torgesen, 2000). Attention to how professionals can most effectively use RTI to identify children with reading disabilities, including specific subgroups of children, will likely dominate the reading-disability literature for the next decade.

Diagnosis using this approach involves providing individuals with quality reading intervention for an extended period of time and charting their rate of growth in reading and reading-related processes. Special types of assessment tools, called *progress-monitoring measures,* are used to chart growth and to identify when the rate of growth is sufficiently poor so as to signify a disability.

Describing Reading Ability and Disability

Assessment for reading disability involves diagnosing the presence of a reading disability and carefully describing an individual's reading ability and areas of disability. Regardless of age, persons who have reading disabilities are remarkably heterogeneous in their reading abilities; for assessment results to be useful, they ought to describe an individual's abilities so that intervention can be carefully tailored to build upon existing capabilities and help an individual progress as a reader. The description of reading abilities afforded by a comprehensive assessment addresses, at the least, the following seven areas, as shown in Table 8.3: (1) processing abilities, (2) word recognition and decoding, (3) vocabulary knowledge, (4) reading comprehension, (5) reading fluency, (6) reading motivation, and (7) writing and spelling.

TABLE 8.3   Reading abilities described in comprehensive reading assessment

Reading Ability Area	Description/Goal
Processing abilities	Document performance on measures of phonological processing (e.g., phonemic awareness), short-term memory, rapid naming, vision, hearing
Word recognition and decoding	Document performance on measures of function words, grade-level words (Dolch word lists), nonsense words (word attack), and recognition of words varying in orthographic patterns and complexity (word recognition)
Vocabulary knowledge	Document performance on measures of basic single-word receptive and expressive vocabulary, abstract vocabulary words, curriculum-based vocabulary words
Reading comprehension	Document performance on reading comprehension tasks for grade-level passages and for passages matched to reading ability (if individual is not reading at grade level), comprehension of information presented explicitly in text and information presented implicitly
Reading fluency	Document the rate and accuracy of reading silently and aloud for grade-level passages and for passages matched to reading ability (if individual is not reading at grade level)
Reading motivation	Document feelings about and motivation toward reading, reading interests, amount of pleasure reading, and reading for instructional purposes
Writing and spelling	Document written composition at preplanning and planning stages, expository and fictional composition, language content (e.g., syntax, word choices), spelling

Sources: Catts & Kamhi (2005); Spafford & Grosser (2006).

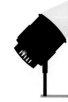

SPOTLIGHT ON TECHNOLOGY

Handheld Assessment Devices for Reading Interventions

Reading interventionists are increasingly using handheld assessment devices to monitor children's progress in reading interventions delivered in schools and clinics. The need for real-time data input and analyses on reading assessments is driven by the growing interest in studying children's responsiveness to intervention, in which children's growth within reading interventions is monitored very closely so that adjustments can be made if necessary (e.g., increasing the intensity of intervention, changing goals of instruction). It is increasingly common to see a teacher, reading specialist, or speech-language pathologist use a handheld assessment device to conduct a quick probe of children's reading skills, such as their fluency in reading nonsense words. The specialist enters the child's raw performance data into the handheld device, which provides real-time calculations of scores, graphs of pupil growth over time, and recommendations for specific types of activities based on those scores.

HOW ARE READING DISABILITIES TREATED? ◉

DISCUSSION POINT:

The involvement of many professionals to address reading disabilities requires close collaboration. What factors contribute to high-quality collaboration among professionals?

The treatment of reading disabilities is complex because it may involve many professionals, including general educators, special educators, speech-language pathologists, reading specialists, clinical/school psychologists, adult literacy educators, and neuropsychologists. The treatment of reading disabilities may occur in many settings, including public schools, independent schools designed solely for children with reading disabilities, outpatient clinics, university clinics, and adult literacy programs. Treatment programs for reading disabilities can look very different depending upon who is delivering the treatment and where the treatment is occurring. Regardless, the goals of any treatment for reading disabilities should be explicitly focused upon helping individuals become automatic and fluent readers who can comprehend what they read; the strategies used to achieve these goals should reflect the accumulated scientific findings regarding how to effectively reach these goals.

TREATMENT GOALS AND APPROACHES

Treatment goals and methods for reading disabilities should be functional in nature and designed to lead to explicit improvements in one's ability to read and to comprehend. Given the Simple View of Reading discussed previously, in which skilled reading is considered the multiplicative product of decoding and comprehension, treatment goals should address skills that support achievements in both decoding and comprehension. For the child who is not yet reading—the prereader—treatment goals are designed to support the development of precursors to decoding and comprehension. For the child who is a reader, treatment goals are designed to support ongoing improvements in decoding and comprehension. It is important to keep in mind that the treatment described in this chapter is applicable to all struggling readers, not only those with reading disabilities. Children with reading disabilities are not a qualitatively different group from other struggling readers; rather, they differ from them in the severity of difficulty with regard to key areas of reading (e.g., decoding, comprehension; Shaywitz, Shaywitz, & Fletcher, 1992). Thus, intervention efforts will not be qualitatively different from those recommended for other struggling readers but will differ in intensity.

Treatment Goals and Methods for Prereaders

Some children show delays in acquiring skills that serve as a foundation for the later development of decoding and comprehension skills. Foundational skills related to later achievements in decoding include phonological awareness, alphabet knowledge, print-concepts knowledge, and early writing skill (National Early Literacy Panel, 2004; Whitehurst & Lonigan, 1998); foundational skills related to later achievements in comprehension include grammar, vocabulary, and narrative (Justice, Sofka, & McGinty, 2007; Pankratz et al., 2007). Many children acquire these foundational skills with relatively little difficulty and without any direct instruction; these children are poised for success in beginning reading instruction, which begins around 6 years of age. However, some children show delays in acquiring these skills; delays are commonly associated with a language impairment or cognitive disability (Justice, Bowles, & Skibbe, 2006) as well as lack of home support for literacy (Roberts, Jurgens, & Burchinal, 2005). Prereading interventions offered to children with early delays in prereading skills are designed to increase the likelihood that they will be ready for, and therefore be successful in, beginning reading instruction. In this regard, interventions for prereaders are considered *preventive* in nature, designed to keep children who exhibit early risk indicators from progressing toward a reading disability (Snow et al., 1998).

Foundational Skills Related to Decoding

Phonological Awareness.   Children who start beginning reading instruction with sensitivity to the sound structure of spoken language are likely to be successful acquiring the alphabetic principle and knowledge of sound-letter correspondences (Storch & Whitehurst, 2002). In fact, low levels of phonological awareness are seen as a major impediment to children's success in beginning reading instruction. Intervention for prereaders will include explicit attention to building phonological awareness—for example, teaching awareness of rhyme patterns (e.g., *bike/hike*), syllabic composition of words (*bi-cy-cle*), onset and rime boundary in single-syllable words (e.g., *b/ike*), and initial sounds in words (b̲ike).

Many approaches may be used to provide effective phonological awareness intervention, including use of relatively low-cost commercial curricula such as *Phonemic Awareness in Young Children* (PAYC; Adams, Foorman, Lundberg, & Beeler, 1998). This curriculum contains a comprehensive set of activities that can be readily implemented in the classroom, clinic, or even home environment to build children's phonological awareness. The games are relatively fun for children too. For example, in one activity, children pull objects out of a basket with their eyes closed, say the name of the object, and identify how many syllables are in the word.

Alphabet Knowledge.   Children who are successful in beginning reading instruction have well-developed knowledge of the alphabet letters. Children whose knowledge of alphabet letters is limited will receive treatment to improve this knowledge, including increasing knowledge of many (if not all) of the uppercase letters, some uppercase/lowercase letter correspondences (e.g., N/n), and some letter-sound correspondences (e.g., $N = /\eta/$). Many approaches are available to teaching alphabet knowledge to prereaders, ranging from use of songs to direct instruction with worksheets. However, to ensure that children learn the alphabet letters in a meaningful way, some researchers advocate use of **print referencing** during shared storybook reading as a way to address alphabet knowledge goals (Justice & Ezell, 2004). When reading storybooks with young children, adults can explicitly reference letters by pointing to them and commenting on them, particularly when reading storybooks in which the narrative print is relatively large or when letters are an object of attention, as with alphabet books. When adults call attention to letters by pointing or commenting, children look more often at letters and show increases in their alphabet knowledge in relatively short periods of time (Justice & Ezell, 2000; Justice, Pullen, & Pence, 2008).

Print-Concepts Knowledge. Children who become successful readers arrive at beginning reading instruction with knowledge about the rules that govern print; this includes knowledge of how books are organized (e.g., cover page, author name depiction), the functions of print in various genres (e.g., lists, invitations), and major print units (e.g., letter, word, punctuation devices). Building children's knowledge of print concepts, including those listed in Table 8.4, can be readily addressed using the print-referencing technique discussed previously. When reading storybooks with children, professionals can pause explicitly to draw attention to certain features or functions of print, as in the following:

DISCUSSION POINT:
Identify several specific print references you could use when reading with a young child to increase her attention to print in the storybook.

> Speech-language pathologist: The sign on this crate says "danger" (runs finger along the word). This word says danger because the crate contains a lion. Let's look at this word "danger." What is the first letter in the word "danger"?

Repeatedly reading books with children and highlighting attention to print is an effective way to promote their knowledge of various print concepts (Justice & Ezell, 2000).

Early Writing. Supporting prereaders' early development of writing skills can serve to promote their knowledge not only of writing but also of skill areas that are closely associated with writing, including phonological awareness, alphabet knowledge, and print-concepts knowledge (Aram & Biron, 2004). This is because the production of writing, even early writing efforts (see Figure 8.1), requires children to encode their knowledge of print and sounds. Interventions for prereaders will often include a writing component to increase their knowledge of

TABLE 8.4	Print concepts targeted in prereading interventions
Book cover	Understanding the difference between the front (cover) and the back of book
Page order	Understanding that pages turn from front to back of book
Book title	Understanding where the title of the book is located and the purpose it serves
Book author and illustrator	Understanding where the name of the author and illustrator are located and the roles they play in preparing a book
Page organization	Understanding that print on a page is read from top to bottom
Print directionality	Understanding that print on a page is read from left to right
Concept of letter	Understanding that a letter is a distinctive unit of print
Concept of word	Understanding that a word is a distinctive unit of print
Letter-word relationship	Understanding that words are composed of letters
Narrative print	Understanding that narrative print provides the storyline of a book

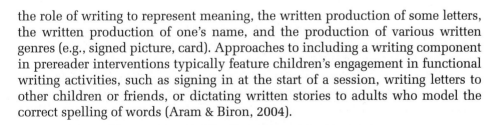

SPOTLIGHT ON RESEARCH AND PRACTICE

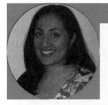

NAME: SONIA Q. CABELL

PROFESSION/TITLE
Research Coordinator, Preschool Language and Literacy Lab, University of Virginia

PROFESSIONAL RESPONSIBILITIES
As Research Coordinator, I oversee the federally funded research activities conducted in the lab. These activities focus on early language and literacy development as well as teacher training. I also engage in collaborative research projects and serve as a resource to others.

A DAY AT WORK
A typical day may begin with a meeting with colleagues about research projects or data management. Throughout the day, I supervise research assistants as they enter or code data. In addition, I am involved in data analysis and manuscript preparation for a variety of research projects.

HOW INTERESTS IN COMMUNICATION SCIENCES AND DISORDERS BEGAN
Prior to pursuing my doctoral degree, I served as a second-grade teacher and a reading specialist in the public school system. Because the training I received thus far did not include courses in child language, this important piece was missing from my knowledge base. While a doctoral student at UVA, I focused specifically on preschool literacy, which requires an interdisciplinary knowledge of language and reading. My work in the lab began as a research associate of a project designed to enhance the oral language abilities of preschoolers. As my appreciation for the contribution of language to reading grew, my interests shifted to examining the intersection of language and reading problems. Specifically, I undertook research projects focusing on preschoolers with specific language impairment (SLI).

CURRENT RESEARCH AND PRACTICE INTERESTS
I am currently exploring the heterogeneity of emergent literacy skills among children with SLI by identifying subgroups of children who display different patterns of performance with regard to print concepts, alphabet knowledge, emergent writing, and rhyme awareness.

MOST EXCITING/INTERESTING PROFESSIONAL ACCOMPLISHMENT IN CSD
I led a study that investigated the name-writing abilities of preschoolers with SLI, a first step in the examination of emergent writing within this population.

the role of writing to represent meaning, the written production of some letters, the written production of one's name, and the production of various written genres (e.g., signed picture, card). Approaches to including a writing component in prereader interventions typically feature children's engagement in functional writing activities, such as signing in at the start of a session, writing letters to other children or friends, or dictating written stories to adults who model the correct spelling of words (Aram & Biron, 2004).

Foundational Skills Related to Comprehension

Oral Language Skills: Grammar, Vocabulary, and Narrative. Intervention for prereaders must include attention to those skills that foreshadow decoding success (e.g., phonological awareness, alphabet knowledge) and those oral language skills that provide the foundation for reading comprehension. Prereading intervention will therefore promote such grammar skills as the ability to comprehend and produce elaborated noun phrases (e.g., "The very little dog"), multiclause sentences (e.g., "I don't want that one because it's not pretty"), and a variety of sentence types (e.g., interrogatives, negatives). In the area of vocabulary, attention is directed toward helping the child to comprehend and produce at least 1,000 word roots, to learn morphemes to inflect words (suffixes and prefixes) to expand vocabulary, and to gain the ability to rapidly acquire meaning of new words. In the area of narrative, attention is directed toward helping the child to comprehend and produce a variety of narrative types (e.g., personal accounts, fictional stories), to learn major story grammar elements (e.g., setting, character, conflict), and to identify cohesive devices that tie together narrative events.

Treatment Goals for Readers

Treatment goals for children who have difficulty learning to read in the primary or later grades typically focus on producing functional improvements in reading skill in both decoding and comprehension. Treatment goals generally focus on fostering growth in five areas considered to be essential components of reading instruction (NRP, 2000): phonemic awareness, phonics (word recognition), vocabulary, reading comprehension, and fluency. A quality intervention program for struggling readers will include attention to each of these areas in every intervention session, as shown in the sample lesson plan in Figure 8.7. These 30-minute lessons must be offered with suitable intensity if they are to make a difference in children's reading trajectories. Treatment sessions for kindergarteners should occur two or three times per week, often in small groups, whereas sessions for early primary students should occur daily in a one-on-one format. For older students who have persistent struggles with reading achievement, sessions must be delivered with even greater intensity if intervention is to effectively remediate their reading problems (Torgesen, 2003).

FIGURE 8.7

Sample lesson plan for treatment of reading disability.

5 min	Familiar text-reading activity: Child rereads a familiar text that is at independent reading level (words are read with 95–99% accuracy)
5 min	Phonemic awareness activity: Represent and manipulate sounds using colored blocks for words varying in complexity (consonant-vowel-consonant pattern, consonant-consonant-vowel-consonant pattern, etc.)
2 min	Sight word identification activity: Play a game to practice a bank of words drawn from previously read texts.
8 min	Phonics/word study activity: Word study and sort of words based on analysis of specific phonics patterns
10 min	Guided reading activity: Read a text unfamiliar to child and that is at instructional reading level (words are read with 90–95% accuracy); provide instruction in targeted tier-two vocabulary words, comprehension of text, and use of comprehension strategies

Source: Spafford & Grosser (2006); Vellutino et al. (2006).

Phonemic Awareness.   The achievement of skilled word recognition relies upon, in part, attainment of the alphabetic principle. Phonemic awareness, or the ability to represent each of the individual sounds comprising spoken words, is a prerequisite for mastering the alphabetic principle. As mentioned earlier, phonemic awareness falls under the larger umbrella term of *phonological awareness.*

Consequently, treatment goals will include some attention to developing phonemic awareness if a child's skills in this area are deficient. These goals will focus on fostering the child's ability to identify and blend the individual sounds in words, to segment the individual sounds in words, and to reorganize and manipulate the sounds in words (NRP, 2000). Commercial programs such as the Lindamood Phonemic Sequencing for Reading, Spelling, and Speech can be readily implemented by professionals and are effective for improving phonemic awareness as well as related areas of development, including word recognition and spelling (Torgesen et al., 1999).

Phonics.   To be a skilled reader, one must recognize words rapidly and automatically. Children with dyslexia or mixed comprehension disability have problems with developing word-recognition skills and as a result, their reading progress is stifled, such that the third-grade child with a reading disability may be reading books typical for first graders. Thus, fostering decoding skills is an essential goal of all reading treatment programs, and these will focus on increasing the child's ability to identify and blend individual sound sequences in words, to identify and blend familiar orthographic chunks (e.g., *pre + view*), to recognize words as whole units, and to make analogies from words known (e.g., *sight*) to those unknown (e.g., *fright*) (Torgesen, Al Otaiba, & Grek, 2005).

For word-recognition skills to improve, experts emphasize that intervention must be intensive, explicit, and supportive (Torgesen et al., 2005). Intensive interventions feature high levels of interaction between the therapist and the child by increasing intervention time (e.g., number of sessions per week) and by lowering the therapist-child ratio; explicit instruction involves directly teaching the child strategies to use to engage in successful word recognition; and supportive instruction features strong emotional support coupled with extensive scaffolding designed to help the child succeed in a given task (Torgesen et al., 2005).

Vocabulary.   To be a skilled reader, one must match words read in text to words stored in the lexicon. A word that is read that has no entry in the lexicon cannot be comprehended; consequently, even if a child can successfully decode the word *orchestra* in written material, meaning cannot be attached to the word if it is not stored in the lexicon. Ensuring that children have a sufficient vocabulary in their lexicon to comprehend what they read is an important element of reading treatments. Largely, vocabulary instruction will focus on building the child's base of **tier-two words** (Beck, McKeown, & Kucan, 2002). Tier-two words are those commonly known and used by mature speakers of a language community, and they generally add precision to one's ability to express meaning; these are words children will encounter frequently in written texts. Examples include *predator, hustle, haste,* and *grimace.* These words occur much less commonly than basic-level tier-one words (e.g., *cat, go, fast, sad*) and thus are not often in the repertoire of children who are developing vocabulary knowledge slowly (Beck et al., 2002).

Treatment for reading disabilities should include explicit attention to promoting tier-two vocabulary knowledge for children, with at least seven new words introduced per week. A common approach to delivering vocabulary instruction is through the use of trade books; these contain a great deal of tier-two words that are not commonly heard in everyday conversations. The first few pages of an abridged version of *Frankenstein* (Shelley/McFadden, 2006) include such tier-two words as *reality, company, stubbornly, savage, layers,* and *fainted.* When reading trade books with children, using *elaborated exposures* is an important way to teach these tier-two words (Justice, Meier, & Walpole, 2005). An elaborated exposure involves pausing after the child hears the tier-two word, defining it using a child-friendly definition, extending its meaning beyond the text, and giving the child an opportunity to say the word and discuss it (Beck et al., 2002).

Reading Comprehension.   Successful comprehension of what one reads relies upon well-developed language skills in areas of grammar, vocabulary, and narrative. However, it also requires one to draw upon and integrate knowledge of content area facts and text schemata (Westby, 2005). Content area facts are basic information (e.g., content) presented in a text, such as facts in a science text about the different types of cloud formations. *Text schemata* refer to the way information is hierarchically arranged within various texts. For instance, information is presented in a very particular way within science texts, and the reader who understands the presentation will comprehend the text better than the reader who does not. An important component of effective reading interventions is helping children to learn to read strategically so that they can identify when difficulties with content area facts or schemata have hindered their comprehension. Reading treatments will include helping children to learn to engage in *comprehension monitoring* and to take corrective actions when comprehension has failed (NRP, 2000; Westby, 2005).

Reading Fluency.   Promoting children's ability to read with appropriate rate, expression, and little error is an essential component of reading treatment. Approaches to building reading fluency are based on the premise that practice engaging in a skill is what will build that skill; consequently, to increase reading fluency, a child must practice reading aloud connected text. Effective reading treatments provide dedicated time in every session for children to read text that is aligned with their word-recognition capabilities—text that is not too hard and not too easy. An important skill of the reading interventionist is being able to match readers to texts so that children have time practicing highly fluent and automatic reading of texts at their *independent level* (95 to 99% of words are recognized automatically and comprehension is high) and texts at their *instructional level* (90 to 95% of words are recognized automatically and comprehension is at least 80%). Repeated reading (aloud) of independent-level texts builds reading fluency, whereas repeated reading of instructional-level texts builds word-recognition skills; children with reading disabilities must have ample opportunities to read both types of texts.

   Treatment goals for struggling readers, particularly those who have faced challenges with reading achievement for several years, may also need to include explicit attention toward improving their motivation to read. Additionally, treatment goals for struggling readers may also include attention to any related problems in written composition and spelling.

CHAPTER SUMMARY

SLPs play a supportive role in the treatment and identification of reading disabilities and thus must possess a knowledge base of reading development and disability. According to the Simple View of Reading, reading is the product of adequate decoding/word recognition and language comprehension. Reading disabilities can be classified, using the Simple View, into three categories: dyslexia, specific comprehension disability, or mixed reading disability. Dyslexia is a neurobiologically based and heritable condition that is primarily characterized by a core deficit in phonological processing; persons with dyslexia display adequate language-comprehension abilities. Specific comprehension disability is characterized by difficulty in language comprehension with adequate word-reading abilities. Mixed reading disability involves difficulty in both word recognition and language comprehension.

Screening measures and diagnostic approaches identify the presence of a reading disability and describe the features of the disability. Screening approaches are available for both prereaders—used in prevention activities—and readers. The response to the intervention approach identifies reading disabilities by studying the rate with which an individual responds to high-quality reading instruction.

Interventions for reading disabilities are differentiated in terms of whether an intervention recipient is a prereader or a reader. For the prereader, intervention is designed to promote the child's acquisition of precursory skills predictive of future decoding performance, including alphabet knowledge, print-concepts knowledge, and early writing skill, as well as precursory skills related to later achievements in comprehension of grammar, vocabulary, and narrative. For the child who is a reader, intervention targets functional improvements in reading skill, including enhancing development of phonemic awareness, word recognition through **phonics instruction**, vocabulary, reading comprehension, and reading fluency.

KEY TERMS

Alphabetic principle, p. 251
Alphabet knowledge, p. 261
Decoding, p. 251
Dyslexia, p. 249
Grammatical processing, p. 258
Intraindividual differences
    approach, p. 269
Language comprehension,
    p. 252
Lexical processing, p. 257
Low achievement approach,
    p. 270

Mixed reading disability, p. 260
Orthographic processing, p. 256
Phonics instruction, p. 279
Phonological awareness, p. 255
Phonological memory, p. 255
Phonological processing, p. 254
Phonological retrieval, p. 256
Print-concepts knowledge,
    p. 267
Print referencing, p. 273
Response to intervention (RTI)
    approach, p. 269

Screening assessments, p. 267
Simple View of Reading, p. 251
Specific comprehension
    disability, p. 260
Spelling, p. 253
Tier-two words, p. 277
Treatment resistance, p. 270
Word recognition, p. 252
Writing, p. 253

ON THE WEB

Check out the Companion Website at www .pearsonhighered.com/justice2e! On it, students will find:

• suggested readings
• reflection questions

• a self-study quiz
• links to additional online resources, including current technologies in communication science and disorders

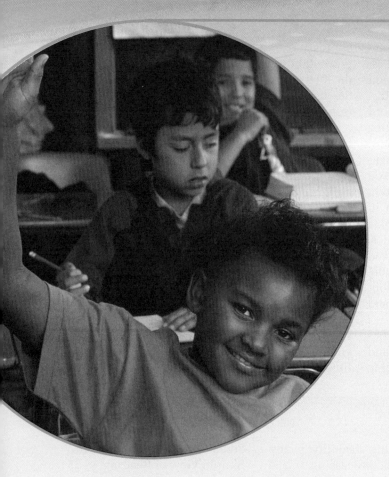

PHONOLOGICAL DISORDERS

FOCUS QUESTIONS

This chapter answers the following questions:

1. What is a phonological disorder?
2. How are phonological disorders classified?
3. What are the defining characteristics of phonological disorders?
4. How are phonological disorders identified and described?
5. How are phonological disorders treated?

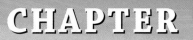
INTRODUCTION

Phonological disorders are one of the most prevalent types of communication impairment among children. Children with phonological disorders have difficulty developing and using the sounds of their native language, a problem commonly known as **speech delay** or speech-sound disorder (SSD). These children produce multiple errors in the articulation of specific sounds and sound patterns and may be unintelligible because they produce a number of sounds in error. Unintelligibility can cause marked frustration in very young children, because they are unable to communicate their needs and interests to important people in their lives. Consider, for instance, the following interaction between Julie and her mother:

> JULIE: e-uh an I o-ah mo-y e ou a be
>
> MOTHER: What? Say it again.
>
> JULIE: e-uh an I o-ah mo-y e ou a be
>
> MOTHER: You want the ear? The mirror? Honey, what?
>
> **Julie starts crying and lies down on the floor.**

In older children, phonological disorders can affect the ability to communicate effectively with peers and teachers and can undermine the ability to learn critical literacy skills, including reading and spelling.

A phonological disorder becomes evident during the developmental period for speech-sound acquisition, from birth through 9 years of age (Shriberg, 1997). During this period, children develop a keen sensitivity to the rules that govern the phonology of their native language and learn to articulate all the sounds of their language to intelligibly produce words and sentences. As children's phonological growth progresses, they often produce interesting renditions of words and sounds that display their yet-to-be-perfected phonological and articulation skills. It would not be surprising, for instance, to hear a 2-year-old refer to a computer as a "moocuter" and a tomato as a "motito," or to hear a 3-year-old say "lellow tun" for *yellow sun* or "over dey-ah" for *over there*. My 18-month-old son currently says "da" for *bath* and "wawa" for *water*. Four- and 5-year-old children might say "dat" for *that* and "wabbit" for *rabbit*. Errors such as these are normal and mark children's ongoing quest to master phonology and articulation. Such errors are systematic, predictable, and typical for this important period of speech-sound development. For roughly 90 to 95% of young children, they do not impact speech intelligibility, nor do they cause breakdowns in children's communication with others.

For a small but consequential portion of children, phonological development proceeds much more slowly, and early achievements in phonology and articulation are marked by great difficulty and unintelligibility. When children's speech is unintelligible, their ability to communicate with those in their lives is compromised, and there can be long-standing consequences for literacy and social performance when they enter school. Although phonological disorders often accompany physical and developmental disabilities, such as hearing impairment and intellectual disability, for the majority of children with significant phonological disorders, the cause is unknown. This chapter provides an overview of the characteristics of phonological disorders and describes assessment and treatment options for children with these disorders. ●●●

CASE STUDY 9.1   Phonological Disorders in Early and Later Childhood

OCTAVIO is a 5-year-old student in Ms. Hudson's kindergarten classroom in San Diego, California. Octavio has only limited proficiency in English, as he comes from a home in which Spanish is spoken exclusively. Octavio speaks few words in English in the classroom and does not interact at all with his peers. He works with an English as a second language (ESL) teacher, Mr. Peras, who is bilingual in Spanish and English. Both Mr. Peras and Ms. Hudson are concerned about Octavio's speech-sound production, noticing that in both Spanish and English he is very hard to understand. In English, for instance, he says "obby" for *doggy* and "aa-oo" for *bathroom*. Mr. Peras and Ms. Hudson have asked the speech-language pathologist to come to the kindergarten classroom and observe Octavio for an evaluation. They have also called for a child-study meeting to begin the process of referral for a formal speech-language evaluation.

Internet research

1. What proportion of children in California's schools speaks Spanish as a first language?

2. Octavio's ESL teacher is bilingual, but his teacher is not. How likely is it that a teacher in an American elementary classroom of primarily Spanish-speaking children would not speak Spanish?

Brainstorm and discussion

1. What strategies can be used to identify whether Octavio's suspected phonological difficulties are the result of a speech difference or a speech disorder?

2. What are some strategies Ms. Hudson might use in the classroom to promote Octavio's successful communication with his classmates?

● ● ●

EMILY is a 9-year-old who has received speech-language therapy for as long as she can remember. She has always struggled with producing certain sounds and still has problems producing /l/ and /r/. Emily has always valued working with the speech-language pathologist at her school and feels that she is making good, although slow, progress. This year, Emily's drama teacher is encouraging her to audition for a role in the school play *Much Ado about Nothing*. Emily is hopeful that by the time auditions come around, her speech problems will be completely resolved. Recently, Emily's parents were informed that she was no longer eligible for speech services at school, as her speech problems did not impact her educational performance. School officials explained that they could not provide services unless the effects of Emily's speech difficulties had clear educational impact. Emily has asked her parents if she can see a speech-language pathologist privately, but they cannot afford it, and their insurance will not cover it. Emily is very concerned about her upcoming audition and is considering backing out.

Internet research

1. How many children receiving special education services at school participate in extracurricular activities such as school plays?

2. What percentage of children in the early elementary grades qualify for special education services? What amount of the federal budget for education is directed toward special education services for children?

3. What does the term *educational impact* mean in schools when determining whether a child is eligible for special education services?

Brainstorm and discussion

1. What does the term *educational impact* mean to you? What are some obvious and less obvious ways that a communication disorder can affect a child's educational performance?

2. Emily's parents are considering appealing to the school to pursue her right to special education services. Do you think they will be successful in their appeal? What factors might affect the likelihood of success?

WHAT IS A PHONOLOGICAL DISORDER? ●

DEFINITION

A **phonological disorder** is an impairment of an individual's phonological system that results in a significant problem with speech-sound production that differs from age- and culturally based expectations. The onset of the disorder occurs prior to 9 years of age, and its cause may be known or unknown (Shriberg, Kwiatkowski, & Gruber, 1994). The term **articulation disorder,** often used interchangeably with *phonological disorder,* emphasizes the impact of the disorder on an individual's ability to articulate certain speech sounds effectively (Bauman-Waengler, 2004). The term *phonological disorder* is preferred when emphasizing that the articulation disturbance results from an impaired phonological system. The term *speech-sound disorder* (SSD) is increasing in popularity given that it does not explicitly imply that an individual's disordered speech is attributable to an impairment of phonology or articulation; it is seen as a neutral term (Shriberg, in press).

Recall from Chapter 1 that phonology is the part of the language system that governs its sound structure. Phonology includes the inventory of sounds used in a particular language and the set of rules governing how these are combined to make meaningful units (e.g., syllables and words; Bauman-Waengler, 2004). As their phonological systems develop, children acquire a representation of each phoneme in their native language as well as the rules that govern how these phonemes are arranged into syllables and words. Children develop boundaries around each phoneme that differentiate the phonemes from one another in the phonological system. For instance, in English, /r/ and /l/ have boundaries that separate them, whereas in Mandarin Chinese, there is no such boundary, and these are considered a single phoneme.

Two important aspects of phonological development are therefore (1) developing a representation for each phoneme in one's language and (2) developing a solid and stable boundary around each phoneme to make it distinct from the other phonemes. The boundary is particularly important for phonemes that are similar, such as /t/ and /d/ and /f/ and /v/. The boundary between these **cognates**—two phonemes that differ by only one characteristic (voicing, for these examples)—needs to be especially solid for their differentiation.

If the phonological system develops too slowly, children experience a delay in the acquisition of internal phonological representations and have difficulty creating boundaries between phonemes (Shriberg et al., 2000). These problems with the phonological system can result in mild to profound problems producing individual speech sounds and using these speech sounds in syllables and words for conversational speech. The most common symptom of this disorder is unintelligibility.

PREVALENCE

Prevalence is an epidemiological term used to describe the number of cases of a condition among the population. Prevalence describes the percentage of persons who exhibit a disorder at a particular point in time (i.e., the number of cases within a population in a given year). The term *lifetime prevalence* describes the percentage of persons who experience the disorder sometime within their lives, whereas *point prevalence* and *period prevalence* identify, respectively, the percentage of persons affected during a short interval (1 day to 1 month) or over a year (1 month to 12 months). The term *incidence* is similar to that of *period prevalence* and is used to specify the number of persons who develop a disorder within a specific period of time, typically during the course of a year. Tracking the incidence of a disorder year to year is useful for determining whether a condition is increasing or decreasing in the population.

Estimates of the prevalence of phonological disorders indicate that 4 to 13% of children are affected, with recent research supporting the lower estimate of about 4 in 100 children (Shriberg, Tomblin, & McSweeney, 1999). Phonological disorders affect boys at slightly higher rates than girls—4.5% versus 3%. Estimates also suggest that African American children exhibit phonological disorders at slightly higher rates (5.3%) than do European American children (3.8%, Shriberg et al., 1999). In 60% of cases, the phonological disorder cannot be attributed to any known cause; about 40% of cases are associated with recurrent middle-ear infections, developmental motor speech disorders (described in Chapter 12), and other developmental disorders, such as Down syndrome (Shriberg, 1997).

DISCUSSION POINT:

Young boys are affected with phonological disorders at slightly higher rates than are girls. Brainstorm some possible explanations for this phenomenon.

TERMINOLOGY

Phonological versus Articulation Disorders

Speech-language pathologists (SLPs) were historically called *speech teachers* because of their focus on treating speech-sound problems. Although much has changed in the treatment of communication disorders over the last several decades, treatment of speech-sound problems remains one of the most common activities of speech-language pathologists. Because of their prevalence, speech-sound problems are also one of the most heavily researched childhood communication disorders.

Changes in the terminology used to describe speech-sound problems mirror our increasing knowledge about the bases for speech delays. Until recently, the terms *articulation disorder* and *speech disorder* prevailed in the literature, describing significant speech-sound problems in children, and these terms are still often used. The use of the term *articulation* emphasized the perspective that speech-sound problems resulted from a motor problem affecting the positioning of the articulators (tongue, lips, teeth, etc.). Consequently, traditional approaches to treatment focused on speech correction—helping children to

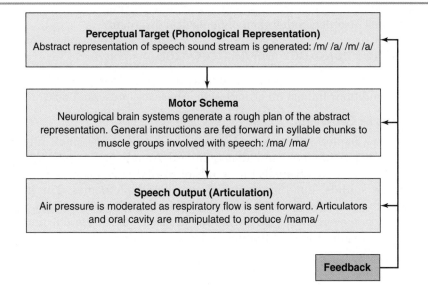

FIGURE 9.1

Model of speech production.

Source: Adapted from Raphael, Borden, & Harris (2007).

improve their articulatory patterns by remediating one sound at a time (van Riper, 1963).

Research in the 1970s increasingly emphasized a linguistic perspective that viewed articulation problems as rooted in the phonological system specifically and the language system more generally (Elbert, 1997). Figure 9.1 provides a contemporary model of speech production that depicts the link between phonological representations and speech output, or articulation. A linguistic perspective of disordered speech views the problem as emerging from the level of phonological representation. Children's faulty phonological representations result in immature but systematic phonological productions. Although on the surface such children have difficulties articulating sounds, the problem results from delays in the maturation of the underlying phonological system. This perspective emphasizes the importance of considering both the **surface representation** and the **underlying representation** of phonology—what we produce (articulation) and the underlying representation (phonology). Increasingly, treatment for phonological disorders focuses on building and reorganizing children's phonological representations rather than improving the surface articulation of specific speech sounds.

These shifting perspectives have influenced the terminology used to describe significant speech disorders affecting children. *Phonological disorder, developmental phonological disorder,* and *phonological impairment* are the current preferred terms (Shriberg, 1997). Likewise, terms used to describe assessment and treatment for speech-sound disorders also emphasize a phonological perspective. These include *phonological assessment* and *phonological analysis,* which describe clinical tools used to evaluate the organization of an individual's phonological system, and *phonological remediation* and *phonological intervention,* which describe the process clinicians use to bring about change in an individual's phonological system.

The term *phonological disorder* does not capture all varieties of speech-sound problems in children. Chapter 12 describes two other prevalent childhood disorders that impact the production of speech sounds: apraxia and dysarthria. Unlike phonological disorders, apraxia and dysarthria are disorders of the motor functions that affect articulation planning and delivery; thus, these are considered motor speech disorders rather than phonological disorders.

DESCRIBING PHONOLOGY AND ARTICULATION

Knowledge of a number of key concepts is necessary to discuss phonological disorders and their impact on articulation. These are presented next.

Phonemes as Contrasts

Recall from Chapter 1 that every language has a relatively small number of sounds, called *phonemes,* and that Standard American English (SAE) uses about 40 phonemes to create its thousands of words. SAE speakers actually use many more sounds, but these are not considered phonemes. For instance, the /p/ in *pig* is subtly different from the /p/ in *map.* Despite being produced differently, however, these two variations of /p/ are not different phonemes; rather, they are allophones. **Allophones** are the variations of a single phoneme.

To be considered a phoneme, a speech sound must be able to signal a contrast in meaning between two words of a language. This property of phonemes is called *contrastiveness.* We know, therefore, that /b/ and /p/ are two different phonemes in English, as they signal a meaning contrast in words that share all other sounds, such as *bat* and *pat, big* and *pig,* and *rip* and *rib.* During the developmental period of speech-sound acquisition, children form an underlying representation of each phoneme—a phonological representation—that establishes its contrast to other phonemes.

DISCUSSION POINT:
This chapter describes the abstract concept of phonological representation, which is a difficult concept for some students to understand. Spend a few moments creating your own definition of this term, and share it with a peer.

The International Phonetic Alphabet

Any discussion of speech sounds and phonological disorders requires at least a basic knowledge of the International Phonetic Alphabet (IPA). The **International Phonetic Alphabet** is a phonetic alphabet that describes and classifies each speech sound on the basis of how and where it is produced in the speech mechanism. The IPA is the most commonly used system to represent the phonemes making up the world's languages. It is used by SLPs, linguists, educators, and others to transcribe children's speech patterns.

The IPA represents each phoneme used in the world's languages—both vowels and consonants—as a specific symbol. When IPA symbols are used to transcribe an individual's speech production, each sound is represented by a symbol, and the transcription is usually placed between slashes (e.g., /bIg/ for *big*). Figure 9.2 provides a list of the IPA symbols used to transcribe the American English consonants.

Articulatory Phonetics

Examination of the IPA chart may reveal some unfamiliar terms, such as *bilabial, labiodental, fricative,* and *trill.* These terms characterize and classify the articulatory features of different phonemes. An articulatory feature serves as a road map to what the articulators are doing when a phoneme is produced. The classification of speech sounds in this way is called **articulatory phonetics.**

One important articulatory feature of a speech sound is whether it is a vowel or a consonant. Vowels and consonants differ primarily in the extent of constriction in the oral cavity when the sound is produced. With a **vowel,** there is relatively little constriction against the airflow in the oral cavity, whereas with a **consonant,** the airflow is constricted in some way—this is their defining feature. For instance, with /t/ and /d/, the constriction occurs when the tongue strikes against the alveolar ridge. With /m/, /b/, and /p/, the constriction occurs

FIGURE 9.2

IPA symbols for consonant phonemes of Standard American English.

b	bat	r	rose
p	pat	s	sun
d	dip	ʃ	shine
t	tip	t	toast
g	give	tʃ	birch
h	hot	θ	think
j	yes	ð	that
k	cat	v	vet
l	lot	w	wash
m	mine	z	zag
n	nose	ʒ	treasure
ŋ	ring	ʤ	jail

when the top and bottom lips press together. With /h/, the constriction occurs in the glottal area near the vocal folds.

Vowels.   Each vowel is characterized by four articulatory features (Lowe, 1994):

1. *Height:* How high is the tongue placed when the vowel is produced? Vowels are classified as high, mid, or low.

2. *Frontness:* How far forward is the tongue placed when the vowel is produced? Vowels are classified as front, central, or back.

3. *Roundness:* Are the lips rounded when the vowel is produced? Vowels are classified as rounded or unrounded. Only vowels characterized as back on the frontness dimension are rounded.

4. *Tension:* Are the articulators tense or lax when the vowel is produced? Vowels are classified as tense or lax. Only tense vowels can serve as open syllables (syllables that end with a vowel rather than a consonant), as with the vowel /o/ in the second syllable of "shallow" and the vowel /i/ in the single-syllable word "flee."

For example, the features for /I/ (as in *pin*) are (1) the tongue is high in the oral cavity, (2) the tongue is forward in the oral cavity, (3) the lips are unrounded, and (4) the articulators are tense. Table 9.1 describes these characteristics for each vowel in the Standard American English vowel system.

Consonants.   Consonants are characterized by three key articulatory features, although the dimensions by which they are classified differ from those of vowels.

1. **Place of articulation:** Where in the oral cavity or vocal tract is the constriction when the consonant is produced? Consonants are classified as bilabial, labio-dental, interdental, alveolar, palatal, velar, or glottal.

2. **Manner of articulation:** How is the consonant produced, or how is the airflow manipulated by the articulators? Consonants are classified as stop, nasal, fricative, affricate, liquid, or glide.

3. **Voicing:** Are the vocal folds vibrating during production of the consonant? Consonants are characterized as voiced or unvoiced.

TABLE 9.1   Vowels, characterized by four articulatory features

Vowel Symbol	Example	Articulatory Features
i	f<u>ee</u>t	high, front, unrounded, tense
ɪ	f<u>i</u>t	high, front, unrounded, lax
e	m<u>a</u>ke	mid, front, unrounded, tense
ɛ	b<u>e</u>t	mid, front, unrounded, lax
æ	c<u>a</u>t	low, front, unrounded, lax
a	f<u>a</u>ther	low, front, unrounded, tense
u	bl<u>ue</u>	high, back, rounded, tense
ʊ	h<u>oo</u>f	high, back, rounded, lax
ɔ	b<u>ough</u>t	mid, back, rounded, tense
o	g<u>o</u>	mid, back, rounded, tense
ɑ	b<u>o</u>x	low, back, unrounded, tense
ʌ	b<u>u</u>g	mid, central, unrounded, lax
ə	<u>a</u>round	mid, central, unrounded, lax
ɝ	b<u>ir</u>d	mid, central, unrounded, tense
ɚ	fath<u>er</u>	mid, central, unrounded, lax

Table 9.2 depicts the consonants of Standard American English on these features, and Figure 9.3 is a guide to thinking about these characteristics for the consonant /s/.

Children's Acquisition of Consonants

Children follow a fairly predictable path in acquiring the English phonemes, as discussed in Chapter 2. Table 9.3 summarizes this order of acquisition. The 24 consonant phonemes of English can be further divided into three groups on the basis of when they are typically acquired: Early 8, Middle 8, and Late 8 (see Table 9.4; Shriberg et al., 1994). Children who are developing their phonology normally master the Early 8 phonemes by about age 3, the Middle 8 phonemes by about age 4, and the Late 8 phonemes by age 6½. For children exhibiting speech delays, progress is much slower; for instance, although typically developing children have mastered the Early 8 phonemes by about 3 years of age, children with phonological disorders may not achieve mastery until age 7 (Shriberg et al., 1994).

Sounds and Syllables

Assessment and treatment of phonological disorders often focus on describing how a child produces (or doesn't produce) individual sounds, but it is also necessary to consider how sounds are used in syllables, words, and sentences. This is the context, or the phonological environment in which a sound is used.

The phonological system enables children to unlock the alphabet code.

TABLE 9.2   Place, manner, and voicing features of consonants

Consonant Feature	Categories	Description	Phonemes in English
Place of Articulation			
	Labial	Lips are site of constriction	p, b, m
	Dental	Teeth are site of constriction	f, v, θ, ð
	Alveolar	Alveolar ridge is site of constriction	t, d, n, r, s, z, l
	Palatal	Hard palate is site of constriction	ʃ, ʒ, tʃ, ʤ, j
	Velar	Soft palate is site of constriction	k, g, ŋ
	Glottal	Glottis in the vocal fold area is site of constriction	h
Manner of Articulation			
	Stop (Plosive)	Airflow is completely stopped somewhere in the vocal tract; air pressure builds up to be released in a quick burst; also called *plosives*.	p, b, t, d, k, g
	Fricative	Airflow is continually forced through a tiny fissure in the vocal tract	ʄ, v, θð, s, z, ʃ, ʒ
	Nasal	Airflow is channeled into the nasal cavity by lowering the velum (soft palate)	m, n, ŋ
	Affricate	Airflow is completely stopped in the vocal tract; air pressure is built up and then released in a continuous stream through a tiny fissure in the vocal tract (a stop followed by a fricative)	tʃ, ʤ
	Glide	Articulators are held more open than for other consonants; in their production, articulators glide from a constricted to a more open position; also called *approximants*	w, j
	Liquid	Tongue is held tight at midline with openings laterally; airflow moves around the sides of the tongue.	l, r
Voicing			
	Voiced	The vocal folds vibrate when airflow is pushed over the vocal folds during speech.	b, m, v, ð, d, z, n, r, l, ʒ, ʤ, ŋ
	Unvoiced	The vocal folds do not vibrate and are held open (are approximated) when airflow is pushed over the vocal folds during speech.	p, f, θ, t, s, ʃ, tʃ, h

Often, the context in which a sound is used influences how it is produced. For instance, the /t/ in *tea* is produced differently than the /t/ in *too;* note how the /t/ in *tea* is produced with the lips drawn back into a smile (influenced by the high, front, unrounded features of the vowel), whereas the /t/ in *too* is produced with rounded lips (influenced by the high, mid, rounded features of the vowel). These two variations of the /t/ phoneme occur because of coarticulation. **Coarticulation** explains how the articulatory characteristics of phonemes vary according to context and how sounds overlap one another during articulation (Liberman, 1998). Although we might think that speech production involves producing a series of discrete, individual

FIGURE 9.3

Thinking about place, manner, and voicing for consonant production.

1. Locate the place of articulation for /s/, or where the constriction occurs in the vocal tract when /s/ is produced. Produce a few other sounds, such as /m/ and /g/, to think about where different sounds are produced. The constriction for /s/ occurs at the site where the tongue rests against the alveolar ridge whether you produce /s/ with the tongue tip up or down (this can vary). By comparison, the constriction for /m/ occurs forward at the lips and for /g/ occurs back on the soft palate. Sounds that are created at the alveolar ridge are called *alveolars;* accordingly, /s/ is an alveolar phoneme. Can you think of any other sounds in English that are created by making a constriction at the alveolar ridge?

2. Identify the manner of articulation for /s/, or how it is produced. It might be helpful to compare the production of /s/ with other sounds, such as /t/ and /m/. Notice that when producing /s/, a tight constriction is formed in the mouth and the airflow is channeled through this constriction. Sounds that are produced this way are called *fricatives,* of which /s/ is one. (By contrast, /t/ is produced by forcing a complete stoppage of air followed by a quick release, whereas /m/ is produced by forcing a vibrating column of air into the nasal cavity.)

3. Determine whether your vocal folds are vibrating for /s/. Is it a voiced sound? Or is it unvoiced? The easiest way to identify whether /s/ is voiced or unvoiced is by holding your palm across the front of your throat and producing a long "ssss." In doing so, you will not feel any vibration of the vocal folds, showing /s/ to be an unvoiced consonant. By contrast, produce a long "zzzz" to feel the vocal folds' vibration, and note that /z/ is a voiced sound.

Now, do the same activity for several more phonemes. Work with a peer to describe place, manner, and voicing for /d/, /m/, and /t/. Do you arrive at the description provided in Table 9.2 for these consonants?

DISCUSSION POINT:

Phonological disorders and reading problems appear to co-occur in a number of children. Consider the case of Octavio in Case Study 9.1. If he has a phonological disorder, how would you expect it to impact his reading development in kindergarten and first grade?

sounds (e.g., /t/ + /I/ + /p/) that are linked to make words, in articulation these sounds are smeared across the entire word (Liberman, 1998).

Assimilation is another concept important to understanding phonology, and it also describes a phenomenon involving the influence of context on the production of specific sounds. **Assimilation** describes how the features of one sound take on the features of neighboring sounds. In the word *man,* for instance, the vowel /æ/ is influenced by the nasal features of the surrounding /m/ and /n/, and it becomes nasalized. When children are developing their phonology, they make many errors that are attributable to assimilation, such as saying "goggy" for *doggie* and "lellow" for *yellow.* The sound substitutions (/g/ for /d/ and /l/ for /j/) mirror other sounds in the words—the result of assimilation.

TABLE 9.3   Development of phonetic inventory during early childhood

Birth to 24 months	p, b, m, n, w, t, d, h
24 months to 30 months	k, g, ŋ
30 months to 42 months	f, s, j
42 months and beyond	y, z, r, l, ʃ, θ, ð, ʒ, d ʒ, t ʃ

Source: Adapted from: Grunwell (1987), Sander (1972).

TABLE 9.4 Three groups of phonemes

Phoneme Group	Phonemes	Age of Mastery for Group	
		Typical Children	Speech Delay
Early 8	m, b, j, n, w, d, p, h	3 years	7 years
Middle 8	t, ŋ, k, g, f, v, tʃ, ʤ	4 years	8 years
Late 8	ʃ, s, z, θ, ð, r, ʒ	6.5 years	>12 years

Source: Adapted with permission from Shriberg, L. D., Kwiatkowski, J., & Gruber, F. A. (1994). Developmental phonological disorders: II Short-term speech-sound normalization. Journal of Speech and Hearing Research, 37, *1127–1150.*

SPOTLIGHT ON LITERACY

Phonology and Literacy

As discussed in Chapter 8, to learn to read, children must unlock the alphabetic code that forms the basis for written English. The **alphabetic code** is the symbolic relationships between letters of the alphabet and the sounds of spoken language that they represent. The sound-symbol relationship between letters and sounds (for instance, the letter *k* and the sound it makes, /k/) is called **grapheme-phoneme correspondence.** The instruction children receive to help them learn about sound-symbol relationships is called **phonics.** Phonics is a necessary part of a balanced literacy program and is particularly critical for children who have difficulties unlocking the alphabetic code on their own.

Phonics instruction typically begins in kindergarten and continues into first and second grade. It gives children the tools they need to decode words. Decoding is the child's use of knowledge about grapheme-phoneme correspondence to read words. To profit from phonics instruction, children must have adequate sensitivity to the phonology of their language, and they must have knowledge of the print system used to represent that phonology, which for English is the alphabet. **Phonological awareness** is the child's awareness of how running speech can be broken into smaller phonological components (Justice & Schuele, 2004). For instance, the spoken string *I am hungry* consists of three words, four syllables, and eight phonemes. At about 3 or 4 years of age, children become sensitive to the word and syllable segments of speech. For instance, a 3-year-old child might break the word *butterfly* into three syllables, showing awareness of phonological units of words. At about 5 or 6 years of age, children recognize the phonemic nature of spoken language—that words and syllables can be broken into phonemes (e.g., *cat* is made up of three sounds). Children with underdeveloped phonological awareness often struggle during phonics instruction and consequently develop reading skills more slowly than other children. This puts children at risk for reading disabilities and academic difficulty (Gillon, 2004).

The relationship among phonological disorders, problems with speech-sound production, and difficulties with phonological awareness is not straightforward. On the one hand, some children with phonological disorders do not have problems developing phonological awareness. On the other hand, some children have difficulties with phonological awareness but do not have a problem with speech-sound production (Dodd et al., 1995). Despite the lack of clear overlap between these two types of developmental challenges, both stem from an underlying problem with the development of phonological representations. In some cases, the weak phonological representations result in a problem with speech-sound production; in others, they produce a problem with phonological awareness. For some children, problems in both areas occur. Monitoring the development of phonological awareness for all children, including those with phonological disorders, is important for ensuring that children are able to develop reading skills and phonics knowledge as effortlessly and fluently as possible.

HOW ARE PHONOLOGICAL DISORDERS CLASSIFIED? ●

DIFFERENTIATING PHONOLOGICAL DISORDERS FROM OTHER SPEECH-SOUND DISORDERS

The primary symptom of many communication disorders is a problem with speech-sound production. Not all instances of speech-sound problems result from a faulty phonological system; some result, for instance, from motor and muscular disturbances. The two major indicators of a defective phonological system are

1. Immature or inaccurate representations of individual phonemes or groups of phonemes

2. Immature or ineffective organization of phonemes within the larger phonological system

Obviously, we cannot look at the representations and organization of the phonological system, as they are deeply hidden within the brain and are only discernible with complex technologies. Thus, we must look for four major symptoms often associated with a faulty phonological system:

1. *Expressive phonology:* Difficulties producing specific speech sounds or groups of speech sounds and delays suppressing the normal errors (phonological processes) of early phonological production. These problems result in decreased intelligibility and are a hallmark of a phonological disorder.

2. *Phonological awareness:* A lack of sensitivity to the phonological units of spoken language, such as how syllables make up words and how phonemes make up syllables. This problem undermines a child's ability to learn to read (Gillon, 2004).

3. *Phonological processing:* Difficulties retaining and retrieving phonological information, which reflect one's underlying ability to process phonological stimuli, can reveal weaknesses in the phonological system. A sample task is having individuals to repeat a series of spoken single- and multisyllable nonwords (e.g., *naib, doif, noitouf;* Dollaghan & Campbell, 1998). To do this task, an individual must hold a string of phonologically coded speech sounds in sequence within working memory and then translate these into speech (Dollaghan & Campbell, 1998).

4. *Word learning and word retrieval:* Problems accessing and retrieving words from one's language system in which words are organized as phonological representations. Problems with the phonological system can slow a child's learning of new words (word learning) and can affect the ability to efficiently retrieve words from the language system (word retrieval, Storkel & Morrisette, 2002).

Children who show speech-sound production problems (symptom 1) but who do not show any of the other three signs of a faulty phonological system may not have a phonological disorder. Rather, these children may have a motor-speech disorder (see Chapter 12), or they may have an articulation disorder resulting from a structural problem with the articulators (e.g., palate or teeth).

TYPES OF SPEECH-SOUND DISORDERS

Relatively large numbers of children exhibit problems with speech-sound production, yet not all have a developmental phonological disorder. A developmental phonological disorder—or *phonological disorder,* as it is called in this chapter—is an impairment of the phonological system sufficient to impact speech intelligibility with onset prior to age 9. A phonological disorder causes problems with expressive phonological production—the production of speech sounds—and the underlying phonological representations that may potentially impact phonological awareness, verbal working memory, and word learning and retrieval. Developmental phonological disorders must be distinguished from nondevelopmental speech disorders and speech differences (Shriberg et al., 1997a). Nondevelopmental speech disorders are those that occur after age 9, perhaps as a result of illness, trauma, or accident. A *speech difference* refers to speech-sound distinctions attributable to linguistic or cultural factors (Shriberg et al., 1997a). Speech differences are the speech patterns of an individual that reflect a native language or a regional or cultural dialect. In the United States, there are many regional and cultural dialects that vary in systematic ways from the Standard American English dialect, including the regional dialect of Appalachia and the dialect of some African American communities. These should not be mistaken for speech disorders, as they represent naturally occurring cultural or geographic variations of a language.

The Speech Disorders Classification System (SDCS; Shriberg et al., 1997a) is one system commonly used to classify children's speech-sound disorders. The SDCS is also helpful for differentiating developmental phonological disorders from other disorders that affect speech-sound production. The SDCS differentiates developmental phonological disorders into three descriptive subtypes: speech delay, questionable residual errors, and residual errors.

Descriptive Subtypes

Speech Delay.   The term *speech delay* describes a subtype of phonological disorders in which children who are between 2 and 9 years of age (2:00 to 8:11 years) exhibit developmental phonological impairment characterized by low intelligibility and a high frequency of errors in their speech production. The etiology is unknown, although recent genetic research shows strong familial linkages in many cases of speech delay.

While children less than 2 years of age can show delayed speech development, and such delays are important indicators of later risk for phonological disorder, children are typically not diagnosed as truly delayed in speech development until 2 to 3 years of age. The term *delay,* as used here, implies that many children with speech-sound disorders, perhaps as many as 75%, will develop normal speech production by age 6 with treatment (Shriberg, 1997; Shriberg, in press). Consequently, their achievement of normal speech occurs in a delayed manner relative to other children. Not all children with speech delay completely resolve their speech difficulties. As a result, additional descriptive subtypes are included in this system to identify groups of children with early speech delay who continue to show persistent speech errors, termed **residual errors,** even with treatment.

Questionable Residual Errors.   This subtype describes children between 6 and 9 years of age (6:00 to 8:11 years) who show subtle errors in speech production. These errors do not typically affect intelligibility and include sound substitutions, such as using /w/ for /r/; sound distortions, such as lateralizing the sound /s/, and sound omissions, such as dropping one or more sounds in consonant clusters (e.g., the /r/ in *strong*).

Residual Errors.   This subtype describes children 9 years of age or older who persist in producing errors in speech production; many of these children have a history of speech delay. These residual errors include distortions, omissions, and substitutions of sounds, particularly for Late 8 sounds (see Table 9.4).

Etiology Classification

Phonological disorders may also be organized based on suspected or known etiology, as presented in the SDCS (Shriberg et al., 1997). Five distinct etiological classifications are presented here.

Speech Delay: Unknown Origin.   This subtype describes children with phonological disorders for which there is no known cause, also called a *functional phonological disorder.* This is the most prevalent type of phonological disorder, accounting for up to 60% of cases of childhood speech delay (Shriberg, 1997). Many cases of unknown etiology are likely to have genetic origins. Accumulating research in behavioral genetics has shown that for many children, a liability for poor phonological development that manifests itself in speech, language, or reading disabilities is inherited (Shriberg, in press). Children with an affected immediate family member are five to six times more likely than other children to develop a phonological disorder (Felsenfeld, McGue, & Broen, 1995), and children who have several nuclear family members affected tend to have relatively more severe speech-sound production problems (Shriberg, in press). One study found that 25% of 7-year-olds for whom one or both parents had a history of speech difficulties failed a speech screening at age 7, compared to 9% of children with no family history (Felsenfeld & Plomin, 1997).

Speech Delay: Otitis Media with Effusion.   Chronic infections of the middle-ear cavity, particularly those that involve the persistent presence of a serous, thick fluid within the middle-ear space, can delay children's phonological development (Nittrouer, 1996). Otitis media with effusion (OME) is caused by such microorganisms as pneumococcus, hemophilus influenza, and streptococcus, which infect and inflame the middle-ear space via the eustachian tube, typically the result of a respiratory infection (Hall & Mueller, 1997). Phonological development can be impaired when children have recurrent infections during infancy and toddlerhood (Shriberg, 1997). Presence of OME appears to hinder children's development of robust phonological representations and may account for up to 30% of speech-sound disorders in children (Shriberg, in press). One study found an increased rate of phonological disorder observed among poor children with histories of OME compared to children with no such history; such findings suggest that when risk factors accumulate in a child (e.g., OME combined with poverty), the likelihood of a negative impact of OME on phonology may be exacerbated (Shriberg et al., 2000).

However, the relationship between chronic OME and difficulties with phonological development is not straightforward. Many well-conducted studies have failed to find a direct causal relationship between early chronic OME and an increased risk for speech delay and phonological problems in young children (Miccio, Yont, Clemons, & Vernon-Feagans, 2002; Shriberg, Flipsen, Kwiatkowski, & McSweeny, 2003). Although the current body of science on ear infections and phonology suggests an increased rate of speech deficits in children with histories of chronic OME not all children with chronic OME will experience phonological difficulties.

DISCUSSION POINT:

The occurrence of otitis media among young children appears to be increasing. Brainstorm some reasons that might explain why this is happening.

Speech Delay: Developmental Apraxia of Speech.   This subtype describes disorders of speech production that result from an underlying problem with the motor or muscular processes associated with speech-sound production. *Apraxia of speech* is a disorder of speech production that accounts for 3 to 5% of cases of childhood speech disorder (Shriberg, 1997). Apraxia of speech is not a phonological impairment per se; rather, it is an impairment of the motor system that plans and sequences the delivery of speech sounds (see Chapter 12). **Myofunctional disorders** describe a type of speech production problem resulting from inaccurate or unusual learned movements of the articulators. For instance, *tongue thrust* is a myofunctional disorder in which the tongue is pushed forward through the teeth for alveolor speech sounds, resulting in a type of lisp; therefore, /s/ is produced more like *th*. Tongue thrust, like apraxia of speech, is not a phonological disorder, as the underlying phonological system is intact.

Speech Delay: Developmental Psychosocial Involvement.   An estimated 7 to 12% of cases of speech-sound disorders may reflect psychosocial factors related to temperament and personality (Shriberg, 1997; in press). These types of speech-sound problems do not result from a faulty phonological system per se, but rather seem to reflect temperamental characteristics of the child, such as being more withdrawn or prone to avoidance. Although this subtype accounts for a substantial number of cases of speech-sound disorders, it is not well understood.

Speech Delay: Special Populations.   Phonological disorders are a common symptom of several developmental disorders that affect the language system, the hearing system, or both. Three special populations of children in which the phonological system appears particularly vulnerable include those with hearing loss, Down syndrome, or cleft palate.

Children with hearing loss have an organic disorder of the hearing system resulting in mild to profound hearing loss. The impact of this loss on the acquisition of phonology can range from minimal to severe. Children with Down syndrome often have significant delays in the development of phonology, as Down syndrome frequently affects both the language system, of which phonology is a part, and the hearing system; hearing loss is commonly associated with this syndrome. Cleft palate, which describes a genetic anomaly of the palate's development, often results in problems with articulation of specific sounds. Possibly because of these difficulties with articulation, children with cleft palate are prone to delays in phonological development (Broen & Moller, 1993).

> **DISCUSSION POINT:**
>
> Consider the case of Emily in Case Study 9.1. Which of the subtypes best describes Emily's condition?

WHAT ARE THE DEFINING CHARACTERISTICS OF PHONOLOGICAL DISORDERS? ●

This section discusses the defining characteristics, causes, and risk factors for phonological disorders of unknown origin, as well as those associated with otitis media and such special conditions, such as cleft palate.

PHONOLOGICAL DISORDER OF UNKNOWN ORIGIN

Defining Characteristics

Children with a phonological disorder of unknown origin exhibit delayed development of the phonological system for reasons that cannot be unequivocally identified. This disorder affects more boys than girls, with a ratio of about

1.5 boys to 1 girl (Shriberg et al., 1999). Overall, about 4% of preschool-to-kindergarten-age children experience this disorder.

The defining characteristic of phonological disorders of unknown origin is a significant delay in development of the phonological system, which affects a child's speech-sound production and intelligibility. Characteristics of the delay in speech development include the following (GrunWell, 1997):

1. *Small phonetic inventory:* The child with a phonological disorder has a smaller set of phonemes and phonemic contrasts compared to other children. For instance, a 2-year-old child with a phonological disorder might use only four consonant sounds consistently at the beginning of words, whereas same-age peers would be using 10 sounds in this position.

2. *Phoneme collapse:* Phoneme collapse occurs when several phonemes are represented by only a single phoneme, common for children with a small phonetic inventory (Williams, 2000). For instance, a child may collapse seven phonemes into a single phoneme, as illustrated in Figure 9.4. In this figure, seven phonemes are represented by a child as the phoneme /d/, significantly affecting the child's intelligibility.

3. *Target-Substitute Relationship:* There is a systematic phonetic resemblance between the phonetic target and the child's substitute for that target (e.g., the child's production of /d/ for /g/), such that there is "order to the disorder" (Williams, personal communication, March 3, 2008). Consider the phoneme collapse presented in Figure 9.5, where a child uses a single phoneme to represent seven different phonemes. While some of these error substitutions may seem unusual (e.g., /d/ for /l/), closer examination will show that all of the phonetic targets (d, t, s, k, g, l, n) share the same place of articulation (alveolar) with the child's error substitute /d/. This phonetic resemblance between phonetic targets and the child's substitutes for those targets is a hallmark of phonological disorder. Professionals who work frequently with children with phonological disorder will be able to recognize these orderly patterns even when others do not.

4. *Reduced intelligibility:* A smaller phonetic inventory combined with phoneme collapses to make the final characteristic of phonological disorders—reduced intelligibility. **Intelligibility** refers to the degree to which a child's speech is understood by a naive or unfamiliar listener; conversely,

FIGURE 9.4

Collapse of seven phonemes into one phoneme.

Source: Williams, L. (1993).

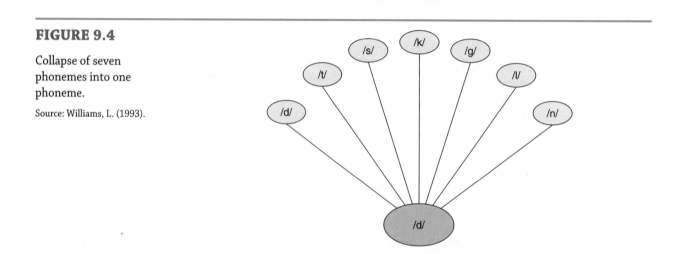

unintelligibility generally represents the percentage of speech that is not understood. It ranges from mild to severe (Fudala & Reynolds, 2000):

- Mild: speech is understood but contains noticeable errors.
- Moderate: speech is difficult to understand.
- Severe: speech cannot be understood at all.

Usually, unintelligibility relates to the number of errors a child makes in producing sounds, with more errors resulting in greater unintelligibility. About one-third of children with phonological disorders have severe unintelligibility (Shriberg & Kwiatkowski, 1994).

About 30% of children with a speech delay also have a significant language impairment that affects vocabulary, grammar development, or both (Shriberg et al., 1999). Children who experience language disorders concomitant with speech delay experience more significant problems with social and academic performance compared to children with only phonological disorders.

Causes and Risk Factors

The cause of this subtype of phonological disorders, as the name suggests, is unknown. In general, difficulties with motor skills, intelligence, and home environment do not serve as specific risk factors in the development of phonological disorders (Bernthal & Bankson, 2004). There is, however, a tendency for phonological disorders to run in families, suggesting that most children experience phonological impairment as a result of a specific inherited weakness of the phonological system (Felsenfeld et al., 1995). This same underlying weakness is also implicated in **dyslexia,** which is a significant disability in learning how to decode words using the alphabetic principle. Children with a weak phonological system, including those with phonological disorders, seem particularly vulnerable for developing dyslexia, as discussed in Chapter 8.

Children with phonological disorders are also at significant risk for having more generalized difficulties with language development. Comorbidity is when two disorders coexist in a person. Comorbidity estimates vary widely, but more recent estimates suggest that about 30 to 40% of children with phonological disorder will also experience language disorder (Shriberg et al., 1999). Among children with language impairment, about 10% will also have phonological disorder (Shriberg et al., 1999).

> **DISCUSSION POINT:**
> Adults with severe reading problems may have a weak underlying phonological system. Why would underlying problems with phonology be difficult to identify?

PHONOLOGICAL DISORDER: OTITIS MEDIA WITH EFFUSION

Defining Characteristics

The defining characteristics of a phonological disorder resulting from otitis media with effusion (OME) are the same as those of the unknown subtype: (1) small phonemic inventory, (2) phonemic collapse, (3) target-substitute relationship, and (4) reduced intelligibility. As with the other subtype, these characteristics stem from poorly established phonological representations within the child's language system. In the case of OME, however, the problems with the development of phonological representations result from periods of **auditory deprivation**—a lack of input to the auditory system that occurs when a child has fluid in the middle ear for a sustained period of time. The risk for problems with phonological development is heightened when OME recurs repeatedly; OME is considered recurrent when children experience at least six episodes in the first 3 years of life (Shriberg, 1997).

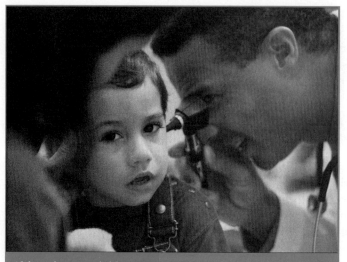

Although many children are resilient to the impact of ear infections on the phonological system, some children are not.

Research on children with recurrent OME suggest specific markers of this type of phonological disorder, which include (1) delayed onset of babbling during the first year of life, (2) delayed onset of the use of meaningful speech, (3) reduced intelligibility compared to children with phonological disorders of unknown origin, (4) problems with specific classes of sounds (like *s* and *sh*), and (5) use of nonnatural sound changes (errors that are not expected with the child's native language; Churchill, Hodson, Jones, & Novak, 1988; Miccio et al., 2002; Shriberg, 1997; Shriberg et al., 2003). However, it is important to recognize that the relationship between OME and phonological disorder is not consistently demonstrated in research reports.

Causes and Risk Factors

DISCUSSION POINT:
Otitis media seems to be an equal opportunity disorder in that it knows no geographic or economic boundaries in whom it affects. Survey your friends to find out how many of them were affected by this disorder. Did it have an impact on their development?

Any child can experience otitis media, although it is most common in children who are under 3 years old. This infection of the middle-ear cavity is caused by bacteria, a virus, or allergens. These microorganisms reach the middle-ear space through the eustachian tube and affect hearing in the following ways. First, the middle-ear space, typically filled with air, may fill with a thick fluid, which inhibits the processing of auditory information from the outer ear to the auditory centers of the brain. Second, the microorganisms can degrade and perforate the eardrum, which also negatively affects the processing and relay of auditory information.

Many children experience these passing challenges to the health of the middle-ear cavity with few obvious negative effects. Perhaps someone you know had chronic ear infections during early childhood and appears none the worse for the experience. In such cases, the individual was resilient to the potential negative repercussions of this illness. On the other hand, some individuals are not resilient, and the experience of chronic OME tips the scale toward the negative impact of this disease. Many variables can affect the risk and resilience related to OME, such as poverty, language quality in the home or other caregiving environment, genetic predisposition for language disorders, and other health problems. For children who are not resilient, chronic OME can have a negative impact on phonological development, particularly when infections are recurrent, resistant to treatment, or incompletely treated (Katz, 1994).

Special Populations

Down Syndrome

Down syndrome is a congenital developmental disability that affects about 1 of 700 children (Capone, Roizen, & Rogers, 2008). Common characteristics associated with Down syndrome include mental retardation, small stature, heart defects, hearing loss, small oral cavity, and language delays. Phonological disorders are also prevalent among children with Down syndrome. These children often show delays in early phonological development of a variety of speech sounds, including a limited inventory of phonemes, delayed development of phonological representations, and poor phonological memory (Laws & Bishop, 2003). These basic deficits in phonology may be further compounded by the increased risk for hearing loss and articulation difficulties resulting from dental and oral cavity anomalies among children with Down syndrome.

Causes and Risk Factors.   Down syndrome (also known as *trisomy 21*) results from a chromosomal abnormality and is associated with higher maternal age (Capone et al., 2008). The majority of cases result from a defect in the 21st pair of chromosomes. Early intervention is important for promoting the positive development of children with Down syndrome and can help enhance phonological and communication development.

Hearing Loss

Defining Characteristics.   For children to develop phonological representations of their native language, they must have access to the phonological code of that language via exposure. This exposure need not be oral, as we know from research on children who are deaf who develop phonological representations through their exposure to a signed language (Luetke-Stahlman & Nielsen, 2003). As is explained in greater detail in Chapter 13, children who experience either transient or permanent impairment of their hearing are at significant risk for lack of adequate exposure to the phonology of their language. Inadequate exposure during the first 5 years of life is particularly detrimental, as this is when phonological representations are rapidly being acquired and laying the foundation for reading ability.

Phonological disorders resulting from hearing loss tend to reflect the severity of the hearing loss and the extent to which the child receives intervention to ensure exposure to oral (speech) or manual (sign) phonological representations. Characteristics of phonological development for children with hearing loss are similar to those of children with unknown or other subtypes of phonological disorders and include limited inventory of phonemes and decreased intelligibility. Hearing loss commonly affects a large range of consonant types, including stridents (*s, sh, ch*), velars (*k, g*), nasals (*m, n*), and glides (*y, w*). Speech of affected children includes substitutions of sounds, omissions of sounds, and distortions of sounds (Hodson, 1997), which together can have a significant negative impact on effective and intelligible communication.

Causes and Risk Factors.   Hearing loss occurs prenatally, perinatally, and postnatally. Prenatal causes of hearing loss include chromosomal abnormalities, maternal ingestion of toxins, and medications. Perinatal causes include birth trauma and anoxia, or loss of oxygen to the brain. Postnatal causes include bacterial infections, such as bacterial meningitis, trauma or accident, exposure to noise, and medications. The ear is a fragile and complex mechanism, and many things can impact its sensitivity to sound and its role in the development of phonology. Thus it is critically important to protect children's hearing. Adults who work with young children should watch for seven signs of possible hearing loss (Hall & Mueller, 1997): (1) ear pain or fullness, (2) discharge or bleeding from the ear, (3) sudden or progressive hearing loss, (4) unequal hearing by the ears, (5) hearing loss after an injury or loud sound, (6) slow speech and language

FIGURE 9.5

Unilateral cleft of the lip and palate.

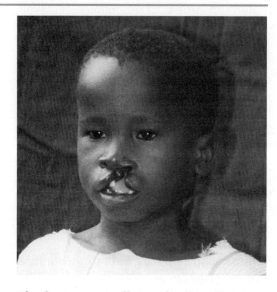

development, and (7) balance disturbance. Chapter 13 provides a more detailed explanation of causes and risk factors in early childhood hearing loss.

Cleft Palate

Defining Characteristics. Cleft palate is a congenital malformation of the palate, or roof of the mouth, that affects about 1 in 700 newborns (Bauman-Waengler, 2004). The name of the condition refers to the fissure or gap that is present in the roof of the mouth when the two sides of the palate do not fuse together during prenatal development. The fissure may affect only the soft palate or both the hard and soft palates, or it may extend to the lip; the latter is called *cleft lip.* The cleft may be unilateral (on one side) or bilateral (affecting both sides of the oral structures). Figure 9.5 illustrates a unilateral cleft of the lip and palate.

Surgery is typically performed to correct clefts within the first year of life, after which the cleft is considered repaired. The average age of children undergoing surgical repair for cleft palate is 12 months (Chapman, Hardin-Jones, & Halter, 2003). Prior to surgical repair, children with cleft palate have a range of articulation difficulties, including problems producing specific sounds and considerable phonological delay. Also involved are problems with managing the valving of sounds and pressure between the nasal and oral cavities. Thus children with cleft palate have particular problems with consonants that require the building up of pressure in the oral cavity, such as the stops /b/ and /p/. Given that earlier surgery for palate repair may contribute to better speech outcomes, some researchers argue that surgery needs to occur much earlier, preferably prior to the onset of babbling (Hardin-Jones, Chapman, & Schulte, 2003).

A child with cleft palate is prone to phonological delays both before and after repair that stem mainly from these challenges with the articulation of specific sounds. Children with cleft palate show preferences for production of certain sounds, such as nasals and glides, with only limited use of other sounds, including those requiring pressure in the oral cavity. Infants and toddlers may also produce a lot of sounds toward the back of the oral cavity, including glottal stops and laryngeal growls (growls produced in the throat). Although infants and toddlers will often produce such sounds, those who have a cleft may continue to use these in place of other sounds that are not emerging (e.g., bilabial sounds, like /b/ and /p/). Experts prompt parents to not encourage these sounds but to focus on increasing the child's phonetic inventory of more conventional sounds (Hardin-Jones, Chapman, & Scherer, 2006). During the months preceding repair, when children with cleft palate begin to babble and use a few words, they practice and receive reinforcement for using a small inventory of preferred sounds and do not practice or receive reinforcement for the use of other phonemes. Even after surgery, children with repaired clefts have a smaller consonant inventory compared to other children (Chapman et al., 2003). Several speech-sound patterns are observed for children with cleft palate:

- Consonant and vowel distortions due to nasal emissions and hypernasality (inappropriate valving of airflow into the nasal cavity during production of consonants and vowels)

- Consonant distortions due to misarticulation (inappropriate placing of articulators when producing some consonants)

- Consonant distortions due to lack of pressure in oral production, particularly /b/, /t/, /d/, /k/, and /g/

Causes and Risk Factors.   The fusion of the palatal structures occurs between the 8th and 12th weeks of gestation (Siren, 2004). There are 400 different syndromes with which cleft palate is associated (Pore & Reed, 1999), including Van der Woude syndrome and Smith-Lemli-Opitz syndrome. Van der Woude syndrome is a chromosomal disorder commonly associated with cleft palate and phonological disorders, although it carries few other physical characteristics. Smith-Lemli-Opitz syndrome is a disorder linked to the X chromosome and thus affects only males. Cleft palate is one of many markers of Smith-Lemli-Opitz syndrome; others include mental retardation and learning disabilities (Siren, 2004).

HOW ARE PHONOLOGICAL DISORDERS IDENTIFIED AND DESCRIBED? ⬤

Speech-language pathologists use a systematic and comprehensive process of assessment to identify phonological disorders in children. To ensure the accuracy of identification, the SLP typically consults with others to gather information about the child, including an audiologist for input on hearing, a pediatrician for input on general development and health history, a psychologist for input on the child's well-being and mental health, classroom teachers for input on the child's learning skills and classroom behaviors, reading specialists for input on reading development, and, most important, the parents for input on the child's communicative performance in the home and elsewhere. Information from all these constituents is crucial for developing an accurate profile of a child's phonological and more general communicative abilities and for understanding the contribution of specific factors of risk and resilience for the child.

> **DISCUSSION POINT:**
> A team approach is beneficial for truly representing a child's phonological capabilities. Consider the case of Octavio in Case Study 9.1. Who should be involved in the study of his phonological performance?

The Assessment Process

Referral

Referral for phonological evaluation is typically made by a parent, a pediatrician, or an early childhood educator. All of these adults are in a good position to note that a child does not appear to be using speech sounds at a level that is age appropriate. For children who are under 2 years of age, signs of a possible phonological delay may include the following:

- Suspected hearing loss or chronic ear infections

- Known physical impairment, particularly of the oral-facial structures, such as cleft palate

- Known mental or cognitive impairment, such as Down syndrome or Prader-Willi syndrome

Specific vocal and verbal behaviors also serve as warning signs and suggest the need for referral:

- Delay in vocal play, babbling, appearance of the first word (expected around 1 year of age) and use of two-word combinations (expected between 18 and 24 months of age)
- Limited repertoire of phonemes (the child should use at least three or four different phonemes by 1 year, such as /b/, /m/, /p/, and /n/)
- Lack of intelligibility of early words for familiar caregivers
- Reliance on nonverbal communication to get needs met, such as gesturing, and inability to use verbal communication for functional purposes (e.g., to request, to reject)

Identifying phonological problems as early as possible may help prevent these problems from growing in severity. In the first few years of life, the difference in phonological skill between a child with a delay and a child without a delay might be quite small. However, over time, this gap grows, and the problems become much more difficult to remediate. To ensure that the gap stays narrow—or, in the best scenario, disappears—two things must happen for children with early phonological delays: (1) they must be identified and (2) they must receive early intervention services focused specifically on building phonological skills.

Most children are not identified as having phonological difficulties until they start using language as a primary means to communicate. In the second year of life, usually between 12 and 18 months, children shift to using spoken communication to get their needs met and to comment on the world around them. They use their slowly emerging vocabulary and phonology, saying such words as *no, night-night, Mommy,* and *milk.* It is normal for some of these productions to be unintelligible. By the time the child turns 2, however, he or she should be intelligible a majority of the time (more than 50%) when communicating. At this age, children should not show persistent frustration when trying to communicate with others, nor should they rely on close caregivers to translate their words so that others can understand them. By 3 years of age, children should be intelligible 75% of the time when talking with a person unfamiliar to them (Vihman & Greenlee, 1987). Children who do not meet these guidelines should be referred to a professional.

Screening

Nearly all children show errors in their sound use during early development, such as omitting the final consonant in words or deleting a sound in consonant clusters. Children also only gradually acquire all of the phonemes of their language; some phonemes are not acquired until kindergarten or first grade. For these reasons, it is sometimes challenging to determine whether a child is showing a delay in phonological development or merely demonstrating phonological errors that are normal.

Screening is a way to take a quick look at a child's phonological development to determine whether a child's speech errors go beyond what is normal and warrant a more comprehensive assessment. It is not used to identify whether a child should receive treatment. Screening can be conducted using informal or formal measures. An informal measure might involve an assessor engaging a child in play for a few minutes to observe communicative patterns during spontaneous speech. The assessor might try to elicit specific sounds or processes that should have been mastered by a child of this age. The assessor might also ask the child to imitate some specific sound targets, for example,

> *I saw seashells on the seashore. I love lollipops and licorice. Rufus the rabbit is really tired.*

Some formal measures an assessor might use as a quick check of phonological performance include the Denver Articulation Screening Test (Drumwright, 1971) and the Quick Screen of Phonology (Bankson & Bernthal, 1990), both of which take just a few minutes to administer. Regardless of whether an informal or a formal protocol is used, the assessor should be familiar with the normal phonological characteristics of children at various stages of development in order to determine whether a child is showing improper phonological development.

Comprehensive Phonological Assessment

For children showing signs of a phonological disorder, a comprehensive assessment is needed. This is administered by a specialist in phonological disorders, usually a speech-language pathologist. This individual must be skilled in administering a variety of assessment procedures, working with children, and phonetically transcribing phonological productions, and must have an arsenal of tools for eliciting the child's speech. A comprehensive assessment is designed to achieve six aims (Miccio, 2002):

1. To characterize the child's general developmental background, including family characteristics
2. To characterize the status of hearing and oral structures and functions
3. To characterize current phonological and language performance
4. To characterize the nature and severity of the phonological disorder
5. To determine the prognosis for phonological outcomes
6. To determine the course of treatment

These aims are met through an assessment lasting as long as 2 hours and including such activities as caregiver interview and case history, oral mechanism screening, hearing screening, language screening or evaluation, and phonological analysis. The assessment usually ends with the professional meeting with a caregiver to present the findings and make recommendations.

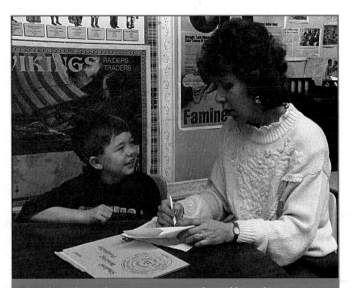

The phonological assessment is conducted by a clinician skilled at enticing children to use speech during informal and formal activities.

Caregiver Interview and Case History.   An interview with a child's primary caregivers, which includes administering a case history, is needed to develop a broad understanding of the child's phonological, social, communicative, and health history. The caregiver interview helps the professional understand the child's communication challenges from the family's perspective (Miccio, 2002). The interview also enables the clinician to (1) recognize

General Topic	Specific Questions
	TABLE 9.5 Questions for caregiver interview during phonological evaluation
Communication	When did the child first begin to babble regularly?
	When did the child first speak three different words? What were they?
	When did the child start saying two- and three-word sentences on a regular basis?
	When did the child begin to speak in sentences, even if some of the words in the sentences were missing?
Birth/Medical	Were there any complications during the pregnancy?
	Was the baby full-term?
	How much did the baby weigh?
	How long was the baby in the hospital after delivery?
	Did the baby have any diagnosed medical conditions?
	Does the child take any medications regularly?
	Has the child ever been hospitalized?
	Has the child ever had an ear infection?
	How is the child's present health?
Social	Who are the members of the child's family?
	Who are the main people with whom the child interacts?
Education	Has the child attended any type of day care or preschool? Did she/he receive any special services?
	Describe the child's current education program and any special services.

Source: From Bleile, K. (2002). Evaluating articulation and phonological disorders when the clock is running. American Journal of Speech-Language Pathology, 11, 243–249. Reprinted with permission.

cultural factors that may influence the assessment, (2) create a familiarity with the family that can facilitate the assessment process, and (3) understand family variables that may complicate or complement the child's phonological development (Miccio, 2002). Table 9.5 details specific questions for an interview with caregivers. Sometimes these questions can be gathered in a telephone interview prior to assessment.

Oral Mechanism Screening.   An **oral mechanism screening** carefully examines the structures and the functions of the systems that are needed for effective speech production. An examination of structures looks at the appearance of the articulators, including the lips, teeth, tongue, jaw, hard palate, soft palate, and tonsils, for any deviations that may impact speech production. The clinical tools for this inspection include surgical gloves, a tongue depressor, cotton swabs, and a flashlight. After examining the structures, the clinician looks at how the speech system functions during speech and nonspeech activities. An example protocol is shown in Table 9.6. In this protocol, the clinician studies lip rounding, lip spreading, tongue movement, lip closure, and mandible movement and looks for possible neuromuscular abnormalities that may contribute to or cause phonological difficulties (Miccio, 2002).

TABLE 9.6 Items for oral mechanism screening

Prompt	Purpose
Show me a kiss	Lip rounding
Say /u/	Lip rounding
Smile	Lip spreading
Say /i/	Lip spreading
Say /i/-/u/	Forward-backward movement of tongue, lip rounding and spreading
Say /ki/-/ku/	Up-down movement of tongue dorsum
Close your lips tight and don't let me open them	Lip closure strength
Say /ib/-/ib/	Lip closure and adduction of vocal folds
Say /bi/-/bi/	Lip closure and adduction of folds
Slowly open your mouth as wide as you can and then close it	Nonspeech mandible lowering and raising
Say /pa/-/pa/	Lowering mandible
Say /ap/-/ap/	Raising mandible
Open your mouth wide	Structural appearance of oral cavity
Say /ab/	Raising the velum
Say /am/	Lowering the velum
Touch your teeth with your tongue	Forward-backward movement of tongue
Say "th"	Forward-backward movement of tongue, contact of teeth and tongue
Touch the tip of your tongue to the ridge behind your teeth	Upward-downward movement of tongue

Source: From Miccio, A. W. (2002). Clinical problem solving: Assessment of phonological disorders. American Journal of Speech-Language Pathology, 11, 221–229. *Reprinted with permission.*

Hearing Screening. A hearing screening is an essential part of phonological assessment to rule out the possibility that a hearing impairment is the cause of any phonological difficulties. The hearing screening is conducted at standard thresholds—typically a loudness of 20 decibels (dB) in each ear at four frequencies (500, 1,000, 2,000, and 4,000 hertz). Careful questioning of caregivers for a history of hearing difficulties, including otitis media, is also important. If a child does not pass the screening, referral to an audiologist for a more comprehensive hearing evaluation is warranted.

Language Screening/Evaluation. Children who exhibit a phonological disorder may also have problems with language development, including grammar and vocabulary (Tyler, Lewis, Haskill, & Tolbert, 2002). Often, a child sees a speech-language pathologist because of poor speech intelligibility. Sometimes, however, the speech-sound problems are just the tip of the iceberg, and the child's phonological problems present a "warning that other linguistic systems need attention" (Khan, 2002, p. 250). For many children, a problem with speech-sound production reveals not only a disorder of phonology, but also a more extensive problem with the language system. Thus, including measures of receptive and expressive language is an important part of phonological assessment. Clinicians often collect measures of spontaneous language use during play and conversation, supplemented by a formal evaluation with a standardized assessment (Williams, 2002). The language sample collected to examine language abilities serves dual purposes, as it will also provide important information about the children's phonological performance within communicative interactions with others (Williams & Elbert, 2003).

Phonological Analysis.   The heart of the phonological assessment is a careful examination of the child's phonological system to determine error patterns. Clinicians use a variety of tools to identify errors in the phonological system, to identify patterns and consistencies in these errors, and to determine the stimulability of certain sounds and patterns. **Stimulability** refers to the extent to which a child can produce a new sound or pattern when given some sort of assistance. The main tools used in phonological analysis include (1) standardized testing, (2) spontaneous speech sampling, and (3) probing.

Standardized testing is used to gather a summary of a child's use of specific sounds and patterns and compare it to similar information for children of the same age. Typically, a child is shown a series of pictures and is asked to name each one. The stimuli are designed to elicit the full range of English phonemes in a variety of different word positions. One popular test is the Goldman-Fristoe Test of Articulation–2 (GFTA; Goldman & Fristoe, 2000), in which the child produces 53 words (e.g., *duck, yellow, finger*), and production errors are recorded on a score sheet. The total number of errors the child makes are summed and translated into a percentile rank, which indicates a child's standing in speech production compared with children of the same age. When a child's percentile rank is sufficiently low (e.g., 10th percentile or lower), a delay or disorder may be indicated.

Standardized testing is also used to examine other aspects of the phonological system, such as phonological awareness and phonological memory. The Phonological Awareness Test (PAT; Robertson & Salter, 1995) is a standardized test that asks children to make rhymes ("What rhymes with *cat*?"), identify the beginning sounds in words ("What is the first sound in *dog*?"), and identify the number of syllables in words ("How many parts are in *pizza*?"), among other tasks. These tasks tap the child's ability to reflect on the phonological structure of language. Phonological memory is tested in the standardized Comprehensive Test of Phonological Processing (CTOPP; Wagner, Torgesen, & Rashotte, 1999). On one task, for instance, children listen to spoken strings of increasing length and must repeat them to an examiner. Tests such as these are useful for comparing a child's phonological capabilities with age-based normative references.

Spontaneous speech sampling is a second critical tool for phonological analysis. By collecting a sample of a child's phonological production across a variety of activities, clinicians can observe the child's consistency of error patterns and overall speech intelligibility in everyday conversational activities. Sometimes children perform very well producing sounds during the structured tasks of standardized tests but cannot communicate intelligibly during naturalistic activities. Experienced clinicians are quite skilled at eliciting children's use of specific sounds during play activities and making sense of patterns observed and how the context influences those patterns.

When collecting spontaneous speech samples to evaluate phonology, clinicians can determine the severity of the phonological disorder by calculating the **Percentage of Consonants Correct** (PCC) metric (Shriberg, Austin, Lewis,

McSweeney et al., 1997a). The PCC is the ratio of the number of consonants produced correctly to the total number of consonants:

$$\frac{\text{Total number of correct consonants produced}}{\text{Total number of consonants produced}} \times 100$$

Thus, a child who produced 500 consonants in a conversation but produced only 288 of them correctly has a PCC of 57.6%, meaning that only about 58 of 100 consonants are produced correctly. The PCC is used to characterize the severity of speech difficulties, and scores are interpreted as (Shriberg et al., 1997a):

>90%	mild
65–85%	mild to moderate
50–65%	moderate to severe
<50%	severe

For the child in our example, whose PCC is about 58%, speech production is severely compromised.

Probing is a third important tool clinicians use for conducting phonological analysis and complements standardized testing and conversational speech sampling. The clinician uses probing to look at how the child performs on specific sounds or patterns. For instance, based on observations during testing and conversation, the clinician may suspect that a child has not developed representations of final consonant sounds. The clinician therefore develops probes to study the child's ability to differentiate words on the basis of final consonants (e.g., *hoe* versus *hope, bow* versus *bone, pop* versus *pod*) and also asks the child to produce a series of real and nonsense words differing only on final consonants (e.g., /plk/, /pIm/, /pIt/, /pIŋ/).

Probing is also used to determine stimulability. Once a child is shown *not* to have a particular sound or pattern, such as final consonant sounds, the clinician studies how much and what type of support is needed for the child to produce that sound or pattern. This is called *stimulability testing,* and it helps a clinician select sounds and patterns for therapy and identify specific techniques that may be useful for bringing about change.

> **DISCUSSION POINT:**
> What is the added benefit of using probing? Why wouldn't a clinician rely solely on standardized testing to study a child's phonology?

Describing Phonological Performance

A key outcome of the comprehensive assessment activities is that it facilitates a thorough description of the child's phonological system in terms of predominant error patterns. The clinician will have collected a variety of speech and language samples as well as test data that are then carefully studied to discern and document patterns of error. Two types of analyses are used (Davis, 2005). *Independent analysis* develops a description of the child's unique self-contained phonological system, without reference to what a mature phonological system looks like (Williams & Elbert, 2003). This type of analysis identifies the consonants, consonant clusters, and vowels the child uses, including how often these occur and in what position of words and syllables (e.g., initial sound, medial sound). Attention is also directed toward the syllable shapes that predominate and the prosodic features of speech, such as pitch, loudness, and rate. An independent analysis might show, for instance, that a 15-month-old child uses four different consonants, no consonant clusters, three vowels, and primarily one syllable shape (consonant-vowel-consonant) to communicate. *Relational analysis* develops a description of the child's phonological system as it compares to a mature phonological system. This includes calculating a PCC and identifying and interpreting specific error patterns using any one of several systems, including nonlinear phonological theory (see Bernhardt & Stoel-Gammon, 1994) and optimality theory (see Barlow, 2001). In relational analysis, the speech-language pathologist identifies the specific patterns of error present in a child's phonological system by identifying why and when these errors take place. For instance, the clinician who documents a child's use of "seep" for *sweep* and "ca-" for *cat* will identify these errors as instances of cluster reduction and final consonant deletion, respectively, two phonological processes discussed in Chapter 2. The clinician will use phonological theories to determine why these errors occur and what treatment approach makes the most sense for the child.

Diagnosis

Diagnosis of a phonological disorder is made by considering the cumulative evidence from the comprehensive evaluation. A phonological disorder is present if the child's phonological system is developing at a rate sufficiently different from age-based expectations; if the phonological differences are not accounted for by cultural or linguistic factors, such as dialect; and if the phonological difference has an impact on the child's ability to effectively communicate for social or academic purposes. The extent of the disorder can range from mild to severe. Children with a mild disorder make only a few distortions of sounds, which do not affect intelligibility, such as saying *f* for *th*. This type of problem is sometimes seen in adolescents who as children had severe phonological problems but who now have mild residual errors. Children with a moderate disorder show some sound substitutions and sound omissions, with an occasional impact on intelligibility. Children with a severe disorder also use substitutions and omissions, and intelligibility is often compromised. Children with a profound disorder are unable to effectively communicate their needs, because sound substitutions and omissions are extensive, and they have few speech sounds to use (Hodson & Paden, 1991).

DISCUSSION POINT:
Consider the case of Emily in Case Study 9.1. Her difficulties are probably consistent with a mild impairment. In what ways might a mild impairment affect a child's educational performance?

HOW ARE PHONOLOGICAL DISORDERS TREATED? ●

INTERVENTION APPROACHES

This chapter has emphasized the phonological basis for the majority of cases of speech delay in young children, which represents a paradigm shift in speech-language pathology. Since the 1990s, treatment paradigms have moved away from therapies emphasizing the child's learning of better articulatory movements toward phonologically oriented therapies, which emphasize the child's achievement of distinct, underlying representations for each phoneme. The more traditional motor- and articulatory-oriented therapies emphasized the child's gradual learning of improved ways to produce specific sounds, typically one at a time. In the traditional approach, the clinician would select a sound and help the child to improve production of it over time through a series of highly controlled drill-like activities. In a given session, the client might produce the target sound in isolation ten times with reinforcement, then produce the sound in different contexts (e.g., at the beginning of words, at the end of words) multiple times, and perhaps complete some motor exercises with a mirror to study how the tongue moves during production of the sound.

Clinicians are gradually shifting from these traditional techniques to more phonologically oriented approaches, which seem more effective for many children (Klein, 1996). The principal governing phonologically oriented approach is to achieve a change in the child's underlying phonological knowledge rather than surface behaviors (Gierut, 2005). Some of the governing principles of phonologically oriented approaches follow (Bauman-Waengler, 2004):

1. *Phonological processes or rules are treated, rather than the individual sounds.* The clinician identifies patterns or processes that explain the child's errors. For instance, the child who leaves out the /s/ at the beginning of such words as *star, skunk,* and *spot* is using the process of cluster reduction. Rather than training the child to use the /s/ sound, the clinician remediates the underlying pattern of cluster reduction.

2. *The contrasts between phonemes are emphasized.* Therapy emphasizes the child's development of an awareness of how phonemes signal changes in meaning, as with the minimal pairs *swipe* and *wipe,* in which the inclusion of the /s/ in the first word signals a difference in meaning from the second. Accordingly, in phonologically based therapies, words, phrases, and sentences are used to train children to recognize contrasts between phonemes; a focus on training children to produce individual sounds accurately in isolation is rare.

3. *Efforts to enhance language and communication are included.* Many children with phonological disorders also have impairments in other domains of language, including morphology, syntax, and vocabulary. Children with phonological disorders are also at risk for problems developing important literacy skills, such as phonological awareness and reading abilities. Phonologically oriented therapies emphasize the role of phonology in communication and move away from drill-like activities focused on sounds in isolation that do not feature authentic communication. Phonologically oriented therapies also often incorporate attention to other linguistic targets, such as improved morphology and the child's development of phonological awareness (Tyler, Lewis, Haskill, & Tolbert, 2003).

The following sections provide a brief overview of five common approaches to phonological intervention: minimal opposition contrast therapy, multiple oppositions therapy, cycles therapy, maximal oppositions therapy, and phonological awareness therapy.

Minimal Opposition Contrast Therapy

Minimal opposition contrast therapy trains children to recognize and produce the phonemic contrasts between words that differ by only a single phoneme (Bauman-Waengler, 2004). The word *minimal* in the name of this approach emphasizes the focus on helping children become aware of minimal differences among words that are marked by phonemes, and *opposition contrast* emphasizes the focus on teaching through contrasts. The purpose of this therapy is to help children develop representations of phonemes or phonological rules that are not yet present in their underlying phonology. It does so by training children to be conceptually aware of the phonemic differences among words that differ by only a single contrast. For instance, when a child does not represent final consonants in words—known as *final consonant deletion*—a clinician trains this pattern by teaching the child to sort words into those that have a final consonant and those that do not (e.g., *bow, bone, boat*).

DISCUSSION POINT:

For a child whose intelligibility is compromised by consonant cluster reduction, what are some minimal pairs that might be used in treatment to build use of consonant clusters?

SPOTLIGHT ON TECHNOLOGY

Many treatment approaches for phonological disorders use contrasts to build children's phonological knowledge. For instance, to treat a phoneme collapse in which a child produces /g/ for /k/, /d/, /f/, and /s/, the clinician will develop contrastive word pairs that distinguish the child's production (go, gate, gown) and the target production (doe, date, and down for the *g/d* collapse). Pictures of these words (e.g., *gate* versus *date*) are used in therapy to provide the child with practice producing and hearing the targeted contrasts. It can be very challenging to develop lists of words that provide meaningful contrasts tailored to an individual child's phonological system and treatment goals, and then find pictures that represent these words. The computer program Sound Contrasts in Phonology (SCIP; Williams, 2006) is a new technology available to clinicians that will develop individualized sets of contrasts for children based on whatever contrastive approach to therapy is being used (e.g., minimal opposition contrast therapy, multiple oppositions therapy, maximal oppositions therapy, as discussed in this chapter). Although the computer software is not a replacement for therapy, it can save the clinician a great deal of time in generating therapy materials. A sample screenshot is provided below, which depicts a multiple oppositions contrast of a child's error substitute, [t], for the target sounds /k, s, tS, tr/ in the initial position of words. The contrasted sounds are highlighted and underlined in the printed words next to each illustration to focus the child's attention to the sound contrasts that make a difference in the words. SCIP tracks the child's performance by a click of the mouse to indicate accuracy of production. In the screenshot, the sunny face indicates that the child produced [tS] correctly in the word *chew*. The data from each therapy session are then graphed and can be displayed on the screen, printed out, or imported into a clinical report.

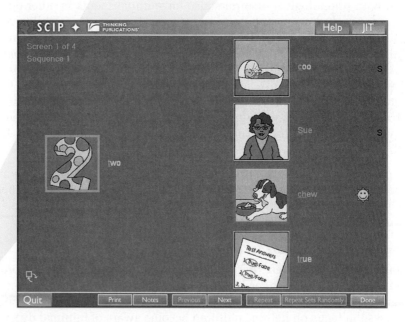

Source: Williams, L. (2006). *Sound contrasts in phonology [Computer Software]*. Eau Claire, WI: Thinking Publications. Reprinted with permission.

Multiple Oppositions Therapy

Multiple oppositions therapy is also based on the principle of teaching children to focus on the contrasts, or oppositions, between words (Williams, 2005). This therapy builds contrasts within a phonemic collapse. Recall from earlier in this chapter that a phonemic collapse is when a number of phonemes are produced as a single phoneme. To build up the child's phonology, multiple oppositions therapy focuses on several targets from the phoneme collapse, or rule set. Thus, for a child who collapses /t/, /k/, /g/, and /z/ into /d/, training will build contrasts between /d/ and /t/, /d/ and /k/, /d/ and /g/, and /d/ and /z/.

Cycles Therapy

Cycles therapy is a popular phonologically based approach that tries to stimulate children's use of certain phonemes or patterns by treating them in cycles. A cycle is a period of therapy, usually about 2 to 6 hours over several weeks, in which a small set of phonemes or patterns are exclusively targeted (Hodson & Paden, 1991). At the end of the cycle, the therapist selects a new set of phonemes or patterns to target. Phonemes and patterns that are not resolved within a cycle are recycled and addressed in a future cycle. For a child with severe unintelligibility who uses many different processes, cycle 1 might focus on final consonant deletion, cycle 2 might focus on consonant cluster reduction, cycle 3 might recycle final consonant deletion in addition to focusing on weak syllable deletion, and so forth. The principle of cycles training is to stimulate the emergence of a particular phoneme or pattern rather than targeting it until mastery is reached. By cycling through many different targets, children's speech skills may improve more quickly than they would using approaches that focus on several targets at once over a lengthy period of time.

Maximal Oppositions Therapy

Maximal oppositions therapy is based on the premise that treating complex phonological targets will bring about the greatest amount of change in a child's phonological system, as the focus on complex targets will generalize to less complex targets (Gierut, 2005). As an example, affricates are considered to be more complex sounds than fricatives. For a child who uses neither fricatives nor affricates, it would seem intuitive to treat first the least complex target— fricatives—and then gradually move to the more complex target. However, some research findings show that treating more complex targets first, like affricates, can have a positive effect on untreated, less complex sounds. Thus, the efficiency and effectiveness of therapy is improved (Gierut, 2005). Maximal oppositions therapy builds upon this premise by targeting phonemes that are extremely different (or opposed). Whereas minimal opposition targets phonemes that differ minimally (as in big and pig, in which the two words differ only in the voicing applied to the initial sounds), maximal opposition targets contrasts that are maximally opposed, as in the words mat and cat. The initial sounds /m/ and /k/ are maximal oppositions, in that they differ in all aspects of production, including manner (nasal versus stop), place (bilabial versus velar), and voicing (voiced versus unvoiced). By treating more complex contrasts, like /m/ and /k/, it is possible to have positive effects on untreated minimal contrasts, like /b/ and /p/ (Gierut, 1989).

Phonological Awareness Therapy

The significant challenges faced by many children with phonological disorders in the area of phonological awareness argue the need to integrate phonological awareness therapy into phonological interventions. The goal of phonological awareness therapy is to develop the child's sensitivities to the sound structure of language. For children who are under age 5 phonological awareness therapy helps develop recognition of (1) words as sentence units (word awareness); (2) syllables as word units (syllable awareness); and (3) intersyllabic units, such as beginning sounds (e.g., s in sit) and rhyme patterns (e.g., og in bog and hog). As important as these early sensitivities are, what is most crucial is that children come to recognize the phonemic structure of language, or that words and syllables are made up of phonemes. One program that helps children develop this awareness is the Gillon Phonological Awareness Training Program, described in Gillon (2004). In this program, children participate in a range of activities to help them focus on the phonemic elements of words, including blending activities, in which they identify words that are presented as broken segments (e.g., "What word is this: /b/ . . . /I/ . . . /g/?") and segmenting activities, in which children identify the phonemes in a word ("Tell me all the sounds in the word *big.*"). One useful activity for helping children develop these phonemic sensitivities is moving blocks that represent sounds, which makes the phonemes more concrete for children. For instance, given a red block to represent the /I/ sound and a blue block to represent the /z/ sound, the clinician might instruct the child to arrange the blocks to make /Iz/ and then rearrange them to make /zI /.

GOALS AND TARGETS IN PHONOLOGICAL THERAPY

Phonological therapy may last for months or years, depending on the child's age, the severity of the disorder, and the type of treatment used for remediation (Klein, 1996). The time taken for resolution of problems is also related to the goals of therapy and the targets selected for therapy.

A therapy goal is an objective to be reached and may be short-term or long-term. A short-term goal focuses on more immediate change, whereas a long-term goal identifies the end goal of treatment. Effective short-term goals concentrate on eliminating broad patterns rather than on training specific sounds. For instance, a child who never uses /k/ in the final position of words might be using a pattern of final consonant deletion whereby all final consonants in words are omitted. A short-term goal might read something like "Johnny will suppress final consonant deletion in 80% of opportunities during spontaneous speech." When setting short- and long-term goals in phonological therapy, it is important to keep in mind that the principle objective is to improve children's ability to communicate more effectively in social and academic situations.

A target is the phoneme or error that is addressed in a given therapy session. Many children who receive phonological therapy have multiple errors in their speech-sound production and have widespread gaps in their underlying phonological knowledge. Some children may be highly unintelligible when they first begin therapy and may not even be able to communicate their most basic needs and interests. These children (and their family members) might be frustrated and even angry about how hard it is to communicate. Clinicians must select the specific speech-sound targets that will bring about the greatest amount of change in the shortest possible time for these children. In general, five approaches are used to select targets:

1. *Target errors or patterns that most affect intelligibility:* Typically, errors that occur more than 40% of the time affect children's intelligibility.

2. *Target sounds or patterns that are stimulable:* Children show greater progress during therapy on stimulable sounds and patterns than on those that are not stimulable (Rvachew, Rafaat, & Martin, 1999). Some clinicians prefer to target stimulable sounds during therapy to achieve immediate and observable success.

3. *Follow developmental norms and select early-acquired sounds and patterns:* Many clinicians select phonological targets using developmental norms for

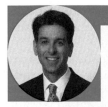

SPOTLIGHT ON RESEARCH AND PRACTICE

NAME: BRIAN A. GOLDSTEIN, PH.D., CCC-SLP

PROFESSION/TITLE
Speech-Language Pathology; Associate Professor, Temple University

PROFESSIONAL RESPONSIBILITIES:
I teach academic courses in assessment, phonological development and disorders, and clinical management of diverse populations, and supervise students in clinical practica. I engage in research activities to further the knowledge base and apply that information to clinical practice. I am active by providing service to the profession (for 3 years, I was editor of *Language, Speech, and Hearing Services in Schools*).

A DAY AT WORK:
Here is a typical Tuesday. When I first arrive at the university, I work on something I can complete before my 8:40 class (e.g., adding slides to an upcoming conference presentation). After class, I hold office hours. If no one shows up for office hours, which is usually the case (why don't students take more advantage of office hours?), I try to focus on research by either analyzing data or writing. I also might complete a service activity such as reviewing an article for a scholarly journal. After that, I meet with the students who work in my research lab where we discuss ongoing projects.

ACADEMIC DEGREES/TRAINING:
B.A. in Linguistics from Brandeis University; M.A. in Speech-Language Pathology from Temple University; Ph.D. in Speech-Language Pathology from Temple University

HOW INTERESTS IN COMMUNICATION SCIENCES AND DISORDERS BEGAN:
I became acquainted with CSD through one of my brothers who received therapy for a phonological disorder. Growing up, however, I didn't want to be a speech-language pathologist (SLP). I wanted to be an actor, but I realized I had neither the temperament nor the skill to be one. Thus, I turned my interest in language and love of Spanish into a degree in Linguistics. Because I was interested in applying knowledge about language, I recalled my brother's work with an SLP and gravitated toward the field of speech-language pathology. During my senior year of college, I completed an internship with an SLP in an elementary school, and I was hooked and still am.

CURRENT RESEARCH AND PRACTICE INTERESTS:
My research focuses on phonological development and disorders in Spanish–English bilingual children. I also supervise graduate students in assessing bilingual children.

MOST EXCITING/INTERESTING PROFESSIONAL ACCOMPLISHMENT IN CSD:
The most exciting accomplishment is to get an article published in a scholarly journal, because it combines a number of exciting tasks: significant and precise planning, coordination with outside agencies, working with students, reading of background material such as books and articles (who wouldn't like to get paid to read?!?), and writing (and rewriting).

FUTURE TRENDS IN CSD:
In CSD, I believe students need specialization in one area of the discipline. Currently, most students in CSD are trained rather broadly. I would like to see a future focus on depth of knowledge that might come through specialization.

the order in which children attain phonemes and the order in which certain error patterns are suppressed. In this paradigm, clinicians select targets according to the pattern of normal phonological development based on the assumption that mastery of earlier-developing phonemes will be easier for children than later-developing phonemes (Gierut, Morrisette, Hughes, & Rowland, 1996).

4. *Target sounds that are more complex:* Some research indicates that greater change occurs to the child's phonological system when phonologically complex targets are chosen (Gierut et al., 1996; Gierut, 2005). For example, one might treat nonstimulable sounds (sounds that cannot be stimulated) so as to effect these sounds, as well as untreated stimulable sounds (Rvachew et al., 1999). Likewise, one might treat late-acquired sounds so as to effect these sounds, as well as untreated early acquired sounds (Gierut, 2005).

5. *Target sounds that impact overall system-wide change:* For children who collapse several target sounds to a single phoneme (i.e., phoneme collapse), choosing up to four targets from that collapse can reduce or eliminate the phoneme collapse and stimulate a system-wide restructuring of the child's phonological system (Williams, 2005).

DISCHARGE

Children are generally discharged from therapy when their speech skills have normalized, usually defined as producing more than 85% of consonants correctly in spontaneous speech and having adultlike speech production (Gruber, 1999). For children who are in school, it is also important that their speech skills do not interfere with educational progress. Some children experience **short-term normalization,** meaning that they achieve articulate and intelligible speech prior to age 6, whereas others experience **long-term normalization,** in which articulate speech is achieved after age 6 (Shriberg, Gruber, & Kwiatkowski, 1994). For children who do not normalize by age 6, problems persist primarily with the *s* sounds (*s, z, sh*), with *r*-influenced vowels (*or, ar, ir*), and with the liquids (*l, r*) (Shriberg et al., 1994). These sorts of residual errors are most common in children with a history of moderate to severe phonological problems during early childhood (Shriberg, Gruber, & Kwiatkowski, 1994).

As a final note, some children may normalize in their speech production and have intelligible, adultlike speech but continue to have phonological problems in areas associated with literacy. These include difficulties with phonological awareness and with applying this awareness to phonics instruction. Although the child's speech production skills have normalized, the history of phonological weakness may have set the child back in important ways that influence literacy and reading development (Gillon, 2004). Intervention may be needed to promote the child's application of phonological skills to literacy activities.

CASE ANALYSIS

Review Kayley's case (Case Study 4 in the Companion Website at www.pearsonhighered .com/justice2e). Reflect on the challenges of a child who cannot speak intelligibly.

● CHAPTER SUMMARY

The term *phonological disorder* describes a condition in which an individual's phonological system is impaired. Children with phonological disorders develop their phonological system slowly and have deficient or immature phonological representations.

This condition affects the production of speech sounds and is most serious when the child's intelligibility is severely compromised, making communication difficult.

The four primary symptoms of phonological disorders are difficulties with expressive phonology, phonological awareness, phonological processing, and word learning and word retrieval. *Expressive phonology* refers to the production of specific speech sounds and patterns and is the hallmark of a phonological disorder. *Phonological awareness* describes an individual's awareness of the segmental aspects of spoken language, such as words, syllables, and phonemes. Many children with phonological disorders have problems with phonological awareness, which is a necessary skill for early reading development. Verbal working memory describes an individual's capacity to hold verbal information in storage for processing. This is important for language comprehension and is commonly weak in children with phonological disorders. *Word learning* and *word retrieval* describe the ability to learn new words and to retrieve words from the mental lexicon; this area, too, is weak in people who have a phonological disorder. Not all children have all four symptoms, but children with a poor underlying phonological system are at risk for difficulties in each area.

Five subtypes of speech delays include three varieties of phonological disorder—phonological disorder–unknown origin, phonological disorder–otitis media with effusion, and phonological disorder–special populations. Additional subtypes of speech delays include motor speech disorders and psychosocial involvement. For most cases of phonological disorders, the cause is unknown.

Treatment of phonological disorders requires early identification. With referral, a child who shows signs of a phonological disorder receives a comprehensive assessment by a specialist that involves case history, parent interview, articulation testing, speech sampling, and language assessment. The specialist identifies whether the phonological system is underdeveloped or disordered and develops a treatment plan for remediation. Phonologically oriented therapies focus on developing the underlying representations of phonology while simultaneously improving the child's intelligibility. Common approaches include minimal opposition contrast therapy, multiple oppositions therapy, and cycles therapy.

● KEY TERMS

allophone, p. 286
alphabetic code, p. 291
articulation disorder, p. 283
articulatory phonetics, p. 286
assimilation, p. 290
auditory deprivation, p. 297
coarticulation, p. 289
cognates, p. 283
consonant, p. 286
cycles therapy, p. 311
dyslexia, p. 297
expressive phonology, p. 292
grapheme-phoneme
    correspondence, p. 291
Intelligibility, p. 296

International Phonetic Alphabet
    p. 286
long-term normalization, p. 314
manner of articulation, p. 287
maximal oppositions therapy,
    p. 311
minimal opposition contrast
    therapy, p. 309
multiple oppositions therapy,
    p. 310
myofunctional disorders, p. 295
oral mechanism screening,
    p. 304
Percentage of Consonants
    Correct, p. 306

phonics, p. 291
phonological awareness, p. 291
phonological disorder, p. 283
place of articulation, p. 287
residual errors, p. 293
short-term normalization, p. 314
speech delay, p. 281
stimulability, p. 306
surface representation, p. 285
underlying representation, p. 285
unintelligibility, p. 297
voicing, p. 287
vowel, p. 286

● ON THE WEB

Check out the Companion Website at www.pearsonhighered.com/justice2e! On it, you will find:

• suggested readings
• reflection questions

• a self-study quiz
• links to additional online resources, including information about current technologies in communication sciences and disorders

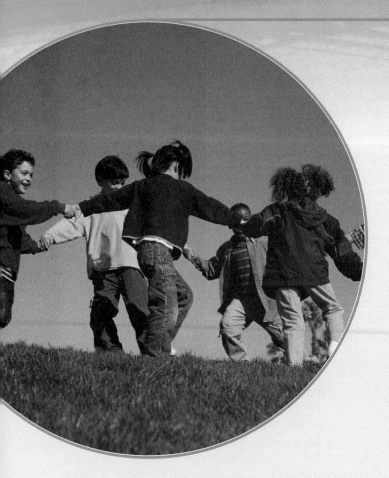

FLUENCY DISORDERS

FOCUS QUESTIONS

This chapter answers the following questions:

1. What is a fluency disorder?

2. How are fluency disorders classified?

3. What are the defining characteristics of fluency disorders?

4. How are fluency disorders identified?

5. How are fluency disorders treated?

CHAPTER 10

INTRODUCTION

This chapter describes disorders of fluency, in which an individual's ability to produce speech effortlessly and automatically is seriously compromised. Fluency disorders are better known as **stuttering,** an onomatopoeic word that well captures the stops, starts, and hesitations in the speech of persons with fluency disorders.

Fluency disorders affect a relatively small number of people, compared to other disorders of communication; about 1 to 2% of the population are affected at any given time (Craig, Hancock, Tran, Craig, et al., 2002). Despite their generally low prevalence, fluency disorders seem to be the communication disorder with which the general population is most familiar—for a variety of reasons:

- Fluency disorders have perhaps the longest documented history of any communication disorder. Bobrick (1995) reports that "stuttering is probably as old as speech itself" (p. 49), with documented reports going back to ancient times. For instance, two famous Greek contemporaries who lived from 384 to 322 B.C., Demosthenes and Aristotle, were both purported to have significant fluency disorders. Obviously, neither Demosthenes, a great orator, nor Aristotle, a revered philosopher and scientist, allowed his speech difficulties to hold him back.

- Fluency disorders have affected some very famous people, including such contemporary celebrities as John Stossel (ABC reporter), Annie Glenn (wife of astronaut and former senator John Glenn), James Earl Jones (film and theater actor), Nicholas Brendon (television actor, known for his role on *Buffy the Vampire Slayer*), and diver Greg Louganis (Stuttering Foundation of America, 2004). Not only have these individuals learned to manage their communication difficulties, but many have also used their positions to advocate for stuttering treatment and research.

- Fluency disorders are often used as a comedic device in the media or, alternatively, as a dramatic, metaphoric technique. A comic example was Adam Sandler's character in the 1998 film *The Waterboy*. (However, one CNN reviewer did not find his stuttering a humorous device: "The biggest impediment to this movie is Sandler's speech. His stammering and stuttering prevents the classic Sandler from shining through" [Rickett, 1998].) A dramatic, metaphoric example is the character Billy Bibbit in Ken Kesey's award-winning *One Flew over the Cuckoo's Nest*. Confined to a mental institution, Bibbit is fearful and anxious, particularly toward his overbearing mother. Kesey seems to use Bibbit's stuttering as a window into his internal psychological turmoil.

DISCUSSION POINT:
What are your perceptions about stuttering? In what ways have you had exposure to persons with fluency disorders?

What the general population may not know, however, are other interesting facts about stuttering: (1) Most young children go through a period of normal disfluency in which as much as 5% of their speech may be disfluent (Ambrose & Yairi, 1999); (2) the majority of stuttering cases in children are resolved either spontaneously or through treatment (Yairi & Ambrose, 1999); and (3) many of the perceptions the public holds about stuttering are not accurate, such as stutterers being timid, fearful, and anxious. This chapter delves into these and other topics concerning fluency disorders in children, adolescents, and adults. ●●●

CASE STUDY 10.1   Fluency Disorders Across the Life Span

KAIMON is a 7-year-old boy just starting second grade in Detroit, Michigan. Kaimon is in the same class as his twin sister, Kaida. Kaimon received treatment for a fluency disorder in kindergarten and first grade but was dismissed from therapy at the end of first grade. (In contrast, Kaida has never shown any problems with fluency.) Kaimon's new second-grade teacher, Mr. Damon, reports to Kaimon's parents that Kaimon is still stuttering and that he thinks Kaimon should be referred to the school speech-language pathologist again.

In their fall conference, Mr. Damon reported that earlier in the day, Kaimon changed seats three times to avoid reading during a round-robin reading activity in which each child in the class read aloud a page of a book. Mr. Damon also reported that Kaimon asked to use the restroom seven times during the day, which he suspects is an avoidance tactic. Kaimon's parents noted that they had not seen these behaviors or indicators of disfluency at home and that Kaimon does not want to go to therapy again, because he is afraid the other kids will make fun of him, and he doesn't want to miss class. In addition, he doesn't think it's fair, since Kaida doesn't have to go to therapy. Mr. Damon agrees to try different strategies in class over the next 3 months, and Kaimon's parents agree to the speech-language referral if the stuttering doesn't decrease by winter.

Internet research

1. Approximately how many second graders in the public school system in the United States receive special services for speech-language disorders? Of these, what proportion of the children receive services specifically for fluency disorders?

2. How likely is it for only one member of a twin set to have a fluency disorder?

3. What is one example of a treatment program available for an elementary-school child who stutters?

Brainstorm and discussion

1. What are some strategies that Mr. Damon might use to promote peer acceptance of children with communication disabilities in his classroom?

2. What are some strategies that Mr. Damon might use to increase Kaimon's fluency and decrease his disfluency within the classroom?

3. Why do you agree or disagree with Kaimon's parents for keeping him out of therapy for the next few months?

● ● ●

MR. CHO is a 39-year-old man who recently had a stroke during heart surgery. Although the heart surgery was successful, the stroke has left Mr. Cho both paralyzed on his right side and significantly impaired in his ability to communicate. Mr. Cho's communicative difficulties include a severe motor-speech disorder, in which he has trouble planning and coordinating the motor movements needed to produce speech, as well as a severe fluency problem marked by frequent pauses, interjections, word and phrase repetitions, and sound prolongations. Fortunately, Mr. Cho has no fear of or embarrassment toward his disfluencies, and he works closely with his daughter to keep track of his disfluencies and to try to decrease their rate. Upon Mr. Cho's recent release from the hospital, his insurance approved him for only 12 sessions of outpatient therapy, including both physical and speech therapy. Mr. Cho decided to use these 12 sessions for physical therapy and to pay out-of-pocket for an experimental treatment offered by a local rehabilitation specialist. His daughter saw the advertised treatment in the newspaper; it reported a 100% cure for acquired stuttering using a 3-month vitamin treatment, which is designed to improve neurological functioning following disease. Mr. Cho purchased the 3-month treatment for $1,200 and is pleased with his decision: 2 months into the treatment, his communication difficulties began to improve.

Internet research

1. What are the policies of major health insurance carriers for coverage of speech-language therapy for acquired disorders of communication?

2. What evidence (if any) supports vitamin therapy as a therapeutic rehabilitation tool for acquired communication disorders, including fluency impairment?

Brainstorm and discussion

1. Do you agree with Mr. Cho's decision to forfeit the outpatient speech therapy in favor of the physical therapy and to pursue the vitamin treatment? Why?

2. Mr. Cho selected a rehabilitation treatment from the newspaper under the guidance of his daughter. How can a consumer differentiate between those treatments that are effective and those that are questionable?

3. What other explanations might explain Mr. Cho's improved fluency following 2 months of a special vitamin regimen?

WHAT IS A FLUENCY DISORDER? ●

DEFINITION

Defining Fluency

Fluency is a descriptive term used to characterize the flow of speech during communication. Speech that is fluent moves along at an appropriate rate with an easy rhythm; it is smooth, effortless, and automatic. By contrast, speech that is disfluent is disrupted in one or more of these elements—rate, rhythm, smoothness, effort, or automaticity. A **disfluency** is the speech behavior that disrupts the fluent forward flow of speech, such as pauses, interjections, and revisions.

The speech of many adults contains a number of typical disfluencies:

> *You know, I think we should, um, well, I know you don't want to, but I really think we should consider giving it—the money—back.*

The speech of young children also often contains a great number of disfluencies:

> *I want, I want ice cream, too. Daddy, Mommy, Daddy, Daddy has ice cream.*

Although the disfluencies in these two snippets seem considerable, they are examples of normal disfluencies that typically do not detract from the communication between two people. These disfluencies reflect a combination of personal dialect ("You know"), hesitation in imparting an idea ("I know you don't want to"), and moments of mental processing or thought gathering ("um, well" or "I want, I want"), which are entirely normal in the complex process of communication.

Defining a Fluency Disorder

A fluency disorder describes speech with an unusually high rate of stoppages that disrupt the flow of communication and are inappropriate for the speaker's age, culture, and linguistic background, including dialect. The disorder must be significant enough that it impacts social communication and educational or occupational performance (APA, 1994; Guitar, 2005). Formal definitions of fluency disorders emphasize the presence of both these features:

- Disturbance in the normal fluency and timing patterns of speech that is inappropriate for the person's age and is characterized by at least one of the following: sound and syllable repetitions, sound prolongations, interjections, words broken by pauses, pauses in speech (i.e., blocks), word substitutions to avoid problematic words, and excess physical tension in producing speech
- Disturbance in social communication, academic performance, or occupational achievement as a result of the fluency disturbance

An important point regarding these definitions is that disorders of fluency are constrained to speech and communication and do *not* involve an impairment in language functioning. While some children and adults with fluency disorders may have concomitant disorders of language, this is not the case for the majority of persons who stutter. In fact, studies convincingly have shown that among children and adults who stutter, the prevalence of language disorders is similar to what is seen in the general population (Nippold, 1990; 2001; Watkins, Yairi, & Ambrose, 1999). Although linguistic factors may influence stuttering, in that individuals may be more likely to stutter on a grammatically complex sentence compared to a simple sentence, this does not mean that their language abilities are less developed than or more impaired than those who do not stutter (Watkins & Johnson, 2004).

Identifying Core and Secondary Features

Speech disfluencies are the **core features,** or primary characteristics, of a fluency disorder. Three types of disfluencies predominate: repetitions, prolongations, and blocks. A **repetition** occurs when a sound, syllable, or word is repeated several times to the point of interrupting the flow of speech, as in "I want-want-want more milk." A **prolongation** refers to a sound being held longer than is normal. With a prolongation, the airflow continues but the articulators seem to be stuck, as in "I wwwwwant more cake." A **block** occurs when the airflow and the articulatory movement completely stop during production of a sound; the block can last as long as 5 seconds (Guitar, 2005).

Accompanying these core features are the **secondary features,** which are also important characteristics of a fluency disorder. These result from an individual's excessive mental and physical efforts to promote fluent speech and to disrupt disfluent speech (Guitar, 2005). They are called secondary, associated, or concomitant features because they emerge in response to the core behaviors. A person with a fluency disorder develops secondary features to avoid and escape moments of disfluency. Common secondary features include physical/motor behaviors such as eye blinks, lip tremors, and head jerks and speaking behaviors such as fillers, pauses, and word changes.

Another secondary feature is negative feelings and attitudes, which reflect an individual's emotional reactions to disfluency. People who stutter may have negative feelings about speaking; they worry about speaking situations, view speaking as difficult, and believe that others do not like the way they talk (Vanryckeghem & Brutten, 1997). These negative feelings and attitudes reflect the everyday challenges that accompany communication for someone with a fluency disorder. An adult whose fluency disorder resolved after an intensive 3-week

DISCUSSION POINT:

Consider the case of Kaimon in Case Study 10.1. What signs suggest that he is already manifesting some negative feelings about communication?

treatment program described it this way (Anderson & Felsenfeld, 2003): "You just feel naked, you just feel so vulnerable, especially when you are in the midst of the speaking problem" (p. 248).

TERMINOLOGY

Stuttering and *stutterer* are two terms that are used to describe a fluency disorder and the person exhibiting it. However, in describing anyone affected by a disorder or a condition, the use of person-first language helps to give the individual primacy over the disorder. Thus, Kaimon, in Case Study 10.1, is not described as the *stutterer* or the *stuttering child* but as the *child who stutters.*

Discussion of stuttering and fluency requires careful use of vocabulary. Some key descriptors are explained in Table 10.1.

PREVALENCE AND INCIDENCE

Fluency disorders affect relatively few individuals, with a prevalence rate of about 1 in 100 persons and an incidence rate of about 5 in 100 persons (Månsson, 2000). Thus, although about 5% of people have stuttered sometime in their lives, only about 1% have a fluency disorder at the present time. Fluency disorders affect children most between 2 and 10 years of age, with estimates showing a prevalence rate of about 1.5% for children under 10 as compared to about 0.5 to 0.7% for adolescents and adults (Craig et al., 2002). Boys are affected at higher rates than girls, with a ratio of about three or four boys to every one girl affected (Craig et al., 2002).

> **DISCUSSION POINT:**
> Did you or any family member go through a period of stuttering? How long did it last?

TABLE 10.1	**Terminology used with fluency disorders**
Term	**Explanation**
Block	A complete pause in the production of a syllable or a word; the airflow stops and the articulators become stuck in place. A block can last 1 to 5 seconds and may be accompanied by jaw tremors. A block is represented in writing with a #, as in "He was #wrong," with a block occurring before the word *wrong.*
Broken word	A word interrupted by a pause, prolongation, or block; the location of the break in the word is notated with a #, as in "My name is Lau#ra."
Circumlocution	Talking around a word or substituting another word or phrase for it, as in "We went to the, uh, the, uh, the city where they make cars," in which the word *Detroit* is avoided.
Filler word, interjection	A word(s) inserted into utterances or phrases, such as *um, uh, I mean,* and *like* ("I, like, think we should go").
Prolongation	A consonant or vowel sound held for a longer-than-normal time, ranging from a fleeting moment to several seconds. During a prolongation, the airflow continues, but the articulators seem stuck in place. Prolongations are represented in writing as a repeated letter, as in *"thaaaat"* or *"mmmmommy."*
Rate	An individual's pace of speaking, which is often measured as the total number of words produced in a minute or the total number of syllables produced in a second (Hall, Amir, & Yairi, 1999). Fluency disorders negatively impact rate, with persons who stutter producing fewer words per minute and fewer syllables per second.
Repetition	The replication of a sound (*b-b-b*), a syllable (*an-an-animal*), or a word (*that-that-that*). The repetition of part of a word, as in the first sound, is called a *part-word repetition* (*th-th-that*). The repetition of a whole word (*that-that-that*) is called a *whole-word repetition,* and repetition of a phrase (*I want-I want-I want)* is a *phrase repetition.*
Revision	Changing or abandoning an utterance during its delivery, as in "He cooked/he made me dinner" or "I really can't/I just don't think we should go."

Recovery from Stuttering

The difference between incidence and prevalence estimates indicates that the majority of people who stutter do recover. Some estimates indicate that as many as three-fourths of preschool and early school-age children who exhibit persistent stuttering behaviors (stuttering for 4 years or longer) will recover, and at least some of these cases of recovery occur spontaneously without treatment (Yairi & Ambrose, 1999). Recovery from stuttering that occurs in conjunction with treatment is called *assisted recovery,* whereas the terms *unassisted recovery* and *spontaneous recovery* refer to recovery that occurs without treatment (Ingham, Finn, & Bothe, 2005; Yairi & Ambrose, 1999). Spontaneous recovery among adults is also called *self-managed recovery,* which carries the connotation that some adults facilitate their own recovery using techniques they select or use on their own (e.g., changing their mental attitude toward stuttering, practicing speaking in various situations; Finn, 1996). Although it is unclear how many adolescents and adults experience complete recovery from stuttering, it is not an uncommon occurrence even among adults who have stuttered for years (Finn, 1996).

Given that many cases of stuttering do resolve, it seems reasonable to ask whether treatment should be given to a child who stutters, given that the likelihood of recovery is quite high. Scientists have pursued the answer to this question over many years, using a variety of techniques. The body of research is complicated by a lack of consensus on how to define and measure the concept of recovery. For instance, are individuals recovered from a fluency disorder when they have significantly decreased their rate of dysfluencies or when they have achieved essentially normal speech? Similarly, has an individual recovered from a fluency disorder if fluency is improved at 1 month posttreatment or 5 years posttreatment (Ingham et al., 2005)? The concept of spontaneous recovery is also challenging, in that for many children, adolescents, and adults who do recover from stuttering, it is unclear what, exactly, caused the recovery. At least in some cases, it is plausible that what appears to be spontaneous or self-managed recovery may, in fact, be a case of assisted recovery. For instance, for some children who stutter, parents may modify the way they interact with them so that they are, in effect, providing a form of treatment. For some adults who stutter, it is possible that spontaneous recovery reflects effects of treatments received some time prior (Ingham et al., 2005).

In light of evidence regarding the prevalence of spontaneous recovery, some experts argue against the delivery of early intervention for stuttering (e.g., Curlee & Yairi, 1997). However, several points warrant comment. First, research findings show that children who participate in stuttering treatment show a significantly greater reduction in dysfluencies than will occur with natural recovery (Harris, Onslow, Packman, Harrison, et al., 2002). Second, when children begin to stutter, there is no way to know whether they will eventually recover or not. Even though many children do recover, the percentage of those who do not (estimated at 25%) is consequential. The children who do not recover will need ongoing support to develop their communicative skills and to mitigate their negative feelings about communication. Finally, some evidence points to treatment for fluency disorders as being more effective when delivered to children compared to adults (Lincoln & Onslow, 1997). While it is possible that this reflects differences in the severity of fluency disorders among adults versus children, it also underscores the importance of prevention—that is, the goal of preventing a child's fluency disorder from emerging into a lifelong serious impairment of communication.

Therefore, even though we can be optimistic that many persons with persistent stuttering problems will recover from this disorder, this likelihood should not be interpreted to mean that persons with fluency disorders do not need special supports to enhance their recovery, including direct treatment. This is particularly true for young children, for whom early intervention can effectively reduce the rate of dysfluencies and increase the likelihood of achieving lifelong fluency (Yairi & Ambrose, 1999).

HOW ARE FLUENCY DISORDERS CLASSIFIED?●

Fluency disorders are typically classified according to etiology. Etiology-focused classification focuses on the cause of the fluency disorder. An overview of types of fluency disorders based on etiology is presented in Table 10.2.

DEVELOPMENTAL FLUENCY DISORDERS

For the majority of people who experience a fluency disorder, it emerges in early childhood, and its cause is unknown. When stuttering emerges in early childhood, typically when children are between 2 and 5 years of age, it is called a *developmental disorder of fluency,* or **developmental stuttering** (Einarsdóttir & Ingham, 2005). Children who exhibit developmental stuttering may stutter for only several months, or they may stutter for several years. The

TABLE 10.2 Types of fluency disorders by etiology	Developmental Fluency Disorders	Acquired Fluency Disorders
Time of onset	Childhood	Adulthood
Type of onset	Gradual or sudden	Sudden
Circumstances at onset	Variable, typically unattributable to specific circumstances	Neurological impairment or psycho-emotional distress
Frequency of stuttering	Ranges from mild to severe	Ranges from mild to severe
Types of stuttering behaviors	Variety of disfluency types; usually core disfluencies near onset	Variety of disfluency types, syllable repetitions common with psychogenic etiology
Secondary or concomitant behaviors	Secondary behaviors present; difficulty with eye contact common	Secondary characteristics uncommon; normal eye contact
Location of disfluencies in speech	Disfluencies typical in initial position of words and utterances; disfluencies at end of syllables or words are rare	Disfluencies occur throughout an utterance
Variability of stuttering	Stuttering appears to be variable across situations (occurs more frequently in some situations)	Stuttering relatively constant across situations
Emotional response to stuttering	Attitudes of anxiousness or avoidance related to speech or stuttering	Feels annoyed but not anxious or fearful about stuttering; for psychogenic etiology, may feel indifferent toward stuttering

Source: Adapted from Seery, C. H. (2005). Differential diagnosis of stuttering for forensic purposes. American Journal of Speech-Language Pathology, 14, 284–297.

SPOTLIGHT ON LITERACY

Fluency and Fluency

Fluency as described in this chapter refers to qualitative aspects of the flow of speech, and disfluencies are disruptions to the flow of speech, such as repetitions, prolongations, and blocks. *Fluency* is a term often used in the field of reading assessment and intervention, but it means something somewhat different. *Fluency* as used in the reading field refers to reading with appropriate (1) speed, (2) accuracy, and (3) expression (Spafford & Grosser, 2005). Speed of reading is generally an index of one's automaticity in word recognition and can vary across different types of texts (e.g., a textbook versus a pleasure book), physical conditions (e.g., lighting, noise), and one's motivation. Adults may read highly technical content at about 100 to 200 words per minute (Richardson & Morgan, 1994). When people read very slowly, it may mean that they do not process many of the words in the text automatically and, by extension, that the text is too difficult. Reading specialists often examine oral reading rate across different levels of texts to document a person's reading rate. *Accuracy of reading* generally refers to reading without error such that most if not all words are processed correctly. Reading specialists use a technique called *miscue analysis,* which looks at the number and types of errors that readers make when reading orally. These miscues (i.e., errors) provide important indications of how a reader is processing what is read and can help to determine if a text is the right level of difficulty for a reader. If a reader makes more than five miscues on a page, the text is probably too difficult (Spafford & Grosser, 2005). *Expression* generally refers to such qualitative dimensions of reading as pausing, pitch changes, and loudness. An individual who is struggling with a text (i.e., the text is too difficult) may show reduced expression; the same is true for children with dyslexia, as they may be so focused on reading without error that expression suffers as a result.

longer a child's stuttering persists, the less likely it is that the stuttering problem will be resolved on its own (Yairi & Ambrose, 1999). Roughly 25% of children who exhibit developmental stuttering will continue to have a fluency disorder 4 years following its onset (Yairi & Ambrose, 1999); the other 75% of children will resolve their stuttering within 4 years either spontaneously or as a result of treatment.

Developmental stuttering needs to be differentiated from the normal disfluencies seen in most young children. Nearly all children go through a period in which disfluencies are prevalent in their speech, particularly during the toddler and preschool years. The key to differentiating between developmental stuttering and normal disfluencies in young children is to examine the type of disfluencies that are present. Developmental stuttering is characterized by the appearance of **stuttering-like disfluencies** (SLDs), which include (1) part-word repetitions, (2) single-syllable-word repetitions, (3) sound prolongations, (4) blocks, and (5) broken words. For children who exhibit developmental stuttering, SLDs are seen at higher rates than for children who are developing typically. For instance, children with developmental stuttering produce about 5 part-word and 3 single-syllable-word repetitions per 100 spoken syllables, as compared to about 0.5 and 0.7, respectively, for other children (Ambrose & Yairi, 1999).

As a general rule of thumb, part- and single-syllable-word repetitions are viewed as a hallmark of developmental stuttering, particularly when 3 or more are seen within 100 words of conversational speech (Zackheim & Conture, 2003). Children without developmental stuttering may occasionally produce part-word and single-syllable-word repetitions, but they do so relatively infrequently. Table 10.3 gives examples of stuttering-like disfluencies

TABLE 10.3 The rate of stuttering-like disfluencies in 2- to 5-year-old children		
	Rate of Occurrence	
Type of Disfluency	Typical Children	Children Who Stutter
Single-syllable-word repetitions ("I want-want-want lemonade")	0.7 per 100 syllables	3.3 per 100 syllables
Part-word repetitions ("Give me the pu-pu-puzzle")	0.5 per 100 syllables	5.3 per 100 syllables
Prolongations ("That's my mmmmommy") and blocks ("Here it i#s")	0.09 per 100 syllables	1.8 per 100 syllables
Total stuttering-like disfluencies	1.3 per 100 syllables	10.4 per 100 syllables

Source: From "Normative Disfluency Data for Early Childhood Stuttering" by N. G. Ambrose and E. Yairi, 1999, Journal of Speech, Language, and Hearing Research, 42, 895–909. Copyright 1999 by ASHA. Reprinted with permission.

and indicates their rate of occurrence in children with and without developmental stuttering.

In contrast, other types of disfluencies in the speech of young children are considered to be quite normal. These include interjections, revisions, and multisyllabic word and phrase repetitions, as shown in Table 10.4. These types of disfluencies can occur at high rates for young children, averaging about 4 per 100 spoken syllables. The most common type of normal disfluency is the interjection, which is seen on average in 2 of 100 spoken syllables (Yairi & Ambrose, 1999).

Preschoolers with Fluency Disorders

When stuttering first emerges in a child, often between the ages of 2 and 5 years of age, they typically exhibit all three characteristics of stuttering, including core behaviors, secondary behaviors, and the emergence of negative feelings

TABLE 10.4 The rate of normal disfluencies in 2- to 5-year-old children		
	Rate of Occurrence	
Type of Disfluency	Typical Children	Children Who Stutter
Interjection ("I want, uh, that one")	2.1 per 100 syllables	2.5 per 100 syllables
Revision ("It's on yellow, red paper")	1.8 per 100 syllables	2 per 100 syllables
Multisyllable word repetition ("It's the elephant-elephant") or phrase repetition ("I want the I want the blue one")	0.4 per 100 syllables	0.9 per 100 syllables
Total normal disfluencies	4.3 per 100 syllables	5.4 per 100 syllables

Source: From "Normative Disfluency Data for Early Childhood Stuttering" by N. G. Ambrose and E. Yairi, 1999, Journal of Speech, Language, and Hearing Research, 42, 895–909. Copyright 1999 by ASHA. Reprinted with permission.

and attitudes about stuttering. Core behaviors most commonly seen are repetitions of words and sounds, sound prolongations, and perhaps some blocking. You may recall that a block is a speech disfluency characterized by a complete stoppage of the airflow and the articulators. For the preschooler who stutters, these blocks may not last long and may be hardly noticeable. The severity of the disorder, often characterized by the number of disfluencies per 100 words and by qualitative ratings, can be quite diverse among children. Some children may be perceived to stutter quite severely, whereas others will be perceived to stutter mildly (Yairi et al., 1993).

In addition to these core behaviors, the preschooler who stutters also will show some secondary behaviors to escape and avoid moments of disfluency. These include, for instance, head nods, eye blinks, and interjections. These core and secondary behaviors may prompt the beginning of negative emotions and feelings, such as frustration toward stuttering and communication.

School-age Children with Fluency Disorders

School-age children who have stuttered for a prolonged period of time, for one or several years, are described by some as being at an "intermediate level" of stuttering (Guitar, 2005). The core disfluencies of the school-age child who stutters include prolongations and blocks, with blocks becoming increasingly prevalent and lasting up to several seconds. Secondary behaviors that help the child to avoid a block (e.g., substituting words or phrases) and to escape a block (e.g., nodding the head and blinking the eyes) become more evident and habitual. A hallmark of stuttering for school-age children is that they have had to live with this speech impairment for several years and have developed fear of and frustration with stuttering. They may increasingly fear and avoid situations in which they are called upon to talk, which can bring about feelings of helplessness and embarrassment.

Adolescents and Adults with Fluency Disorders

Some experts have used the term *advanced stuttering* to describe the fluency disorders of adolescents and adults (Guitar, 2005). Adolescents and adults with fluency disorders have lived with speech difficulties for some time and have likely had a range of experiences attempting to remediate or compensate for their speech difficulties; these experiences may be self-managed or other-managed (e.g., managed by a speech-language pathologist) and, in some cases, will not be perceived as being very helpful (Finn, 1996). The core and secondary behaviors of the adolescent and adult who stutters are similar to those of the school-age child who stutters. For some adolescents and adults, core behaviors are not very evident, for they have honed their secondary behaviors to completely avoid or escape the appearance of prolongations and blocks.

Acquired Fluency Disorders

Unlike developmental disorders of fluency, acquired fluency disorders do not necessarily emerge in early childhood. Rather, they can emerge at any time across the life span, resulting from illness, trauma, or accident affecting the brain or, occasionally, from psychological trauma. Stuttering that results from brain injury or neurological insult is called **neurogenic stuttering,** whereas stuttering resulting from psychological trauma is called **psychogenic stuttering.** Both occur less frequently than developmental stuttering, with psychogenic stuttering being the rarest of the three types. Possible causes of neurogenic stut-

SPOTLIGHT ON TECHNOLOGY

Manipulating Auditory Feedback

When individuals speak, they hear their voice in real time as it occurs, referred to as *auditory feedback*. (You can experience real-time auditory feedback right now by saying something out loud.) There are ways to manipulate this auditory feedback so that there is a slight delay introduced, called *delayed auditory feedback* (DAF), or a change in frequency, called *frequency altered feedback* (FAF). When feedback involves both a delay and a frequency alteration, it is called *altered auditory feedback* (AAF). Whether DAF, FAF, or AAF, the result is that individuals hear their voice as slightly different than it actually sounds. For some persons who stutter, DAF, FAF, and AAF can greatly reduce the rate of disfluencies in certain speaking situations. One study showed that stuttering was reduced among persons with fluency disorders by 79% and 71% for DAF and FAF, respectively (Kalinowski, Armson, Roland-Mieszkowski, Stuart, et al., 1993). SpeechEasy is a commercial device—called a *fluency tool*—that capitalizes upon such findings by making AAF available to individuals for everyday use. SpeechEasy looks like a hearing aid, with the feedback technology fitted to a size small enough to sit completely in one's ear canal or, if preferred, behind the ear. AAF technologies are specifically patented for the SpeechEasy, such as the Intelligent Noise Attenuation Strategy, designed to analyze incoming sounds to identify that which is noise, so that noise can be attenuated (rather than accentuated). Several drawbacks to the SpeechEasy are of note. First, the device is expensive ($4,100–$4,900), and, because it is a relatively new product, most insurance companies may not cover this expense. Second, the device is not efficacious for all users, with some persons experiencing noticeable benefits and others experiencing marginal benefits (Armson, Kiefte, Mason, & DeCroos, 2006). Third, there is relatively little evidence showing its long-term effectiveness, and the available evidence (while promising) is largely confined to adults. Use of the SpeechEasy with children is not recommended presently, until more information on its potential benefits with this population is available (Yaruss & Gabel, 2005).

tering include stroke, traumatic brain injury, brain infections (e.g., meningitis), and brain tumors (Mysak, 1989). Possible causes of psychogenic stuttering include serious abuse and conflict (Roth, Aronson, & Davis, 1989).

Acquired disorders of fluency show many of the same symptoms seen in developmental stuttering, but their onset is more dramatic. Also, neurogenic disorders of fluency are often accompanied by other disorders of communication, such as aphasia (an acquired impairment of language functioning) or dysarthria (an acquired impairment of speech functioning). When accompanied by significant brain damage, as may be the case following a stroke, people with neurogenic stuttering may be unaware of their disfluencies and thus may not exhibit the associated emotional reactions seen in individuals with developmental disorders of fluency.

When adults have a sudden onset of stuttering, it is necessary to determine whether its etiology is neurogenic (e.g., due to stroke) or psychogenic (e.g., due to acute anxiety; Roth et al., 1989). Neurogenic and psychogenic disorders of fluency have several key similarities, making differential diagnosis difficult: (1) The fluency of speech is seriously disrupted, (2) the disfluencies in speech occur involuntarily and cannot be controlled, and (3) the disfluencies are sometimes accompanied by physical secondary behaviors (e.g., head nods; Roth et al., 1989). A primary difference between the two etiologies for acquired fluency disorders is that those of psychogenic origin are typically provoked by a significant stressor.

DISCUSSION POINT:
Consider the cases of Kaimon and Mr. Cho in Case Study 10.1. Characterize each as having either a developmental or an acquired disorder of fluency.

WHAT ARE THE DEFINING CHARACTERISTICS OF FLUENCY DISORDERS? ⬤

The most readily apparent characteristic of a fluency disorder is the disruption of speech with disfluencies, which for the intermediate and advanced stutterer include primarily sound and word repetitions, sound prolongations, and blocks. These speech disfluencies represent the core features of a fluency disorder. As discussed previously, however, secondary features also emerge—escape and avoidance behaviors such as head nods and word substitutions, as well as negative feelings and attitudes about disfluency and communication. This section provides greater detail on core and secondary features and describes the causes of and risk factors for stuttering.

CORE FEATURES

Their Dynamic Nature

The core features of fluency disorders are the speech disfluencies that disrupt an individual's ability to effectively communicate at home, school, work, and in the community. For most persons with a fluency disorder, the disorder emerges during the toddler and preschool years, and for those who do not resolve the impairment either spontaneously or through treatment, the symptoms of the disorder will gradually change.

The hallmark characteristic of stuttering is the presence of an abnormally high rate of speech disfluencies and the presence of specific types of disfluencies, namely sound repetitions and sound prolongations. As stuttering progresses from beginning to intermediate stuttering, the types of disfluencies are dynamic, changing to reflect the individual's physical and cognitive maturation, self-awareness of stuttering, and development of compensatory strategies to avoid and escape moments of stuttering. The early sound repetitions and brief sound prolongations give way to longer sound prolongations and serious blocks. For individuals who reach the level of advanced stuttering, these disfluencies may all but disappear as they learn to avoid and escape the majority of speech disfluencies (Peters & Guitar, 1991).

Description of Core Features

The term *core feature,* or *core behavior,* emphasizes speech disfluencies as the original and primary source of communicative difficulty experienced by individuals with fluency disorders (Guitar, 1998). Core features represent the original manifestation of the speech impairment, which may give way to secondary features if the core features are not resolved. For children who exhibit beginning stuttering, core features are often called *stuttering-like disfluencies* (SLDs; Ambrose & Yairi, 1999). Although this term is controversial—the word *like* emphasizes a resemblance to stuttering rather than stuttering per se (Wingate, 2001)—it is often used to differentiate the disfluencies of stuttering from normal disfluencies.

The core features of fluency disorders include four types of speech disruptions (Ambrose & Yairi, 1999; Pellowski & Conture, 2002):

1. *Part-word repetition.* During part-word repetitions, part of a word, typically a sound or a syllable, is repeated, as in "It's my b-b-b-baby," "Judy is my ba-ba-ba-baby," or "Thi-thi-this is my baby." For young children who are borderline or beginning stutterers, part-word repetitions represent about one-third

of all disfluencies, occurring at a rate of about 5 times in 100 syllables (Ambrose & Yairi, 1999). In contrast, part-word repetitions are only one-tenth of all disfluencies seen in typically developing children, occurring at a rate of about 0.5 times in 100 syllables. The number of part-word repetitions in a single moment of stuttering—referred to as *repetition units*—ranges from 2 to 4, with an average of about 2.5 units (Zebrowski, 1994).

2. *Single-syllable-word repetition.* In a single-syllable-word repetition, a single-syllable word is repeated two or more times, as in "My-my-my-my friend is here" or "and-and-and-and-and then we went on." Although single-syllable-word repetitions characterize a normal speech disfluency seen in children, this type of disfluency occurs at much higher rates for children who are borderline or beginning stutterers. Children who stutter average more than 3 word repetitions in 100 syllables, as compared to typical children, who produce fewer than 1 per 100 syllables (Ambrose & Yairi, 1999). Nonetheless, it is important to note that this type of disfluency is common in young children, comprising about 12% of speech disfluencies for typical children. Thus, the occurrence of single-syllable-word repetitions in the speech of a young child is not necessarily cause for alarm, although it is a core feature of a fluency disorder.

3. *Sound prolongation.* A sound prolongation occurs when the duration of a speech sound is lengthened. During the prolongation, the movement of one or more of the articulators stops in its place, but the airflow serving as the source of the speech sound continues (Guitar, 1998). For instance, in the prolongation of the sound /r/ in "He went to rrrrrun," the mandible and the tongue are held in place while the /r/ sound continues for half a second or longer. This type of core behavior includes both inaudible and audible prolongations. For the former, the speech sound is prolonged quietly and inaudibly followed by a hard attack when the sound is forced forward. For the latter, the speech sound is prolonged constantly and audibly. Persons who stutter produce both types of prolongations about equally.

This type of disfluency can occur fairly frequently in the speech of those who stutter. For instance, one study recorded an average of 31 prolongations during 45 minutes of speech for 14 children with fluency disorders (Zebrowski, 1994). The sound prolongations of those who stutter range in duration from about .4 seconds to 1 second, with an average duration of .7 seconds (Zebrowski, 1994). Sound prolongations are unusual as a normal disfluency and represent an important and early sign that a child is stuttering.

4. *Block.* Blocks represent the core behavior most frequently associated with stuttering. In a block, the articulators and airflow completely stop during the production of a sound, syllable, or word. Blocks can last for less than a second or for several seconds, and the duration and severity of blocks can increase as stuttering develops (Guitar, 2005). The block can also be accompanied by physical tension, including tremors of the jaw or the neck. Blocks are not typically seen in beginning stuttering but are a core feature of intermediate and advanced stuttering. Many adolescents and adults who stutter learn to compensate for blocks by avoiding them with word substitutions and pauses or escaping them through various means.

Within-Word and Between-Word Disfluencies

The types of core features just described are quite different from speech disfluencies that are not stuttering-like (Yaruss, 1997). Researchers classify disfluencies in two categories: (1) those that are stuttering-like, or of a stuttering type, and (2) those that are normal-like, or of a normal type (Yaruss, 1997). The best way to differentiate between disfluencies is to consider whether the disfluency affects the internal structure of a word. Those that do are called **within-word disfluencies;** these include sound repetitions, sound prolongations, and blocks. These disfluencies characterize problematic speech behaviors, or stuttering. When a disfluency does not affect the internal structure of a word, it is called a **between-word disfluency**—that is, the disfluency occurs between words rather than within a word. Between-word disfluencies include phrase repetitions (e.g., "He is in the—in the—in the house"), interjections (e.g., "Put it in the, uh, um, drawer"), and revisions (e.g., "I gave it to, uh, wait a minute, I gave it to Frances"). These types of disfluencies are perfectly normal unless they occur at inappropriately high rates, characteristic of cluttering.

Note that the core feature of single-syllable-word repetition was not included in either the within-word or the between-word category. Single-syllable-word repetitions technically fall into the between-word category, which is more or less synonymous with normal disfluencies. Single-syllable-word repetitions *are* a normal disfluency, but when seen at higher than expected rates in young children, they are also characteristic of borderline and beginning stuttering. Thus, some researchers place single-syllable-word repetitions in the category of within-word disfluencies (e.g., Conture, 1990).

SECONDARY FEATURES

As an individual's stuttering progresses, secondary features emerge. Secondary features include **escape behaviors,** which an individual develops to get out of a moment of stuttering; **avoidance behaviors,** which an individual develops to evade moments of stuttering; and feelings and attitudes about stuttering, which develop over time with the experience of stuttering. Because these behaviors develop secondarily, they tend not to be seen until people have experienced the core features for a period of time. For those with intermediate and advanced stuttering who have stuttered for years and for whom secondary features are well developed, secondary features can be even more prominent and difficult to treat than the core disfluencies.

Escape Behaviors

Escape behaviors develop in a person with a fluency disorder as a response to moments of stuttering. These are, in essence, volitional strategies to cope with disfluencies. Whereas stuttering itself seems to be involuntary, escape behaviors are within a person's control, used strategically to break out of a disfluency. Typical escape behaviors include head nods, eye blinks, hand tensing, and leg movements. These and some other physical behaviors used to escape disfluencies are listed in Figure 10.1. Sometimes physical behaviors are combined with verbal behaviors, such as interjections.

Escape behaviors tend to change over time as their effectiveness decreases. Bobrick (1995) provides an apt description of how escape behaviors change over time:

There was a student at Harvard, for example, who discovered one day that he could break his blocks by stamping on the

FIGURE 10.1

Examples of physical escape behaviors.

Blinking eyes
Closing eyes
Shifting eyes (up/down)
Widening eyes
Flaring nostrils
Wrinkling nose
Licking lips
Pursing lips
Tensing lips
Trembling lips
Clicking tongue
Clenching jaw
Trembling jaw
Nodding head
Shaking head
Rubbing fingers
Tapping fingers
Clenching hands
Tapping foot
Crossing/uncrossing legs
Bunching shoulders

Sources: Based on Guitar (2005); Shipley and McAfee (1998); Zebrowski (2000).

floor. It worked for a while, we are told, but then he found he had to stamp harder and longer to release a word. Finally, the whole house in which he lived seemed to shake from his pounding. (pp. 33–34)

For persons who are very experienced at stuttering, escape behaviors can be molded to look like natural speaking behaviors.

It is not hard to imagine how escape behaviors might emerge. Consider, for instance, what you might do if you were introducing yourself to someone unfamiliar and became stuck on the first sound in your name. In my own simulation, I can see myself extending my hand to introduce myself to the friend of a friend: "Good to meet you, I'm L# . . . ." As I put myself through this, blocking on the /l/ in my name for several seconds, I can feel the air swell in my chest, my neck tense, my eyes bulge, and my jaw jut forward as I try to push the sound out. I am embarrassed and feel as if I might pass out as my friend and her friend look at me. Nothing happens—the block doesn't give. Suddenly, I jerk my head to the side, and finally the block is released. Thus, I have developed a strategy that seems to dislodge the block, and it is adopted for future use.

Avoidance Behaviors

Although escape behaviors might be useful for breaking out of a moment of stuttering, you can imagine that a person with a fluency disorder would prefer to simply avoid those moments of stuttering altogether. People who stutter are often able to anticipate moments of stuttering, based on their experiences in certain speaking situations or with certain words or phrases; they might be more likely to stutter on certain sounds or words. For instance, some people might always stutter on words that start with /m/ or on the name of their hometown, perhaps Chicago. Knowing this and not wanting to subject themselves to a moment of stuttering, these individuals might try to avoid their probable pitfalls. Avoidance behaviors commonly used include both word and sound avoidance and situation avoidance (Guitar, 2005).

Word and Sound Avoidance.   With **word avoidance** and **sound avoidance,** a person with a fluency disorder uses several strategies to avoid a disfluency (Guitar, 1998; Van Riper, 1982). A substitution occurs when a word or phrase is substituted to avoid a word or sound. For example, the person who stutters on the word *Chicago* might say, "I am from Ch-Ch . . . the Windy City." A **circumlocution** occurs when a person tries to delay a potential disfluency by putting it off or avoid it by talking around it, as in "He told me, uh, when we met, uh, we were at the mall, and . . ." With a postponement, the person pauses or uses filler words prior to producing a potential disfluency, as in "I would like . . . (pause) bacon."

Situation Avoidance.   Few people find public speaking easy and enjoyable; some of us may even find it frightening or anxiety producing. This is not uncommon, particularly in demand situations, when we are put on the spot, as on the first day of a class when we all have to introduce ourselves to the group. For people who stutter, one strategy that emerges as a secondary feature is **situation avoidance,** in which the individual steers clear of circumstances in which stuttering is probable. The number of such situations is endless—answering the phone at home, introducing oneself at a party, ordering food in a restaurant, asking a price in a store, asking for directions when lost.

Avoiding situations that cause discomfort is a common, if not normal, behavior among children (e.g., going to the dentist), adolescents (e.g., calling someone for a date), and even adults (e.g., sending food back at a restaurant). But for

> **DISCUSSION POINT:**
> What are some opportunities an individual might lose out on because of situation avoidance?

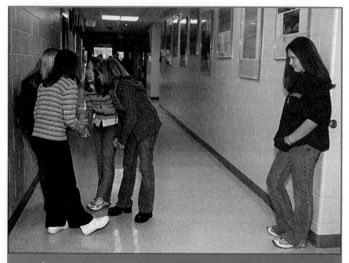

Avoiding situations that require speaking can have a negative impact on the social and educational achievement of an adolescent who stutters.

people who stutter, situation avoidance can have an extraordinarily negative impact on their achievements at home, school, and work, and in the community. Anxiety, mood disturbances, and stress can all result as a function of chronic avoidances (Blood, Blood, Bennett, Simpson, et al., 1994).

Feelings and Attitudes

It is probably not surprising that people with long-term fluency disorders may develop negative feelings toward communication. Those who stutter may feel fear, frustration, and embarrassment, both within and beyond direct communicative activities. As the experience of stuttering accumulates, "these experiences pile up like cars in a demolition derby to create the entanglement of fear, embarrassment, and shame that accompanies moments of stuttering" (Peters & Guitar, 1991, p. 99). Peters and Guitar note that negative feelings toward stuttering increase as fluency problems move from being "an annoyance to a serious problem" (p. 99), illustrated by this adult's description of her own experiences with stuttering:

> I just couldn't get anything out, but you could tell that my mouth was trying. It would be like my cheeks were puffed like I was trying to blow a trombone without any air coming out. . . . And you could see my jaw tightening and my lips tightening, but not any word would come out. (Anderson & Felsenfeld, 2003, p. 248)

It is through the accumulation of disfluent experiences that stress, tension, and negative emotions emerge (Ezrati-Vinacour et al., 2001). This is not to say that young children do not recognize stuttering; even children as young as 3 are able to differentiate between fluent and disfluent speech, preferring fluent speech over disfluent speech (Ezrati-Vinacour et al., 2001). However, as an interesting tribute to the sensibilities of 3-year-old children, they are no more likely to choose a friend who is fluent over a friend who is disfluent. But by 4 and 7 years of age, 69% and 94% of children, respectively, would choose a friend who is fluent over one who is disfluent (Ezrati-Vinacour et al., 2001).

DISCUSSION POINT:
Strong negative feelings toward speaking can emerge with the repeated experience of stuttering. Why do you think Mr. Cho in Case Study 10.1 doesn't seem to have these feelings?

Adolescents and adults who have stuttered for years are likely to identify themselves as stutterers, to view communication with negativity, and to use a myriad of techniques to avoid speaking situations. They may have experienced people laughing at them, treating them harshly, or avoiding talking to them altogether because of their stuttering. Surveys do suggest that the general public has negative attitudes toward people who stutter, viewing them as tense, anxious, withdrawn, fearful, and emotional (Kalinowski, Stuart, & Armson, 1996). Although these perceptions may stem from the tensions inherent in moments of stuttering, they are not appropriate descriptions of the character of those who stutter (Kalinowski et al., 1996).

Causes and Risk Factors

What causes the emergence of the core features of fluency disorders, which lead to secondary features? This question has long been a focus of researchers who study stuttering, particularly those who study developmental stuttering.

Nonetheless, the cause of developmental stuttering remains very elusive. In fact, for the majority of children, stuttering begins for no obvious reason. Van Riper (1973), a researcher who spent most of his career studying the development of stuttering in children, noted that for most children, "stuttering seemed to begin under quite normal conditions of living and communicating" (p. 81), with no apparent conflicts, illnesses, shocks, or other types of disturbances to explain the fluency disorder.

The inability of researchers, practitioners, and parents to pinpoint a cause is likely because stuttering does not result from a single identifiable cause. Rather, stuttering results from the complex interaction of a variety of predisposing and precipitating factors (Peters & Guitar, 1991), which emphasize an integrated model of stuttering development (Guitar, 1998). **Predisposing factors** are constitutional factors that make an individual susceptible to a fluency disorder, such as carrying a genetic trait (Yairi, Ambrose, & Cox, 1996) or having an overly sensitive temperament (Guitar, 1998). **Precipitating factors** include both developmental and environmental factors that can worsen stuttering, such as age or stress. These two sets of factors must interact in such a way as to disturb the developmental trajectory of a child, with predisposing factors accounting for about 70% of the likelihood to stutter and precipitating factors accounting for 30% of the liability (Andrews, Morris-Yates, Howie, & Martin, 1991). Thus, an individual may have one or more significant predisposing factors for a fluency disorder, yet not develop one. Or an individual may experience several salient precipitating factors and not develop a disorder. Figure 10.2 identifies key predisposing and precipitating factors in fluency disorders. We discuss these here but remind the reader that to date, we do not know why a person develops a fluency disorder.

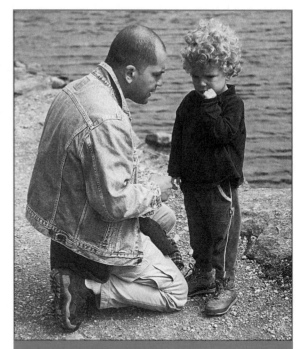

About 50% of young children who stutter have an immediate family member who also stutters, such as a sibling or a parent.

FIGURE 10.2

Key predisposing and precipitating factors in the development of fluency disorders.

Predisposing factors	Family history/Genetic predisposition
	Gender
	Neuroanatomical differences
	Motor-speech coordination
Precipitating factors	Age
	Stressful adult speech models
	Stressful speaking situations
	Stressful life events
	Self-awareness/temperament

Source: Based on Guitar (1998).

Predisposing Factors

Predisposing factors, also called *constitutional factors,* make a child more susceptible than other children to developing a fluency disorder. Considered here are four important predisposing factors: family history, gender, neuroanatomical differences and motor speech coordination.

Family History.   Fluency disorders tend to run in families, suggesting that genetics are a particularly important predisposing factor. Of young children who stutter, nearly half have an immediate family member who stutters, and about 70% have an extended family member who stutters (e.g., grandmother, uncle; Yairi et al., 1996). A genetic transmission is also suggested by twin studies, which show that when one twin stutters, there is an increased likelihood (estimates range from 20 to 90%) that the other twin will also stutter (Yairi et al., 1996). Given this genetic linkage, one might wonder whether stuttering is perhaps a gene-linked dominant or recessive trait. Although this may be too simplistic a picture, studies from the 1990s have suggested that a susceptibility to stuttering may be linked to a single specific gene (Ambrose, Yairi, & Cox, 1993).

Gender.   Gender is a second predisposing feature, with boys more likely to develop a fluency disorder than girls. Among children in the early stages of developmental stuttering, the gender ratio is about 3 boys to 1 girl (Ambrose, Cox, & Yairi, 1997). Among adolescents and adults who have not resolved their stuttering, the gender ratio shifts to about 7 boys to 1 girl affected. Therefore, while boys are not only more likely to experience a fluency disorder, they are also more likely to persist in the disorder once it is manifested. And about 77% of boys who stutter will recover, as compared to 87% of girls (Ambrose et al., 1997). Reasons for these gender differences have been explored for decades, focusing on environmental differences in social pressures on boys and girls. More recent data suggest that explanations may be found in genetic research examining how girls and boys may vary in their susceptibility to an expression of genetic traits (Ambrose et al., 1997).

Neuroanatomical Differences in Brain Morphology.   Recent advances in brain imaging show there to be significant differences in the brain morphology of adults who stutter compared to those who do not. These seem to reflect differences in cerebral lateralization of speech and language functions, with relatively *less* asymmetry in anatomically important regions of language processing among adults who stutter (Foundas, Bollich, Corey, Hurley, et al., 2001). Recall from Chapter 3 that the regions of the brain linked to language processing are largely lateralized to the left hemisphere, giving rise to leftward anatomical asymmetry that corresponds to its functional importance. Among adults who stutter, there is more symmetry (and less asymmetry) in the regions of the left hemisphere important to language relative to the same location in the right hemisphere. Within the brains of adults who stutter, there also appear to be more gyri and greater variability in gyri patterns, which may disrupt the flow of information among the speech-language areas of the brain (Foundas et al., 2001). Although we can speculate that these anatomical differences found in the brains of those who stutter emerge very early in development, perhaps prenatally or in early childhood during cellular pruning, it is also possible that these anatomical differences emerge as a response to stuttering.

Motor Speech Coordination.   People who stutter may have an underlying difficulty in coordinating and timing the motor activities required to produce fluent speech (McClean & Runyan, 2000). Observations of differences in various aspects of speech timing (e.g., rate of tongue movement) and coordination (e.g., movement of tongue in relation to lips) suggest that difficulties in motor speech production may make persons who stutter vulnerable for fluency breakdowns (Kleinow & Smith, 2000; McClean & Runyan, 2000). However, research on whether timing problems cause stuttering are generally inconclusive (Max & Gracco, 2005).

Unlike the other predisposing conditions described, this one is located directly within the motor speech apparatus itself, placing the cause of the fluency problem somewhere in the muscular or articulatory systems involved with fluent speech production. However, the exact site of the breakdown remains speculative, with research continuing to rule out possibilities. For instance, theories that the muscles of the larynx are overactivated (or hyperactive) during stuttering, and thus a cause of disfluencies, have not held up in laboratory studies (Smith, Denny, Shaffer, Kelly, et al., 1996).

It is possible that early in the development of stuttering, the rate and coordination of these children's speech exceed their capacity to produce fluent speech, resulting in disfluencies (van Lieshout, Hulstijn, & Peters, 1996). This predisposing factor emphasizes discrepancies between a child's demands on coordination and timing for speech production (potentially fueled by a desire to communicate) and the capacity of the speech system. This early disruption in the coordination and timing of the speech system may undermine the development of well-coordinated and well-timed speech, setting the stage for ongoing problems with fluency.

Precipitating Factors

For an individual to develop stuttering, a predisposing factor must be present, which may account for as much as 70% of the likelihood that a child develops stuttering (Yairi et al., 1996). But what about the other 30%? It represents the precipitating factors, which influence whether an individual's predisposition, or susceptibility, to stuttering will actually manifest itself as a fluency disorder. Many children may have a constitutional predisposition to a fluency disorder but may nonetheless follow a path to healthy fluency development. Predisposing and precipitating forces must align in a way that steers a child onto the path to stuttering. Three categories of precipitating factors may contribute to the likelihood of developing a fluency disorder: age, developmental stressors, and self-awareness.

Age.   Age is a significant risk factor in the development of a fluency disorder. In one study of children with fluency disorders, the average age of stuttering emergence was 3 years for boys and 2.5 years for girls (Yaruss, LaSalle, & Conture, 1998). The likelihood of developing a fluency disorder beyond 6 years is negligible; thus, it seems safe to say that everyone reading this book need not worry about this particular precipitating factor.

To understand why age is a significant risk factor, let's consider the normal challenges for a young child in achieving fluent speech and language. About 2 years after birth, children move into a period of remarkable speech and language growth, in which their ever-developing urge to communicate is accompanied by a dramatic increase in speech and language capabilities. As children produce more phonologically complicated words (e.g., *hippopotamus*) and more syntactically complex utterances (e.g., "Mommy sit here and Daddy sit there"), the speech and language mechanisms are repeatedly taxed, compromising the fluency of communicative acts. The challenges of picking precise words, conveying appropriate intent, organizing sentence structure, and articulating strings of sounds result in considerable disfluency in the speech of most youngsters—about 6 disfluencies in 100 syllables (Ambrose & Yairi, 1999).

Now let's consider the child who is genetically susceptible to stuttering. For reasons that remain unknown, this child's communicative system is already vulnerable to a weakness in fluency. With the repeated taxing of the system that occurs between 2 and 5 years, the systems of a number of these children give way to a more serious problem with disfluencies than other children experience. These children produce about 16 disfluencies in 100 syllables (Ambrose & Yairi, 1999). Fortunately, the majority of these children—about 75%—will not stutter into adulthood, although their stuttering may last for months, if not years. The longer the child's stuttering continues, the less likely it is to be resolved and the more likely it is to increase in severity (Ambrose & Yairi, 1999; Pellowski & Conture, 2002).

Developmental Stressors.   Stress does not promote fluency, as we have all probably experienced at least once in our lives. Accordingly, some evidence suggests that a variety of developmental stressors may serve as precipitating factors in the emergence of stuttering in children, specifically for those who are already susceptible to a fluency disorder. Yaruss, Coleman, and Hammer (2006) present three categories of stressors that can influence stuttering in children: communicative stressors, interpersonal stressors, and child factors. *Communicative stressors* describe children's participation in communicative exchanges that are not well tuned to their speech, language, or cognitive capabilities.

Features that may be stressful include a rapid speech rate, use of complex syntax and complicated vocabulary, interruptions of child speech, overuse of questions and directives, and short wait times following questions (Rustin & Cook, 1995).

Developmental researchers have long shown the value of parental speech and language input that is sensitive and well-tuned to a child's developmental functioning. Well-tuned parental input is not too simple nor too challenging; rather, it mirrors and is sensitive to a child's own capabilities. Exposure to sensitive and well-adjusted speech models serves as a powerful accelerant to children's early speech and language development (e.g., Hoff, 2003). However, consistently exposing children with a susceptibility to fluency disorders to adult speech in the home or other caregiving environment that is too demanding or complicated may precipitate disfluencies. Yet, there is little evidence showing that parents of children who stutter are overly or inappropriately demanding of their children during communicative activities. Indeed, many parents of children who stutter are sensitive to the communicative skills of their children and adjust their own language accordingly (Miles & Bernstein Ratner, 2001).

Communicative stressors also involve competing to speak, hurrying when speaking, and having many things to say (Yaruss et al., 2006). Although these stressors can be influenced by external events, such as being interrupted often when speaking or being asked many questions, it seems more likely that these stressors arise from internal sources within the child. For instance, a child may be trying to hurry and share a thought but may not have the capacity to meet that demand. Or a child may be producing a particularly long sentence and again may not have the capacity to produce it fluently. *Cross-talk* describes the challenge to the child's developing but still immature nervous system when the expression of emotion interfaces with speech and language production (Guitar, 1998). In such cases, fluent speech production can become compromised and over time may result in chronic fluency breakdowns.

Interpersonal stressors are a second precipitating factor in fluency disorders. Possible stressors include moving, divorce of parents, loss of a parent or close family member, illness, or accident (Guitar, 1998). Transitions such as these may impact development of any young child in a variety of ways, fluency abilities notwithstanding. For some children, these and other types of stressors can provide the catalyst for the emergence of stuttering.

Self-Awareness. Child factors are a third category of stressor that can influence stuttering in children. These may include temperamentally based attributes, such as being particularly sensitive or having a genetic predisposition to stutter. Self-awareness is increasingly receiving attention as a possible precipitating factor in stuttering. Researchers and clinicians have longed viewed young children as being unaware of their own disfluencies, even children who are borderline and beginning stutterers. A newer perspective of the last 2 decades is that children who stutter are aware of their disfluencies at an early age (Ezrati-Vinacour et al., 2001). Researchers Rustin and Cook (1995) of London, England, describe an interview with a 4-year-old who stuttered, in which she noted, "Oh, it's so hard sometimes; the words won't come out." In this same interview, the child reported that the one thing she would change about herself if given some magic would be to "make her voice better" (p. 130). By 6 years of age, children who stutter have more negative attitudes toward their speech than do children who do not stutter (Vanryckeghem & Brutten, 1997).

Some experts believe that children who stutter have an atypically high awareness of their own disfluencies (Bernstein Ratner, 1997), which may serve as a precipitating factor in the emergence of fluency disorders. For children with a predisposition to fluency disorders, this atypically heightened awareness of their own fluency may create a tension toward communication that builds with each disfluency.

> **DISCUSSION POINT:**
> What are some possible precipitating factors in the case of Kaimon in Case Study 10.1?

Can Stuttering Be Induced?

The discussion of potential precipitating factors in the previous sections could lead one to believe that stuttering can be induced or caused. This is not the case. While we currently do not know what causes stuttering to persist in a child, it is most likely that there are interactions among predisposing factors (e.g., genetic predisposition) and precipitating factors (e.g., stressful life events).

Historically, some experts strongly believed that stuttering was induced in children when negative attention was paid to their normal disfluencies. This theory—the diagnosogenic theory of stuttering—implied that disfluencies among children should be ignored and should not be treated, as this would precipitate development of a fluency disorder. Unlike many theories regarding what may or may not cause stuttering, this one was directly tested in an experiment of questionable ethics (now known as the Monster Study), conducted in 1939 by Professor Wendell Johnson and his student Mary Tudor at the University of Iowa (Ambrose & Yairi, 2002). In this study involving 22 orphans in an Iowa orphanage, for 6 months, the experimenters and orphanage staff (by instruction of the experimentors) treated a select group of six 5- to 15-year-old children who did not stutter as if they did stutter. These children were told that

> "you have a great deal of trouble with your speech. The type of interruptions that you have are very undesirable. These interruptions indicate stuttering. . . . You must try to stop yourself immediately. Use your willpower. Make up your mind that you are going to speak without a single interruption. It's absolutely necessary that you do this. . . . Don't ever speak unless you can do it right. . . . You see how (the name of a child in the institution who stutters very severely) stutters, don't you? Well, he undoubtedly started this very same way you are starting. (Tudor, 1939, pp. 10–11, as cited in Ambrose & Yairi, 2002)

Tudor reported that they were able to induce persistent stuttering through these methods, although a recent reanalysis of the original data indicated that none of the six children developed persistent stuttering as a result of the experiment (Ambrose & Yairi, 2002). The six children did, however, show some increases in certain types of disfluencies, notably interjections and pauses, although these are "normal" types of disfluencies seen in most children's speech. It seems that the experiment may have induced certain types of disfluencies and an increased hesitation to or discomfort in communicating but did not induce stuttering per se. Part of the controversy surrounding this experiment is that the children were never told that they were part of an experiment and found out only through media reports that surfaced in 2001. The university issued a formal apology in 2001, and the state of Iowa settled a lawsuit in 2007 brought by several plaintiffs for $925,000.

HOW ARE FLUENCY DISORDERS IDENTIFIED? ●

The identification of fluency disorders is complicated by the fact that nearly all persons are disfluent in their speech at least some of the time. Thus, professionals must carefully study an individual's disfluencies to determine whether their quality or quantity is significantly different from what is normal.

As an exercise in studying the quality and quantity of disfluencies, you can record yourself during a conversation with a friend and then count the number of disfluencies in your speech. Count the number of sound and word repetitions, prolongations, blocks, interjections, revisions, and longer-than-normal pauses or hesitations. You can then calculate two common metrics to arrive at an estimate of your level of disfluency:

1. *Average number of disfluencies per 100 words:* Count the total number of disfluencies produced, divide this by the total number of words, and then multiply the result by 100. For example, a sample of 300 words containing 22 disfluencies results in an average number of 7.3 disfluencies per 100 words.

2. *Average number of disfluencies per 100 syllables:* Count the total number of disfluencies produced, divide this by the total number of syllables, and then multiply the result by 100. For example, a sample of 622 syllables containing 34 disfluencies results in an average number of 5.5 disfluencies per 100 syllables.

You should also examine the quality or type of disfluency. For most students, I would expect that interjections and revisions will predominate and that repetitions, prolongations, and blocks will be infrequent, if not nonexistent.

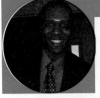

SPOTLIGHT ON RESEARCH AND PRACTICE

NAME: JOHN SPRUILL, III

PROFESSION/TITLE
Dual-title Doctoral Student (Speech, Language and Hearing Sciences-Gerontology)

PROFESSIONAL RESPONSIBILITIES
My professional responsibilities include assisting students as needed, as I am the most senior doctoral student in the lab, and performing what is required in order to complete my dissertation work.

A DAY AT WORK
A day at work consists of providing the necessary guidance to students performing research in the lab, and collecting/analyzing data for my dissertation.

ACADEMIC DEGREES/TRAINING
I currently have a Master of Arts degree in Communicative Sciences and Disorders.

HOW INTEREST IN COMMUNICATION SCIENCES AND DISORDERS BEGAN
My interest in CSD began in my senior year of undergraduate study. As a political science major, I decided to step outside the box and take "Voice and Stuttering" as an elective, just out of curiosity. While enrolled in the course, I became increasingly more interested in the field of CSD. Following the completion of the course, I was approached by the instructor, also the department chair, about pursuing a master's degree in CSD.

CURRENT RESEARCH AND PRACTICE INTERESTS
My current research focuses on language processing and aging, specifically related to older adults' ability to inhibit irrelevant information with increasing age.

MOST EXCITING/INTERESTING PROFESSIONAL ACCOMPLISHMENT IN CSD
My most exciting professional accomplishment in CSD has been the ability to produce published works while pursuing my doctoral degree.

FUTURE TRENDS IN CSD
I predict that future trends in CSD will manifest themselves in more collaborative work with various disciplines. This could possibly even lead to the creation of new disciplines as a result.

If you prefer to practice on someone other than yourself, have a friend read the following statement of 43 words and calculate the average number of disfluencies per 100 words:

> *Um, yesterday I picked her, uh, up from daycare and we, then, uh, we walked to my office to see if Becky was there, she wasn't, but, um, but uh, oh what's her name, Linda was there and had the key, so, uh we got to pick up the candy.*

This type of careful study of speech disfluencies characterizes the assessment process for identifying fluency disorders.

THE ASSESSMENT PROCESS

Referral

Speech-language pathologists (SLPs) are the professionals who are specially trained for assessing, diagnosing, and treating fluency disorders. Other professionals—such as special and general educators, psychologists, and physicians—often play an important role in referring individuals to SLPs for fluency assessment, informing the diagnostic process, and executing treatment plans. Thus, it is important for these and other professionals to be familiar with the warning signs of possible fluency disorders to make timely and appropriate referrals.

Warning Signs for Developmental Fluency Disorders.   Professionals who work with young children should be aware of the following warning signs of a possible developmental fluency problem, particularly for children between 2 and 6 years of age (Guitar, 1998), the period in which most cases of developmental fluency disorders emerge:

1. Repetition of parts of words, such as the first sound ("b-b-ball") or the first several sounds ("ba-ba-ball"), including repetitions in which the vowel sound "uh" is substituted ("cuh-cuh-cuh-cake")

2. Repetitions of words or parts of words involving three or more repetitions of the unit ("I-I-I-I do it")

3. Prolongation of a sound or appearance of being stuck on a sound ("It is mmmine")

4. Feelings of frustration or embarrassment toward speaking and communication

Professionals who work with young children should also be aware of three epidemiological facts in conjunction with these warning signs. First, fluency disorders tend to run in families, with children more likely to be affected if they have an immediate or extended family member with a fluency disorder. Second, fluency disorders occur more often in boys than in girls. Third, fluency disorders often co-occur with other disorders of communication, such as phonological impairment. Thus, professionals should be particularly vigilant for warning signs in children who have one or more of these general vulnerabilities.

Additionally, professionals should recognize that fluency disorders become less likely to resolve the longer they persist. Although some cases of developmental stuttering do resolve spontaneously without treatment, there is no crystal ball that can identify those fortunate youngsters. Thus, when warning signs are present, consultation with an SLP who can provide further input on the possible disorder and the need for treatment is always the best approach.

Warning Signs for Acquired Fluency Disorders.   Acquired fluency disorders can result from various types of trauma, illness, or injury that affect the brain. For instance, stuttering can follow a brain injury caused by a stroke or dementia from a progressive brain disease. In these persons, stuttering can result from the loss of automaticity in retrieving language (Mysak, 1989). For example, an elderly person with dementia might not be able to remember the word for *table,* thus compromising fluency: "I put it on the, the, the, the . . . I don't know." A small minority of acquired cases of stuttering result from psychological causes, such as severe abuse or a mental illness (National Institutes of Health, 2002). Warning signs for a possible acquired fluency disorder include these:

1. Presence of stuttering-like disfluencies, such as part-word or whole-word repetitions and sound prolongations

2. Presence of cluttering-like disfluencies, such as overuse of interjections, revisions, and abandonment of phrases or sentences (e.g., "He told me he would, uh, uh . . . He said, um . . . Do you want to sit down?")

3. Inability to effectively communicate, which may or may not be coupled with frustration or embarrassment toward communication

DISCUSSION POINT:
Early childhood educators and daycare providers should be well aware of signs of possible fluency disorders. What are some approaches to increase this awareness for these professionals?

Assessment Protocol

Assessment by the speech-language pathologist is designed to answer four main questions (Zebrowski, 2000): (1) Is the individual stuttering or at risk of stuttering? (2) Does the individual exhibit any other communicative risk factors or disabilities? (3) Is therapy for stuttering warranted? (4) What therapy approach would be most beneficial? Answers to these questions are obtained using a variety of different tools, including case history and interview, speech observation, questionnaire and survey, and direct testing.

Case History and Interview.   The case history is an indispensable part of the fluency assessment process; it is a detailed questionnaire and interview in which the clinician gathers information about the individual. As implied by its name, the case history is designed to clarify the history of the perceived fluency problem and place it within the context of the individual's life. For children, the case history informant is typically the primary caregiver; for adolescents and adults, the informant is typically the person experiencing the fluency problem.

A child's case history examines family demographics (e.g., number of siblings); developmental milestones in all areas (e.g., motor, self-care, communication, social, cognitive); medical history; educational history; and history of the fluency problem, including parental perceptions of the child's specific difficulties and the ways the problems have changed over time. The clinician asks the informant to provide details on what was happening in the child's life when the disfluencies were first noticed and to discuss changes in the disfluencies since the problem began. The clinician may use a questionnaire, such as that provided in Figure 10.3, to gather information about stressors that may be contributing to a child's disfluencies. The items on this inventory are designed to explore the presence of precipitating and predisposing factors discussed previously.

The adolescent's and adult's case history is similarly organized but encourages greater detail on how fluency has changed over time and how it affects their lives, including educational and occupational performance. For instance, the informant is asked about specific situations in which fluency becomes more compromised and the details of strategies used in such situations to promote fluency (Guitar, 1998).

Additional informants are often interviewed to complement the case history. For preschool children, the clinician is likely to interview any individual who cares for the child, such as daycare providers. These persons can provide important information on the ways a child's disfluencies are manifested in different environments and the extent to which these affect the child's communicative performance in everyday activities. For older children and adolescents, teachers are likely to be interviewed to determine how disfluencies affect the child's performance in the classroom and whether stuttering interferes with academics. For adults, interviews might be conducted with an individual's family members, including spouses or children, as well as employers and colleagues. Each of these individuals can provide a unique and important perspective in determining the extent to which fluency problems affect a person's life in diverse contexts.

Speech Observation.   Observation of a child's, adolescent's, or adult's speech in a variety of situations is the most important part of the fluency assessment. The clinician observes and records the individual's speech in as many activities as possible, including home, classroom, work, and social situations. The clinician uses a fluency charting grid, which is a tool for counting the total number and

FIGURE 10.3

Stressor inventory for parents.

Personal, Interpersonal, and Communicative Stressor Inventory

Please help us understand the factors that may affect your child's speech by checking those items that you feel apply to your child and your child's environment. Keep in mind that these factors do not *cause* stuttering—they simply contribute to your child's overall communication environment.

Possible Stressors Within the Child
_____ Is sensitive (reacts strongly to life experiences)
_____ Tends to be perfectionistic
_____ Becomes easily frustrated or upset
_____ Has an intense personality
_____ Is highly competitive with others
_____ Demonstrates performance anxiety or fears about speaking
_____ Becomes more disfluent when tired or ill
_____ Exhibits other speech and language or communication difficulties
_____ Has family members or other relatives who have stuttered or who currently stutter

Possible Stressors Within the Environment
_____ Experiences hectic daily routines at home or in other settings
_____ Faces intensive sibling rivalry or competition for talking time
_____ Has limited opportunities for free time or quiet time
_____ Shares communication environment with others who talk fast or interrupt frequently
_____ Has experienced stressful life situations (e.g., divorce, death, etc.)
_____ Experiences high expectations imposed by others (e.g., family members, teachers, etc.)

Source: From Stuttering Center of Western Pennsylvania © 2004. Reprinted with permission.

different types of disfluencies that occur within a speech sample. By calculating the number of disfluencies within a sample, the clinician can estimate the percentage of disfluent speech in a given speaking situation. For instance, in a sample of 500 words during play with a peer, if a child produces 30 repetitions, 10 sound prolongations, and 4 blocks, the clinician's calculations can show that about 9% of the child's speech is disfluent in peer-play context. The sample grid in Figure 10.4 can be used to calculate the percentage of stuttered disfluencies (word repetitions, sound/syllable repetitions, prolongations, and blocks) for 4 100-word samples.

By calculating the exact amount and type of disfluent speech, the clinician can then determine whether it is sufficiently different from normal expectations *and* whether it sufficiently detracts from effective communication. If one or both of these conditions exist, a fluency disorder may be present. The clinician can also use the speech observation to determine the presence of secondary features (e.g., escape and avoidance behaviors). These emerge as stuttering progresses and thus may provide a useful index of the extent of the problem.

When working with parents, it may be helpful for them to gather evidence on children's disfluencies in the home environment. The chart presented in Figure 10.5 is one example of a tool parents can use at home. To use this chart, parents observe between five and ten instances of their children's speech at home and document aspects of the interaction, such as who the child was speaking to and what the child was trying to convey, as well as features of the child's disfluencies (Yaruss et al., 2006). A tool such as this is useful for

Stuttering Center of Western Pennsylvania

Speech Disfluency Count Sheet

Name: _____

DOB: _____ DOE: _____ Age: _____

Situation: _____ Clinician: _____

Overall Frequency / Severity: _____

Stuttered Disfl. %: _____ Types: _____

Non-stutt. Disfl. %: _____ Types: _____

Type	#
I	
Rv	
Rp	
Rw	
Rs	
P	
B	
O	
%	

Type	#
I	
Rv	
Rp	
Rw	
Rs	
P	
B	
O	
%	

Type	#
I	
Rv	
Rp	
Rw	
Rs	
P	
B	
O	
%	

Type	#
I	
Rv	
Rp	
Rw	
Rs	
P	
B	
O	
%	

Notes: _____

"Nonstutt." Disfl.	"Stuttered" Disfl.	#	NonStutt	Stutt
I Interjection	Rw Word Rep.	1		
Rv Revision	Rs Sound/syllable rep.	2		
Rp Phrase rep.	P Prolongation	3		
O Other (Specify)	B Block	4		

Sample Fluency Charting Grid.

FIGURE 10.4

Source: From Stuttering Center of Western Pennsylvania © 2004. Reprinted with permission.

gathering data on children's patterns of disfluency and is important in treatment approaches that involve parents, discussed later in this chapter.

Questionnaire and Survey.   The clinician uses questionnaires and surveys to study an individual's feelings and attitudes about stuttering and communication. These instruments are an important component of the assessment process because of their focus on health-related quality of life (HRQL). HRQL refers to an individual's quality of life specifically with respect to impairments and injuries they may experience. It considers an individual's perceptions for physical functioning, social functioning, role functioning, and mental health (Franic & Bothe, 2008). These questionnaires are particularly helpful for estimating the extent to which experiences with stuttering have resulted in the accumulation of negative feelings about speaking. One such questionnaire is the Communication Attitude Test by Brutton (1985; cited in Vanryckeghem & Brutten, 1997). It contains 35 true/false statements that explore an individual's attitudes toward communication; examples include "I like to talk" and "People don't seem to like the way I talk." By

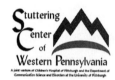

**HOME CHARTING
EXERCISE**

With whom was the child speaking?	What was the child's *message*?	What types of disfluencies were observed?	Was the child aware of the disfluencies?	What was the listener's reaction?	What was the child's reaction?	Describe the speaking situation.

FIGURE 10.5　　　　Sample Home Charting Exercise.

Source: From Stuttering Center of Western Pennsylvania © 2004. Reprinted with permission.

6 years of age, children who stutter have more negative attitudes toward communication than do other children, and these tend to increase in magnitude for older children (Vanryckeghem & Brutten, 1997). The Adolescent Communication Questionnaire (Bray, Kehle, Lawless, & Theodore, 2003) examines adolescents' confidence and sense of self-efficacy related to specific communication activities, such as ordering food at a restaurant or telling a joke. This questionnaire is shown in Figure 10.6. Adolescents who stutter give lower ratings on individual items on this questionnaire than do adolescents who do not stutter (average 3.5 vs. 4.6; Bray et al., 2003).

Direct Testing.　　The clinician also uses formal norm- and criterion-referenced tests to study an individual's speech and language skills. Such tests examine an individual's skills in syntax, vocabulary, phonology, and pragmatics and compare performance against expectations. Speech and language performance is an important part of the fluency assessment; as for some children and adults, speech-language impairments can coexist with fluency disorders.

Diagnosis

After the clinician administers a comprehensive fluency assessment, a diagnosis is made, based on all of the accumulated evidence. As a general rule, a fluency disorder is more likely to be diagnosed when the following are observed during assessment (Guitar, 2005):

FIGURE 10.6

Adolescent communication questionnaire.

We are interested in learning more about your speaking ability. Your responses are confidential.

DIRECTIONS: How much confidence do you have about doing each of the behaviors listed below? Circle the number that best represents your confidence.

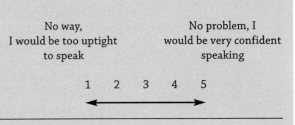

No way, I would be too uptight to speak

No problem, I would be very confident speaking

1   2   3   4   5

No way	No problem		No way	No problem	
1 2 3 4 5	1. Talking with a parent about a movie.		1 2 3 4 5	19. Asking a sales clerk how much an item costs.
1 2 3 4 5	2. Talking to a brother or sister at the dinner table.		1 2 3 4 5	20. Telling a police officer your home address.
1 2 3 4 5	3. Talking with three friends during lunch at school.		1 2 3 4 5	21. Calling a store to find out what time it opens.
1 2 3 4 5	4. Talking with a large group of friends during lunch at school.		1 2 3 4 5	22. Talking to a teacher alone after class.
1 2 3 4 5	5. Answering the telephone.		1 2 3 4 5	23. Reading aloud to a whole class.
1 2 3 4 5	6. Talking with the teacher during class.		1 2 3 4 5	24. Reading aloud to 5 classmates.
1 2 3 4 5	7. Talking with the principal.		1 2 3 4 5	25. Reading aloud to your family.
1 2 3 4 5	8. Asking a friend to come to your house after school.		1 2 3 4 5	26. Speaking to your pet.
1 2 3 4 5	9. Arguing with a brother or sister.		1 2 3 4 5	27. Raising your hand to ask the teacher a question.
1 2 3 4 5	10. Asking a parent if you can spend the night at a friend's house.		1 2 3 4 5	28. Answering a question in class.
1 2 3 4 5	11. Telling a new friend about your family.		1 2 3 4 5	29. Asking a question in class.
1 2 3 4 5	12. Telling your teacher your birth date.		1 2 3 4 5	30. Ordering food at a restaurant.
1 2 3 4 5	13. Calling your friend on the telephone.		1 2 3 4 5	31. Telling a joke.
1 2 3 4 5	14. Asking your parent if you can go to bed later than usual.		1 2 3 4 5	32. Giving a book report in front of the class.
1 2 3 4 5	15. Talking to a family member on the telephone.		1 2 3 4 5	33. Taking a speaking part in a school play.
1 2 3 4 5	16. Explaining how to play a game to your friends.		1 2 3 4 5	34. Reading aloud just to your teacher.
			1 2 3 4 5	35. Talking with a large group of your friends.
1 2 3 4 5	17. Asking a librarian for help in finding a book.		1 2 3 4 5	36. Talking aloud to yourself with no one else there.
1 2 3 4 5	18. Talking with a friend alone.		1 2 3 4 5	37. Talking with the school secretary.
			1 2 3 4 5	38. Reading a book aloud with no one else in the room.
			1 2 3 4 5	39. Talking to your teacher on the telephone.

Source: From "The relationship of self-efficacy and depression to stuttering" by M. A. Bray, T. J. Kehle, K. A. Lawless, and L. A. Theodore, 2003, *American Journal of Speech-Language Pathology, 12,* 425–431. Copyright 2003 by ASHA. Reprinted with permission.

1. Ten or more total disfluencies in 100 words
2. Three or more stuttering-like disfluencies in 100 words, summed across monosyllabic word repetitions, sound repetitions, prolongations, and blocks
3. Physical escape behaviors, such as head nods and eye blinks
4. Verbal avoidance behaviors, such as word substitutions

In addition to determining whether a disorder is present, assessment findings also characterize the severity of the disorder. A common estimate of stuttering severity is the Stuttering Severity Index (SSI; Riley, 1972). It estimates severity based on three variables, to each of which the clinician assigns points.

The first variable is the frequency of disfluencies—the percentage of disfluencies within a 100-word sample. Frequency estimates range from 1% (2 points) to more than 29% (18 points). The second variable is duration of blocks, ranging from none (0 points) to longer than 60 seconds (7 points). The third variable is physical concomitants, which encompass distracting sounds (e.g., sniffing), facial grimaces (e.g., jaw jerking), head movements (e.g., turning away), and extremity movements (e.g., foot tapping). To each, the clinician assigns points, ranging from none (0 points) to severe (5 points). The clinician then sums the points allocated to each variable and produces an SSI score and a severity rating: very mild, mild, moderate, severe, or very severe.

Prognosis

The prognosis describes the likelihood that the symptoms of a disorder will be resolved with time or treatment. A good prognosis predicts that a disorder will be resolved or will reverse its course, whereas a poor prognosis predicts that resolution is unlikely. The prognosis is a subjective decision made by the clinician, based on careful scrutiny of the complex body of information aggregated through the assessment process. For fluency disorders prognosis is complicated; the likelihood of resolution relates to many factors, including the age of stuttering onset, length of time since onset, type and number of core features, type and number of secondary features, and presence of such individual risk factors as gender, family history, coexisting speech and language disorders, and available support systems.

Treatment Recommendations

DISCUSSION POINT:
To what extent would you consider the treatment pursued by Mr. Cho in Case Study 10.1 to be evidence-based?

When a fluency disorder is diagnosed, the SLP recommends a specific course of action derived from (1) in-depth knowledge of the client, (2) clinical experience with fluency disorders, and (3) knowledge of the current scientific research on fluency disorders. Treatment recommendations derived from these information sources are called **evidence-based practice** (Ingham, 2003; Justice & Fey, 2004), a term that emphasizes the clinician's use of the scientific literature when making treatment decisions.

HOW ARE FLUENCY DISORDERS TREATED? ●

The pursuit of effective approaches to eliminating stuttering has a long history. As described so colorfully in Bobrick's (1995) *Knotted Tongues: Stuttering in History and the Quest for a Cure,* historical treatments included Demosthenes' placement of stones in his mouth to reduce his stuttering, which was undoubtedly less painful than the bloodletting of the tongue practiced by physicians in the Middle Ages. Other treatments included electroshock therapy, tongue lozenges, beetroot nose drops, tongue wrapping, and immersion of the head in cold water followed by eating and vomiting horseradish. Many of these historical treatments were based on faulty understanding of both fluency and disfluency. For instance, one treatment approach from more than 1,000 years ago involved drying out the person who stuttered, because experts thought that excess moisture and humidity caused stuttering (Bobrick, 1995). In one approach to drying out, the tongue was rubbed with salt, honey, and sage, and the neck and ears were cauterized and blistered.

Fortunately, scientific knowledge of stuttering causes and treatments continues to grow, and the tenets of scientific reasoning and empirical evidence have become the norm when making treatment decisions for fluency disorders.

Described here are illustrative examples of treatment approaches for children, adolescents, and adults.

TREATMENT FOR CHILDREN

As mentioned earlier, there is some controversy as to whether young children who show characteristics of borderline stuttering should be provided with treatment and early intervention or whether a wait-and-see approach is more appropriate. This argument focuses specifically on children who are between 2 and 5 years of age and who show stuttering-like disfluencies in their speech but are not advanced in stuttering beyond borderline characteristics (Curlee & Yairi, 1997).

Professionals who argue for early intervention for these children emphasize that treatment is needed to prevent them from progressing to more advanced levels of stuttering. These professionals stress that (1) it is impossible to know for sure which children will recover from early stuttering without treatment, (2) the consequences of an established stuttering disorder can be both devastating and consequential to the life of the child and the family, and (3) early treatments do no harm and are more likely to be effective than later treatments are (Zebrowski, 1997).

Other professionals advocate withholding treatment for 6 months or longer after stuttering begins (Curlee & Yairi, 1997). These experts emphasize research showing that (1) the majority of children spontaneously recover from stuttering within a year or two after onset, (2) little evidence supports the effectiveness of earlier rather than later treatment, and (3) treatment should be based on clear indicators that a child is likely to progress as a stutterer (Curlee & Yairi, 1997). This wait-and-see approach is not a new concept: as Bobrick reported (1995), Mercurialis' 1583 *Treatise on the Disease of Children* argued that children should not be treated for stuttering until at least 7 years of age "since before that time it cannot be known whether their speech is defective or not" and many children are spontaneously cured.

> **DISCUSSION POINT:**
> As you might guess, the debate over early treatment versus wait-and-see is a heated one. If you were a parent, which would be your preference? If you were a clinician, which would you endorse? Why?

Because of the enormous personal and societal costs of a persistent fluency disorder, and in light of recent data showing that treatment of stuttering among young children reduces disfluencies at rates greater than occurs with spontaneous recovery (Harris et al., 2002), the provision of early intervention is the current gold standard of practice. Treatment with children will often involve a variety of approaches, including parent-implemented treatments that take advantage of the home environment as well as direct treatment by a therapist. Parent-implemented treatment should be offered in conjunction with direct treatment, not as an alternative.

Parent-Implemented Treatment

Treatments implemented by parents within the home environment, often used in conjunction with clinician-implemented treatment, are frequently used for young children. These parent-implemented treatments are often called *indirect treatment*, because the clinician provides the treatment indirectly through the parents. Two popular models of indirect treatment are environmental modification and operant training.

Environmental modification models emphasize reduction of the mismatch between environmental demands and the child's capacity for fluent speech. These models typically involve training parents to both reduce environmental demands and promote fluency models. Parents are counseled about ways to reduce demands on fluency, such as frequent interruptions, questions, and a lack of listening, especially when children are fatigued, excited, or anxious (Gottwald & Starkweather, 1995; Rustin & Cook, 1995). Clinicians provide parents with specific suggestions:

- Avoid putting the child on the spot during social situations
- Repeat what the child says to show that you are listening
- Make comments when talking with the child rather than asking questions
- Modify activities that seem particularly stressful to the child (Nelson, 1985)

By offering these suggestions to parents, the goal is not to limit children's opportunities to communicate, but rather to reduce pressures that may surround communicative interactions (Yaruss et al., 2006). Thus, helping parents to maintain a high level of communicative engagement with their children is essential. They may be taught how to substitute comments ("I notice that the red chicken is limping") for questions ("What's wrong with the red chicken?"), the former providing greater freedom to children in whether and how to respond.

Clinicians are also likely to provide parents a set of specific techniques that help them to provide improved models of fluency for their children. Two such techniques include easy talking and reflecting/rephrasing (Yaruss et al., 2006). Parents use these techniques in periods of sustained interaction with their children. With easy talking, the parent uses a slowed rate of speech with lengthened pauses (up to 1 second) between words and phrases; these changes are to be subtle, so that communication proceeds naturally and the parents' speech appears normal and relaxed (Yaruss et al., 2006). Yaruss and colleagues use the television personality Mister Rogers as a good example of easy talking. The goal of easy talking is for children to participate in communicative interactions that move along at an easy and relaxed pace. Parents use the reflecting/rephrasing technique in conjunction with easy talking; with this technique, parents reflect what children say during communicative interactions using a slightly slower and relaxed manner of speaking. For example, a parental reflection of the child utterance, "I-I-I-I wa-wa-want this guy oooover here" might be "Oh . . . you want the guy . . . over there" (Yaruss et al., 2006, p. 125). The goal of reflecting is for children to receive appropriate fluency models that reflect an easy, relaxed speaking style. Parents who participate in training programs that help them learn these techniques rate them as very helpful (Yaruss et al., 2006).

To assist the parent in making these changes, the clinician is likely to provide ongoing and periodic support to the family. The clinician might see the family monthly to monitor the child's fluency, discuss progress in the home treatment, and counsel the parent, particularly if the parent is anxious about the child's fluency (Zebrowski, 1997). Some families might participate in a parent fluency group, in which parents share the strategies they use to promote fluency.

Operant training models take a different approach, viewing stuttering as a learned behavior that can be eliminated through contingent stimulation (Onslow, Andrews, & Lincoln, 1994). *Contingent stimulation* refers to the way in which adults respond to children's disfluencies and uses these responses to stimulate children's production of fluent speech. In operant training models, such as the Lidcombe Program of Sydney, Australia, parents receive training in three techniques they use to shape their child's use of fluent speech (Onslow et al., 1994):

1. *Identify disfluencies and provide positive input:* Parents learn to identify disfluencies and to correct disfluent speech in a nonpunitive and positive manner, as in "Oops, that was a bumpy word" (Onslow et al., 1994, p. 1246). Parents also learn to praise fluent speech, as in "You said that very smoothly."

2. *Prompt fluent speech:* Parents prompt the child to produce fluent speech in normal everyday speaking situations, as in "Let's see if you can have really smooth speech while we are at the grocery store."

3. *Prompt self-correction:* Parents help the child identify when disfluencies occur and self-correct, as in "I heard a bumpy word. Did you hear it? See if you can say it again."

When used with children between 2 and 5 years of age, operant training programs appear to be effective in reducing the likelihood of ongoing fluency problems (Lincoln & Onslow, 1997).

CLINICIAN-IMPLEMENTED TREATMENTS

Current Approaches to Stuttering Treatment

Two approaches to stuttering treatment predominate in the field today (Guitar, 2005): stuttering modification therapy and fluency shaping therapy. These two approaches differ not only in the methods used to treat fluency disorders, but also in the overall goal of treatment (see Table 10.5). The goal of **stuttering modification** therapy is to help the person who stutters to better manage the moment of stuttering—that moment when an individual repeats, prolongs, or blocks on a sound. As stuttering progresses, these moments become more intense and long-lasting; they are what the person with a fluency disorder fears and strives to avoid or escape. Stuttering modification therapy focuses on helping the individual manage these moments and stutter more effortlessly and less tensely. Thus, the outcome of treatment is *controlled stuttering,* coupled with careful attention to feelings and emotions toward stuttering and communication. The end goal is for moments of stuttering to be hardly noticeable and completely manageable. Disfluency is viewed as a problem that one can learn to manage.

The goal of **fluency shaping** therapy is to help the person who stutters produce fluent speech more often, potentially eradicating disfluencies completely. This therapy focuses on increasing the amount of fluent speech produced as an individual progresses through a highly structured program. Fluency shaping pays little attention to the individual's feelings and emotions toward stuttering; the end goal is for fluent speech to predominate and moments of stuttering to

TABLE 10.5	Key principles in stuttering modification and fluency shaping therapy	
	Stuttering Modification	**Fluency Shaping**
Goal	To manage and modify the moment of stuttering (i.e., controlled stuttering) and reduce fear and anxiety associated with stuttering	To increase the amount of fluent speech and eliminate moments of stuttering (i.e., controlled fluency)
Focus	To teach how to modify disfluencies using cancellations and pull-outs, to reduce escape and avoidance behaviors, and to reduce anxiety and fear	To establish fluent speech by using a slower speech rate, more relaxed breathing, easy onsets into speech, and soft contact while speaking
Approach	Involves counseling; loosely structured; practice with different techniques in clinic and then in different settings	Highly structured; practice with different techniques in clinic and then in different settings

Source: Based on B. Guitar (1998).

disappear, resulting in *controlled fluency*. Completely fluent speech is the therapeutic goal.

Stuttering Modification.   Charles Van Riper, who died in 1994 at the age of 88, was one of the greatest authorities on stuttering and the original champion of stuttering modification. For this reason, this approach is sometimes called the Van Riper method. Stuttering modification used with beginning stutterers emphasizes positive fluency models, fluency-building techniques, and desensitization (Guitar, 1998; Van Riper, 1973). The therapist provides positive fluency models during comfortable, well-paced interactions in which the therapist uses simple words and phrases intermixed with generous pauses and - periods of silence. The therapist introduces the child to fluency-building techniques through games focused on improving the child's rhythm and timing during talking, such as chanting familiar rhymes. The therapist also focuses on desensitizing the child to disruptors of smooth speech and increasing the child's ability to manage disfluencies. The therapist uses specific exercises designed by Van Riper that build the capacity to handle fluency disruptors.

Fluency Shaping.   Like stuttering modification, fluency shaping focuses on building the beginning stutterer's capacity for and experience with fluent speech. However, fluency shaping uses different techniques to reach this goal. The Lidcombe Program described earlier is an example of a fluency shaping approach based on operant procedures; it emphasizes positive reinforcement of fluency and negative reinforcement, or correction, of disfluencies. Parents or therapists provide regular reinforcement of periods or instances of good fluency (e.g., "That was terrific—you didn't stutter at all") in conjunction with correction of disfluencies (e.g., "That word was bumpy—say it again for me"; Lincoln & Onslow, 1997). Over time, with appropriate amounts of reinforcement, the child's production of fluent speech increases and disfluent speech decreases (Jones, Onslow, Harrison, & Packman, 2000). Children who participate in the Lidcombe Program show significant reductions in the rate of disfluencies. In one recent study, 10 children who received the program for 12 weeks (one treatment per week at a clinic) reduced the percentage of syllables stuttered from an average of 8.6% to 3.5%; by comparison, children in a control group who received no treatment showed a reduction from 8.4% to 5.8%. Although children in the control group showed a substantial reduction in disfluency rates over the 3-month period, the reductions were doubled for those who received treatment (Harris et al., 2002).

TREATMENT FOR ADOLESCENTS

Providing stuttering treatment to adolescents who are intermediate or advanced stutterers is not for the fainthearted. A number of experts have commented on the challenge of working with adolescents who stutter, noting that these are among the toughest clinical cases (Daly, Simon, & Burnett-Stolnack, 1995). In addition to the well-known social, academic, psychological, and physical challenges of the adolescent period, stuttering therapies are complicated by the fact that the most well-established therapies were designed for either children or adults, not for adolescents (Blood, 1995). The treatments for adolescents need to contend with the specific challenges of this period of life—peer pressure, time commitments, the drive for autonomy and individuality, academic demands, self-doubt, self-esteem, and the like (Blood, 1995; Daly et al., 1995). Several important considerations are listed in Figure 10.7.

FIGURE 10.7

Suggestions for delivering stuttering treatment to adolescents.

- Improve the adolescent's knowledge of stuttering, including what causes it and how it is treated
- Teach cognitive and self-instructional strategies that promote the adolescent's awareness of and responsibility for treatment outcomes
- Introduce relaxation strategies to promote awareness and use of relaxation techniques
- Use mental imagery in which the adolescent pictures himself or herself in different speaking situations, communicating fluently
- Model the use of positive self-talk and the use of positive language when describing self
- Teach positive coping strategies, such as how to express negative emotions and how to recover after stuttering episodes
- Introduce assertiveness training and emphasize alternative means of asserting oneself, such as art, exercise, and writing
- Identify social support systems available to the adolescent, including friends, teachers, and family members

Sources: Based on Blood (1995); Daly, Simon, and Burnett-Stolnack (1995).

Both stuttering modification and fluency shaping approaches are useful for adolescents (see Ramig & Bennett, 1995). Stuttering modification emphasizes teaching the adolescent about stuttering (i.e., getting to know your stuttering) to demystify the disorder. This approach teaches adolescents how to work through instances of disfluency, using different techniques such as cancellations and pull-outs. In cancellations, individuals pause after a word containing a disfluency, wait until they have control, and then repeat the word with a gentle, easy stutter, as in "He said he w-w-w-wanted . . . wanted it." In pull-outs, individuals stop during a disfluency, wait until they have control, and then gradually and lightly produce the rest of the word. With both cancellations and pull-outs, the individual practices moving easily, gently, and voluntarily through disfluencies (Guitar, 1998). While learning these skills, an adolescent also learns to reduce anxiety, fear, and tension about stuttering.

One example of a stuttering modification program used with adolescents and adults is the Successful Stuttering Management Program (SSMP; Blomgren, Roy, Callister, & Merrill, 2005). SSMP is an intensive 3-week residential program in which hundreds of people have participated in the United States and abroad. Individuals participate in group and individual therapy each afternoon for 3.5 hours and complete a variety of speaking tasks in the morning, such as conducting surveys. SSPM involves three phases (Blomgren et al., 2005):

Phase 1: confrontation of stuttering (about 2 weeks)

Phase 2: modification of stuttering (1 week)

Phase 3: maintenance (2 days)

Phase 1 activities focus on modifying the participants' attitudes toward stuttering, and treatment activities focus on eliminating avoidance strategies. Individuals "advertise" their stuttering in many different speaking situations and analyze their own moments of stuttering. Phase 2 activities involve learning specific techniques that help to lessen severity of stuttering moments, such as pull-outs and cancellations. Phase 3 activities involve developing an individualized maintenance plan that would help them continue to use stuttering modification techniques behind the SSMP. Recent research findings suggest that the positive impacts of the SSMP are largely confined to reducing individuals' avoidance behaviors and anxieties toward stuttering rather than reducing core behaviors, including severity of stuttering (Blomgren et al., 2005).

Fluency shaping with adolescents, sometimes called *smooth speech treatment,* emphasizes an increase in fluent speech using a combination of operant conditioning techniques (Craig et al., 2002). Fluent speech is promoted by training the adolescent to use several techniques characteristic of smooth, or fluent, speech, including easy onset, soft contact, and continuous airflow. With *easy onset,* an individual releases a soft flow of air prior to initiating a word or phrase, providing a gentle entrance into speaking. *Soft contact* describes the use of gentle and soft movement of the articulators, including their contact with one another (e.g., a soft touch of the tongue to the teeth when producing the first sound in *to*). With *continuous airflow,* the airflow continues across phrases and words, decreasing the stops and starts of normal airflow for speech. These and other techniques are used to increase the adolescent's production of fluent speech and elimination of disfluencies.

TREATMENT FOR ADULTS

Treatment of stuttering in adults utilizes both stuttering modification and fluency shaping approaches or an integration of the two. For the adult who may have experienced stuttering for years, treatment emphasizes the following:

1. *Knowledge about stuttering:* Treatment helps adults understand and confront the disorder of stuttering. They can examine their own core and secondary features and even confront their own stuttering in a mirror or video to develop an intimate catalog of their own behaviors.

2. *Reduction of negative feelings:* Treatment helps adults reduce their fear, embarrassment, and discomfort with stuttering. They are guided to view their stuttering with interest and curiosity, to discuss stuttering openly and honestly, and to resist word and situation avoidances.

3. *Fluency building:* Treatment helps adults increase their use of fluency-enhancing strategies and work through moments of stuttering. Strategies to increase fluency include talking at a slower rate and using easy onsets and soft contact. Strategies to help adults work through moments of stuttering—or to stutter more easily—include using cancellations and pull-outs. Treatment helps adults maintain improvements outside the therapy room (Guitar, 1998).

As a complement to these approaches, pharmaceutical intervention is increasingly being explored for stuttering treatment. Several medications used in the treatment of anxiety and depression have been shown to reduce stuttering symptoms, including several selective-serotonin reuptake inhibitors (SSRIs; Costa & Kroll, 2000; Riley et al., 2001). The use of medication provides a promising and interesting avenue for future research on fluency disorders.

CASE ANALYSIS

Review Harry's case (Case Study 5 in the Companion Website at www.pearsonhighered.com/justice2e). Reflect on factors in Harry's life that may promote a healthy resolution of his fluency problems.

● CHAPTER SUMMARY

A fluency disorder occurs when a person's ability to produce speech effortlessly and automatically is significantly compromised by the presence of disfluencies, specifically sound and word repetitions, sound prolongations, and blocks. When these core features persist over time, the individual with a fluency disorder develops secondary features as well, including escape and avoidance behaviors and negative feelings toward speaking, including fear.

The majority of fluency disorders emerge during early childhood and are referred to as *developmental fluency disorders* or *developmental stuttering.* Although about 5% of the population has experienced developmental stuttering at some time, only about 1% of the population continues to experience stuttering in adolescence and adulthood. For the others, stuttering is resolved either therapeutically or spontaneously. Acquired fluency disorders occur less frequently than developmental fluency disorders but may occur at any time as a result of trauma, disease, or illness.

Assessment of fluency disorders is the domain of the speech-language pathologist, who carefully studies an individual's speech in a variety of situations to determine the type and number of disfluencies. The SLP also carefully identifies any secondary features, including physical behaviors, that signal escape from and avoidance of moments of stuttering, as well as the individual's feelings toward stuttering. When the fluency assessment is completed, the SLP provides an estimate of severity, for which one common metric is the Stuttering Severity Index. Fluency disorders range from very mild to very severe.

Treatment of fluency disorders involves a variety of different evidence-based techniques, most commonly differentiated into those treatments that emphasize stuttering modification and those that emphasize fluency shaping. Stuttering modification focuses on helping the individual work through and modify the moment of stuttering, whereas fluency shaping focuses on reducing disfluencies and promoting overall speaking fluency. Both approaches are useful; selection is usually determined by the SLP and client preferences.

● KEY TERMS

avoidance behaviors, p. 330
between-word disfluency, p. 330
block, p. 320
circumlocution, p. 331
core features, p. 320
developmental stuttering, p. 323
disfluency, p. 319
escape behaviors, p. 330
evidence-based practice, p. 346

fluency, p. 319
fluency shaping, p. 349
neurogenic stuttering, p. 326
precipitating factors, p. 333
predisposing factors, p. 333
prolongation, p. 320
psychogenic stuttering, p. 326
repetition, p. 320
secondary features, p. 320

situation avoidance, p. 331
sound avoidance, p. 331
stuttering, p. 317
stuttering-like disfluencies,
    p. 324
stuttering modification, p. 349
within-word disfluency, p. 330
word avoidance, p. 331

● ON THE WEB

Check out the Companion Website at www .pearsonhighered.com/justice2e! On it you will find

- suggested readings
- reflection questions
- a self-study quiz

- discussion of hot topics in fluency disorders
- description of current technological innovations in fluency disorders
- links to additional online resources

VOICE DISORDERS

FOCUS QUESTIONS

This chapter answers the following questions:

1. What is a voice disorder?

2. How are voice disorders classified?

3. What are the defining characteristics of voice disorders?

4. How are voice disorders identified?

5. How are voice disorders treated?

CHAPTER 11

INTRODUCTION

You may recall from Chapter 3 that the larynx sits deep in the neck at the base of the pharynx; it cannot be seen without some type of technological assistance. Prior to the advent of these technologies, knowledge of the larynx required dissections of human cadavers, which obviously did not permit scientists or physicians to see the larynx at work or to study its function. The well-hidden larynx avoided careful scrutiny until the sixteenth century.

The first book on laryngeal structures appeared in 1600, and by the eighteenth century, scholars had achieved a relatively well-developed understanding of the way in which the vocal folds vibrate to produce the human voice (Karmody, 1996). Technological innovations furthered this understanding in the early nineteenth century. The **glottiscope,** invented in 1829, coupled a tongue retractor with a mirror to provide a crude glimpse of the laryngeal cavity. An 1853 improvement attached a gaslight to a more sophisticated glottiscope to project a beam of light down onto the vocal folds (see Figure 11.1). The most elegant, novel, and simple innovation, which contributed to a vast improvement in understanding the laryngeal function, occurred in 1854 when voice teacher Manual Garcia devised the concept of the laryngeal mirror, also called a *laryngoscope*. A **laryngeal mirror** is essentially a small, round dental mirror that is placed at the back of the oral cavity to look down on an individual's vocal folds.

These early technologies gave way to increasingly sophisticated approaches to looking at the larynx and its structures in action, including the twenty-first century's embrace of *endoscopy* and *videostroboscopy*. These tools, discussed later in the chapter, allow clinicians and scientists to watch the vocal folds in action by lowering a flexible tube through the oral and nasal cavity into the laryngeal area.

Long ago, clinicians and scientists had few resources to study a person's larynx compared to those available today. In 1888, Friedrich III, who reigned only briefly as Germany's emperor, died of laryngeal cancer. The professionals then relied on subjective acoustic evaluation (listening to the emperor's hoarse voice quality) and indirect examination of the laryngeal cavity with a laryngeal mirror (Karmody, 1996). Now, clinicians and scientists have numerous resources to study the larynx.

This chapter describes disorders of voice, in which an individual's vocal quality is in some way compromised. Some voice disorders are mild and transient and require no treatment, as you may have experienced after a night of cheering for your favorite sports team. In other cases, voice disorders are severe and persistent, and require ongoing treatment. In the most serious cases, an individual's larynx may need to be removed, as is sometimes required with laryngeal cancer.

● ● ●

DISCUSSION POINT:
Consider your own voice. How would you characterize it? Is its pitch high or low? Is its loudness loud or soft? What gives it your own vocal signature?

FIGURE 11.1

The nineteenth-century glottiscope.

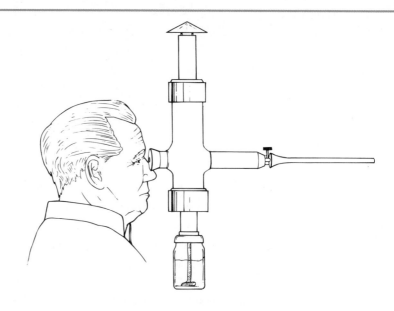

WHAT IS A VOICE DISORDER? ●

DEFINITION

Defining Voice

Voice is the complex, dynamic product of vocal fold vibration that allows us to vocalize (i.e., make sounds) and verbalize (i.e., produce language through speech). An essential tool for both speech and communication, voice is also a major tool for personal expression, creativity, and art. Consider the opera singer, the actress, the professor, the minister, the talk show host, the stock trader, the politician. Could these professions exist without voice?

The human voice resides in the vibratory patterns of the larynx's tiny vocal folds. Humans can volitionally set their vocal folds into a vibratory pattern, referred to as *phonation,* using airflow from the lungs as fuel. Pause for a moment to phonate—try "ooo" and "ahh." Contrast these two sounds with some that are *not* phonated in their production, such as "sss" and "fff." Now take a moment to compare whispering with talking. Whisper a short phrase, such as "My dog is brown," followed by the same phrase at a conversational level. Think about your voice and where and how it is produced.

As you may recall from earlier chapters, phonation is one of several systems critical to the process of speech production. To phonate, the vocal folds must be closed, or *adducted,* at midline. Such a state is called **adduction.** (When not producing voice, the vocal folds rest in an open, or *abducted,* position so that one can breathe—a state called **abduction.**) For phonation to occur, air is exhaled from the respiratory system upward against the adducted vocal folds, which are then blown apart and set into a rapid vibratory pattern. Once voice is produced, it is modified as it travels up through the pharynx, or throat, and into the oral and nasal cavity, a process called *resonation.* **Resonance** refers to the actual vibration of the air within the pharyngeal column, which impacts the quality of the voice. The voice is also manipulated within the oral cavity in a process of *articulation.*

Individual voices seem very distinct. When familiar people call us on the telephone, they often do not have to introduce themselves because we know their voices so well. Our voices arise from the complex interaction of three vocal characteristics: frequency, intensity, and phonatory quality (Stemple, Glaze, & Gerdeman, 1995).

Frequency is the rate of vocal fold vibration, expressed as cycles per second, or hertz (Hz). Frequency is an objective, physical measurement of vibratory rate, whereas **pitch** is the psychological or perceptual equivalent. When the vocal folds vibrate, they actually do so at several different frequencies simultaneously. *Fundamental frequency,* notated as F_0, is the arithmetic mean of the rates of vibration for the vocal folds (Robb & Smith, 2002). If an individual's vocal folds vibrate 250 times in a second, the F_0 is 250 Hz, which is the average F_0 for kindergarten girls and boys (Awan & Mueller, 1996). For adult

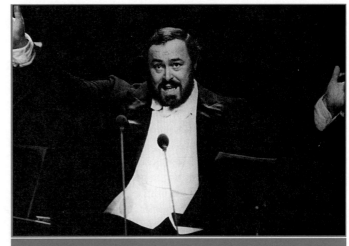

Voice is a tool not only for communication but also for art and creativity.

women, the F_0 ranges from about 180 to 220 Hz, and for adult men, the F_0 ranges from about 120 to 140 Hz (Morris, Brown, Hicks, & Howell, 1995; Russell, Penny, & Pemberton, 1995).

A person's fundamental frequency relates to three characteristics of the vocal folds:

1. *Length:* Longer vocal folds contribute to a lower F_0.
2. *Mass:* Thicker vocal fold mass contributes to a lower F_0.
3. *Tension:* Greater tension contributes to a higher F_0 (Case, 2002).

A potentially confusing point is the importance of differentiating the concept of *length of vocal folds* from *lengthened vocal folds.* While it is true that longer vocal folds, as in the adult male, are associated with a lower fundamental frequency than are shorter vocal folds, as in the adult female, it is also true that lengthened vocal folds are associated with an increase in fundamental frequency due to increased tension of the folds. As individuals stretch and lengthen their vocal folds, the speed of vibration tends to increase, thereby contributing to an increase in fundamental frequency. An adult male's voice may have a relatively low fundamental frequency compared to an adult female because of longer vocal folds, but by stretching and lengthening his vocal folds, he can increase his fundamental frequency.

The fundamental frequency of our voices changes as we age because of the impact of physical growth and change on the length, mass, and tension of the vocal folds. The greatest amount of change occurs between birth and puberty, when the vocal folds lengthen from 2 mm to an average of 9 mm for females and 16 mm for males (Titze, 1994). As these physical changes occur, fundamental frequency decreases, most significantly for males. Fundamental frequency then plateaus for several years, but at midlife it begins to decrease again, particularly for women. Toward the end of the life span, a woman's fundamental frequency has decreased from an average of 220 Hz to 180 Hz (Russell et al., 1995).

Intensity is the physical measurement of sound pressure reported in decibels (dB); the perceptual correlate of intensity is **loudness.** Intensity of voice production is determined by how far the vocal folds separate laterally and how

CASE STUDY 11.1	**Voice Disorders Across the Life Span**

Ms. Chin is a 42-year-old television personality in Houston, Texas. She is the co-anchor for the 5:00 PM news show on the local CBS affiliate, a position that she reached after about 18 years at the station. Ms. Chin has begun to experience intermittent problems with her voice; it seems to start and stop and feel strangled. Three times while on the air, she had to stop what she was saying and allow her co-anchor to take over. On the not-so-gentle advice of her producer, Ms. Chin consulted her primary care physician, who referred her to an otolaryngologist at the Houston Medical Center. During the appointment, her voice never broke down, but the otolaryngologist made a preliminary diagnosis of spasmodic dysphonia (SD). The otolaryngologist did not know any local speech-language pathologists who specialized in SD but referred her to a therapist who had treated his child's vocal nodules. Ms. Chin has an appointment next week to discuss treatment options. Meanwhile, Ms. Chin's producer has suggested that she take a disability leave or at least be reassigned until her voice problems are resolved.

Internet research

1 How many people are affected annually by spasmodic dysphonia? Does it affect women and men at similar rates?

2 What other media personalities have been affected by voice problems? How did this impact their careers?

Brainstorm and discussion

1 Do you agree with Ms. Chin's producer that she should be off the air until her voice problem resolves?

2 Ms. Chin has an appointment soon with a speech-language pathologist who may not be skilled in treating spasmodic dysphonia. How important is it to see a clinician who has worked with this condition before?

3 What other professionals should be involved with Ms. Chin's voice treatment?

● ● ●

Kate Mitchell, M.D., is a 46-year-old former trauma surgeon and mother of four in Salt Lake City, Utah. Dr. Mitchell was in a car accident 2 years ago after a night of emergency surgery. She swerved to avoid a deer, suffered a severe spinal cord injury, and became a quadriplegic. Dr. Mitchell is unable to breathe on her own and is ventilator dependent. She was extremely depressed and did not speak for over a year, even when a speaking valve was placed on the ventilator. However, after 1 year, Dr. Mitchell began to work with a speech-language pathologist and a psychologist to use her voice. She began to speak at home to her four daughters and her husband and then increasingly used her voice in public. She recently gave a brief speech to members of the trauma surgery department, who held a ceremony on her behalf. Dr. Mitchell's speech-language pathologist has set up a voice-activated computer so that eventually Dr. Mitchell can use the

speaking valve to interact with the computer for typing and even accessing the Internet.

Internet research

1 Annually, how many vehicular accidents result in severe spinal cord injuries?

2 Dr. Mitchell received a Passy-Muir ventilator speaking valve. How many different kinds of speaking valves are on the market?

Brainstorm and discussion

1 What community activities might be possible for Dr. Mitchell, now that she uses her voice?

2 How might Dr. Mitchell be involved with her profession as a quadriplegic?

quickly they come back together in a vibratory cycle. *Intensity* relates to two features of vocal production: (1) the amount of airflow from the lungs and (2) the amount of resistance to the airflow by the vocal folds (Case, 2002). An increase in airflow from the lungs results in increased intensity (perceived as greater loudness); shouting is a good example. When you shout, you first take a large gulp of air, which is then exhaled forcefully through the vocal folds. The greater volume of air results in a wider excursion, or separation, of the vocal folds, contributing to a loud shout. Increased resistance by the vocal folds—achieved through compression of the vocal folds at the midline—also results in increased loudness. You can experience this by clenching together the vocal folds, as if you were about to lift something heavy. This tightening creates resistance to the air pressure under the vocal folds; when the pressure is released, it is louder than it would have been without the resistance. Even though vocal loudness is under volitional control, every individual has a baseline intensity level that characterizes that person's conversational speech.

Phonatory quality is a more difficult concept to define but is no less important in constructing a definition of voice. As Case (2002) notes, the numerous terms used to describe phonatory quality suggest its importance: *mellow, rich, harmonious, velvety, reedy, whispery, whining, harsh, shrill, flat, breathy, pleasing.*

Phonatory quality relates to how well the two vocal folds work during the vibratory cycle (Stemple et al., 1995). When the vocal folds work together symmetrically and harmoniously, the voice is pleasant, clear, and unremarkable. When the relationship between the two folds is compromised in some way, phonatory quality is also compromised. For instance, a growth on one of the two vocal folds impedes the union of the two folds as they come together, resulting in a breathy or hoarse quality.

Phonatory quality can also be influenced by the resonation of the voice as it travels up from the vocal folds through the pharynx and into the oral and nasal cavities. Fran Drescher's character in the long-running television sit-com *The Nanny* had an unmistakably nasal voice quality, which Drescher made an essential part of her character's personality. She produced that quality by manipulating the column of air in her nasal cavity.

Defining a Voice Disorder

Individuals exhibit a voice disorder when their pitch, loudness, or phonatory quality differs significantly from that of persons of a similar age, gender, cultural background, and racial or ethnic group (Stemple et al., 1995). The difference must be serious enough to draw attention and to detract in some way from performance in ecological contexts, such as school, home, community, or work.

Many people exhibit vocal characteristics that differ significantly from those of peers. We all vary in our pitch, loudness, and other vocal qualities, and this variation gives us our unique voices. For some public personalities, unique vocal characteristics are an intrinsic part of their personae. For instance, former president Bill Clinton often had a hoarse vocal quality, resulting from both innate laryngeal characteristics and constant overuse of his voice. Actresses Kathleen Turner and Marilyn Monroe and singers Jamie O'Neal and Billie Holiday are also well known by their breathy or hoarse vocal qualities. Thus, when an individual's voice qualities differ from those of others, it does not always signal a disorder. For a disorder to be present, the voice should call attention to the speaker in a negative way and should detract from the person's ability to function in society.

For some public personalities, severe breathiness and hoarseness resulted in a loss of livelihood. Julie Andrews, whose voice became world famous from her role in *The Sound of Music,* lost her singing voice after surgery on her vocal folds in 1997 to remove vocal nodules that were restricting her range and

DISCUSSION POINT:
Consider other terms used to describe variations in voice. For each term you come up with, decide whether it references frequency, intensity, or phonatory quality.

DISCUSSION POINT:
Why is a voice disturbance considered attractive in some cases, as with Marilyn Monroe, but detrimental in other cases, as with Ms. Chin in Case Study 11.1?

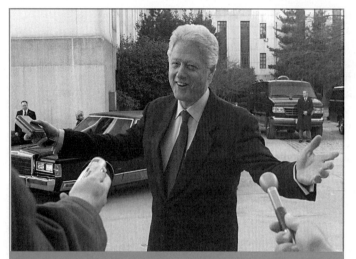

Former president Bill Clinton is an example of a public personality with a well-known and unique vocal signature.

voice quality. The surgery further compromised the elasticity of her vocal folds, and Andrews did not perform publicly for several years after the surgery. Diane Rehm, host of the *Diane Rehm Show* on National Public Radio, developed **spasmodic dysphonia,** a voice problem characterized by a strained, broken, and breathy quality. Rehm is currently treated with Botox injections into her vocal folds, which allow her to maintain her daily radio program. (Rehm shares her experience in the 1999 memoir *Finding My Voice.*)

TERMINOLOGY

Voice Quality

Numerous terms are available to describe aberrations in vocal quality. **Dysphonia** is the umbrella term used to refer to a voice that is disordered in some way (*dys-* is a common prefix meaning "abnormal or impaired," and -*phonia* refers to voice). **Aphonia** refers to the total loss or lack of voice. In addition, many other terms are used to describe the ways in which a voice differs from the norm. Most of these terms are subjective—terms like *breathy, hoarse,* and *rough.* These and other less familiar terms are described in Table 11.1. Some of these terms describe variations in pitch and frequency, such as *jitter* and *diplophonic.* Other terms focus on loudness and intensity, such as *pressed* or *strident,* whereas some focus specifically on resonance, such as *nasal* and *ringing.* Some terms focus more broadly on general phonatory quality, describing voices that *flutter* or *creak.* All of these terms provide more precise ways of describing dysphonia and aphonia.

Vocal Fold Functioning

Many problems with vocal quality result from a malfunctioning of the vocal folds in which the relationship of the folds during vocal production is undermined in some way (Case, 1996). Two terms that describe the most common malfunction are *hypofunction* and *hyperfunction.* **Hypofunction** describes vocal folds that are underfunctioning and have inadequate tension. With hypofunction, the vocal folds do not come together adequately or evenly, allowing air to escape through the vocal folds and resulting in a breathiness or hoarseness. With complete hypofunction, no voice is produced at all, and the person either does not speak or must whisper. In some voice disorders, hypofunction affects only one vocal fold and the other works normally.

The opposite of hypofunction is **hyperfunction.** Hyperfunctioning vocal folds are overly tense and compress together too tightly. Thus, the hyperfunctioning voice may sound too loud, too high, or too strained. Excessive tension in the neck or jaw may accompany the hyperfunctioning voice. In some cases, the hyperfunctioning vocal cords completely impede the production of voice, resulting in *spasticity,* in which the voice stops and starts intermittently.

Diplophonia is a particularly interesting type of vocal fold malfunction. *Diplophonia* means "double pitch" and describes a vocal quality in which the vocal folds produce two different pitches simultaneously. The primary cause of

TABLE 11.1	Terms used to describe voice and its many variations
Descriptive Term	**Perception**
aphonic	No sound or little sound; may cut out or whisper
biphonic or diplophonic	Two pitches produced simultaneously
breathy	Excessive air escaping voice folds
covered	Muffled sound
creaky	Sounding like two hard surfaces rubbing against one another
glottal attack	Harsh, rapid initiation of voicing at beginning of words
glottal fry	Voice pulsing in and out at low frequency; rough, low-pitched, tense voice quality
hoarse (raspy)	Harsh, grating, bumpy sound
honky/hypernasal	Excessive nasality; nasal emissions possible
hyponasal	Reduced nasal resonance; sounds flat
jitter	Rough-sounding pitch
monotonic	No variation in pitch or loudness
pressed/strident	Harsh, loud quality
rough	Noisy, uneven, bumpy vocal fold vibration
shimmer	Crackly, buzzy
soft	Difficult to hear; sounds fatigued
strained	Effortful, hyperfunctioning; neck and jaw perhaps appearing tense
tremorous	Voice shaking during phonation
twangy or ringing	Sharp, bright sound
wheezy	Turbulent airflow when inhaling or exhaling; may sound like asthma or troubled breathing
wobble	Wavering or irregular variation

Sources: Based on Lee, Stemple, and Glaze (2003); National Center for Voice and Speech (2004).

diplophonia is that the two vocal folds have different mass characteristics and therefore vibrate at different rates. It can also occur if one vocal fold is paralyzed or hypofunctioning.

Voice without a Larynx

A **laryngectomy** is a procedure in which a person's larynx is surgically removed. It occurs typically because a person is diagnosed with laryngeal cancer or has received trauma to the larynx. Benign tumors of the larynx can be removed surgically, and the laryngeal structures and their functions typically can be preserved (Nishimura, Satoh, Maesawa, Ishijima, et al., 2007). However, when a laryngeal tumor is cancerous, surgical removal of the larynx (partially or totally) combined with radiation therapy is a likely course of treatment, particularly for cancers that affect multiple membranes of the larynx. Laryngeal cancer is one of the most serious causes of voice disorders, affecting an estimated 12,000 persons and causing nearly 4,000 deaths each year (National Cancer Institute, 2008). Surgical removal of the larynx also may occur for individuals who sustain severe

DISCUSSION POINT

Smoking accounts for 87% of lung cancer deaths, yet 45 million Americans are currently smokers. Why do so many people smoke despite tobacco's association with increased risk of cancer?

trauma to the larynx, as can occur in a car accident. The larynx may be removed if it is too damaged to protect the respiratory system or if the damage impedes breathing. People who have no larynx must develop an alternative way to produce speech, which is called **alaryngeal communication** and is discussed later in this chapter.

PREVALENCE AND INCIDENCE

Voice Disorders in Adults

The prevalence and incidence of voice disorders in both children and adults are relatively high compared to other disorders of communication. Epidemiological research on the rate of voice disorders among adults indicates incidence and prevalence rates of about 29% and 6%, respectively (Roy, Merrill, Thibeault, Parsa, et al., 2004). These rates show that the number of persons who have ever exhibited voice disorders is relatively high, although at a given point in time only about 6 in 100 persons exhibit a voice disorder. Incidence rates are higher for women (7%) compared to men (5%); they tend to peak between the ages of 40 and 60 years; and they are significantly higher among persons with frequent respiratory allergies, asthma, colds, and sinus infections (Roy et al., 2004).

The most common causes of adult voice disorders include vocal nodules (22% of cases), edema/swelling (14%), polyps (11%), carcinoma (10%), and vocal fold paralysis (8%); in about 10% of cases, the cause is unknown (Herrington-Hall, Lee, Stemple, Niemi, et al., 1988). Many more adults experience recurrent but short-term problems with vocal quality or production. Consider Mr. Grey, a fourth-grade teacher in Albuquerque, New Mexico. Mr. Grey has experienced a 3-week bout of laryngitis each of the last three winters, during which time he has had no voice at all. His laryngitis typically accompanies colds and respiratory infections. Of the nearly one-third of adults who have experienced voice disorders, most cases resemble that of Mr. Grey—a short-term problem that appears on several occasions.

Mr. Grey's case also brings up an interesting point about voice disorders: People in some professions exhibit much higher rates of voice disorders (Roy et al., 2004). Whereas about 29% of the general adult population reports a voice disorder at some time, the rate doubles to 58% for teachers. Studies consistently show that some work conditions are causally linked to an increased rate of vocal problems (e.g., Sala, Laine, Simberg, Pentti, et al., 2001). The combination of constant voice use (or overuse) and a noisy environment seems to pose the greatest risk of vocal problems. The Center for the Voice at the New York Eye and Ear Infirmary reports that the most frequently seen professionals in that clinic, other than teachers, are vocal performers, sales representatives, customer service personnel, restaurant workers, police officers, and machine shop or factory workers (Center for the Voice, 2004).

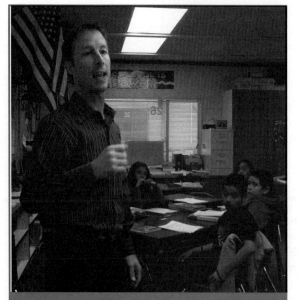

People such as teachers who must use their voices to perform their jobs often experience short-term but recurrent voice problems.

Voice Disorders in Children

Epidemiological studies are highly variable in their estimates of the prevalence and incidence of voice disorders among children. Relatively recent findings show that somewhere between 4 and 6% of children have significant problems with their voice. One study of voice problems among preschoolers found that nearly 4% of 2- to 6-year-olds had significant hoarseness (Duff, Proctor, & Yairi, 2004); another study, looking more generally at presence of childhood dysphonia among 8-year-olds, found that 6% of children were affected, with more boys having dysphonia (7.4%) than girls (4.6%; Carding, Roulstone, Northstone, & ALSPAC Study Team, 2006). For some of these cases, the voice problem reflects a congenital issue with the vocal apparatus, such as vocal fold paralysis. For a larger number of children, the problem is acquired, resulting from overuse or misuse of the voice. The most common cause of voice dysfunction in children stems from **vocal nodules,** which affect more than 1 million children annually (von Leden, 1985). A recent study that involved direct laryngoscopic examination of the vocal folds of 617 children aged 7 to 16 years provides the best estimate of the prevalence of vocal nodules (Kiliç, Okur, Yildirim, & Güzelsoy, 2004). In this study, nearly one-fifth (17%) of the children had vocal nodules; substantially higher number of males (22%) had nodules compared to females (12%). The nodules, or protuberances, that appear bilaterally on children's vocal folds impede the smooth meeting of the folds at midline, typically resulting in a breathy or hoarse vocal quality and, in some cases, complete loss of voice. Vocal nodules can result from physiological factors—such as gastroesophageal reflux, low blood circulation, dehydration, and laryngeal tension—but are most often associated with psychological and social factors, such as anger, anxiety, distractibility, frustration, interpersonal problems, hyperactivity, and loud talking (Sapienza, Ruddy, & Baker, 2004).

Prevalence and Treatment

Although the rate of voice disorders is relatively high, many of these cases go undiagnosed and untreated. For instance, although estimates show that 17% of schoolchildren may have vocal nodules, only one-third of school speech-language pathologists report working with children with voice disorders and, among those who do, report treating an average of only two children (ASHA, 2006). Given that voice disturbances sometimes serve as the outward manifestation of a significant life-threatening disease, such as carcinoma, voice professionals work hard to raise the public's awareness of the importance of diagnosis and treatment for voice problems.

Experts point to several reasons that children and adults with voice disorders may not receive treatment. The first relates to treatment access. Even though children with communication disorders can receive voice therapy through their school's speech-language pathologist, they might not be eligible for treatment if the disorder does not adversely impact educational performance. Also, when a voice disorder is suspected, the SLP will typically request a medical evaluation that includes direct laryngoscopic examination to gather information on what may be causing voice problems. School-based SLPs have expressed some difficulties in acquiring these examinations, including lack of parental follow-up, lack of physical referral, and lack of family financial resources (e.g., insurance; Hooper, 2004).

The second reason for nontreatment relates to knowledge. Some individuals may believe that voice difficulties will disappear spontaneously (Andrews & Summers, 2002). Further, the general public may not be well informed about voice disorders and may not understand how the voice works or that treatment can correct vocal problems. This is particularly true for children. Experts argue that a child's early abuse and misuse of the voice, such as being habitually loud, can trap the child in inappropriate habits that result in negative listener reactions and can greatly impact later life ambitions (Andrews & Summers, 2002).

For adults, voice problems can undermine many aspects of life, including work performance, employment opportunities, and communication with friends and family. Vocal problems can also impact how others perceive us: "[A] voice that draws attention to itself and results in negative listener reactions is a significant lifetime handicap, although at times an insidious one" (Andrews & Summers, 2002, p. 63). Providing the general public with information about how the voice works and how treatment can improve vocal quality is important for ensuring that people who need treatment are able to access it.

The third reason for nontreatment relates to social perceptions about vocal quality. In American society, a breathy or hoarse vocal quality is sometimes considered an attractive attribute, particularly for women. Marilyn Monroe's breathy voice quality was one of her most frequently acknowledged assets. A breathy voice quality is also viewed as a social marker of the female gender (Hillenbrand, Cleveland, & Erickson, 1994). Thus, a breathy voice quality may bring an individual positive social attention, which is quite different from the possibly negative impact of other communication disorders. However, a breathy vocal quality is also one of the most prominent features of serious voice pathologies, including vocal fold paralysis and carcinoma (Hillenbrand et al., 1994).

HOW ARE VOICE DISORDERS CLASSIFIED? ●

Experts typically classify voice disorders according to their cause. This etiological classification organizes disorders into four different causal categories (Case, 1996): vocal abuse, neurogenic disorders, psychogenic disorders, and alaryngeal communication.

VOCAL ABUSE

The vocal folds are a well-used part of the human body; in a given minute of speaking, the vocal folds strike together over 9,000 times. And even when we are not speaking, the vocal folds are often hard at work, as Case (1996) points out in describing the "aerodynamic turmoil" of coughing:

> The tissues of the larynx are tossed about as though caught in a hurricane. The arytenoid cartilages are in chaotic and frenzied motion, matched by the turbulent actions of the vocal folds. . . . It is impossible to watch this coughing episode without realizing how vulnerable laryngeal tissues are to this and other forms of abuse. (p. 127)

The vulnerability of the laryngeal tissues is readily apparent in the regular appearance of scratchy voices during flu season, congested voices during allergy season, and even the loss of voice (laryngitis) during basketball season.

The most common cause of voice disorders in both children and adults is **vocal abuse,** which describes the chronic or intermittent overuse or misuse of the vocal apparatus. Consider your own experience with these vocally abusive behaviors (Case, 2002; Shipley & McAfee, 1998):

- Talking in noisy environments
- Coughing or clearing the throat frequently
- Using caffeine products

DISCUSSION POINT:
Consider the two cases in Case Study 11.1. What could these individuals do to raise public awareness about their particular voice disorders?

DISCUSSION POINT:
We all misuse our voices sometimes. What are some ways you have misused your voice? Do any of these ways occur chronically? If so, brainstorm some strategies for eliminating your own chronic voice misuse.

SPOTLIGHT ON LITERACY

Health Literacy

Health literacy refers to an individual's capacity to obtain, process, and understand basic health information and services, all of which are important to making appropriate decisions about one's health (U.S. Department of Health and Human Services, 2005). In *Healthy People 2010*—the U.S. government's set of objectives regarding health promotion for its citizens over the first decade of the new century—promoting health literacy is a principal goal. Estimates indicate that over one-half of U.S. adults do not have adequate levels of health literacy, including the ability to comprehend and analyze information about health and prevention; analyze symbols, charts, and graphs; and weigh costs and benefits (Agency for Healthcare Research and Quality, 2004). In contrast, only about 10% of U.S. adults have proficient health literacy. This is not particularly surprising given how common low literacy is among U.S. adults, with 40 million scoring at the lowest level on a measure of basic adult literacy skills (Agency for Healthcare Research and Quality, 2004). A recent review of research on the connections between literacy levels of adults and their knowledge of specific health care services, including mammography and cervical cancer screening, showed that less knowledge was associated with lower literacy levels (Agency for Healthcare Research and Quality, 2004). Lower levels of literacy also are associated with higher rates of smoking and alcohol misuse.

In this chapter, we discussed the importance of seeking professional assistance when vocal problems are suspected. If one experiences hoarseness, for instance, for several weeks, it is imperative that a physician be consulted so that the larynx can be studied to identify whether a structural cause, such as a tumor, may be causing the dysphonia. However, individuals with low health literacy may not have access to information about voice disorders, and if they do, they may not be able to fully weigh the costs and benefits of seeking further assistance and evaluation, or they may not understand how to access these services within their community.

There are many ways to promote health literacy. One strategy is improving the usability of health information. It is crucial that information made available to individuals is appropriate in terms of the words selected, the information presented, and the messages conveyed. Guidelines are available to help persons ensure the usability of health information, but the most important guideline is to use plain language, which involves (U. S. Department of Health and Human Services, 2005)

1. organizing information so that the key points come first,
2. breaking complex information into smaller chunks,
3. avoiding technical jargon, and
4. using active (rather than passive) voice.

Look for some health-promotion materials on the Internet, and evaluate them in terms of plain language. You'll likely find a great deal of variety. Materials that achieve the above principles of plain language were likely prepared by individuals who were invested in promoting health literacy.

- Yelling, screaming, and cheering
- Giving speeches or lectures
- Spending time in smoky environments

Figure 11.2 provides a list of the more common misuses and abuses of the voice. Common conditions associated with vocal abuse include vocal nodules, contact ulcers, and granuloma.

Vocal Nodules

Sometimes called *teacher's nodules* and *singer's nodules* because of their increased prevalence among these professionals, vocal nodules are small, bilateral protuberances or calloused growths on the inner edges of the vocal folds (see Figure 11.3). Described for the first time in the 1880s, vocal nodules are

FIGURE 11.2

Common misuses and abuses of the voice.

Yelling and screaming	Alcohol use
Hard glottal attack	Excessive speaking
Abusive singing	Inadequate breath support
Hydration concerns	Laughing hard
Speaking over noise	Aspirin (drugs)
Coughing/throat clearing	Cheerleading, aerobics instruction, pep clubs
Grunting in exercise	Making toy/animal noises
Calling at a distance	Athletic activity (coaching, etc.)
Inappropriate pitch	Intense personality
Excessive talking with allergy or upper-respiratory infection	Arguing
Muscular tension	
Smoking factor	

Source: From *Clinical management of voice disorders* (4th ed.) by G. L. Case, 2002, Austin, TX: Pro-Ed. Copyright 2002 by Pro-Ed. Adapted with permission.

one of the most frequent causes of hoarseness in adults and children (Benjamin & Croxson, 1987; Goldman, Hargrave, Hillman, Holmberg, et al., 1996). Among the estimated 23% of children who have experienced chronic hoarseness at some time in their lives, vocal nodules are to blame in the majority of cases (Benjamin & Croxson, 1987).

Vocal nodules come in two varieties—acute and chronic. Acute nodules are essentially bruises on the vocal folds, which over time will thicken and harden as they become a chronic condition and advance to becoming fibrous protuberances. Vocal nodules represent the body's response to an irritant, which in this case is the vocal folds' repeated hard contact at midline. The protuberances

FIGURE 11.3

Vocal nodules.

Source: From "Laryngeal structure and function in the pediatric larynx: Clinical applications" by C. M. Sapienza, B. H. Ruddy, and S. Baker, 2004, *Language, Speech, and Hearing Services in Schools, 35,* p. 303. Copyright 2004 by ASHA. Reprinted with permission.

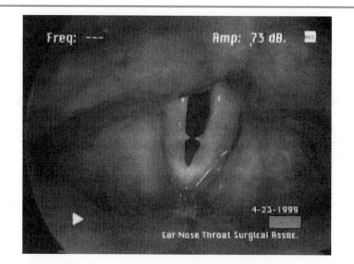

impede the vocal folds from seamless contact and allow air to escape during phonation, resulting in a breathy or hoarse vocal quality.

Nodules are most prevalent in young children and in adults who engage in vocal overuse and misuse (Holmberg, Hillman, Hammarberg, Södersten, et al., 2001). Research on high school and college cheerleaders described by Case (1996) found that nearly 50% of high school cheerleaders showed emerging vocal nodules after a 1-week cheerleading camp (none had any evidence of vocal pathology before the camp started), and 75% of the college cheerleaders had emerging nodules after only several weeks of practice. The characteristics of cheerleaders who developed nodules included excessive laryngeal tension when cheering, hard glottal attacks when beginning a cheer, cheering at too low or too high a pitch, and general misuse of voice (e.g., cheering during a cold or infection). An individual's temperament and general health may also come into play in elevating the risk of nodules. Adults with vocal nodules have greater anxiety and bodily complaints, such as trouble sleeping or stomach ailments (Goldman et al., 1996).

Contact Ulcers and Granuloma

Contact ulcers are inflamed lesions, or ulcers, that develop on the arytenoid cartilages in the posterior region of the larynx. These lesions develop from repeated forceful contact of the vocal folds and progress from tissue irritation to necrosis, or death of the tissue. The body's healing process then generates a mass of tissue, or *granuloma,* at the site of the ulcer (see Figure 11.4). Contact ulcers and granuloma, which typically result in a breathy, low voice quality, affect both men and women in a ratio of roughly 4:1 (Watterson, Hansen-Magorian, & McFarlane, 1990). The ulcers can result from persistent vocal abuse and overuse and can affect persons in a variety of professions. Case (1996) reports that he has treated vocal nodules in a Buddhist chanter, a school superintendent, a high school physical education teacher, and a politician—all of whom rely on voice in their everyday life and work.

Contact ulcers and granuloma can also result from acidic irritation to the laryngeal areas because of chronic reflux. Gastroesophageal reflux disease, also called *GERD* (and, more commonly, *heartburn, indigestion,* and *acid reflux disease*) is a condition in which acid from the stomach backs up into the

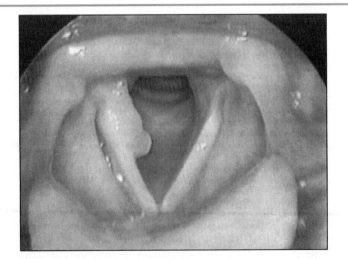

FIGURE 11.4

A contact ulcer with granuloma.

Source: From *Clinical management of voice disorders* (4th ed., p. 171) by J. L. Case, 2002, Austin, TX: Pro-Ed. Copyright 2002 by Pro-Ed. Reprinted with permission.

esophagus. Because of the neuroanatomical proximity of the larynx to the esophagus, the acidic regurgitation can have a host of negative effects on the larynx's functions and structures, including vocal nodules, contact ulcers, and granuloma (Toohill & Kuhn, 1997). Although these are benign conditions, they can contribute to a variety of problems with voice quality (hoarseness, voice breaks) as well as chronic irritation of the laryngeal area. The constant throat clearing associated with GERD is likely the culprit for the ulcers and granuloma that appear on the arytenoid cartileges.

NEUROGENIC DISORDERS

Neurogenic voice disorders result from illness, damage, or disease to the neurological systems associated with voice production. Both the central nervous system (CNS) and the peripheral nervous system (PNS) are involved in managing the motor and sensory functions of the larynx, and damage to either can cause dysfunction of the vocal mechanisms. Figure 11.5 illustrates the complex interplay of the CNS, the PNS, and the larynx. One of the most important nerves involved in the smooth functioning of the larynx is the **vagus nerve** of the PNS, also described as *cranial nerve X.* The vagus (which means "wandering") nerve runs from the cranium down and around the heart and has several branches departing from the main nerve to innervate the pharynx and the larynx. The first branch is the pharyngeal nerve, which communicates sensory and motor information to the pharynx and the soft palate. The next branch is the superior laryngeal nerve (LN), which departs from the vagus above the larynx to innervate parts of the tongue, pharynx, and larynx. Yet another branch, the recurrent laryngeal nerve, departs from the vagus below the larynx to innervate the larynx, esophagus, and trachea (Zemlin, 1997).

FIGURE 11.5

The nervous system and voice production.

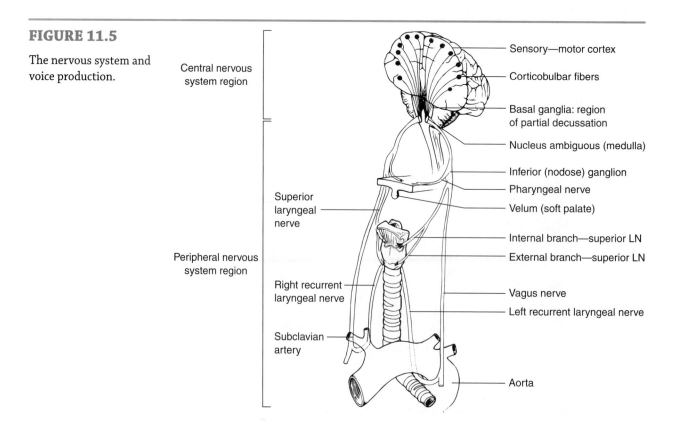

If the nerves of the CNS or PNS that innervate the voice-production system are disrupted in some way, a voice disorder can result. Disorders of this type are called *neurogenic,* because their etiology stems from neurological malfunctioning. Several of the more well-known types of neurogenic voice disorders are described here.

Vagus Nerve Lesions

Lesions to the vagus nerve can occur for a variety of reasons, including surgical damage (particularly thyroid surgery), trauma, and viral infections (Case, 2002). The most serious outcome of vagus nerve damage is vocal fold paralysis, which typically is unilateral, affecting only one vocal fold. When the vocal fold is paralyzed in an adducted position—called *abduction paralysis* because the vocal fold cannot open—the voice is usually not affected because the other fold can press against it to phonate. However, in these cases, a person will struggle with breathing because of the closed position of one fold. When the vocal fold is paralyzed in an abducted position—called *adduction paralysis* because the vocal fold does not close—vocal production is compromised because the two vocal folds do not meet at midline. This causes a hoarse or breathy vocal quality. In some cases of vagus nerve damage, complete paralysis of the vocal folds occurs, leaving them completely opened or completely blocking the airway. In the latter case, a **tracheostomy** is performed, in which an artificial airway is placed below the larynx so the individual can breathe.

Spasmodic Dysphonia

Spasmodic dysphonia (SD), also called *spastic dysphonia,* is a disorder affecting motor control of the larynx. Vocal spasms that result in intermittent voice stoppages are the hallmark of this disorder. A diagnosis of SD has these characteristics:

- An occasionally normal voice
- Intermittent breaks in voicing
- A normal-sounding whisper
- Improved voice at high pitches
- Worsening voice with stress
- Periods of significant dysphonia (Cannito et al., 1997)

Terms used to describe the voices of people with SD include *jerky, grunting, squeezed, groaning,* and *stuttering-like* (Aronson, 1990). Although SD was historically viewed as a voice disorder of psychological origin—early described as nervous hoarseness (Cannito et al., 1997)—current theories recognize SD as a neurologically based **laryngeal dystonia,** which affects the movement patterns of the laryngeal muscles (Brin, Fahn, Blitzer, Ramig, et al., 1992). *Dystonia* describes abnormal movements of the body (Case, 1996), and *laryngeal dystonia* identifies this condition as it affects the larynx. For people with laryngeal dystonia, vocal tremors are common.

SD appears in several different forms and can range from mild to severe. The adductor type is the most common, representing about half of SD cases (Blitzer & Brin, 1992; Cannito et al., 1997). In this type, a person exhibits a hyperfunctioning voice that seems strangled, strained, and squeezing (Cannito et al., 1997). The abductor type of SD is less common and features a hypofunctioning voice that is breathy and open. Some people show a mixed SD, in which they intermittently experience both adductor and abductor characteristics.

ALS

Amyotrophic lateral sclerosis (ALS), also called Lou Gehrig's disease, is a progressive, degenerative, neuromuscular disease resulting in muscular weakness, fatigue, and atrophy as well as muscular spasms, tremors, and cramping (Renout, Leeper, Bandur, & Hudson, 1995). The cause is unknown, and the impact of the disease is significant, with most individuals surviving fewer than 10 years (Case, 1996). Because of its widespread impact on muscular functioning, voice disorders are a common symptom of ALS, and voice functioning deteriorates over time (Strand, Buder, Yorkston, & Ramig, 1994). The voice of an individual with ALS is usually soft, breathy, low in pitch and loudness with limited variability, and hypernasal. In addition to voice disturbances, people with ALS have difficulty clearly articulating speech sounds, because they cannot precisely and strongly coordinate the motor processes needed to articulate (Case, 1996).

As Case (1996) notes, the cognitive abilities of people with ALS remain intact even while muscular processes are rapidly deteriorating. In the later stages of the disease, a person is unable to produce voice or speech yet is aware of this loss of function. Augmentative communication devices, such as those described in Chapter 5, can provide a person with ALS an alternative way to communicate with others.

PARKINSON'S DISEASE

Parkinson's disease is another progressive, degenerative neurological disease, one that is caused by dopamine depletion (Ramig, Countryman, Thompson, & Horii, 1995). The majority of people with Parkinson's disease exhibit impaired communication abilities, including a significant disorder of voice, which occurs because of the disease's impact on the respiratory and laryngeal systems. A person with Parkinson's disease is unable to produce a strong voice because of a weakened respiratory system, resulting in reduced loudness and a breathy, weak voice. The disease also creates a more rigid muscular tone, which restricts the movement of the laryngeal muscles so that the vocal folds can no longer forcefully adduct (Ramig & Dromey, 1996), resulting in hoarseness and a monotonic pitch. The Lee Silverman voice treatment program (Ramig, Pawlas, & Countryman, 1995) is effective in improving respiratory strength and vocal fold adduction for people with Parkinson's disease, helping them have a stronger voice even as the disease progresses.

Iatrogenic Etiology

Some voice disorders result from surgery or other treatments. Symptoms or disorders that result from medical or clinical treatments are called *iatrogenic.* It is unclear how many voice disorders result from iatrogenic causes, but because of the proximity of the larynx to the chest, pharynx, and oral cavity, surgical procedures directed toward these areas can negatively affect the functioning of the larynx and, in turn, one's voice quality. Vocal fold movement impairment (VPMI) is one disorder of laryngeal functioning for which nearly half of cases are attributable to iatrogenic causes (Merati, Shemirani, Smith, & Toohill, 2006). VPMI is present when one or both of the vocal folds functions poorly (e.g., incomplete closure at midline). VPMI can result from surgery to the spine, chest, and thyroid as well as intubation procedures used during surgery.

A striking example of a disorder with iatrogenic etiology was described in the *American Journal of Otolaryngology—Head and Neck Medicine and Surgery* (Ozer, Ozer, Sener, & Yavuz, 2007). A case report was presented in which an 11-year-old boy was admitted to the hospital due to chronic mouth breathing, foul-smelling rhinorrhea (discharge from the nose), and complete nasal obstruction presumably resulting in significant hyponasality. An endoscopic examination of the nasal cavity showed that a gauze pack was lodged deeply in the cavity, causing total obstruction. In this case, the foreign object had been left behind during a 6-month prior tonsillectomy (Ozer et al., 2007). This case stresses the importance of thoroughness when evaluating an individual's vocal structures and functions.

Vocal Tics and Tourette Syndrome

Two additional conditions that can impact voice production are vocal tic disorder and Tourette syndrome. Individuals with **vocal tic disorder** produce sudden, rapid, recurrent vocalizations, including clicks, yelps, snorts, and coughs. These can occur many times per day for longer than 1 year, causing significant stress and impairment in key areas of functioning, including interpersonal relationships and occupational or academic performance (APA, 1994). With *Tourette syndrome,* vocal tics occur simultaneously with other motor tics affecting the head, torso, and extremities. These might include such things as eye blinking, twirling, or deep knee bends (APA, 1994). The vocal tics seen in both vocal tic disorder and Tourette syndrome are not linked to any known physical cause, but recent research shows the disorder to relate to central nervous system dysfunction. These disorders appear to affect about 1 to 2% of the population (Khalifa & von Knorring, 2003).

PSYCHOGENIC DISORDERS

Our voices often carry information about our emotional and psychological states, as when we speak angrily and produce voice forcefully with tightly contracted muscles or when we speak tenderly and produce voice with smooth and light contact of the vocal folds (Andrews & Summers, 2002). Most of us can remember a time when our voices gave our feelings away, perhaps conveying our excitement, fear, anxiety, or shock. The human voice also serves as a more permanent marker of our personalities. For instance, consider the macho, tough personality of Tony Soprano in the HBO hit show *The Sopranos* and the way his vocal characteristics convey this part of his personality. The voices of individuals who experience significant disorders of personality or psychological health can be impacted. **Psychogenic disorders** of voice, also called *nonorganic disorders,* result from or are linked to emotional and psychological characteristics. *Psychogenic dysphonia* is the diagnostic term used to describe disordered voice quality that results from an emotional or psychological event.

DISCUSSION POINT:
Consider the case of Dr. Mitchell in Case Study 11.1. What are some explanations for her psychological response to the loss of voice?

Psychological or Emotional Triggers

Some individuals develop a chronic voice disorder as a result of a vocal injury. People who rely on their voice professionally—such as actors, singers, and teachers—are particularly vulnerable to a vocal injury. However, once the injury is resolved, these individuals may experience a sense of vulnerability and anxiety about their voice, which can translate into hypochondria and chronic worry that a brief lapse is the signal of a serious disorder. The anxiety that can follow a vocal injury can result in disturbances in memory, concentration, and emotional well-being, all of which can then further exacerbate vocal problems (Rosen & Sataloff, 1997).

Voice disorders can also result from traumatic experiences, such as being treated for cancer, being robbed or raped, or having throat surgery (Case, 1996;

Rosen & Sataloff, 1997; Stemple et al., 1995). Case (1996) describes his work with a 45-year-old woman who exhibited dysphonia for several months, stemming from an intense fear of having laryngeal cancer. Delving into the patient's history, Case found that she had already been treated for uterine cancer and breast cancer and had a friend who was diagnosed with laryngeal cancer. Although her fears were understandable given these circumstances, examination of her larynx showed them to be unfounded, and her dysphonia resolved soon after.

Psychopathology

A variety of psychopathological conditions can also affect the quality of the voice. Several of the more common psychological disturbances—such as stress, anxiety, and depression—can detract from voice quality, as can more serious disturbances, such as conversion disorder.

Stress, Anxiety, and Depression. Stress, anxiety, and depression are relatively well-known psychological disturbances, which, in their more severe forms, can have a significant impact on an individual's well-being. Sometimes an individual's vocal patterns provide the first clue of severe stress, anxiety, or depression. *Acute stress disorder* develops within 1 month of a traumatic experience, such as a sexual or violent assault or diagnosis of a life-threatening illness (APA,1994) The chronic distress that results involves a cluster of symptoms, including exaggerated startle responses, motor restlessness, and irritability, all of which can be reflected in a person's voice.

Anxiety conditions, such as generalized anxiety disorder and performance anxiety, are generally less serious psychological disturbances but can also be reflected in vocal characteristics. A person with *generalized anxiety disorder* is excessively anxious and worried, is easily fatigued and irritable, and experiences long periods of general restlessness (APA, 1994). Common symptoms also include muscle tension, which results in trembling, twitching, shakiness, and muscular aches, all of which can extend to the muscles of the larynx. Someone with *performance anxiety,* also called *stage fright,* experiences anxiety in the context of specific triggers, such as speaking to a large group of people or performing a task (e.g., surgery) in front of an audience. The context triggers a fight-or-flight response that features heart palpitations, sweatiness, vocal tremors, and voice breakages. Successful treatment for stress, anxiety, and depression can alleviate voice-related symptoms as a by-product of resolving the primary disorder, although in some cases specific targeting of communication and voice production is beneficial.

Conversion Disorder. **Conversion disorder** is a psychological disturbance in which an individual exhibits symptoms of a physical disease or disorder. The physical symptoms reflect emotional stress or conflict. One possible symptom of conversion disorder is dysphonia or aphonia, characterized by a weak, breathy voice with little or no voicing. A person with conversion disorder is not malingering, or feigning illness; rather it appears the physical symptoms result from severe anxiety or stress (APA, 1994). Some experts suggest that the loss of voice for people with conversion disorder provides them a way to reduce communication with persons of importance—such as parents, spouse, or others—particularly if communication is psychologically painful (Case, 1996). Despite the serious impact of conversion disorder, the person affected may be indifferent to vocal problems (called *la belle indifference*) or may exhibit a dramatic or histrionic response (APA, 1994).

Mutational Falsetto and Juvenile Voice

Two additional categories of psychogenic voice disturbances require mention; both describe vocal characteristics that are inconsistent with an individual's age and gender. **Mutational falsetto,** also called **puberphonia,** describes a male child or adolescent who exhibits an inappropriately high voice. During puberty, hormonal changes greatly impact the male voice, and fairly sudden and dramatic changes in voice quality and pitch occur. However, for some boys, the changes do not occur easily, and their voices maintain an unusually high pitch, which may resemble or even exceed that of prepuberty. Voice therapy is usually quite effective in helping the adolescent male shift his voice to a more appropriate pitch. When specific organic factors, such as undergrowth of the larynx or endocrine imbalance, are to blame for an overly high pitch in adolescent or adult males, the condition is considered an *organic mutational falsetto,* and medical treatment may be needed (Lim et al., 2007).

Juvenile voice disorder, in which women maintain a juvenile voice into adulthood, is the female companion to mutational falsetto. The female voice also changes dramatically during puberty, reducing its pitch to a more adultlike level. Juvenile voice disorder describes cases in which females do not drop their pitch but maintain the pitch of a child. Often accompanying the childlike pitch is a low intensity, nasality, and breathiness (Stemple et al., 1995).

ALARYNGEAL COMMUNICATION

Some individuals must produce voice without the benefit of a larynx; theirs is called *alaryngeal communication,* which most often results from a tracheostomy or a laryngectomy.

Tracheostomy

When a person's respiratory system is compromised, mechanical ventilation and respiration are needed to preserve life. The most common reasons for mechanical ventilation are progressive neuromuscular conditions, spinal cord injury, genetic syndromes, and premature birth. A tracheostomy is a surgical procedure in which a tracheostomy tube, or trach, is inserted through the neck below the vocal folds to direct air into the lungs (see Figure 11.6). Some people receive a trach because their vocal folds are not functioning well, as in the case of laryngeal cancer and bilateral vocal fold paralysis. These individuals are at risk of aspiration or penetration of substances into the lungs, increasing the risk of pneumonia and other respiratory ailments.

A person with a trach is unable to talk, because the air that is typically expelled over the vocal folds to produce phonation is directed outward through the trach tube. As you can imagine, this creates a "multitude of adverse physical and psychological experiences for the critically ill patient" (Bergbom-Engberg & Haljamae, 1989), not the least being the inability to communicate. One study of adults who had received respiratory treatment showed that their inability to talk was second only to general anxiety and fear in their list of discomforts (Bergbom-Engberg & Haljamae, 1989). For children, being on a trach for an extended period of time can undermine their ability to develop

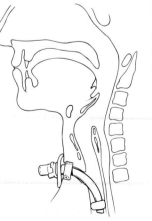

FIGURE 11.6

A standard tracheostomy tube placed in the upper airway.

FIGURE 11.7

A child fitted with a Passy-Muir speaking valve and tracheostomy tube.

Source: Courtesy of Passy-Muir, Inc.

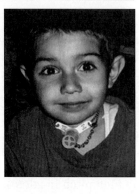

speech, language, and communication abilities. This is particularly true for children who receive a trach at birth and have never been able to use their voices.

Fortunately for these children and adults, David Muir, a young man with muscular dystrophy, invented a speaking valve that enabled him to produce speech while on a trach tube. Now commercially available as the Passy-Muir tracheostomy speaking valve, it uses a valving system that sends air downward into the pulmonary system during inhalation but directs exhaled air over the vocal folds to produce speech. Thus, the valve allows adults to speak while ventilated and allows infants (see Figure 11.7) to vocalize and communicate (Torres & Sirbegovic, 2004).

Laryngectomy

For adults, the most common reason for alaryngeal communication is the removal of the larynx. This can occur because of trauma, such as a car accident in which the larynx is seriously damaged, but commonly the larynx is removed because of laryngeal cancer. To prevent the spread of cancer or to treat an advanced cancer, the larynx is removed in a procedure called *laryngectomy;* a person whose larynx has been removed is called a **laryngectomee.** Speaking and voicing is possible through a variety of procedures described later in this chapter. Here is an overview of the etiology, symptoms, and treatment of laryngeal cancer.

Etiology.   Laryngeal cancer is an aggressive cancer with high mortality rates. It accounts for about 1 to 2% of all cancers and for about 30 to 50% of head and neck cancers; it occurs at a rate of 12,000 cases annually in the United States. It affects men at much higher rates than women (Surveillance, Epidemiology, and End Results [SEER], 2004) and older African American males at the highest rates. In general, the rate of laryngeal cancer has declined since the 1970s, most dramatically for African American and European American men. However, current rates of diagnosis remain high for men, affecting about 11 in 100,000 African American men and 6 in 100,000 European American men, as compared to about 1.5 to 2 per 100,000 African American and European American women (SEER, 2004).

Laryngeal cancer is linked to tobacco use; as tobacco use goes up, so does the risk of developing laryngeal cancer (Cann, Rothman, & Fried, 1996). About 15 of 100,000 smokers develop this form of cancer, as compared to fewer than 1 of 100,000 nonsmokers (Cann et al., 1996). Alcohol use also increases the risk of laryngeal cancer; that risk is elevated exponentially when alcohol and tobacco use are combined (Cann et al., 1996). Additional risks include nutritional inadequacies and occupational exposures, particularly exposure to asbestos and certain man-made fibers, like glass wool production.

Some studies have suggested that there is a causal relationship between GERD and laryngeal cancer. In part, this relates to the established associations among GERD, alcohol and tobacco use, and laryngeal cancer, in that all three seem to co-occur at rates greater than expected by chance (Qadeer, Colabianchi, Strome, & Vaezi, 2006). Given these shared associations, some experts suggest that GERD is a cause of laryngeal cancer, as shown in Panel (1) of Figure 11.8. Yet other experts hypothesize that the association occurs due to the causal contribution of alcohol and tobacco use to both GERD and laryngeal cancer, as shown in Panel (2). In this scenario, the relationship between GERD and laryngeal cancer is based solely on

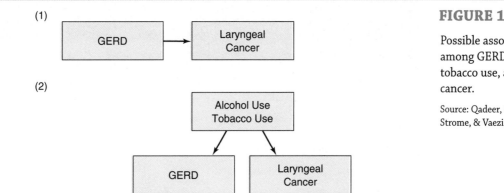

FIGURE 11.8

Possible associations among GERD, alcohol and tobacco use, and laryngeal cancer.

Source: Qadeer, Colabianchi, Strome, & Vaezi (2006).

a shared etiology. A third possibility is that GERD is a co-carcinogen, in that its presence amplifies the odds of developing laryngeal cancer among users of alcohol and tobacco. Presently, the relationship between GERD and laryngeal cancer is unclear. Consequently, experts indicate that GERD should be aggressively treated and alcohol and tobacco use eliminated among those at risk for laryngeal cancer, including those with chronic laryngitis (Qadeer et al., 2006).

Symptoms. Successful treatment of laryngeal cancer requires early identification. The most consistent early symptom is hoarseness. As a general rule, no one should ever allow hoarseness to continue for longer than 2 weeks without a medical evaluation (Brodnitz, 1988). Additional symptoms that may emerge as cancer progresses include *stridor* (i.e., hearing the voice when inhaling), laryngeal pain, discharge, and swelling in the neck (Case, 1996).

Treatment. The first goal in cancer treatment is always to rid the body of the malignancy. The second goal is to maintain the body's functions and structures. With laryngeal cancer, it is likely that some of the body's functions and structures will be adversely impacted, because the malignancy sits squarely in the path of breathing and speaking (Fried & Lauretano, 1996). When the malignancy is removed surgically, most often the surgery affects one or both of these abilities.

Many oncologists use *conservation approaches* when treating laryngeal cancer to preserve the larynx as much as possible. With a conservation approach, the larynx remains, with portions of it removed. With *cordectomy,* one of the vocal folds is surgically removed, and with *hemilaryngectomy,* portions of the laryngeal cartilages are removed. When the larynx cannot be conserved, it is removed in a near-total or total laryngectomy. Alternative ways of communicating are then possible, although they will never replicate the quality of the natural voice.

DISCUSSION POINT:
Consider the two cases in Case Study 11.1. Identify the etiology, or cause, of each type of voice disorder.

WHAT ARE THE DEFINING CHARACTERISTICS OF VOICE DISORDERS? ●

A voice disorder impacts one or more of the following perceptual characteristics of voice: resonance, loudness and pitch, or phonatory quality. Table 11.2 identifies the perceptual aspects of voice affected by the specific voice disorders described in this chapter.

			Pitch/	Phonatory
TABLE 11.2	**The impact of specific voice etiologies and disorders on perceptual characteristics of voice**			
Etiology	**Specific Disorder**	**Resonance**	**Loudness**	**Quality**
Vocal abuse	Vocal nodules		X	X
	Contact ulcers/ granuloma		X	X
Neurogenic	Vagus nerve lesion		X	X
	Spasmodic dysphonia		X	X
	ALS	X	X	X
	Parkinson's disease		X	X
	Iatrogenic	X	X	X
	Vocal tics			X
Psychogenic	Psychological/ emotional experience		X	X
	Psychopathology	X	X	X
	Mutational falsetto/ juvenile voice	X	X	

RESONANCE

As the voice travels up from the vocal folds, it vibrates as a column of air within the nasal and oral cavities. The extent to which the column of air is allowed to enter the nasal and oral cavities is controlled at the **velopharyngeal port,** or the back of the oral cavity where the oral and nasal cavities meet. The velopharyngeal mechanism is the coupling of the velum, or soft palate, and the back of the pharynx to channel the vibrating air into the oral and nasal cavities. The velopharyngeal port typically rests in an open position with the velum lowered, as it is when we are breathing through the nose. When we speak, the velum rises to close the port, channeling the airflow and voice into the oral cavity, with no airflow released into the nasal cavity. Only during the production of the three nasal consonants—/n/, /m/, and /ŋ/—and adjacent vowels is the velopharyngeal port open to allow air into the nasal cavity.

Resonance disorders result from problems with control of the velopharyngeal port due to velopharyngeal inadequacy. **Velopharyngeal inadequacy** occurs when there is imperfect closure of the port because of structural or muscular problems (Case, 1996). There are several common causes of velopharyngeal inadequacy:

1. *Cleft palate and craniofacial anomalies:* This congenital malformation often affects the functioning of the velopharyngeal port. Even after surgical repair, the velum may be weakened or stiff because of scar tissue.

2. *Iatrogenic problems:* These result from surgery, particularly removal of the tonsils and adenoid tissues, which are located in the velopharyngeal region.

3. *Allergies:* Allergic rhinitis can cause hyponasal speech and can impact the smooth functioning of the velopharyngeal port through swelling and congestion.

4. *Neuromuscular impairment:* Disorders that undermine neuromuscular functioning often affect control of the velopharyngeal port. Common causes of neuromuscular disturbance include cerebral palsy, head injuries, meningitis, tumors, neck trauma, nerve trauma, and muscular dystrophy (Dworkin, Marunick, & Krouse, 2004).

Velopharyngeal inadequacy causes either hypernasality or hyponasality. With hypernasality, the velopharyngeal port remains open, allowing too much resonance in the nasal cavity. Often, nasal emissions are present—that is, air emits from the nose during speech. The lowered pressure in the oral cavity also degrades the production of some oral speech sounds, particularly the pressure consonants—such as /b/, /p/, and /t/—which require a large buildup of air for their production.

Hyponasality describes a condition in which there is too little nasal resonance. When the nasal cavity is blocked in some way and thus is not available to serve as a resonating chamber, sounds that require nasal resonation, such as /m/, become denasalized. These are some conditions that can cause hyponasality:

- *Acute rhinitis:* Nasal inflammation and congestion, both of which are symptoms of the common cold
- *Allergic rhinitis:* Nasal inflammation due to environmental allergies
- *Papilloma:* Wartlike growths, potentially caused by a virus, that grow in the nasal cavity
- *Tonsillitis:* Inflamed tonsillar tissue due to infection (Case, 1996)

These and other conditions can make it difficult to breathe through the nose and to use the nasal cavity for the production of speech. In such cases, the voice may sound denasalized, stuffy, and congested.

PITCH AND LOUDNESS

Appropriate vocal pitch and loudness—corresponding, respectively, to the physical characteristics of frequency and intensity—relate directly to how well the vocal and speech production mechanisms work together as a system. Too much or too little tension or force in voice production can result in aberrational pitch or loudness, such as a voice that is too loud, too soft, too high, or too low. Pitch changes are one of the most common symptoms of vocal pathologies (Stemple et al., 1995).

Pitch

When vocal pitch is aberrational, it brings undesirable attention to the voice of the speaker. For instance, when a young adult male speaks with a functional falsetto voice or a young adult female speaks with a juvenile voice, both pitches are inappropriately high, with hyperfunctioning laryngeal muscles. More common is the pitch disturbance described as **glottal fry,** in which the pitch is unusually and chronically low, produced on tightly approximated vocal folds and sounding like a "poorly tuned motorboat engine" (Stemple et al., 1995, p. 50).

SPOTLIGHT ON TECHNOLOGY

The Flexible Endoscope

Professionals who assess and treat voice disorders often use the flexible endoscope to carefully examine the structures and functions of the nasal, pharyngeal, and laryngeal areas. When designed specifically for these purposes, this specialized endoscope is sometimes called a *nasopharyngoscope,* shown in the picture below. An endoscope is essentially a tube that is inserted into the interior surfaces of the body and that allows one to inspect these areas. The flexible endoscope is able to bend, whereas a rigid one cannot. Typically a light is attached to one end. Any procedure that uses an endoscope is called *endoscopy.* To look at the vocal folds, the endoscope is usually passed through the nasal cavity to focus down upon the larynx. The patient will then make various vocalizations so that the vocal folds can be observed for various functions (e.g., high pitch/low pitch). The endoscope can also be used to look at the esophagus and stomach, important for identifying such things as potential causes for reflux disorder. In these instances, an individual swallows the endoscope after the throat is sprayed with a numbing solution.

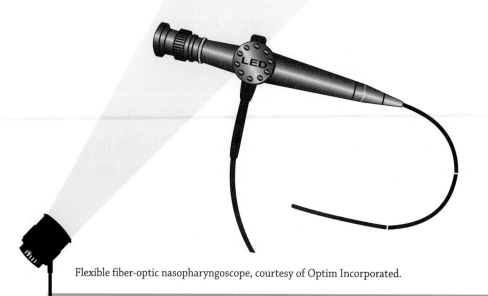

Flexible fiber-optic nasopharyngoscope, courtesy of Optim Incorporated.

Several concepts are important in understanding pitch disturbances:

1. **Habitual pitch:** Also called *vocal idle,* the pitch used in normal speaking situations without applying any extra physiological effort

2. **Optimal pitch:** The pitch at which one's voice is the least abusive, least effortful, and most efficient

3. **Basal pitch:** The lowest steady pitch a person can produce without pitch breakages or glottal fry.

4. **Ceiling pitch:** The highest pitch at which a voice can be sustained without pitch breakages

5. **Vocal range:** The difference between a basal and a ceiling pitch, normally covering two to three octaves (Case, 2002)

A pitch disturbance is present when a person's habitual pitch differs significantly from the optimal pitch or when vocal range is overly limited.

Loudness

Voice disorders can also affect loudness, resulting in a voice that is insufficiently or overly loud or one in which loudness does not vary, referred to as **monotonic.** Excessive shouting, loud talking, and screaming are several types of vocal abuses that are overloud. To produce an overly loud voice, the air pressure under the vocal folds must build up. Excessive loudness is sometimes seen in persons who are deaf or hard of hearing, because they are unable to monitor the loudness of their voices.

Other people are not loud enough, and listeners must strain to hear them. Underloudness can result from a lack of respiratory force due to neurological injury or disease, such as traumatic brain injury, Parkinson's disease, or multiple sclerosis, all of which can undermine the muscular processes required to produce a strong voice. Researchers Solomon, McKee, and Garcia-Barry (2001) described a 23-year-old man, JN, who sustained a severe traumatic brain injury in a motor vehicle accident. In addition to other cognitive, language, and speech problems, JN's neurological damage compromised his ability to produce a loud, strong voice: "In connected speech, [JN's] vocal quality was breathy and rough, accompanied by decreased vocal pitch and mono-pitch/monoloudness" (p. 54).

Underloudness can also occur for social or psychogenic reasons. Some homes value quietness, and children may develop early patterns of speaking softly. Other reports suggest that underloudness can occur for psychological reasons. Case (1996) reports a case in which a woman was virtually aphonic (i.e., unable to produce an audible voice) because of a traumatic incident in which she was robbed at knifepoint. In less obvious cases, an adult or a child might experience serious vocal or throat pain and then be hesitant to exert the pressure needed to produce a strong voice. Like overloudness, speaking too softly is a type of vocal abuse; persistent underloudness can cause vocal strain and fatigue, because the vocal muscles must work harder, given the inadequate force of the airstream.

PHONATORY QUALITY

Phonation is the production of voice via the vocal folds. The vocal folds must work together easily and harmoniously to produce a normal voice quality that does not draw attention to itself. Several of the more common disturbances to phonatory quality are described here:

1. *Hard glottal attack:* Voice is produced with a hard vocal burst, created by building up air pressure below the vocal folds and tensing them together, after which they burst apart and then bang back together.

2. *Glottal fry:* Referenced previously as a pitch disorder, glottal fry also represents a disordered phonatory quality in which pitch is held at an unusually low level and is produced on tightly approximated vocal folds.

3. *Breathy phonation:* Voice is produced without complete closure or approximation of the vocal folds, resulting in a weak and breathy voice.

4. *Spasticity:* Voice is produced with too much vocal tension and effort, resulting in intermittent stoppage of the voice.

5. *Hoarseness:* Voice is produced with noise introduced into the sound spectrum and a loss of the higher frequencies (Stemple et al., 1995).

HOW ARE VOICE DISORDERS IDENTIFIED? ●

THE VOICE CARE TEAM

The identification and management of voice disorders require the close collaboration of a variety of professionals, called the *voice care team* (Harvey, 1996). Voice management is a holistic process that requires close attention to an individual's physical health and psychological well-being. The professional team includes medical professionals, including the primary care physician (PCP) and an otolaryngologist, as well as allied health professionals, including a speech-language pathologist and perhaps a psychologist or psychiatrist. For children, educators are essential members of the voice care team, including classroom teachers and special educators. For patients who use their voices professionally for performance art, including singers and actors, the voice care team may involve a voice teacher and a voice coach (Harvey, 1996).

Involving a range of professionals in the management of voice disorders results in a more accurate and thorough diagnosis of the voice disorder and a more comprehensive description of how the voice disorder affects the individual both physiologically and psychologically. It also enhances the design of comprehensive and coordinated treatment approaches (Nuss, Hillman, & Eavey, 1996).

THE ASSESSMENT PROCESS

The assessment process for a voice disorder begins with identifying the warning signs of a possible disturbance of resonance, pitch, loudness, or phonatory quality. It is important for professionals who work with children (e.g., general and special educators) and those who work with adults (e.g., primary care physicians and nurses) to be aware of warning signs of voice disorders.

Warning Signs of Voice Disorders

Figure 11.9 presents a comprehensive list of warning signs of possible voice disorders in children and adolescents. Some of these warning signs are indicative of vocally abusive behaviors, such as "yells, screams, or cries frequently." Other warning signs suggest that an underlying medical condition may warrant attention; for example, "loses his/her voice every time s/he has a cold" or "uses a lot of effort to talk." Several warning signs focus on the child's psychological well-being (e.g., "seems tired or unhappy a lot of the time"), acknowledging the intricate relationship between an individual's psychological and physical health.

For adults, the warning signs include many of those identified for children and adolescents. However, adults are better able than children to notice changes in resonance, pitch, loudness, and phonatory quality on their own— even though they will not necessarily seek treatment for those problems! Many adults may assume that a disturbance in voice quality will go away on its own, or they may fail to recognize that the disturbance could signal a more serious underlying problem. Whenever a change in the resonance, pitch, loudness, or general phonatory quality of an individual's voice lasts for longer than 2 weeks, consultation with a primary care physician (PCP) is needed.

The PCP will examine the quality of the voice and likely make two referrals. The first is to an otolaryngologist, who will take a careful look at the

FIGURE 11.9

Warning signs of possible voice disorders in children and adolescents.

Coughs, clears throat, or chokes frequently

Has difficulty breathing or swallowing

Complains of a sore throat often

Voice sounds rough, hoarse, breathy, weak, or strained

Loses his/her voice every time s/he has a cold

Always sounds "stuffed up," like during a cold; or sounds like s/he is talking "through the nose"

Voice sounds worse at different times of the day (morning, after school, evening)

Sounds different from his/her friends of the same age and gender

Voice sounds worse after shouting, singing, playing outside, or talking for a long time

Uses a lot of effort to talk; or complains of vocal fatigue

Yells, screams, or cries frequently

Likes to sing and perform often; participates in acting and/or singing groups

Participates in sports activities or cheerleading activities that require yelling and calling

Has difficulty being understood by unfamiliar listeners

Can't be heard easily in the classroom or when there is background noise

Talks more loudly than others in the family or classroom

Voice problem is interfering with his/her performance at school

Doesn't like the sound of his/her voice; or is teased for the sound of his/her voice

Attends many loud social events (parties, concerts, sports games)

Seems tired or unhappy a lot of the time

Is facing difficult changes, such as death, divorce, household financial problems

Does not express his/her feelings to anyone

Lives with a family that uses loud voices frequently

Smokes, or is exposed to smoke at home or at a job

Uses alcohol

Eats "junk food" frequently; or complains of heartburn or sour taste in the mouth

Drinks beverages that contain caffeine; or drinks little water

Has allergies, respiratory disease, or frequent upper respiratory infections

Has hearing loss or frequent ear infections

Takes prescription medications

Has a history of injuries to the head, neck, or throat

Has had surgeries

Was intubated at birth or later

Has a chronic illness or disease

Source: From *Functional indicators of voice disorders in children and adolescents,* by L. Lee, J. C. Stemple, and L. Glaze, 2003, Gainesville, FL: Communicare. Copyright 2003 by Communicare. Adapted with permission.

structures of the laryngeal system and determine whether a potentially serious underlying medical condition exists. The second referral is to a speech-language pathologist who specializes in voice treatment. This professional will work closely with the individual to assess and treat cases of vocal abuse or misuse, neurogenic voice disorders, psychogenic voice disorders, and alaryngeal communication.

DISCUSSION POINT:
Sometimes a person may exhibit warning signs of a voice disorder but may resist seeking a medical evaluation. What are some ways to raise public awareness of how important it is to get a medical evaluation?

Assessment Protocol

This section focuses on the assessment completed by the speech-language pathologist, even though other professionals, such as the otolaryngologist, will also complete an assessment using a variety of complementary but different techniques. The speech-language pathologist's role in assessment is to

(1) characterize the general features of the voice (i.e., resonance, pitch, loudness, and phonatory quality), (2) establish whether any of these features differ significantly from normal, (3) identify the cause of any disorder, and (4) identify the most beneficial approach to improving the client's voice. Clinicians use a variety of different tools, including case history and interview, oral-motor examination, clinical voice observation, and instrumental voice observation.

Case History and Interview.   The case history and interview with the client are indispensable in learning more about the client, including how the voice is used for daily living activities and how the client perceives the voice in terms of resonance, pitch, loudness, and phonatory quality. The clinician carefully questions the client about the entire history of voice use, including the following:

- The client's medical history
- The chronological history of the problem
- The symptoms and possible etiology of the problem
- The way in which the client uses the voice at home, school, or work and in the community
- The client's motivation for seeking help (Stemple et al., 1995)

For young children who cannot reliably serve as informants, their primary caregivers are carefully questioned.

Another important consideration in the assessment process is gathering information concerning the psychosocial consequences of a voice disorder. This refers to the level of "handicap" a person experiences as a result of voice problems and is specific to a given person based on how they use and need their voice in their daily life. One tool for assessing the psychosocial consequences of a voice disorder is the Voice Handicap Index (VHI; Jacobson et al., 1997), reproduced in Figure 11.10.

Oral-Motor Examination.   The oral-motor examination is used to rule out or identify a structural problem—to identify the condition of the structures involved in speech production, study the amount of tension and sensation involved in speech and voicing, and examine possible swallowing problems. As the client engages in oral-motor activities, the clinician carefully studies the motion of all the articulators and questions the client about any sensations associated with these motions, such as tickling, burning, or aching (Sapienza et al., 2004).

Given the importance of the velum and the velopharyngeal port for modulating resonance, the clinician carefully studies the appearance and functioning of the velum, examining it for symmetry and signs of atrophy, edema, or swelling. The clinician may ask the client to engage in a few oral-motor activities (e.g., saying "ahh") to see that the velum does not deviate to the right or left or show signs of weakness (Dworkin et al., 2004). The clinician also determines whether the velopharyngeal port is closed to nasal airflow by holding a laryngeal mirror under the nostrils while the client produces speech that should not produce nasal emissions (Dworkin et al., 2004). The clinician attends carefully to any abnormal nasal emissions or snorting-like sounds that suggest velopharyngeal insuffiency.

FIGURE 11.10

Voice Handicap Index

Instructions: These are statements that many people have used to describe their voices and the effects of their voices on their lives. Circle the response that indicates how frequently you have the same experience.

F1. My voice makes it difficult for people to hear me.
P2. I run out of air when I talk.
F3. People have difficulty understanding me in a noisy room.
P4. The sound of my voice varies throughout the day.
F5. My family has difficulty hearing me when I call them throughout the house.
F6. I use the phone less often than I would like.
E7. I'm tense when talking with others because of my voice.
F8. I tend to avoid groups of people because of my voice.
E9. People seem irritated with my voice.
P10. People ask, "What's wrong with your voice?"
F11. I speak with friends, neighbors, or relatives less often because of my voice.
F12. People ask me to repeat myself when speaking face-to-face.

P13. My voice sounds creaky and dry.
P14. I feel as though I have to strain to produce voice.
E15. I find other people don't understand my voice problem.
F16. My voice difficulties restrict my personal and social life.
P17. The clarity of my voice is unpredictable.
P18. I try to change my voice to sound different.
F19. I feel left out of conversations because of my voice.
P20. I use a great deal of effort to speak.
P21. My voice is worse in the evening.
F22. My voice problem causes me to lose income.
E23. My voice problem upsets me.
E24. I am less outgoing because of my voice problem.
E25. My voice makes me feel handicapped.
P26. My voice "gives out" on me in the middle of speaking.
E27. I feel annoyed when people ask me to repeat.
E28. I feel embarrassed when people ask me to repeat.
E29. My voice makes me feel incompetent.
E30. I'm ashamed of my voice problem.

Note. The letter preceding each item number corresponds to the subscale (E = emotional subscale, F = functional subscale, P = physical subscale).

Note: Each item is scored on a 4-point scale, whereby 0 = never, 1 = almost never, 2 = sometimes, 3 = almost always, 4 = always. Add points for each item to determine VHI score. A score of 0–30 is low (minimal handicap), a score of 31–60 is moderate (moderate handicap), and a score of > 60 is high (serious handicap).

Source: Jacobsen, B., Johnson, A., Grywalski, C., Silbergleit, A., Jacobson, G., et al. (1997). The Voice Handicap Index: Development and validation. *American Journal of Speech-Language Pathology, 6,* 66–70.

Clinical Observation.   The voice specialist carefully studies the client's voice during a variety of speaking and vocal activities to document the characteristics of the voice. Also called *perceptual observation,* the clinical observation documents how the client's voice sounds. Figure 11.11 provides one tool that clinicians use to document the voice across a variety of measures, including pitch and loudness. Because many of the descriptive terms on this rating scale are highly subjective, relying heavily on the listener's ear, it is important that the clinician be knowledgeable and experienced in working with voice clients so that the subjective observations are valid. (Recall from Chapter 4 that *validity* describes the certainty of findings.) The validity of subjective observations of voice quality is improved when clinicians bring a wealth of experience to their observation, allowing them to differentiate between normal and abnormal voice characteristics.

The clinical observation examines the client's voice in a variety of activities designed to elicit different vocal behaviors, such as the following:

1. Counting from 1 to 40 softly and then loudly
2. Sustaining the vowel /a/ for as long as possible
3. Sustaining the consonants /s/ and /z/ for as long as possible
4. Humming at different pitches

FIGURE 11.11

A rating scale for clinical observation of voice characteristics.

	1	2	3	4	5	6	7	8	9	
High pitch	1	2	3	4	5	6	7	8	9	Low pitch
Loud	1	2	3	4	5	6	7	8	9	Soft
Strong	1	2	3	4	5	6	7	8	9	Weak
Smooth	1	2	3	4	5	6	7	8	9	Rough
Pleasant	1	2	3	4	5	6	7	8	9	Unpleasant
Resonant	1	2	3	4	5	6	7	8	9	Shrill
Clear	1	2	3	4	5	6	7	8	9	Hoarse
Unforced	1	2	3	4	5	6	7	8	9	Strained
Soothing	1	2	3	4	5	6	7	8	9	Harsh
Melodious	1	2	3	4	5	6	7	8	9	Raspy
Breathy voice	1	2	3	4	5	6	7	8	9	Full voice
Excessive nasal	1	2	3	4	5	6	7	8	9	Insufficient nasal
Animated	1	2	3	4	5	6	7	8	9	Monotonous
Steady	1	2	3	4	5	6	7	8	9	Shaky
Young	1	2	3	4	5	6	7	8	9	Old
Slow rate	1	2	3	4	5	6	7	8	9	Rapid rate
I like/voice	1	2	3	4	5	6	7	8	9	Don't like/voice

Source: From *Clinical management of voice disorders* (4th ed., p. 180) by J. L. Case, 2002, Austin, TX: Pro-Ed. Copyright 2002 by Pro-Ed. Reprinted with permission.

5. Repeating multisyllabic words (e.g., *Mississippi*)
6. Repeating sentences that do and do not contain nasal sounds (e.g., "She keeps cheese chips" versus "My mommy makes me mad") (Andrews & Summers, 2002)

The clinician also engages the client in conversations on various topics to study vocal quality during normal speaking situations. Children might be asked to describe an ideal pet or a perfect birthday party, whereas adults might be questioned about what they would do if they won the lottery. On the basis of these observations, the clinician can document ways in which voice is disordered in resonance, pitch, loudness, and phonatory quality.

In 2002, several experts in the study of voice and the treatment of voice disorders convened in Pittsburgh to develop guidelines for and improve consistency in perceptual assessments of voice, particularly concerning severity of voice problems (Voice Disorders Special Interest Division, 2002). The tool that resulted from this consensus meeting—the Consensus Auditory-Perceptual Evaluation of Voice (CAPE-V)—is currently undergoing field review. To use this tool, an individual completes three activities: sustained production of the vowels /a/ and /i/ for 3 to 5 seconds, production of six sentences (e.g., "How hard did he hit him?"), and production of at least 20 seconds of conversational speech in response to prompts (e.g., "Tell me about your voice problem"). The clinician rates the overall severity of any perceived voice problems as well as severity for five attributes of the individual's voice (Voice Disorders Special Interest Division, 2002):

1. Roughness: Is there any perceived irregularity in the voice?
2. Breathiness: Is there any perceived audible air escape in the voice?
3. Strain: Is there any perceived excessive effort in the voice?
4. Pitch: Is there any deviation in pitch in reference to gender, age, and culture?
5. Loudness: Is there any deviation in pitch in reference to gender, age, and culture?

Efforts such as this one, which is supported by the Voice Disorders Special Interest Division of ASHA, are important for improving the consistency of assessment procedures used throughout the field of communication disorders that rely largely on perceptual observations.

The clinician also studies the systems that support vocal production, particularly respiration. The clinician observes how long the client can sustain inhalation and exhalation during different tasks. The client might be asked to inhale as long as possible to keep a piece of tissue on the end of a straw or to exhale through a straw into a glass of water for as long as possible. The clinician also studies how the client modulates breath support when speaking to determine whether inhalation and exhalation are appropriately coordinated and whether airflow is adequate to support phonation.

Instrumental Observation. Objective measures of vocal functioning are an essential part of the clinical voice assessment and complement more subjective procedures. Objective evaluation uses four types of clinical instrumentation to examine how the larynx is functioning during phonation and other speech activities: acoustic assessment, aerodynamic assessment, electroglottography, and videostroboscopy (Nuss et al., 1996).

Acoustic assessment documents the frequency (pitch) and intensity (loudness) of the voice, including the maximal range and habitual levels of each. It also documents **jitter** and **shimmer,** which refer, respectively, to perturbations (or changes) in frequency and intensity in a phonatory cycle. In addition, acoustic assessment can document nasal and oral sound pressure during speaking to quantitatively characterize a client's resonance. Clinicians must be comfortable with the technologies used for acoustic assessment (see Figure 11.12). The information obtained can help determine whether frequency, intensity, and resonance characteristics differ from normative references.

Aerodynamic assessment provides an objective measure of airflow, air pressure, and vocal fold resistance against airflow from the lungs, called *subglottal airflow.* Several devices are commercially available for this assessment, in which clients wear a face mask and have their airflow carefully studied by a computer (Case, 2002). The data provided tell about the flow of air through the laryngeal mechanism and how well the vocal folds resist the airflow.

Electroglottography, or EGG, provides an objective examination of vocal fold contact during voicing (Nuss et al., 1996). The clinician places electrodes on the surface of the client's neck to monitor voltage changes in the vocal folds as they vibrate. The EGG provides a graphic representation of the vocal folds as they close and open to show whether contact is normal, overadducted (too

FIGURE 11.12

Clinical instrumentation for objective voice assessment.

Source: Photo courtesy of Kay Elemetrics.

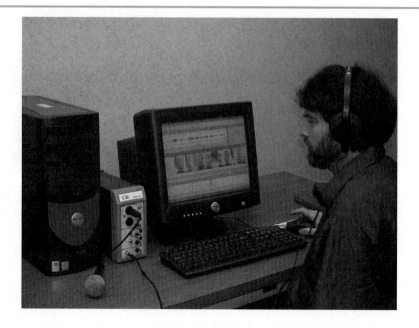

tightly pressed together), or underadducted (inadequately pressed together; Nuss et al., 1996).

Laryngoscopy is the examination of the vocal folds and laryngeal system using a flexible endoscope passed through the nasal cavity. The endoscope is connected to a camera to present the images of the larynx on a color monitor. Laryngoscopy is an important tool, because it provides a close-up view of the vocal folds, allows several people to study the larynx simultaneously, and provides permanent video documentation to monitor change of the vocal mechanism over time (Nuss et al., 1996). Even with this technology, however, the human eye cannot see how the vocal folds move, because they vibrate so quickly—as many as 1,000 cycles per second. But by coupling endoscopy with a pulsing light directed onto the vocal folds—a procedure called **videostroboscopy**—vocal fold movement is slowed down, and the vibratory cycle can be closely observed. Videostroboscopy is used by both speech-language pathologists and otolaryngologists. The otolaryngologist uses it to study the structures of the larynx, whereas the speech-language pathologist studies how the larynx functions and how that function might be improved through therapy (Nuss et al., 1996).

HOW ARE VOICE DISORDERS TREATED?

A voice assessment provides a speech-language pathologist with essential information concerning both the etiology of an individual's voice disorder and the perceptual features of the disorder. Whenever possible, treatment goals target the etiology to eliminate the cause of the disorder, which, in turn, should eliminate the disordered features of voice. Such a goal may be attainable in the case of vocal abuse, but in other cases the cause of the disorder may not be so easily resolved. For people who have had their larynx removed or for those who have spasmodic dysphonia, for instance, the SLP must help the individual compensate for a cause that is not easily eliminated. In those cases, the SLP works with the individual to

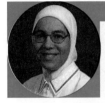

SPOTLIGHT ON RESEARCH AND PRACTICE

ALIAA ALI KHIDR, M.D., PH.D, CCC-SLP

PROFESSION/TITLE
Professor, Phoniatrics Department, Medical School, Ain Shams University, Cairo, Egypt; Faculty, Department of Communication Disorders, Curry School of Education, University of Virginia; Director of the Voice Lab, University of Virginia Medical Center, Charlottesville, Virginia

HOW INTERESTS IN COMMUNICATION SCIENCES AND DISORDERS BEGAN
In my final years in Ain Shams Medical School, I shadowed one of the world pioneers of phoniatrics, Dr. Nasser Kotby. His enthusiasm for providing state-of-the-art services to patients with communication disorders in the Middle East as well as searching for answers for pressing issues in our field was a huge drive for me. Right after graduation, as I joined the department of phoniatrics as a junior faculty, I became a member of the international family of enthusiastic scientists and clinicians who find voice and singing to be one of the most rewarding and celebrated pleasures of life.

CURRENT RESEARCH AND PRACTICE INTERESTS
My passion has always been to develop a means for clinicians to be more reliable and consistent in rating laryngeal observations and vocal parameters. Throughout my career, I have been part of many clinical research teams in Ain Shams University, University of Madison-Wisconsin, Cleveland Clinics, and the University of Virginia. My efforts are part of an international workforce that aims to achieve a common protocol that can be used to accurately describe clients' findings and measure outcomes of therapy. My research addressed these concerns in patients with different laryngeal disorders such as sulcus vocalis, unilateral vocal fold paralysis (UVFP) treated by surgical medialization, UVFP treated by behavioral voice therapy, and reflux laryngitis treated by medical therapy.

My professional interests extend to seeking practical and reliable ways for singers to evaluate physiological parameters that are critical for the production and longevity of the singing voice, such as breath support. Today, most singers, singing teachers, and voice clinicians use totally different subjective ratings to evaluate breath support. I am currently working with great colleagues to evaluate breath support in a group of singers. Abdominal and chest wall displacement measures together with other subjective and objective parameters will be used to quantify changes in their breath support. Finding the best way to evaluate breath support in singers is needed to evaluate the outcomes of voice therapy targeting breath support in singers with functional voice disorders.

And last but not least, one of my professional missions has been establishing multiple digital learning materials and hands-on workshops to make the Smith Accent Voice Therapy Technique more accessible for voice clinicians. This is one of the few holistic voice therapy techniques that provides a clear hierarchy for optimizing breath support as an integral part of voice production for both speaking and singing.

develop improved or alternative ways to produce voice. Often, the speech-language pathologist works closely with other professionals as medical solutions are pursued, such as placement of a voice prosthesis for laryngectomized patients or the use of Botox injections for individuals with spasmodic dysphonia.

In general, treatment for voice disorders has three possible goals:

1. To teach a vocal behavior that is absent
2. To substitute an appropriate vocal behavior for an inappropriate one
3. To strengthen vocal behaviors that are weak or inconsistent (Andrews & Summers, 2002)

To achieve these general goals, the SLP first develops a treatment plan to identify a set of short-term goals and one or more long-term goals, or terminal objectives (Andrews & Summers, 2002). The long-term goal is the functional, meaningful, and concrete outcome of treatment—for example, "Melissa will use a pitch level that is appropriate for her age and gender when speaking spontaneously with others." The set of short-term goals is the carefully arranged hierarchy of steps needed to achieve the long-term goal.

TREATMENT FOR VOCAL ABUSE

The symptoms of vocal abuse—such as vocal nodules and contact ulcers—can be treated through surgery on the vocal folds. If a person has no voice or a severely disordered voice, surgery may provide the most efficient route to improvement (Mori, 1999). However, individuals can often avoid surgery by completing treatment programs that promote better vocal behaviors and improved knowledge about the voice. For adults, voice treatment that focuses on changing vocal behaviors is typically at least as successful as surgical intervention for vocal nodules and ulcers (Ramig & Verdolini, 1998). These *vocal hygiene programs* guide the individual to identify each specific vocal abuse; understand its effect on the voice; identify specific occurrences of the abuse; and then modify, replace, or eliminate the behavior (Stemple et al., 1995).

Specific voice therapies that incorporate laryngeal massage, biofeedback, voice-production exercises, and counseling are often coupled with general vocal hygiene treatment, all of which are effective ways to promote better voice use (Ramig & Verdolini, 1998). Some clinicians use computer programs designed specifically to provide feedback on voice behaviors, such as the rate of airflow (Blood, 1994). Computer software provides an objective way to monitor progress toward certain goals, such as "demonstrating correct breathing patterns during speech" (Blood, 1994, p. 65).

Speech-language pathologists often develop comprehensive voice treatment programs that involve a range of strategies. For instance, 11 women aged 19 to 35, all of whom had bilateral vocal nodules, participated in a program involving five specific components (Holmberg et al., 2001):

1. *Vocal hygiene:* client education about how voice is produced as well as common abuses

2. *Respiration exercises:* exercises focused on better management of air supply when speaking and resting

3. *Loudness reduction:* computer-based exercises to discriminate and produce speech at varying levels of loudness

4. *Relaxation training:* techniques focused on increasing relaxation

5. *Carryover activities:* techniques focused on using newly learned vocal behaviors in various contexts

Voice therapies that systematically train improved vocal behaviors seem especially important for children, for whom teaching general vocal hygiene does not seem to have great effect. In contrast, completing a course of voice therapy, typically three to six sessions, results in an improved or normal voice quality for about 50% of children (Mori, 1999). Even for people who choose surgical treatment for the symptoms of vocal abuse, treatment focused on better use of voice is essential to keep those symptoms from reappearing.

TREATMENT FOR NEUROGENIC DISORDERS

Neurogenic voice disorders result from a specific physiological cause that negatively impacts the voice-production system in some way. Those disorders are often treated with a combination of medical interventions and voice therapy. Medical intervention focused on the improvement, alteration, or restoration of the voice is called *phonosurgery* (Ford, 1996). One type of phonosurgery is *thyroplasty,* which involves modification of the thyroid cartilage of the larynx. This impacts the tension and position of the vocal folds and provides a way to improve their functioning in some cases (Ford, 1996). Thyroplasty is the prevailing surgical approach for treatment of breathy dysphonias resulting from vocal fold paralysis or other vocal fold damage (e.g., scarred folds or bowed folds; Ford, 1996). Vocal outcomes are excellent with this surgery, resulting often in improved vocal intensity and frequency. Although surgical complications of thyroplasty occur relatively infrequently (10% of cases), they can be serious and even life-threatening (Ford, 1996).

Injecting botulinum toxin Type A (Botox) into the vocal folds is also used to treat vocal fold disturbances, such as spasmodic dysphonia (Fisher, Scherer, Guo, & Owen, 1996). A disadvantage of Botox is that its effects are temporary, necessitating regular reinjections (Ford, 1996).

Whether or not surgical intervention is used, voice therapy is an essential part of voice management. This helps an individual cope with voice disturbances and develop compensatory or alternative ways to produce a better voice. One of the better-known programs for treatment of neurogenic voice disorders is the Lee Silverman voice treatment (LSVT) program. LSVT is an intensive 1-month program using repeated exercises informed by theories of motor learning. It is designed to improve the phonatory strength of people with Parkinson's disease, although positive effects are seen in other populations as well (e.g., stroke, multiple sclerosis; Fox, Morrison, Ramig, & Sapir, 2002). This treatment increases the intensity and frequency of the voice and the general rate and articulation of speech.

TREATMENT FOR PSYCHOGENIC DISORDERS

Persons who exhibit psychogenic voice disorders require a multidisciplinary treatment program involving a speech-language pathologist and other mental health professionals. Therapy focuses on determining the emotional and psychosocial cause of the voice disturbance, as resolution of the cause may reduce the voice disturbance (Stemple et al., 1995). Therapy focuses primarily on counseling, reducing tension, and eliminating any voice abuses or misuses (Ramig & Verdolini, 1998).

ALARYNGEAL COMMUNICATION

Individuals whose larynx has been removed must develop alternative ways to produce voice. When the larynx is removed, the airway between the lungs and the mouth is closed, and the airflow is shunted out the front of the neck via a *stoma,* or hole in the neck (see Figure 11.13). An essential aspect of treatment for alaryngeal communication is communication counseling, which explores all the options possible for voice and helps clients make the best choices for their needs and interests (Wagner, 1996). Typically, an artificial larynx is introduced

FIGURE 11.13

Anatomy of the larynx following a laryngectomy.

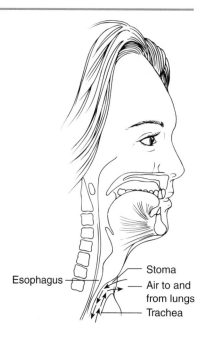

Esophagus

Stoma

Air to and from lungs

Trachea

immediately to provide at least a temporary solution. An artificial larynx is a vibrating power source placed against the neck or in the mouth; sound is shaped through articulation. Some users do not like the artificial larynx because of its mechanical sound and its poor differentiation of similar-sounding consonants, such as *f* and *v, b,* and *p* (Wagner, 1996).

The most commonly used alternative for alaryngeal communication is **esophageal speech,** with which the individual traps air in the esophagus and then uses that air to produce voice. However, it is not easy to get enough air into the esophagus to produce voicing, and learning to use esophageal speech can be very difficult for some people. Consequently, a surgical procedure called a *tracheoesophageal puncture* can be used to create a channel between the trachea and the esophagus, into which a prosthetic device is inserted. The individual then takes a deep breath, covers the stoma, and forces the air into the esophagus, providing an air source for speaking. This type of speech is called **tracheoesophageal speech** and allows an individual to speak longer and more loudly as compared to esophageal speech (Wagner, 1996).

CASE ANALYSIS

Study the case of Arthur (Case Study 6 in the Companion Website at www .pearsonhighered.com/justice2e). Reflect on his prognosis for resolving his voice difficulties.

● CHAPTER SUMMARY

The human voice is a complex, dynamic product of the vocal folds. It is also an essential tool for personal expression, creativity, and art. The human voice is characterized by four different parameters: resonance, loudness, pitch, and phonatory quality. When one or more of these vary significantly from normal, based on age and gender, a disorder may be present.

Voice disorders are relatively common, affecting about 29% of the population at one time or another. In many cases, disorders are transient, resulting from respiratory problems, colds, sinus infections, and the like. Some professionals, such as teachers and singers, experience voice disorders at relatively higher rates than others do.

Experts classify voice disorders in four causal categories. First, vocal abuse describes the chronic or intermittent overuse or misuse of the vocal apparatus. Common abuses include talking in noisy environments; coughing or clearing the throat frequently; and yelling, screaming, and cheering. Second, neurogenic disorders result from illness, damage, or disease to the neurological systems associated with voice production. Spasmodic dysphonia and vocal fold paralysis are two examples of neurogenic voice disorders. Third, psychogenic voice disorders describe disorders that stem from a psychological or emotional cause. Examples are conversion disorder and generalized anxiety disorder. And fourth, alaryngeal communication describes voice without a larynx. The most common reason for removing the larynx is laryngeal cancer. Regardless of etiology, the defining characteristics of voice disorders include aberrational resonance, pitch, loudness, or phonatory quality.

Treatment for voice disorders is a multidisciplinary process. Those involved typically include a speech-language pathologist, a primary care physician, medical specialists such as an otolaryngologist, mental health specialists such as a psychologist, and educators. The speech-language pathologist's assessment focuses on vocal function and ways it might be improved through treatment. The comprehensive assessment process includes case history and interview, oral-motor examination, clinical voice observation, and instrumental voice observation.

Treatment for voice disorders differs based on etiology. In general, three goals are addressed: (1) to teach a vocal behavior that is absent, (2) to substitute an appropriate vocal behavior for an inappropriate behavior, and (3) to strengthen weak or inconsistent vocal behaviors. Treatment for vocal abuse emphasizes vocal hygiene and modifying or eliminating vocally abusive behaviors. Treatment for neurogenic disorders may include medical management, such as thyroplasty, coupled with intensive therapy designed to improve phonatory behaviors. Treatment for psychogenic disorders uses counseling to address the underlying emotional issues. Individuals who require alaryngeal communication receive therapy to teach them alternative means of producing speech, including the use of an artificial larynx, esophageal speech, or tracheoesophageal speech.

● KEY TERMS

abduction, p. 356
acoustic assessment, p. 385
adduction, p. 356
aerodynamic assessment, p. 385
alaryngeal communication, p. 362
aphonia, p. 360
basal pitch, p. 378
ceiling pitch, p. 378
contact ulcers, p. 367
conversion disorder, p. 372
diplophonia, p. 360
dysphonia, p. 360
electroglottography, p. 385
esophageal speech, p. 390
frequency, p. 357
glottal fry, p. 377
glottiscope, p. 355
habitual pitch, p. 378

hyperfunction, p. 360
hypofunction, p. 360
intensity, p. 357
jitter, p. 385
laryngeal dystonia, p. 369
laryngeal mirror, p. 355
laryngectomee, p. 374
laryngectomy, p. 361
loudness, p. 357
monotonic, p. 379
mutational falsetto, p. 373
neurogenic voice disorders, p. 368
optimal pitch, p. 378
phonatory quality, p. 359
pitch, p. 357
psychogenic disorders, p. 371

puberphonia, p. 373
resonance, p. 356
shimmer, p. 385
spasmodic dysphonia, p. 360
tracheoesophageal speech, p. 390
tracheostomy, p. 369
vagus nerve, p. 368
velopharyngeal inadequacy, p. 376
velopharyngeal port, p. 376
videostroboscopy, p. 386
vocal abuse, p. 364
vocal nodules, p. 363
vocal range, p. 378
vocal tic disorder, p. 371
voice, p. 356

● ON THE WEB

Check out the Companion Website at www .pearsonhighered.com/justice2e! On it you will find:

- suggested readings
- reflection questions

- a self-study quiz
- links to additional online resources, including current technologies in communication sciences and disorders

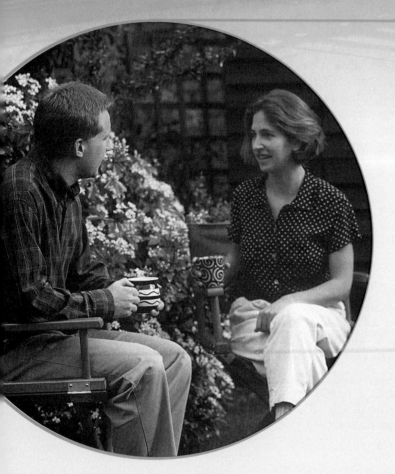

MOTOR SPEECH DISORDERS
APRAXIA AND DYSARTHRIA

Edwin Maas and
Donald A. Robin

FOCUS QUESTIONS

This chapter answers the following questions:

1. What is a motor speech disorder?

2. How are motor speech disorders classified?

3. What are the defining characteristics of prevalent types of motor speech disorders?

4. How are motor speech disorders identified?

5. How are motor speech disorders treated?

CHAPTER 12

INTRODUCTION

Speech production is the most effective way to communicate. It is also one of the most impressive motor skills possessed by the human species. Speech production involves the rapid and fine-tuned coordination of many muscles and muscle groups in a fluent, continuous manner. A difference in the onset of muscle contractions of as little as 40 to 50 milliseconds can mean the difference between two sounds (e.g., /b/ versus /p/); thus, accuracy in motor production is critical for effective communication. The fact that speakers can reliably produce such small differences in timing indicates the degree of control speakers must and can exert over the coordination of muscle contractions. An individual's control over the muscular coordination involved with producing speech is called **speech motor control.**

Speech motor control follows a course of development that begins at birth and continues to about age 12. During these years, children's speech movements are less accurate and show greater variability compared to those of adult speakers (Goffman, Gerken, & Lucchesi, 2007; Smith & Zelaznik, 2004). By adolescence, most children exhibit adultlike speech motor control (Smith & Zelaznik, 2004).

However, some children have great difficulty acquiring the degree of speech motor control seen in adult speakers or other typically developing children. These children have difficulty articulating the stream of speech needed to accurately and consistently have a conversation. Although in many cases the exact cause of children's problems with speech motor control is unknown, most experts agree that such problems are related to neurological difficulties. Adults also can experience difficulty with speech motor control, particularly after injuries or illnesses that affect the brain regions linked to speech motor control. This chapter discusses these disorders of communication, called *motor speech disorders,* from a life span perspective. The two major categories of motor speech disorders are apraxia of speech and dysarthria, both of which can affect children and adults. ●●●

WHAT IS A MOTOR SPEECH DISORDER? ●

DEFINITION

A **motor speech disorder** is an impairment of speech production caused by defects of the neuromuscular system, the motor control system, or both (Duffy, 2005). With a motor speech disorder, defects in these underlying systems involved with planning, programming, and executing speech result in significant

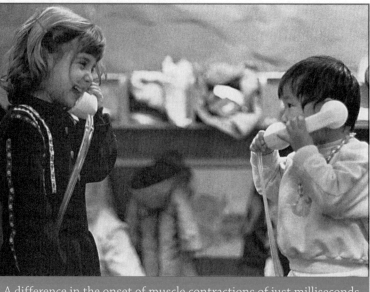

A difference in the onset of muscle contractions of just milliseconds means the difference between a /b/ and a /p/.

difficulties producing fluent, intelligible speech. A motor speech disorder does not result from and cannot be explained by other disorders, such as language impairment or phonological disorders, although these types of communication disorders may co-occur with a motor speech disorder. People with motor speech disorders may also exhibit difficulties with other functions that involve oral movements aside from speech, such as chewing and smiling, since the impairment affects the motor system.

TERMINOLOGY

This section presents concepts and terminology required to understand breakdowns in the control of motor speech. We first describe four systems involved with speech production—the respiratory, phonatory, resonatory, and articulatory systems—and offer a review of concepts presented in Chapter 3. We next describe key concepts for understanding motor control, including motor units; motor planning, programming, and execution; and motor learning.

Systems of Speech Production

Speech production involves the coordination in space and time of muscles and muscle groups from four major systems—the respiratory, phonatory, resonatory, and articulatory systems (see Table 12.1). Three of these systems (respiration,

TABLE 12.1	The four systems of speech production	
System	**Key Structures**	**Muscles and Articulators**
Respiratory	Lungs	Respiratory and postural muscles
Phonatory	Larynx	Vocal folds
Resonatory	Velopharyngeal port, pharynx	Velum, pharynx
Articulatory	Oral cavity	Jaw, lips, tongue

phonation, and articulation) were described in Chapter 1. The resonatory system is introduced here. Each system includes many muscles, which must be carefully coordinated temporally and spatially with other muscles within and across subsystems.

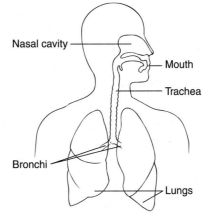

FIGURE 12.1

Respiratory system.

Respiratory System. Speech production requires airflow to produce sound. The airflow for speech may be ingressive (going in) or egressive (going out), but most languages, including English, rely on egressive airflow for sound production (Ladefoged, 2001). The most important mechanism for producing airflow is the pulmonary mechanism, including the lungs, which creates airflow by pushing air out of the lungs through the trachea, or windpipe, using various muscle groups (see Figure 12.1). The pulmonary mechanism is a major structure in the **respiratory system,** which regulates the inhalation-exhalation cycle for passive breathing and for producing speech.

To produce fluent speech, an individual must carefully control the exhalation cycle so that it extends the length of an utterance in a controlled and coordinated manner. In passive breathing, the duration of inhalation versus exhalation corresponds to a ratio of approximately 1:1, but in speech production, this ratio ranges from about 1:6 to 1:9 (Yorkston, Beukelman, Strand, & Bell, 1999). When speaking, people inhale briefly, typically at clause boundaries, and extend the exhalation period to the end of the utterance (Winkworth, Davis, Adams, & Ellis, 1995). For instance, to produce a brief narrative such as that presented below, the speaker pauses at clauses (marked here with a #) to inhale for continued airflow:

> When we received the letter in the mail# we immediately contacted our insurance agent# to let them know about our concerns# they didn't seem too worried# so we didn't pursue the matter. . . .

To further complicate speech production, utterances require stress assignment on some syllables and words. For instance, in the example presented here, the words *letter* and *mail* in the first utterance are emphasized relative to the other words. This means that the exhalation cycle needs to be extended in time for speech production and must be manipulated to produce stress. In short, breath support is crucial for oxygen intake as well as for speech production.

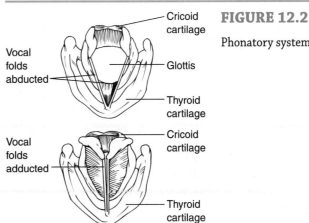

FIGURE 12.2

Phonatory system.

Phonatory System. Humans produce speech sounds by modulating or changing the airflow in various ways and at various points along the vocal tract. One major source of sound is the vibration of the vocal folds that sit within the larynx, as discussed in Chapter 3 and shown in Figure 12.2.

The various muscles and structures in the larynx, including the vocal folds, form the phonatory system of speech production. The **phonatory system** regulates the production of voice and the prosodic, or intonational, aspects of speech. To produce many of the consonant sounds (e.g., /m/, /b/, /z/) and all the vowel sounds, the vocal folds are brought close together (adduction) by various muscle groups so that the airflow causes them to vibrate. The vocal folds are stretched lengthwise to manipulate the frequency or pitch of the voice, which carries both linguistic and nonlinguistic information. The opening between the vocal folds is the glottis, and the buildup of sufficient air pressure below the glottis, called *subglottal air pressure,* sets the vocal folds into cycles of vibration. The phonatory system coordinates with the respiratory system, which provides the airflow needed for phonation. In short, the phonatory system is essential for producing both voiced and voiceless sounds and for modifying word stress, intonation, and other aspects of prosody.

CASE STUDY 12.1   Motor Speech Disorders Across the Life Span

BOB is a 42-year-old bank vice president in the Midwest. He is married, has four children, and is bilingual, speaking both English and Spanish fluently. He travels regularly to visit family in Mexico, California, and Texas. Until recently, Bob coached a children's soccer team and was involved in church and town activities. In 2003, however, he began to have difficulty walking and started to have shaky hands. He also began to speak more softly, making it more difficult for his family to understand him. When he finally saw a neurologist for an assessment, the physician ordered a series of tests, which revealed that Bob had Parkinson's disease. Bob now takes medication to control the symptoms of this degenerative disease, and speech therapy was recommended to improve his communication with his family. Despite the medication and speech therapy, his speech is currently moderately to severely impaired, with estimates of about 30% intelligibility by those close to him, and continues to slowly decline.

Internet research

1. According to current estimates, how many Spanish-English bilingual speakers live in the United States?

2. What percentage of speech-language pathologists are fluent in both Spanish and English?

3. What is the incidence and prevalence of Parkinson's disease in the United States?

4. What are some common interventions (medical and behavioral) for Parkinson's disease?

Brainstorm and discussion

1. What are some ways in which Bob's current motor difficulties affect his participation in life at home and in the community?

2. What types of strategies might you suggest to improve Bob's participation in life?

● ● ●

HIKARU is a 5-year-old boy who came to the United States from Japan with his family when he was 2. Hikaru attends an English-only public school, because that is the only option in his state. Expressively, he is primarily an English user, but receptively, he also understands Japanese because it is used at home. His mother referred him for a speech and language evaluation because of concerns about articulation difficulties. She reported that Hikaru was slow to talk and has always drooled a lot while talking. During the evaluation, the clinician observed that Hikaru had social skills appropriate for the North American culture and interacted well with the

clinician. Hikaru's communication strategies included the use of gestures, facial expressions, changes in prosody, and verbal expression using both English and Japanese words. Hikaru exhibited severe delays in expressive language, particularly in syntax (reduced utterance length) and phonology (sound substitutions and deletions). His speech production was imprecise and appeared weak, consistent with flaccid dysarthria. Based on the evaluation, these motor difficulties seemed largely restricted to the articulatory system. Hikaru's mother is concerned about his speech difficulties and is considering delaying his entry into first grade by a year.

Internet research

1. How many states have adopted legislation that mandates public schools to provide English-only education?

2. What proportion of children in the United States is bilingual?

Brainstorm and discussion

1. What are some possible reasons Hikaru's parents did not pursue an evaluation earlier in light of Hikaru's history of speech problems (e.g., drooling)?

2. The Japanese language does not have consonant clusters and syllable-final consonants (as in *truck*). How relevant is this to the speech evaluation? What other differences between Japanese and English might be relevant for fully understanding Hikaru's problems?

3. In your opinion, will holding Hikaru back from first grade be an advantage or a detriment to his development? After stating your opinion, investigate research on the topic to see what researchers say about the advantages and detriments of grade retention.

Resonatory System. The **resonatory system** regulates the resonation or vibration of the airflow as it moves from the pharynx into the oral or nasal cavities. *Resonance* refers to the effect of the shape and size of the vocal tract on sound quality, and an important aspect of vocal resonance is whether the nasal cavity is used as a vibrating chamber. This is determined by the state of the **velopharyngeal port,** which is the opening between the velum (soft palate) and the back of the pharynx wall (see Figure 12.3). When the velum is raised, the velopharyngeal port is closed (the velum touches the back wall of the pharynx), and air flows out through and resonates only within the oral cavity. When the velum is lowered, the velopharyngeal port is open, and air flows out through both the oral and nasal cavities, affecting the quality of the sound (nasality). Regulation of the velopharyngeal port is important for producing the difference between oral and nasal sounds (e.g., /b/ and /m/) and for ensuring a normal sound quality. The resonatory system must be carefully timed and coordinated with the respiratory and phonatory systems for fluent speech production.

Articulatory System. The fourth system of speech is the **articulatory system,** which regulates the control of the articulators within the oral cavity to

FIGURE 12.3

Resonatory and articulatory systems.

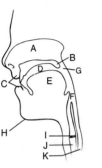
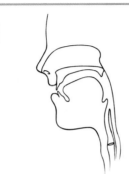

In the left panel the velum (B) is lowered, opening the velopharyngeal port (G) to produce a nasal sound; in the right panel, the velum is raised and the velopharyngeal port closed, to produce an oral sound. A = nasal cavity; B = velum; C = upper and lower lips; D = oral cavity; E = tongue; F = pharynx; G = velopharyngeal port; H = jaw; I = larynx; J = trachea; K = esophagus.

FIGURE 12.4

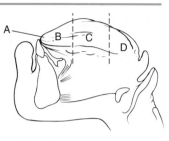

Subdivisions of the tongue.
A = tip or apex; B = blade
or front; C = center;
D = dorsum or back.

manipulate the outgoing airflow in different ways, usually at very high speeds. The major structures involved in articulation are the lower jaw and lips for opening and closing movements and for creating constrictions at the end of the oral cavity. The tongue is also an important structure for creating constrictions and obstructions within the oral cavity (see Figure 12.3). In fact, the tongue is probably the most important articulator because of its flexibility and capacity for high-speed motion. The tongue is a muscular hydrostat, which means that it does not contain bone or cartilage and that it maintains its volume regardless of muscle contractions (Kent, 1997). The tongue comprises many muscles and muscle groups, and these are categorized as *intrinsic muscles,* which originate within the tongue, and *extrinsic muscles,* which originate outside the tongue. The intrinsic muscles regulate the tongue's more fine-tuned movements. The extrinsic muscles regulate coarser movements, such as tongue protrusion, tongue retraction, tongue elevation, and tongue depression (Kent, 1997). Contractions of these muscle groups create constrictions of varying degrees and locations within the oral cavity. The tongue is sometimes divided into four sections: the apex (tip of the tongue), the lamina or blade (front of tongue), the center (middle part of tongue), and the dorsum (back of tongue). These sections are shown in Figure 12.4.

Changes in the positions and shapes of the tongue and other articulators result in different speech sounds. At a very general level, speech sounds are divided into consonants and vowels, as discussed in Chapter 9. To review, *consonants* are a group of speech sounds that involve a constriction in the vocal tract; *vowels* are a group of speech sounds that involve relatively little or no constriction of the vocal tract but a modulation of the oral cavity's shape by the tongue, lips, and jaw.

For consonants, the constriction may be a complete obstruction of airflow, as in the case of stop consonants, such as /p/ (obstruction at lips), /d/ (obstruction at tongue tip), and /k/ (obstruction at tongue dorsum), and nasal consonants, such as /m/ (obstruction at lips), /n/ (obstruction at tongue tip), and /ŋ/ (obstruction at tongue dorsum). Some consonants involve a partial constriction, such as /f/, /z/, and /ð/, for which a narrow constriction is created to push a turbulent airflow through the constriction location. For some sounds, such as /w/, /r/, and /l/, the constriction is wider, so the airflow is smoother and continuous rather than turbulent.

For vowels (at least in English), the airflow is never turbulent, and the continuous airflow is manipulated by the tongue in the oral cavity to create the varying vowel sounds. Diphthongs are an interesting variety of vowels that involve a gliding movement in the production of the sound, as in *oy.*

In producing the consonants and vowels, the actions of the tongue and the articulatory system must work seamlessly with the other systems—respiratory, phonatory, and resonatory—to produce well-articulated speech that unfolds fluently over time.

This brief overview of the motor systems involved in speech production demonstrates the complexity of speech as a motor skill and the requirement for fine-tuned and rapid coordination of the four systems involved with speech production. Given this complexity, it is not surprising that both children and adults may experience failures in motor speech coordination. Sometimes the four individual systems are poorly coordinated, resulting in breakdowns in the larger motor speech production system. Or, deficits in the coordination of the muscles and muscle groups within a specific system may cause the entire system to break down because of the complex interrelationships among the four systems.

Speech Motor Control

Production of fluent speech requires the rapid coordination of muscle activity across a wide range of muscle groups within the four systems. To maintain speed and fluency when speaking, and to maintain accuracy of movements, the sequences of movements are programmed together as a single unit. If we consider the vast number of muscles and muscle groups involved in fluent articulation, and thus the large number of degrees of freedom (the number of elements, such as muscles, that can be independently controlled), the magnitude of the challenge facing the speaker becomes apparent. One way to contend with the challenge of controlling all these different muscles in a coordinated and fluent manner is to reduce the number of degrees of freedom by organizing motor actions into motor units (Kent, Adams, & Turner, 1996). A motor unit is a single control mechanism that controls more than one degree of freedom.

Motor Units.   A **motor unit,** sometimes called a **motor program** or *muscle synergy,* is an abstract representation of a relatively invariant movement pattern that can be scaled in size and time to meet the demands of the particular situation (Schmidt & Lee, 2005). Motor units are those aspects of a movement that remain constant over repeated productions in different contexts and therefore seem to be planned and executed as a whole, although timing and force can vary across executions.

Consider the following as an example. In order to kick a ball, you must swing your leg backward, using muscles in the back of your thigh, and then reverse to swing your leg forward, using muscles in the front of your thigh. The timing and force of these two aspects of the movement are closely related, so when your leg swings backward, it must also swing forward at least the same distance to hit the ball. The relative force and timing of the muscle contractions with respect to each other are organized as a whole. The actual absolute force produced by these muscles depends on other factors, such as the distance between kicker and ball, the size and weight of the ball, and how far the ball is to be kicked. However, the basic pattern of the movement components remains constant, while more specific aspects of the movements (e.g., muscle contractions) are influenced by the specific circumstances.

Speech production is even more complicated than kicking a ball. When speaking, an individual is producing linguistic units—phrases, words, syllables, and phonemes—and is simultaneously producing acoustic events—pitch and loudness variations—that map onto the linguistic units. It is not clear whether the motor units produced during speech correspond to the linguistic units or the acoustic events (Ballard, Granier, & Robin, 2000; Folkins & Bleile, 1990; Smith, 2006). What this means is that the relationship between the linguistic and motor systems involved with speech production is not completely understood (Kent et al., 1996; Smith, 2006). However, experts generally agree that the linguistic system provides input to the motor system in speech production, as discussed in the model of speech production presented in Chapter 1 (Guenther,

2006; Levelt, Roelofs, & Meyer, 1999; Van der Merwe, 2007). It is also clear that speech motor control involves a tight integration and coordination of various muscle groups and systems (Abbs, Gracco, & Cole, 1984; Gomi, Honda, Ito, & Murano, 2002; Shaiman & Gracco, 2002). This coordination involves programming particular patterns of muscle activity into single motor units to ensure accurate and fluent articulation.

Motor Planning, Programming, and Execution. Planning and programming a motor unit are different from executing a motor act (Schmidt & Lee, 2005). Motor planning and programming are aspects of motor control that occur *before* initiation of movement, whereas execution occurs *at* or *after* initiation. For example, when a person produces a sentence, intonation typically declines across the sentence so the sentence ends at a lower pitch than it began. This change occurs in part because of the decreasing breath support at the end of the exhalation phase as the speaker runs out of air. We might consider this lowering of pitch as an effect of motor execution or the biomechanical relation between higher lung volume and associated subglottal pressure at the beginning of the utterance that influences vocal fold vibration (e.g., Watson, Ciccia, & Weismer, 2003). In addition, however, speakers usually start at a higher pitch when producing a longer sentence than when producing a shorter one. This phenomenon provides evidence that speakers plan how they will modulate intonation over a whole sentence. In other words, speakers spread out the exhalation across the entire utterance so they do not have to pause for inhalation, and when they inhale, they typically do so at clause boundaries (Winkworth et al., 1995). The higher pitch and lung volume at the beginning of longer utterances is actually a phenomenon of motor planning (Cooper & Klouda, 1987; Winkworth et al., 1995).

Motor planning and programming—which happen prior to executing a movement—are important aspects of motor behavior that professionals must consider when they work with individuals experiencing motor problems. Professionals must determine whether a breakdown in motor performance occurs in the planning and programming or in the execution of the motor act. The exact nature of the processes involved in motor planning and programming are not totally understood (McNeil, Doyle, & Wambaugh, 2000), but experts do recognize that aspects of a movement are planned, or preprogrammed, based on central processes and without any external feedback since the movement has yet to be executed (e.g., Abbs et al., 1984; Klapp, 2003; Perkell et al., 2000; Schmidt & Lee, 2005). Of course, feedback is not ignored, and speakers have been shown to use sensory and auditory feedback rapidly in controlling their speech movements (e.g., Gomi et al., 2002; Tourville, Reilly, & Guenther, 2008).

On the basis of this background, the remainder of this chapter will use the following terminology to describe motor speech control:

- **Motor planning** refers to the processes that define and sequence articulatory goals (e.g., lip closure, onset of voicing) prior to their occurrence.
- **Motor programming** refers to the processes responsible for establishing and preparing the flow of motor information across muscles for speech production and specifying the timing and force required for the movements.
- **Motor execution** refers to the processes responsible for activating relevant muscles during the movements used in speech production (Van der Merwe, 2007).

It is sometimes difficult for experts to tease apart motor planning and motor programming; therefore, motor planning and programming will be considered together throughout this chapter.

Motor Learning.   The ability to effectively plan and program speech movements requires extensive practice to achieve the stability and flexibility that characterizes skilled speech production. Extensive practice using speech is needed to learn and develop motor control through motor learning. **Motor learning** is the way in which practice or experience leads to "relatively permanent changes in the capability for movement" (Schmidt & Lee, 2005), and it is an important concept for understanding normal and disordered speech motor control.

When considering normal and abnormal development of speech motor control, an important question is how the motor speech system learns to form the appropriate units to ensure fluent and accurate execution of movements during speech. One concept to describe this learning is called *schema theory,* which suggests that individuals develop **schemas**—memory representations of relationships between various sources of information (Schmidt, 1975; Schmidt & Lee, 2005; Shea & Wulf, 2005). These schemas represent the relations between motor specifications, the initial state of the muscles or structures, and the outcome of the movement, and they are used to generate the appropriate instructions to the muscles to achieve the goal. A schema becomes stronger with experience, because information about the movements and muscle configurations is stored after every movement. For future movements, the person can then use the stored schema to produce the corresponding motor specifications that will lead to the desired outcome.

Stable and accurate schemas for speech movements allow for the production of precise, rapid, and intelligible speech. For individuals with motor speech disorders, the schemas may be unstable or damaged, resulting in imprecise or slow speech with reduced intelligibility. In addition, impairments of neuromuscular function (e.g., muscle weakness) may impede the execution of otherwise intact schemas. In both cases, existing schemas may need to be modified or new schemas may have to be learned to improve speech motor control.

> **DISCUSSION POINT:**
> Ask a peer to tell you about something he or she did recently, such as going on a trip. Examine how your peer's pitch changes over utterances, and consider how many of these changes were planned in advance.

PREVALENCE AND INCIDENCE

Reliable estimates of prevalence and incidence for specific motor speech disorders are rare. One estimate comes from a study of 10,444 patients seen in the Mayo Clinic for acquired neurogenic communication disorders. This study found that motor speech disorders accounted for almost 60% of these communication disorders; 54% were diagnosed with dysarthria, and 4% were diagnosed with apraxia of speech (Duffy, 2005). At least at the Mayo Clinic, the prevalence of motor speech disorders among those who seek treatment for acquired neurogenic communication disorders is quite high.

Among children, estimates of prevalence for motor speech disorders are also hard to come by. Speech delays affect about 4% of children (Shriberg et al., 1999); however, what number of these children exhibit speech delays because of a motor speech disorder is not clear. No comprehensive investigation of incidence or prevalence of motor speech disorders among children is available at present, primarily because of difficulties identifying specific motor speech disorders and long-standing debates over the tools and criteria used to identify motor speech problems in children.

SPOTLIGHT ON LITERACY

In societies in which the writing system is related to the spoken language, as with the alphabetic system for English, one might expect that difficulty with speaking may create difficulties for learning the written symbols that represent the speech sounds. For instance, if a child cannot reliably discriminate between a /p/ and a /b/ in her productions, then she might have a hard time decoding the letters p and b in relation to the sounds they represent. However, this reasoning presupposes that knowing how a speech sound is *produced* is necessary or helpful for *decoding* written symbols, and it is not clear that this is the case. As long as the child can *perceive* the relevant distinctions in other people's speech, she should be able to learn the associations between visual symbols (letters) and auditory signals (speech sounds). Thus, if the speech problem is exclusively one of speech motor production, and not of perception or of the underlying phonological knowledge (e.g., representations of phonemes), then there is no reason to expect reading difficulties.

While it has been reported that children with CAS may also have reading difficulties (Lewis, Freebairn, Hansen, Iyengar, et al., 2004; Moriarty & Gillon, 2006; Stackhouse & Snowling, 1992), such reports do not establish a causal role of CAS for these difficulties, and the children in these studies often have language disorders concomitant with CAS. Evidence about reading disorders in children with speech disorders but without co-occurring language disorders is mixed, with some studies showing normal reading abilities (e.g., Lewis et al., 2004; Nathan, Stackhouse, Goulandris, & Snowling, 2004) and others reporting presence of reading disorders (e.g., Raitano, Pennington, Tunick, Boada, et al., 2004).

Of course, if normal speech production is necessary for the development of phonological knowledge, then a motor speech disorder may indirectly impede literacy development, because phonological knowledge and awareness are known to be important predictors for literacy development (e.g., Hogan, Catts, & Little, 2005). Although it may be possible in principle to develop a normal phonological system in the context of a motor speech disorder (based on the ability to *perceive* phonological contrasts), it does appear that phonological development suffers when a child has difficulty producing speech sounds, either due to speech sound disorder (e.g., Raitano et al., 2004) or even to more peripheral, structural problems such as cleft palate (e.g., Konst, Rietveld, Peters, & Prahl-Andersen, 2003). Thus, it is now often assumed that the ability to accurately produce speech sounds aids in the development of phonological representations (Raitano et al., 2004), which in turn can affect literacy development. Evidence is beginning to emerge that children who have CAS and a phonological disorder benefit from treatment that includes a phonological awareness component (Gillon, 2002; Moriarty & Gillon, 2006).

HOW ARE MOTOR SPEECH DISORDERS CLASSIFIED? ●

ETIOLOGY

DISCUSSION POINT:
Consider each of the cases in Case Study 12.1. Characterize each motor speech disorder in terms of acquired versus developmental, and identify the cause of each.

Motor speech disorders may be acquired or developmental. Acquired motor speech disorders result from damage to a previously intact nervous system, most often caused by cerebrovascular accidents (CVAs) or strokes, degenerative diseases such as Parkinson's disease and amyotrophic lateral sclerosis, brain tumors, and traumatic brain injury (TBI).

Developmental motor speech disorders result from abnormal development of the nervous system or from damage to the nervous system in its early development (Thompson & Robin, 1993). Abnormal development may result from various congenital diseases, including cerebral palsy and a variety of genetic syndromes such as fragile X and Down syndrome. Damage to the developing nervous system may be caused by TBI, brain tumors, and CVAs.

MANIFESTATION

Motor speech disorders are divided into impairments of motor planning and programming and impairments of motor execution. For fluent, articulate speech, the individual systems and muscles of speech production, as well as the coordination of muscle contractions within and among systems, must be intact. Breakdowns at all levels of the motor speech system are possible.

Sometimes breakdowns occur at the level of execution, as with disruptions of muscle physiology. For example, paralysis of the tongue will seriously impede speech production, regardless of whether speech is planned and programmed normally or not. Similarly, speech production will be affected by involuntary movements (e.g., tremors) of muscles and by reductions in range, speed, and consistency of movement. In such cases, the speech motor problem results from difficulties or impairment with speech execution.

Breakdowns can also occur at the planning and programming level. In such cases, muscle physiology and movement abilities (e.g., range, speed, and direction of movement) are intact, but the coordination of the relevant muscles and muscle groups (within and among systems) for a given speech target is disrupted. For instance, the individual may not experience paralysis of the tongue but may have difficulty moving the tongue in the right way at the right moment in time for

Children with cerebral palsy, because of its impact on neuromuscular functioning, often exhibit motor speech disorders.

a given speech target. This situation would be consistent with a disruption at a level of processing prior to execution, namely at the motor planning and programming levels.

SEVERITY

Motor speech disorders, whether developmental or acquired, or whether affecting children or adults, range from mild to severe. The degree of severity is determined not only by the symptoms, but also, and more importantly, by how the disorder affects the person's participation in life. An individual may have a motor speech disorder that profoundly affects intelligibility but does not have any impact on daily living activities. What is most critical to consider when determining a disorder's severity is the distinction between different levels of disorder. The World Health Organization (WHO) distinguishes between four aspects of a disorder—body structure, body function, activity/participation, and contextual factors (Threats, 2006; WHO, 2001):

> **DISCUSSION POINT:**
> Consider the case of Bob in Case Study 12.1. In what ways has his impairment impacted his life? Have these impacts been serious or mild?

- *Body structure* refers to the underlying anatomical aspects of a condition that impedes performance. For motor speech disorders, the anatomical structure that is affected is the central and/or peripheral nervous system.
- *Body function* refers to the physiological and psychological functions that are disrupted in a disorder. For motor speech disorders, the function that is impaired is the ability to plan or execute speech movements.

- *Activity/participation* refers to the limitations that the affected body function has on performance and on a person's quality of life as defined by that person (Clark, Stierwalt, & Robin, 2000). For motor speech disorders, the most important indices of activity are speech intelligibility and fluency or naturalness, and **participation in life** is indicated by how the speech impairment impacts an individual's performance at home, at school, at work, and in the community.

- *Contextual factors* include both personal factors, such as attitudes, values, and coping strategies, and wider environmental factors, such as the social support system and resources available to the person, the legal environment, and social and cultural beliefs (e.g., Threats, 2006). The impact of a motor speech disorder depends to a large extent on these personal and cultural factors.

Professionals who work with individuals with motor speech disorders must consider the severity of the disorder in relation to all four aspects: body structure, body function, activity/participation, and contextual factors. A person may have severe symptoms of the body function but be relatively unaffected in terms of activity/participation. On the other hand, the body structure impairment and its symptoms may appear relatively mild but may greatly impact the person's activity and participation. By considering severity using the WHO scales, professionals are able to focus more holistically on motor speech disorders, taking into account the symptoms as well as how those symptoms affect an individual's life at home, at school, at work, and in the community (see Eadie, Yorkston, Klasner, Dudgeon, et al., 2006, for a review of instruments that include assessment of activity/participation in speech-language pathology).

DISCUSSION POINT:
Hikaru, described in Case Study 12.1, has a motor speech disorder. What were some early indicators of this disability?

CHARACTERIZING INDIVIDUAL DIFFERENCES

As is the case with many abilities and disorders, a range of individual differences occur for motor speech disorders. The effects of a neurological disease on an individual differ from person to person, even if the cause and severity of the disease are similar. Individuals differ in their ability to compensate for a motor or muscle physiology problem, their ability to use unimpaired systems to take over for the loss of the impaired system, and their general life response to major medical problems. In addition, treatment of motor speech disorders produces widely varying results, depending on several factors, such as the person's perceptions of functioning, their family support systems, their adherence to intervention activities, and their desire to improve, among others.

WHAT ARE THE DEFINING CHARACTERISTICS OF PREVALENT TYPES OF MOTOR SPEECH DISORDERS? ●

As stated earlier, motor speech disorders are divided into disorders of motor planning and programming and disorders of motor execution (Darley, Aronson, & Brown, 1975; Duffy, 2005; Van der Merwe, 2007). **Motor planning and programming disorders** are caused by an inability to group and sequence the relevant muscles in order to plan or program a movement. **Motor execution disorders** are caused by deficits or inefficiencies in basic physiological or movement characteristics of the musculature, such as muscle tone, movement speed, and movement range. Impairments of the speech motor system may also affect other oral motor behaviors, such as smiling or swallowing (e.g., Folkins, Moon, Luschei, Robin, et al., 1995). An overview of important characteristics of these motor speech disorders and how they affect speech production is provided in Table 12.2.

MOTOR PROGRAMMING AND PLANNING DISORDERS AND ACQUIRED APRAXIA OF SPEECH (AOS)

Defining Characteristics

Apraxia of speech (AOS) is an impairment of motor programming and planning that involves an inability to transform a linguistic representation into the appropriate coordinated movements of the articulators (Maas, Robin, Wright, & Ballard, 2008; McNeil, Robin, & Schmidt, 2007); it is not the result of a language disturbance or an impairment of the neuromuscular system (e.g., muscle weakness, spasticity, abnormal reflexes). Thus, a speaker may have the linguistic representation of the word *cup* well formed in the language systems but be unable to transform this representation into fluent and well-articulated motor sequences. AOS affects primarily the articulatory system of speech production and prosody, whereas the resonatory, phonatory, and respiratory systems are relatively intact (Duffy, 2005; McNeil et al., 2007).

The speech of individuals with AOS is marked by certain salient characteristics (Wambaugh, Duffy, McNeil, Robin, et al., 2006):

- Effortful, slow speech with increased pauses between syllables and sounds and sound prolongations
- Distortions of speech sounds
- Impaired prosody, including a reduction of differences in pitch, duration, and loudness between stressed and unstressed syllables
- Errors that are consistent in type (i.e., distortion) and location *within* an utterance, although the presence of error may vary from attempt to attempt (McNeil, Odell, Miller, & Hunter, 1995; but see Shuster & Wambaugh, 2008)

Additional characteristics of AOS that may occur include difficulties with initiating speech, groping of the articulators when producing speech, and sensitivity to the automaticity of the utterance (Kent & Rosenbek, 1983; McNeil et al., 2007; 2000), although these features are not specific to AOS (McNeil et al., 2007; 2000; Wambaugh et al., 2006). For example, a patient may be unable to say the phrase "Bless you" when explicitly asked to do so in a structured assessment task, but the same patient may spontaneously and without error produce the phrase in response to the assessor's sneeze. Initiation difficulties may reflect programming difficulties rather than problems with activating muscle commands (Maas et al., 2008). Errors of serial order (e.g., saying "can-pake" instead of *pancake*) are more characteristic of phonological disorders associated with aphasia (Wambaugh et al., 2006). Finally, normal or fast speech rate and normal prosody are considered exclusionary features (Wambaugh et al., 2006).

Causes and Risk Factors

Acquired apraxia of speech occurs as a result of neurological damage. The precise location of the lesion responsible for AOS remains subject of debate. Several brain regions have been reported to be associated with AOS (see Robin,

TABLE 12.2   Characteristics of various motor speech disorders

	Apraxia of Speech	Spastic Dysarthria	Flaccid Dysarthria	Hypokinetic Dysarthria	Hyperkinetic Dysarthria	Ataxic Dysarthria	Unilateral Upper Motor Neuron Dysarthria
Impairment	Motor planning for speech, groping and posturing of the articulators	Excessive muscle tone, muscular weakness	Weakness, atrophy, low muscle tone	Slow movement, rigidity, tremors	Variable muscle tone, involuntary movements	Incoordination, tremors, overshooting and undershooting movements	Unilateral facial or tongue weakness
Respiration	Typically normal	Reduced respiratory support and control for speech	Reduced respiratory support for speech	Shallow breaths, reduced breath support	Sudden and irregular respiratory patterns	Irregular respiratory patterns	Typically normal
Phonation	Typically normal, some irregular changes in pitch or loudness	Strained and strangled voice quality, reduced pitch, reduced variations of loudness	Breathiness, monoloudness, monopitch	Reduced loudness	Sudden changes in pitch, loudness, and voice quality	Hoarse or breathy voice quality, irregular pitch, loudness changes	Harsh voice quality, reduced loudness
Resonation	Typically normal	Hypernasal	Hypernasal	Typically normal	Typically normal	Typically normal	Typically normal
Articulation	Sound distortions, distorted substitutions, omissions, and additions; groping of the articulators	Reduced precision of articulators	Reduced precision of articulators	Reduced precision of articulators, reduced range of motion	Sudden, irregular breakdowns in precision of articulators	Reduced and irregular precision of articulators	Reduced precision of articulators, irregular motion rates
Prosody	Slow rate, irregular prolongations and pauses, reduction in stress difference between stressed and unstressed syllables (dysprosody)	Excess stress and/or equal stress, short phrases	Short phrases	Rapid bursts of speech, long pauses	Rapid bursts of speech, inappropriate phrasing	Irregular pitch and loudness changes, irregular speech rhythm	Typically normal

Source: Clark, H. M., Stierwalt, J. A. G., & Robin, D. A. (2000). Motor speech disorders. In J. B. Tomblin, H. L. Morris, & D. C. Spriestersbach (Eds.). Diagnosis in speech language pathology (2nd ed., pp. 337–352). Reprinted with permission of Delmar Learning, a division of Thomson Learning: www.thomsonrights.com.

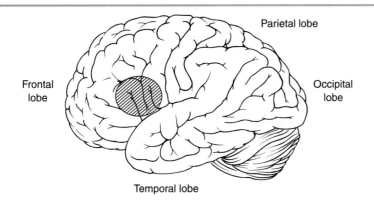

FIGURE 12.5

One suspected location of brain damage in apraxia of speech.

Jacks, & Ramage, 2008), including the left frontal cortex in the area surrounding Broca's area, the darkened region in Figure 12.5 (Duffy, 2005; Hillis, Work, Barker, Jacobs, et al., 2004); the parietal cortex (e.g., McNeil, Weismer, Adams, & Mulligan, 1990; Square, Darley, & Sommers, 1982); the anterior insula (Dronkers, 1996; Ogar, Willock, Baldo, Wilkins, Ludy, & Dronkers, 2006); the basal ganglia (Jones, Peach, & Schneck, 2003; Seddoh, Robin, Sim, Hageman, et al., 1996); and the right frontal cortex and basal ganglia structures (Balasubramanian & Max, 2004). Common causes include stroke, in which the loss of oxygen to the brain causes tissue damage or death; traumatic brain injuries; infections; and neuro-degenerative disease (e.g., Duffy, 2006).

CHILDHOOD APRAXIA OF SPEECH (CAS)

Defining Characteristics

Childhood apraxia of speech (CAS) is a phonetic-motoric disorder of speech production. Children with CAS are unable to translate linguistic or phonetic information concerning speech production into accurate motor behaviors or are unable to learn the motor behaviors to execute planned speech. The symptoms of CAS are the same as those of AOS, including effortful and slow speech, prolonged durations of speech sounds, speech-sound distortions, reduced prosody, and errors that vary across utterances or productions (e.g., Davis, Jakielski, & Marquardt, 1998; Strand, Stoeckel, & Baas, 2006). Children with CAS often show considerable delays in their development of speech produc-tion and have a limited sound inventory when producing syllables and words (Davis et al., 1998). They also typically have severe unintelligibility and progress slowly in speech therapy (Campbell, 1999; Strand et al., 2006).

Causes and Risk Factors

The causes of CAS are not well understood. Experts recognize that some chil-dren have enormous difficulty in planning, programming, and executing speech movements and that these difficulties stem from a motor disorder rather than a phonological disorder (discussed in Chapter 7). Although the incidence of CAS is relatively low, children with CAS struggle greatly with speech pro-duction, highlighting the need for experts to better understand what causes this disorder. Some research shows a hereditary component to the developmental form of CAS for some individuals (Alcock, Passingham, Watkins, & Vargha-Kadem, 2000; Shriberg, Lewis, Tomblin, McSweeny, et al., 2005), and certain genetic disorders such as fragile X syndrome have been suggested as another risk factor (Hall, 2007a; Paul, Cohen, Breg, Watson, et al., 1984). For some cases, CAS results from stroke or traumatic brain injury, but for many cases, there is no evidence of specific neurological damage (Hall, 2007b).

ACQUIRED DYSARTHRIA

Defining Characteristics

Dysarthria is a group of speech disorders caused by disturbances of neuromuscular control of the speech production systems (Darley et al., 1975; Duffy, 2005). In contrast to apraxia of speech, dysarthria is not an impairment of planning and programming of speech movements, but rather is a disruption in the execution of speech movements. Dysarthria results from underlying neuromuscular disturbances to muscle tone, reflexes, and kinematic aspects of movement, such as speed, range, accuracy, and steadiness (Duffy, 2005). Any or all of the systems of speech production may be affected. As with AOS, dysarthria may be accompanied by language disturbances. Dysarthric speech is generally more consistent in type and presence of errors and amount of intelligibility compared to apraxic speech.

Several concepts are important for understanding dysarthria and neuromuscular impairments: muscle tone, muscle strength, movement steadiness, movement speed, movement range, and movement coordination (Duffy, 2005). These describe ways in which the muscles and motor functions are affected and are used to describe various dysarthria types (e.g., Duffy, 2005; see also Table 12.2). **Muscle tone** refers to the resistance to passive movement and reflects sustained muscle activity that provides postural support for active movements. Tone may be abnormally reduced, as in flaccid dysarthria, or abnormally increased, as in spastic dysarthria. **Muscle strength** refers to the ability of the muscle to contract to a desired level and may be reduced, as in flaccid dysarthria. Such weakness may affect any or all the speech production subsystems, depending on the lesion, and may lead to increased fatigability, as in myasthenia gravis. **Movement steadiness** refers to the ability of the muscles to generate steady movements and may be disrupted by involuntary movements. There are two broad classes or involuntary movements, namely tremor and hyperkinesis. Tremor is a relatively rhythmic, repetitive movement, such as may be observed in hypokinetic dysarthria in Parkinson's disease. Hyperkinesis can take many different forms but generally involves relatively arrhythmic and unpredictable movements that may or may not be repetitive. **Movement speed** is important for speech production, which involves many rapid articulator movements, and may be reduced, as in spastic dysarthria; increased, as in some speakers with hypokinetic dysarthria; or variable, as in speakers with hyperkinetic dysarthria. **Movement range** refers to how far a structure such as the tongue or jaw can move, and this range may be reduced, as in hypokinetic dysarthria. Reductions of range of movement can have serious effects on speech, because many speech sounds require a very specific distance to be traveled (e.g., failure to move the tongue tip all the way to the alveolar ridge for the stop /t/ may result in the fricative /s/). **Movement coordination** refers to the ability to precisely time muscle contractions so that each articulator moves the intended distance and direction at exactly the right time. Movement coordination is very important in speech production, as languages use very subtle differences in timing and articulator position to distinguish speech sounds (e.g., recall voice onset time differences between /p/ and /b/). The ability to coordinate movements may be impaired, as in ataxic dysarthria.

The dysarthria types described below are primarily applicable to adults with acquired dysarthria; some have argued that children who become dysarthric secondary to neurological injury may not easily fit into these categories (e.g., Van Mourik, Catsman-Berrevoets, Paquier, Yousef-Bak, et al., 1997).

Spastic Dysarthria.   Spastic dysarthria is characterized by increased muscle tone (hypertonicity), weakness, reduced speed and range of movement, and a state of hyperreflexes (hyperreflexia). It usually results from bilateral lesions in the motor cortex and its pathways to the lower motor neurons that cause muscle contraction. Spastic dysarthric speech is characterized by reduced speech rate; distorted consonants and vowels; reduced or exaggerated stress; reduced pitch and loudness variation; breathy, harsh, or strained strangled voice quality; and hypernasality (Duffy, 2005; Nishio & Niimi, 2006; Portnoy & Aronson, 1982).

Flaccid Dysarthria.   Flaccid dysarthria involves muscle weakness, atrophy, and hypotonicity. These abnormalities may result in restricted speed and range of movement. Flaccid dysarthria results from damage to the lower motor neurons that are responsible for muscle contraction or damage to the cranial nerves that connect these motor neurons to the muscle. The specific deficits depend on which cranial nerve is affected and may be isolated to a single muscle or may span many muscles and subsystems. Often, the speech associated with flaccid dysarthria is characterized by reduced breath support, breathy voice quality, monoloudness and monopitch, hypernasality, reduced articulatory precision, and reduced utterance length (Cahill, Turner, Stabler, Addis, et al., 2004; Duffy, 2005).

Hypokinetic Dysarthria.   Symptoms of hypokinetic dysarthria include bradykinesia (slowness of movement), rigidity (increased muscle tone), and static tremor (Clark et al., 2000; Duffy, 2005). Although any or all subsystems may be affected, usually the effects are most obvious on phonation, articulation, and prosody. Speech characteristics include reduced breath support; reduced loudness; reduced articulatory precision, often with limited range of movement; and rapid bursts of speech and long pauses (Bunton, 2005; Duffy, 2005; Forrest & Weismer, 1995). Hypokinetic dysarthria results from damage to the basal ganglia, a group of subcortical structures important for movement, and is most often observed with Parkinson's disease, a neurodegenerative disease that disrupts the production of dopamine, an important neurotransmitter.

Hyperkinetic Dysarthria.   Hyperkinetic dysarthria is characterized by variable muscle tone and (slow or fast) involuntary movements, and also results from damage to the basal ganglia. There are many different types of hyperkinetic dysarthria, and the effects may range from a single muscle to a wide range of muscles across subsystems. Speech characteristics may include sudden, irregular breathing patterns; sudden changes in pitch, loudness, and quality; sudden breakdowns in articulatory precision; and rapid bursts of speech and inappropriate phrasing (Clark et al., 2000; Duffy, 2005). Although sometimes a specific disease can be identified as the cause, such as Huntington's disease, most cases of hyperkinetic dysarthria are idiopathic (cause unknown).

DISCUSSION POINT:
Differentiating between the dysarthrias can be difficult for students of communication disorders. Think of a strategy for knowing the major characteristics of each type.

Ataxic Dysarthria.   Ataxic dysarthria results from damage to the cerebellum, causing incoordination, dysmetria (undershooting or overshooting when reaching for a target), and tremors (Clark et al., 2000; Duffy, 2005). Speech characteristics include irregular breathing patterns, hoarse or breathy voice quality, irregular pitch and changes in loudness, reduced and irregular articulatory precision, and irregular speech rhythm (Duffy, 2005; Kent, Kent, Duffy, Thomas, et al., 2000).

Unilateral Upper Motor Neuron Dysarthria.   Unilateral upper motor neuron (UUMN) dysarthria involves weakness of the lower face or tongue on one side (Duffy, 2005) and results from unilateral damage to the motor cortex or its pathways to the lower motor neurons. Breathing for speech is usually normal, but there may be a harsh voice quality, reduced loudness, reduced articulatory precision, and irregular alternating motion rates (Clark et al., 2000; Duffy, 2005).

DEVELOPMENTAL DYSARTHRIA

Defining Characteristics

Developmental dysarthrias are present at birth and usually accompany a known disturbance to neuromuscular functioning, as might occur with anoxia (loss of oxygen to the brain) during birth. The most common types of developmental dysarthria are spastic dysarthria and dyskinetic dysarthria, although other types and mixed spastic-dyskinetic dysarthrias may occur as well (Hardy, 1983; Thompson & Robin, 1993). Cerebral palsy (CP), a nonprogressive movement disorder resulting from pre-, peri-, or postnatal brain damage that can affect motor and cognitive function (Wilson Jones, Morgan, Shelton, & Thorogood, 2007), is often accompanied by dysarthria (e.g., Patel, 2003). CP varies considerably in type and severity of impairment (e.g., Koman, Smith, & Shilt, 2004).

Spastic Dysarthria.   Spastic dysarthria is characterized by hypertonicity (increased muscle tone) and hyperreflexia (increased sensitivity of reflexes). There is considerable variability among children with respect to severity and the systems affected. Many children with spastic dysarthria also have spasticity of upper or lower limbs, or both. As with the acquired version, spastic dysarthric speech has a slow speech rate; distorted consonants and vowels; reduced or exaggerated stress; reduced pitch and loudness variation; a breathy, harsh, or strained strangled voice quality; and hypernasality (Clark et al., 2000; Wit, Maassen, Gabreëls, & Thoonen, 1993). Children with spastic dysarthria may have inadequate breath support for producing speech and may produce speech in short phrases (Solomon & Charron, 1998), although some limited control over prosodic features relevant for certain contrasts (e.g., question versus statement prosody) has been reported (e.g., Patel, 2003; Patel & Salata, 2006).

Dyskinetic Dysarthria.   Dyskinetic dysarthria is characterized by impaired coordination of muscles and involuntary movements, including chorea (sudden fast, flailing, jerking movements) and athetosis (slow, writhing movements). In most children with dyskinetic dysarthria, all four limbs are also affected. As with spastic dysarthria, a great deal of variability exists across children. Those with dyskinetic dysarthria may have a hard time producing speech, and speech may be strained, harsh, and low. Children may make abnormally large jaw movements when producing speech, resulting in imprecise and unintelligible speech (Bauman-Waengler, 2004).

Causes and Risk Factors

Developmental dysarthria results from pre-, peri-, or postnatal damage to the nervous system. Prenatal factors that may lead to abnormal development of the motor system include genetic factors (e.g., blood incompatibilities between mother and child, metabolic disturbances, Gilles de la Tourette syndrome), deficient oxygen supply to the fetus, maternal infections, exposure to chemicals, and other problems occurring during early pregnancy. Perinatal factors that may disrupt normal development of the neuromotor system include head trauma in difficult deliveries, premature and rapid deliveries, and respiratory problems during and following birth. Postnatal causes of developmental dysarthria include infections (meningitis, encephalitis), brain abscesses, tumors, head injuries, and strokes. Neurological developmental disorders affecting the motor system are often labeled *cerebral palsy* in the case of pre- and perinatal factors, but less often in the case of postnatal causes (Thompson & Robin, 1993).

HOW ARE MOTOR SPEECH DISORDERS IDENTIFIED? ⬤

THE ASSESSMENT PROCESS

Professionals use a variety of measurement methods to evaluate motor speech disorders. They examine how the disorder affects the individual's activities and participation in life to determine the most appropriate course for treatment. Although speech may be the most affected motor skill and the reason for the referral, assessment should include measures of nonspeech oral motor performance so that the underlying impairment may be isolated from the overall behavior. Each of the four systems (respiration, phonation, resonation, and articulation) may be impaired to different degrees, influencing speech production in different ways. Since all systems interact to carry out communicative demands in speech production, observations of only speech may obscure these differential contributions of the systems or their coordination in speech production. Thus, assessment of nonspeech oral motor performance designed to isolate a particular system or function is invaluable in determining the underlying impairment.

Measurement Methods

Professionals use perceptual, acoustic, and physiological measures to document motor speech disorders. Perceptual measures are the most common tools used to diagnose motor speech disorders, and these typically involve perceptual judgments of intelligibility, accuracy, and speed in an individual's speech production. The clinician listens to and watches the individual during a variety of speech and nonspeech motor tasks. Perceptual measures help the professional characterize the impact of the disorder on various aspects of speech (e.g., loudness, pitch, breath support) and are crucial for differentiating motor speech disorders. For instance, the professional can likely differentiate spastic dysarthria from flaccid dysarthria through perceptual observations alone.

Acoustic measures involve a visual representation of the speech sound wave (e.g., a spectrogram) and allow for more detailed examination of speech abnormalities that may not be perceptible to the professional's eye and ear. Several computer programs are available that transform the auditory signal into a visual form and include various analysis options, thus providing a relatively accessible measurement method (e.g., PRAAT, see Spotlight on Technology in Chapter 1). Acoustic measures can provide information on a wide range of aspects of speech, including both suprasegmental aspects of loudness, pitch,

DISCUSSION POINT:
Consider the case of Hikaru in Case Study 12.1. The speech evaluation provided detailed information on many aspects of Hikaru's speech and language skills. Consider each finding and whether it was obtained from perceptual, acoustic, physiological, or other measures.

and rate (e.g., Patel, 2003; Shriberg, Campbell, Karlsson, Brown, et al., 2003; Wang, Kent, Duffy, & Thomas, 2005) and segmental aspects of vowel and consonant accuracy and coarticulation (e.g., Ballard, Maas, & Robin, 2007; Nijland, Maassen, Van der Meulen, Gabreëls, et al., 2002).

Physiological measures involve measurement of physiological aspects of the speech motor system, such as muscle strength, endurance, and airflow. Some of these measures involve relatively simple equipment and tasks, such as blowing through a straw in a glass of water to assess breath support (Hixon, Hawley, & Wilson, 1982); others may require more elaborate equipment, such as videofluoroscopy to assess the phonatory and resonatory system (Duffy, 2005) or electropalatography to assess articulatory function (McAuliffe & Ward, 2006).

Complementing these tools are other measures used to examine language performance, as disorders of language frequently co-occur with motor speech disorders. In addition, memory, attention, vision, hearing, and mental health should also be examined to determine an individual's ability to process task instructions and perform and learn speech tasks both inside and outside the therapeutic setting. These assessments may be conducted by the speech-language pathologist or other team members, such as a neuropsychologist.

Referral

Patients are generally referred for a motor speech assessment by health care professionals, typically a pediatrician for children or a family physician for adults. In cases of acute injuries, such as TBI, speech-language pathologists are often part of an inpatient hospital team that evaluates the patient for the presence of motor speech and other communicative impairments. In cases of developmental disabilities that occur at or after birth, such as cerebral palsy, speech-language pathologists are often part of early intervention teams that provide multidisciplinary assessments of all critical areas of development. Some children, however, show signs of CAS only after they begin talking and have no other impairment. These children are often referred through their pediatrician at the request of their parents.

Screening

Screening of general motor speech performance is an important first step when people with suspected motor speech disorders are seen by a professional. The nature of the possible disorder is determined based on interviews with the client and the family. In addition, the person's medical history is obtained to determine the cause, or etiology, of the disorder and factors relevant to its prognosis (e.g., presence of strong social support system, smoking habit, history of depression, hypertension, progressive disease process). For adolescents and adults, it is important to interview both the client and the family, since they may have different perceptions of the disorder (Clark et al., 2000). For instance, an adolescent with suspected dysarthria following a TBI may view his or her speech difficulties as mild or insignificant, whereas family members may see the difficulties as severely detrimental to academic and social performance.

Comprehensive Motor Speech Evaluation

Assessment should include motor control tasks that involve speech and non-speech movements (Clark et al., 2000; Folkins et al., 1995). This practice is important to determine how much the language and motor systems contribute to observed speech difficulties. Often, a language impairment may be present simultaneously with a motor speech disorder, and the effect of the language impairment

DISCUSSION POINT:
Consider the cases of Bob and Hikaru in Case Study 12.1. Which of these individuals likely exhibits a language impairment in addition to a motor speech disorder? What evidence is available to support your view?

on speech production should be identified so that the impairments resulting from motor speech deficits can be identified separately. By definition, motor speech disorders involve an impairment of the motor system and thus cannot be explained by a language impairment. The examination of motor speech tasks that do not involve language (e.g., pursing the lips, smiling, clucking the tongue) should exhibit some degradations of motor control when a motor speech disorder is present, even if these degradations are subtle.

The professional assesses an individual's problems at each level of functioning—body structure, body function, and activity/participation—to determine the impact on daily life and to formulate appropriate therapy goals and strategies. Assessment of participation in life is difficult and typically depends on detailed interviews with the patient and the family. The effects of the speech disorder on daily life may also be observed in real-life situations (e.g., interactions with family, activities at work).

A comprehensive motor speech evaluation should include separate assessments of each of the speech systems to determine the contribution of each system to the overall speech disturbance. An overview of the tasks that may be used in evaluations for each system is provided in Table 12.3.

Respiration.   Motor speech disorders rarely result from isolated impairment of the respiratory system; however, when combined with impairments of the other speech production systems, respiratory difficulties can undermine speech. Symptoms might include short phrasings, reduced syllable repetitions, decreased speech rate, and uncontrolled phonation (Hardy, 1983; Thompson & Robin, 1993). Breathing may be irregular, shallow, or noisy, which may affect the rhythm, loudness, and rate of speech. The motor speech assessment encompasses tasks to examine the respiratory system, including both perceptual measures, such as examining how long the individual can sustain a breath, and physiological measures, such as examining an individual's vital capacity (the total amount of air that can be inspired into the lungs after emptying them fully) and respiratory driving pressure that can be generated to produce speech (i.e., using the technique of blowing into a glass of water with a straw; Hixon et al., 1982).

Phonation.   The motor speech system assessment also involves careful study of the phonatory system. For some people with motor speech disorders, phonation is directly impaired because there is abnormal strength or control of the muscles in the larynx. Or, phonation may be impaired due to deficits in the other speech production systems, particularly respiration. A variety of phonatory problems may be observed in motor speech disorders, including reduced loudness, variable loudness, sudden changes in pitch or reduction in pitch range, and breathy or harsh voice quality (Davis, 1982; Thompson & Robin, 1993). The motor speech assessment examines the phonatory system using perceptual, acoustic, and physiological measures, as described in Table 12.3.

Resonation.   Individuals with motor speech disorders may exhibit an impairment of the functioning of the velum, the pharynx, or both. Either structure may exhibit a decreased range or speed of motion, changes in muscle tone, and abnormal reflexes (Thompson & Robin, 1993). In addition, patients may compensate for slowed movements of the velum by reducing their speech rate. These deficits in functioning typically affect resonatory characteristics—for example, resulting in hypernasality. The motor speech assessment examines resonatory characteristics using perceptual tasks, such as watching the velum functioning

TABLE 12.3	Tasks used to assess motor speech function	
Subsystem	**Method**	**Task**
Respiration	Perceptual	Observe an inhalation-exhalation cycle for a deep breath
		Observe breathing during rest and conversation
		Count words per exhalation during counting
		Observe a prolonged vowel "ah"
		Observe counting from one to ten
	Physiological	Determine vital capacity
		Study body posture during speech
		Determine respiratory pressure and flow during speaking tasks
Phonation	Perceptual	Study voice quality during conversation
		Compare voiced consonant-vowel repetitions (*ba-ba*) to unvoiced consonant-vowel repetitions (*pa-pa*)
		Study ability to vary pitch and loudness during conversation
		Examine ability to vary pitch and loudness from minimum to maximum on vowel sound
	Acoustic	Determine pitch and intensity range during conversation
		Determine fundamental frequency for sustained vowel sounds
	Physiological	Study laryngeal resistance during vowel production
		Study the vibration patterns of vocal folds during vocalization
Resonation	Perceptual	Observe production of prolonged /s/
		Observe counting from one to ten
		Examine for nasal emissions during counting using a dental mirror under the nose
	Physiological	Use nasendoscopy to study palatal movement for sustained vowel sound
		Use videofluoroscopy to study velopharyngeal functioning during conversation
Articulation	Perceptual	Conduct oral mechanism assessment to include all structures and functions
		Examine ability to repeat multisyllable words and sentences of varying complexity
		Examine performance during automatic speech tasks like counting and reciting days of the week
	Physiological	Conduct EMG to study timing of articulatory gestures of lip, jaw, and tongue for different syllables

Sources: Barlow (1999); Clark, Stierwalt, & Robin (2000); Love (1992).

during a sustained "aah" and looking for nasal emissions during production of oral sounds. For instance, when producing a sentence like "Bob took a cookie out of the box," the velum should be raised throughout the sentence (i.e., there should be no perception of nasality). One way to assess nasal airflow is by holding a small mirror under the nose during production of such sentences or prolonged vowels; nasal airflow will fog up the mirror. The assessment may also use physiological measures, such as nasendoscopy, which examines the functioning of the velopharyngeal port when producing speech sounds.

Articulation.   Motor speech disorders often result in abnormal articulation. This can arise from impairments of the other systems, such as the respiratory system. Reduced capacity for breath support, as occurs in some cases of dysarthria, may lead to reduced pressure in the oral cavity necessary for production of, say, stop sounds. However, articulatory abnormalities may also result from impairment of the articulatory system itself. For example, reduced muscle strength of the tongue may impede the ability to produce lingual sounds, including all the vowels and most of the consonants. Depending on the particular muscles involved and the extent of the neuromuscular deficits, a variety of articulatory problems may be observed, including speech-sound substitutions and distortions and reduced speech rate.

When examining the articulatory system, the clinician studies the stability of speech errors under different circumstances. If a motor speech disorder is the result of a basic physiological malfunction of the articulatory system, as in muscle paralysis in some dysarthrias, speech errors are likely to be consistent across repetitions, contexts, and tasks (e.g., in repetition, reading, and spontaneous speech). In contrast, if the motor speech disorder results from a malfunction in the coordination or planning and programming of speech (as in apraxia of speech), errors may be more variable across repetitions, contexts, and tasks. The individual may produce a given sound clearly and accurately in one word but not in another, and performance may vary depending on the context in which the sound is elicited. For instance, a phrase may be produced accurately in an automatic or reflexive response, such as greeting someone entering a room, but the phrase may be degraded in its sounds and intelligibility in a volitional task, as with a greeting that is elicited (e.g., "Say this: 'Hello, Mr. Green. I am happy to see you today'").

The motor speech assessment involves a variety of perceptual, acoustic, and physiological tasks for assessing the articulatory system. Of great importance is the professional's ability to closely study the individual's motor speech performance perceptually during a variety of structured and unstructured tasks. The professional will supplement these perceptual observations of motor speech performance with tools that document intensity and loudness in different speech tasks and that study how well the larynx functions.

Prosody.   Although prosody is not generally considered a separate system of speech production, it is an important aspect of speech that characterizes a person's naturalness when speaking. The ability to produce normal prosody results from a complex interaction of all speech production systems and therefore is critical in understanding and treating motor speech disorders. Specifically, prosody requires the controlled exhalation of air divided across a series of syllables (for assigning relative loudness and duration), coordinated with the phonatory system (for assigning relative pitch differences) and the articulatory system (for extending or shortening articulator movements relative to syllable duration). Disorders of prosody may help differentiate between impairments, because by examining prosodic aspects of speech, the professional can determine what systems of speech production are most affected by the disorder.

Assessment of prosody examines the individual's prosodic variations in different types of language use, such as producing a declarative versus an interrogative sentence (e.g., "This is new" versus "Is this new?"), highlighting contrastive

DISCUSSION POINT:
In the case of Bob in Case Study 12.1, which aspects of prosody might be impaired? Describe some tasks that could be used to test his ability to vary prosody.

SPOTLIGHT ON TECHNOLOGY

EMMA

Assessment of the speech motor system may involve perceptual, acoustic, and physiological measures. Analysis of kinematics (movement trajectory, velocity, and acceleration) can provide further insight into abnormal speech motor execution and planning. One current state-of-the-art technique that allows simultaneous tracking of articulator movements both inside and outside the oral cavity is electromagnetic midsagittal articulography, or EMMA (Perkell, Cohen, Svirsky, Matthies, et al., 1992). Small transducer coils are glued to certain articulators (e.g., tongue blade and dorsum) and produce an electric signal when they move through an alternating magnetic field generated by transmitter coils mounted on the speaker's head (see figure below). The electric signal represents the movement trajectory from which velocity and acceleration can be calculated.

Although EMMA equipment is expensive and requires considerable time and expertise to operate, thus limiting its application in everyday clinical practice, it is being used to study the nature of motor speech disorders (e.g., Murdoch & Goozée, 2003; Van Lieshout, Bose, Square, & Steele, 2007). For example, Murdoch and Goozée (2003) showed that children with dysarthria secondary to TBI (all of whom had perceived slow speech rate) demonstrated different kinematic sources of this perceived rate reduction. EMMA is also being used experimentally to provide biofeedback in treatment of AOS (e.g., Katz, Bharadwaj, & Carstens, 1999); findings to date are promising, in that providing visual feedback of the movement trajectory can enhance relearning of speech production in treatment for AOS.

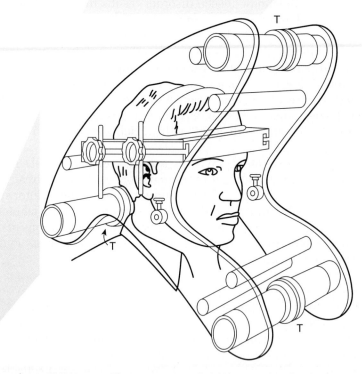

View of speaker in EMMA setup. The transmitter coils (T) that generate the alternating magnetic field are mounted on the three cylinders. Transducer coils on the articulators are not shown (from Perkell et al., 1992).

information (e.g., "She likes the BROWN dog" in response to the question "Does she like the black dog?"), and indicating different emotional states (e.g., happy, angry, surprised; Cheang & Pell, 2007; Seddoh & Robin, 2001). In addition to perceptual observations of prosodic variations, professionals use acoustic measures to provide important information about which aspect of prosody is impaired (e.g., loudness, duration, pitch, rhythm).

Diagnosis

Following the motor speech assessment, the professional interprets findings to arrive at a speech diagnosis. Depending on the findings, a patient may receive a diagnosis of one of the various motor speech disorders discussed previously. A diagnosis that differentiates a person's disorder from other similar disorders—for example, spastic dysarthria from flaccid dysarthria—is called a *differential diagnosis*. It is important to note that a differential diagnosis of a motor speech disorder is based primarily on the perceptual findings and judgment of the clinician, which are derived from extensive experience. No one test can provide a differential diagnosis.

Differential diagnosis in motor speech disorders is important, because the type of treatment depends on the nature of the disorder, and what may be effective for one disorder may not be effective for another. For example, a focus on improving posture and breathing may be useful for patients who have a respiratory system impairment but may not lead to improved speech for patients with aphasia or tongue paralysis.

HOW ARE MOTOR SPEECH DISORDERS TREATED? ●

Individuals with motor speech disorders often have other clinical problems, such as aphasia, limb paralysis, hypertension, or a learning disability. Therefore, treatment options are typically explored and recommended by an interdisciplinary team consisting of physicians, physical therapists, occupational therapists, neuropsychologists, teachers, speech-language pathologists, and the client and their family.

TREATMENT GOALS

Treatment for the motor speech impairment itself is typically provided by the speech-language pathologist through inpatient or outpatient therapy. An important consideration in treatment is clear identification of therapy goals. In motor speech treatment, the goal is to *learn or relearn accurate production of speech* for improved speech intelligibility. In many treatment contexts, professionals face great pressure to achieve maximal progress with limited resources (time, money, staff). Earlier, we defined *motor learning* as the way in which practice or experience leads to relatively *permanent* changes in the *capability* for movement (Schmidt & Lee, 2005; italics added). Accordingly, a primary goal of treatment is that an individual not only learn a new skill, but also maintain that skill over time to show evidence of permanent changes. Thus, it is important to distinguish between temporary performance enhancements observed during treatment (acquisition) and lasting performance enhancements that are maintained after treatment has ended (retention). Evidence from the motor learning literature strongly suggests that improvements during acquisition do not necessarily result in improvements during retention tests (e.g., Schmidt & Bjork, 1992; Schmidt & Lee, 2005). In fact, the factors that enhance acquisition may have negative effects on retention (e.g., Schmidt & Bjork, 1992). This finding has important implications for evaluating the outcomes of motor speech treatment (Maas et al., 2008). In many settings, progress is measured almost exclusively in terms of acquisition, yet the hope is that improvements observed during treatment will continue after treatment ends. Thus, measures of retention must be included to determine the effectiveness of the treatment for permanent improvements.

A second important goal of treatment relates to **generalization,** which refers to application or transfer of a skill to related but untrained movement patterns. In addition to retention, treatment should aim to facilitate an individual's underlying capability for movement so that untrained tasks also improve. Two types of generalizations are desirable (Ballard, 2001; Wambaugh & Nessler, 2004): (1) *response generalization* refers to improvements of untrained behaviors (e.g., speech sounds), and (2) *stimulus generalization* refers to improvement of targeted behaviors in different contexts, tasks, or settings (e.g., in conversational speech versus repetition tasks).

Goals in the treatment of motor speech disorders must thus consider improvements and treatment effectiveness in terms of retention and generalization and not simply measure temporary performance enhancements observed during acquisition.

TARGETS AND STRATEGIES

Treatment Targets

Clinical professionals carefully select treatment targets based on the nature of an individual's speech difficulties and the impact of the speech disorder on daily living function. When deciding on targets for treatment programs, clinicians must answer several questions, including, Should we target speech or nonspeech motor tasks? Should we target simple speech tasks or complex speech tasks? A brief discussion of these important questions follows.

Speech and Nonspeech Tasks.   Some clinicians select both speech and nonspeech treatment targets. For instance, a clinician may target improved intelligibility of certain speech sounds or words while also targeting improved tongue strength and range of motion. The latter types of activities are called *oral motor exercises* (Clark, 2003). The tongue-strength and range-of-motion targets are selected based on the notion that certain basic physiological components (such as muscle strength) must be targeted in isolation in order to be functional in speech production. However, it is important to note that increasing nonspeech motor movements, in this case for a patient with tongue muscle weakness, will not likely improve speech intelligibility. In fact, evidence suggests that practicing oral motor exercises will not result in improved speech production (e.g., Clark, 2003). Since presumably the goal of speech therapy is to improve speech production, it seems reasonable to target speech as an integrated behavior with an emphasis on intelligibility and using speech to communicate functionally.

Some patients may be unable to produce speech in early stages of treatment, particularly after an acute incident, such as stroke. In such cases, targeting isolated speech sounds or articulatory movements may be justified. For instance, an individual may not be able to produce any speech sounds, and the clinician may select specific speech sounds to target (e.g., /b/, /m/). However, given that the goal of speech treatment is to improve speech production, speech targets should be included as early as possible.

Simple and Complex Tasks.   The selection of treatment targets should consider the complexity or difficulty level of the target behavior. For instance, producing sounds intelligibly in a phrase (e.g., "I want some milk") is clearly more complex than producing sounds in isolation (e.g., *m-m-m*). Some experts contend that focusing on more complex targets results in greater learning than does focusing on simpler targets (e.g., Gierut, 2007; Maas, Barlow, Robin, & Shapiro, 2002; Thompson, Ballard, & Shapiro, 1998). Targeting complex sounds, syllables, and sentences leads to improvements in these targeted items and in simpler but untrained items. In contrast, when clinicians target simpler items in therapy, these items improve, but more complex items do not. These recent findings from clinical research show that when a patient is unable to produce either a simple or a complex item, targeting the complex item (e.g., consonant clusters as in *struck*) will improve both simple and complex items (e.g., *struck, truck,* and *tuck*), whereas targeting the simple item (e.g., *tuck*) improves only that simple item. This finding is important clinically, because it suggests that the simpler items do not need to be specifically targeted, which can make treatment more efficient. It is important to note, however, that these recent research findings go against a common approach in clinical treatment that involves beginning with simple items and working up to more complex items.

Treatment Strategies

The goal of treatments for motor speech disorders is generally to improve the accuracy, stability, and intelligibility of speech and its naturalness or fluency. The two primary therapeutic strategies are to (1) improve the impaired system(s) and (2) teach compensatory strategies.

Improvement of individual systems involves focusing on specific functions in relevant speech tasks—for example, by emphasizing the modification of speech breathing patterns, using intonation in utterances, or saying words with specific speech sounds that are difficult. More specific approaches for each system are presented in the next sections.

In addition to directly targeting impaired abilities, teaching compensatory strategies may also be useful. Compensatory strategies may focus on the individual with a motor speech disorder or on the environment and communication partners. These strategies may include slowing down the rate of speech and using gestures, writing, or alternative and augmentative communication devices such as communication books and handheld computers (e.g., Ball, Beukelman, & Pattee, 2004; Van de Sandt-Koenderman, Wiegers, Wielaert, Duivenvoorden, et al., 2007). Clinicians also need to consider the WHO levels of activity/participation and contextual factors by working with family members and other communication partners as well as by making environmental adaptations. Compensatory strategies in this regard may involve environmental modifications (e.g., noise reduction) and communication partner training. For example, communication partners may be instructed to ask more effective yes/no questions.

> **DISCUSSION POINT:**
> For multilingual speakers such as Bob and Hikaru, described in Case Study 12.1, in what language should intervention be provided?

Conditions of Practice and Feedback.   In addition to considering the different levels of functioning based on the WHO model and selecting appropriate treatment targets and strategies, other aspects related to the conditions of practice should also be given careful consideration. A number of principles have been derived from studies on motor learning; in particular, some conditions of practice have been shown to enhance acquisition but impede learning (as measured by retention and transfer), whereas other conditions enhance learning but may not facilitate acquisition to the same extent (e.g., Schmidt & Lee, 2005; Wulf & Shea, 2004). These conditions are relatively easy to implement regardless of the specific treatment program used, and they may have a powerful influence on the extent of learning as revealed through retention and generalization. These conditions can be divided into those related to practice and those related to feedback (see Maas et al., 2008, for a review).

Conditions of Practice.   Conditions of practice refer to factors such as the number of different targets practiced (**practice variability**), the order in which different targets are practiced (**practice schedule**), the number of practice trials (**practice amount**), and how close in time the practice sessions are spaced (**practice distribution**). Evidence from the motor learning literature suggests that learning is greater with a large number of practice trials (e.g., Giuffrida, Shea, & Fairbrother, 2002), consistent with the old adage "practice makes perfect," and when practice sessions or trials are spaced out over time rather than close together (e.g., Shea, Lai, Black, & Park, 2000). For instance, if one plans to do 1,000 practice trials, it might be better for retention and transfer to do these in ten sessions of 100 trials with 2 days between sessions than to do them in two 500-trial sessions on consecutive days. In addition, retention and generalization are expected to be greater when the learner practices multiple targets (variable practice) instead of just one (constant practice; Giuffrida et al., 2002)—for example in shooting a basketball into the basket from different distances instead of the same distance—and when the learner practices targets in random order instead of in blocks (e.g., Shea & Morgan, 1979; Wright, Black, Immink, Brueckner, et al., 2004)—for example, shooting the basketball from different distances in random order rather than in sets of trials from the same distance. This is so even though performance *during the practice session itself* (acquisition) may be better with constant and blocked practice. Thus, the distinction between acquisition and true learning as indicated by retention and generalization is critical and requires professionals to periodically assess retention and generalization of learning.

With respect to treatment of motor speech disorders, particularly AOS, available evidence is generally consistent with the benefits of variable practice and random practice (e.g., Ballard et al., 2007; Knock, Ballard, Robin, & Schmidt, 2000; see Maas et al., 2008, for a review). Variable practice might be implemented by including multiple words with a given target sound, in different word positions—for example *summer, bus,* and *eraser* for /s/, or by including multiple sounds of a given class, such as *zip, voice, fame* for fricatives (e.g., Ballard et al., 2007; Wambaugh, Martinez, McNeil, & Rogers, 1999). Random practice might be implemented by selecting several treatment targets and eliciting them in random order rather than in sets grouped by target (e.g., Knock et al., 2000).

Conditions of Feedback.   A second set of conditions relates to how feedback on performance is provided, including **feedback frequency** (how often the learner receives feedback) and **feedback timing** (how soon after an attempt the learner receives feedback; Wulf & Shea, 2004). For example, providing feedback after each attempt at production (100% feedback) may enhance acquisition relative to providing feedback on fewer attempts, but when one examines retention and generalization, reduced frequency of feedback is found to be more effective (e.g., Bruechert, Lai, & Shea, 2003; Wulf, Schmidt, & Deubel, 1993). Another example relates to the timing of feedback; specifically, it has been found that delaying feedback a few seconds after the attempt results in greater learning than providing immediate feedback (e.g., Swinnen, Schmidt, Nicholson, & Shapiro, 1990). One interpretation of these effects is that reduced frequency feedback and delayed feedback encourage learners to evaluate their own responses and detect errors, thereby strengthening their internal evaluation processes and error-detection mechanisms needed for schema updating. By contrast, 100% feedback and immediate feedback encourage reliance on external, clinician-provided feedback, which may prevent or discourage the development or strengthening of internal error-detection mechanisms. In addition, immediate feedback may disrupt ongoing internal evaluation processes that occur immediately following each movement.

Available evidence regarding speech motor learning in speakers with motor speech disorders is consistent with the findings from the motor learning literature (e.g., Adams, Page, & Jog, 2002; Austermann Hula, Robin, Maas, Ballard, et al., 2008). For example, in two separate studies, Austermann Hula et al. (2008) showed that reducing the frequency of feedback and delaying the provision of feedback enhanced learning in speakers with AOS.

In short, given that these conditions of practice and feedback have been shown to apply in motor learning, it is reasonable to expect them to influence learning in treatment for motor speech disorders as well (e.g., McNeil et al., 1997); indeed, there is evidence that this is the case (Maas et al., 2008). These conditions are independent of the specific treatment targets and can be implemented in any treatment session. Considering their potentially powerful role in speech motor learning, these conditions should be considered in treatment for motor speech disorders.

Pretreatment Considerations.   Treatment is most effective when the clinician pays careful attention to what the client brings to the therapy context. The most influential client characteristics for motor speech treatment include memory, attention, and motivation. Another important consideration relates to establishing a reference of correctness. Descriptions of these considerations are drawn from McNeil and colleagues (1997); much of the following discussion regarding treatment of specific subsystems is based on Duffy (2005) and Yorkston et al. (1999).

> **DISCUSSION POINT:**
> Consider the case of Bob in Case Study 12.1. What indicators are available to suggest that treatment may or may not be effective?

Memory: Since learning involves storing information in long-term memory, it is important to determine whether any memory impairments are present in addition to the motor speech disorder. A memory impairment may impede learning and the potential benefits of therapy.

Attention: If a client has limited capacity to focus and sustain attention, learning may be impeded as well; therapy sessions may be structured in such a way as to maximize attention (e.g., by providing frequent breaks).

Motivation: The client's motivation is important to learning. Understanding the relevance of the therapy task to the goal of improving speech production may help motivate the patient to perform the exercise.

Reference of Correctness: The client needs a reference of correctness to know which productions are considered normal or acceptable and which are not. This reference enables the learner to develop internal error-detection mechanisms.

Treatment of the Respiratory System.   Treatment of the respiratory system may focus on improving respiratory support, modifying inspiration and exhalation and their interrelationship, increasing respiratory flexibility, or a combination of these goals, depending on the nature of the motor speech problem. To improve respiratory support, the clinician works with the client to improve and control the buildup of subglottal air pressure; adjust and improve posture for improved breath support; and if needed, provide a respiratory prosthesis, such as a paddle or a board to push against.

Activities to modify inspiration and exhalation may include increasing the duration of air intake and using various ways of monitoring the duration (e.g., tactile, visual, auditory, torso monitoring). Increasing the inhaled lung volume will also assist exhalation through elastic recoil of the diaphragm. Modifying exhalation can begin with vowel prolongation and counting (e.g., say "ah" for 10 seconds, then 12 seconds, then 15 seconds, etc.), followed by production of larger units of speech, including phrases and sentences (e.g., say "My neighbor," "My neighbor has a dog," "My neighbor has a big black dog," "My neighbor has a big black dog that barks all day"). Since speech breathing involves rapid inhalations with protracted exhalations, it is important to establish or improve the appropriate relationship between these two parts of the respiratory cycle. For example, the clinician can train brief inhalations followed by controlled, slow exhalations in using vowels and then consonants. Furthermore, speakers may be taught where to take inhalations relative to breath groups and clause boundaries, and to hold their breath until exhalation and speech can begin. For instance, if the sentence "My neighbor has a big black dog that barks all day" is too long for a single breath group, then the clinician might indicate appropriate locations for inhalation depending on the clause structure of utterances (e.g., "My neighbor (inhale) has a big black dog (inhale), that barks all day"). Maladaptive respiratory patterns should be eliminated if possible.

Treatment of the Phonatory System.   Treatment of the phonatory system may focus on improving voice quality or on controlling the vocal folds to enhance production of prosodic aspects of speech and thereby enhance the naturalness of speech. Treatment approaches to improving voice quality are described in Chapter 11 and may include postural adjustments and training to increase effort when producing voice. For some individuals with hypokinetic dysarthria secondary to Parkinson's disease, a treatment focused on speaking loudly has been shown to be effective (e.g., Ramig, Sapir, Fox, & Countryman, 2001; Spielman, Ramig, Mahler, Halpern, et al., 2007). In some cases of hyperkinetic dysarthria affecting the laryngeal muscles, medical procedures such as injecting botulinum toxin (Botox) into the laryngeal muscles may be beneficial (e.g., Murry & Woodson, 1995). Treatments to improve prosody are discussed below.

Treatment of the Resonatory System.   Treatment of the strength and control of the velopharyngeal port may involve having the patient view nasal airflow in the form of biofeedback or by practicing nasal versus oral airflow patterns (negative practice). The use of a palatal lift, a device that helps raise the velum, should be considered when resonatory difficulties severely impact intelligibility. For some speakers with flaccid dysarthria affecting the velum, exercises to strengthen the velum-raising muscles in the context of speech production using continuous positive airway pressure (CPAP) may be beneficial (e.g., Cahill et al., 2004). In this treatment, the speaker produces words with nasal sounds followed by non-nasal sounds (e.g., *under*), which requires raising the velum midword; air pressure is supplied into the nose through a mask so as to provide resistance to velar raising.

Treatment of the Articulatory System. Generally, an individual's completion of nonspeech tasks, such as oral motor exercises, has little if any effect on speech production. Therefore, improving speech production requires the use of authentic speech tasks. Exceptions may involve patients whose impairment is so severe as to preclude production of even the simplest speech sounds or utterances. Articulatory treatment should focus the patient's attention on the adequacy of the speech signal. The clinician provides feedback, including modeling the target or using a diagram with a possible articulatory configuration, to guide improved articulation. However, focusing on the speech signal may be more effective than focusing on particular articulator configurations, because a focus on one's body movements may interfere with learning as opposed to a focus on the effects of those movements (e.g., Freedman, Maas, Caligiuri, Wulf, et al., 2007; Wulf, McConnel, Gärtner, & Schwarz, 2002). In addition, the same speech signal can be produced, within certain limits, using different articulatory configurations (for example, think of ventriloquists); some of these may be more easily achieved than others for a given speaker. For example, flaccid paralysis of the lips may prevent production of bilabial sounds, but speakers may produce acceptable "bilabial-sounding" sounds by making a constriction with the tongue and palate, as has been observed in some children with flaccid dysarthria (e.g., DeFeo & Schaefer, 1983; Nelson & Hodge, 2000). Since the goal of speech movements is to produce an adequate auditory signal for the listener (e.g., Guenther, Hampson, & Johnson, 1998), a focus on the speech signal may be more useful than a focus on specific articulator configurations. Visual representations of the acoustic signal may be used to highlight relevant aspects of the signal as a form of biofeedback (e.g., Ballard et al., 2007).

Treatment of Prosody and Rate Control. Prosody is essential for producing natural-sounding speech and involves manipulation of three factors: loudness, pitch, and duration. Impairments of prosody may result from reductions in the range or control of any of these factors. Treatment should include exercises geared toward increasing the range and control of the affected factors. For example, the professional may lead the client through contrastive stress drills, such as producing sets of words or phrases that differ only in stress pattern (e.g., *differ* and *defer* or *a project* and *to project*) and asking questions that elicit differential stress or intonation patterns (e.g., "Is the ball in the red *bag*?" "No, the ball is in the red *box*").

Speech rate contributes significantly to intelligibility, and it may be helpful to reduce the rate of speech, even if it is already slower than normal. There are two types of techniques to improve speech rate: rigid control techniques and nonrigid control techniques (Yorkston et al., 1999). Rigid control techniques disrupt natural prosody; examples include pacing boards and alphabet boards, where the speaker touches a board with every syllable or points to the first

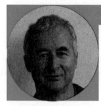

SPOTLIGHT ON RESEARCH AND PRACTICE

NAME: WOLFRAM ZIEGLER

PROFESSION/TITLE
Head of Clinical Neuropsychology Research Group (EKN),
Clinic for Neuropsychology, Bogenhausen Hospital, Munich

PROFESSIONAL RESPONSIBILITIES
My professional responsibilities include primarily (1) design and management of research projects; (2) discussions with students and collaborators on patients, diagnoses, clinical and experimental data, research designs, etc; (3) administrative duties as head of research group; and (4) education of speech therapists and phonetics students.

ACADEMIC DEGREES/TRAINING
Diploma in Mathematics and Computer Science, Technical University, Munich
Ph.D. in Mathematics, Technical University, Munich
"Habilitation" and Associate Professorship for Neurophonetics,
Ludwig-Maximilians University, Munich

HOW INTERESTS IN COMMUNICATION SCIENCES AND DISORDERS BEGAN
As a doctoral student, I received a Ph.D. grant from the Max-Planck Society. After I had finished my thesis, I followed the law of inertia and remained at the institute that had paid for my Ph.D.— Detlev von Cramon's department at the Max-Planck Institute for Psychiatry. As a student assistant, I started developing and implementing computer algorithms for the analysis of pathological speech. I analyzed speech samples from severely dysarthric patients after closed-head injuries. This work attracted my interest in questions relating to the patients and their disorder more than my interest in the computer stuff itself.

CURRENT RESEARCH AND PRACTICE INTERESTS
Apraxia of speech, dysarthria, phonological impairment

MOST EXCITING/INTERESTING PROFESSIONAL ACCOMPLISHMENT
IN COMMUNICATION SCIENCES AND DISORDERS
The work I have done, together with students, on the factors that influence error generation in apraxia of speech and on the modeling of speech errors. In my view, this work may open a window to the understanding of normal speech mechanisms and to new treatment approaches.

FUTURE TRENDS IN COMMUNICATION SCIENCES AND DISORDERS
Instrumental methods will have to find their place in the clinical assessment and treatment of speech disorders. I still believe in the clinical value of auditory methods, in the first place, and of acoustic analyses, in the second. Conceptually, the understanding of the speech motor component in the language production system will change. I don't see the classical, sharp divide between "linguistic" and "motor" to persist in the future.

letter of each word. Nonrigid techniques maintain natural prosody; examples include rhythmic cueing (in which the clinician points to words in a text at a given rate) and computerized cueing (words are presented on the screen one at a time at a given rate, or words in a text are highlighted at a given rate, and the speaker produces only those words).

CASE ANALYSIS

Study the case of Andy Duvall (Case Study 8 on the Companion Website at www .pearsonhighered.com/justice2e). What factors in his life suggest he may resolve his speech difficulties?

CHAPTER SUMMARY

Speech production involves the coordination in space and time of four separate systems of speech production: the respiratory, phonatory, resonatory, and articulatory subsystems. Each of these systems may be impaired independently and to different degrees. These systems exhibit impairments due to deficits at the level of motor planning and preprogramming or at the level of execution.

There are two categories of motor speech disorders, both of which are caused by a neurological impairment of the motor systems involved with speech production. Apraxia of speech results from a disruption of motor planning or programming, whereas dysarthria results from a disruption of basic aspects of the motor system (e.g., muscle weakness, abnormal muscle tone). Both dysarthria and apraxia of speech have acquired and developmental variants, the former describing disorders that result from injury, disease, or illness to the neurological systems and the latter describing disorders present at birth.

Assessment examines motor performance in both nonspeech and speech activities. Assessment of nonspeech oral motor performance is essential to determine the relative contribution of the respiratory, phonatory, articulatory, and resonatory systems to the speech impairment. The functioning of each system and their collective involvement in efficient and intelligible speech is considered at the levels of body structure and function, activity and participation in life, and the environmental context. Assessment may involve perceptual, acoustic, and physiological measures.

The goal of treatment for motor speech disorders is to improve the accuracy, stability, and intelligibility and naturalness of speech. Treatment aims to maximize learning to ensure that effects are maintained over time and to show generalization to other, untrained tasks. Treatment targets should primarily include speech, and the clinician should consider the complexity of targets, as there is evidence suggesting that more complex targets may lead to better learning. Specific approaches are used to treat impairments of the respiratory, phonatory, articulatory, and resonatory systems.

KEY TERMS

apraxia of speech, p. 405
articulatory system, p. 397
dysarthria, p. 408
feedback frequency, p. 420
feedback timing, p. 420
generalization, p. 418
motor execution, p. 400
motor execution disorders, p. 404
motor learning, p. 401
motor planning, p. 400
motor planning and programming
    disorders, p. 404

motor programming, p. 400
motor speech disorder, p. 393
motor unit (motor program),
    p. 399
movement coordination, p. 408
movement range, p. 408
movement speed, p. 408
movement steadiness, p. 408
muscle strength, p. 408
muscle tone, p. 408
participation in life, p. 404
phonatory system, p. 396

practice amount, p. 420
practice distribution, p. 420
practice schedule, p. 420
practice variability, p. 420
resonatory system, p. 397
respiratory system, p. 395
schemas, p. 401
speech motor control, p. 393
velopharyngeal port, p. 397

ON THE WEB

Check out the Companion Website at www .pearsonhighered.com/justice2e. On it, you will find:

- suggested readings
- reflection questions

- a self-study quiz
- links to additional online resources, including information about current technologies in communication sciences and disorders

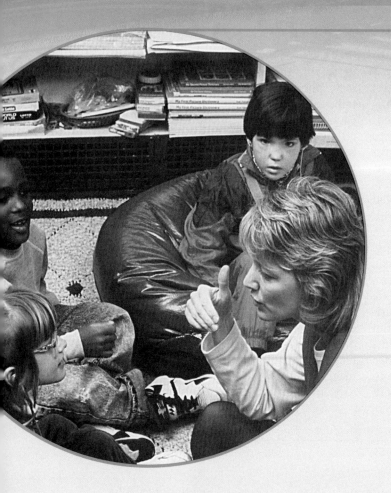

PEDIATRIC HEARING LOSS

L. A. Pakulski

FOCUS QUESTIONS

This chapter answers the following questions:

1 What is pediatric hearing loss?

2 How is pediatric hearing loss classified?

3 What are the defining characteristics of prevalent types of pediatric hearing loss?

4 How is pediatric hearing loss identified?

5 How is pediatric hearing loss treated?

6 What is an auditory processing disorder, and how is it identified and treated?

CHAPTER 13

INTRODUCTION

Deafness is a much worse misfortune [than blindness] for it means the loss of the most vital stimulus—the sound of the voice that brings language, sets thoughts astir, and keeps us in the intellectual company of man. *(Helen Keller, 1933)*

The sense of hearing is miraculous. The ear contains the smallest bones in the human body and has specialized sensory cells that can process sounds ranging from the drop of a pin to the takeoff of an airplane. The human ear can also perceive minute changes in pitch and loudness, recognize a familiar voice on the telephone, and differentiate among the many sounds at an amusement park. In short, hearing links us to the world around us. When an individual's hearing is diminished or lost because of injury, illness, or even genetics, the results are life-altering.

The human auditory system is a complicated mechanism. It is responsible for detecting, categorizing, and comprehending sounds. For instance, it distinguishes speech from nonspeech sounds and then enables comprehension of speech within the language centers. Because of these complexities, impairment of the auditory mechanism is also complex, resulting in many types of hearing problems. Consider the elderly person who complains, "I can hear just fine, if only people wouldn't mumble." This individual is able to detect the overall loudness of sound but misses enough auditory cues to make it difficult to understand what others say.

Speech-language pathologists, audiologists, and educators play important roles in diagnosing and treating children with hearing loss. To work effectively with these children, professionals must understand the auditory mechanism and its disorders, the impact of the disorder on children's social and academic selves, and a variety of intervention strategies to promote children's achievement possibilities. ●●●

WHAT IS PEDIATRIC HEARING LOSS? ●

DEFINITION

A pediatric **hearing loss** refers to a condition in which a child or adolescent is unable to detect or distinguish the range of sounds normally available to the human ear. In some cases, children are born unable to hear at typical levels. In other cases, children's hearing acuity is lost sometime after birth because of an illness, injury, or trauma. Chapter 3 described how the perception and processing of auditory information moves from the outer to the middle to the

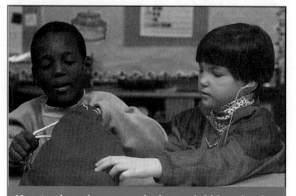

Hearing loss that occurs before a child has developed language is called a *prelingual hearing loss.*

inner ear and then along the auditory nerve to the brain's processing centers. Accordingly, a hearing loss can result from damage to the structures of the outer, middle, or inner ear and occasionally the auditory nerve. Hearing losses resulting from damage to the processing centers of the brain are called **auditory processing disorders** (APD) and are discussed in the final section of this chapter.

Hearing loss among children is highly variable. First, there is variability in the location of damage to the hearing structures. Hearing loss resulting from damage to the outer or middle ear is different from the loss resulting from damage to the inner ear. Second, because humans have two ears, hearing loss varies in whether it affects both ears, called a *bilateral* hearing loss, or whether it affects only one ear, called a *unilateral* hearing loss. Third, hearing loss varies considerably in the extent to which hearing acuity is

CASE STUDY 13.1   Pediatric Hearing Loss

MESHA is a 12-month-old child who was recently diagnosed with profound sensorineural hearing loss. Her father, Michael, also has a significant hearing loss and considers himself Deaf—that is, a member of the Deaf community. Michael was raised in the Deaf community by his parents and grandparents; all of his siblings are Deaf, too. Michael's family and friends communicate with American Sign Language (ASL), e-mail, and instant messaging on the Internet. He feels fortunate to have a full and happy life.

Michael's hearing loss is not as severe as that of his siblings; he attended a mainstream school and learned to speak. However, despite his fine voice and good oral-speaking skills, he chooses not to talk in most circumstances; he considers ASL his primary language. Even though he believes he received a better education than his siblings, who attended a residential school for the deaf, Michael does not want Mesha to grow up conflicted between a hearing and a deaf world. He believes that she should have a strong identity as a Deaf person. Michael's wife, Debra, agrees. Although she does not have a hearing loss, Debra embraces the Deaf community and shares her husband's conviction that Mesha should be raised with her Deaf culture first. Until Mesha was born, Debra did not feel accepted by Michael's family since she herself is not deaf. However, after having a daughter who is deaf, Debra feels that she is becoming a part of the community.

At 12 months, Mesha is signing a few words and actively communicates with her family. Michael and Debra have decided not to get hearing aids for Mesha. For the time being, they are satisfied that she is a well-adjusted child who interacts with her family and is learning new words every day.

Internet research

1. How large is the Deaf community in the United States?

2. How does the Deaf community view amplification devices, such as hearing aids and cochlear implants?

3. As a native user of ASL, Mesha will have what kind of educational programs available to her through the U.S. public school system?

Brainstorm and discussion

1. If you were an interventionist working with Mesha and her parents, would you endorse their decision? Why or why not?

2. What challenges face children who are raised in the Deaf versus the hearing community?

● ● ●

ASHLEY is a 9-year-old girl who was diagnosed with bilateral sensorineural hearing loss in the first few years of life. Like many others, the cause of her hearing loss is unknown. Since Ashley's hearing loss is progressive and because she was born before newborn hearing screening, it is unclear whether she had hearing loss at birth or whether it developed in the first year of life. Her parents noticed that she was not responding to environmental sounds and sought testing. Her hearing loss has progressed to the severe range (70–80 dB). She uses pink bilateral in-the-ear digital hearing aids. Ashley also experiences chronic otitis media with effusion, which contributes to additional fluctuating conductive hearing loss. Currently, Ashley has pressure equalization (PE) tubes that help regulate the pressure in the middle-ear cavity and allow for drainage of any fluid.

Ashley is a bright and articulate young lady who likes animals and school. Her parents have chosen for her to learn to be part of the hearing community, and she is fully included in her school. Ashley's educational concern is that she has to care for her hearing aids and make sure the batteries are working. Her parents must navigate the educational implications in terms of advocating for their daughter's needs, including special resources and intervention activities.

Ashley receives therapeutic intervention that includes auditory and spoken language activities. Her classroom teacher and speech-language pathologist must work cooperatively. For example, Ashley's therapy includes phonemic synthesis tasks that aid her spelling work. Her therapy also includes computer-assisted listening with a software program called Earobics, which provides games requiring Ashley to discriminate and comprehend auditory messages.

Internet research

1. How common is progressive hearing loss?

2. Does progressive hearing loss make it more difficult to identify a problem at an early age?

3. What are the advantages and disadvantages of using computer-assisted software such as Earobics?

Brainstorm and discussion

1. What role can parents of children with hearing loss play in advocating for the needs of individuals with hearing loss?

2. What factors likely contributed to Ashley's positive outcome?

---

impacted. Some children exhibit slight or minimal loss, whereas others have a profound loss in which hearing is not functionally available.

Hearing loss also varies in how long it is present—that is, its *chronicity*. A short-term hearing loss is present for only a brief period of time, as it is with children who have middle-ear infections that resolve in a week or two. A fluctuating hearing loss is essentially a short-term hearing loss that reappears periodically. A permanent hearing loss is a condition that is not going away, and a progressive hearing loss is a condition that grows worse over time. In addition, hearing loss in children varies in its timing. Hearing loss may be present at birth—a **congenital hearing loss.** Other hearing loss occurs soon after birth but before a child has developed language—a **prelingual hearing loss,** which also includes all types of congenital loss. Hearing loss that develops after birth is *acquired,* and if it occurs in later childhood or adolescence after language skills are well established, it is considered a **postlingual hearing loss.**

TERMINOLOGY

Many terms are used to describe hearing loss and the persons affected by this condition. A hearing loss is often called *hearing impairment, hearing disorder, deafness,* or being *hard of hearing.* In this chapter, we use the term *hearing loss* to emphasize the decrease in hearing acuity that is the hallmark of this condition. Terms such as *hearing impairment* and *hearing disorder* imply abnormality of the auditory system or hearing function and indicate the impact of the loss on a person's life. However, not all cases of hearing loss result in disability or disordered functioning. With early identification, a child may have a hearing loss but may not exhibit impaired abilities. Thus, the term *hearing loss* is preferred, because it focuses solely on the physical condition that is present and carries no connotation of handicap.

When describing people with hearing loss, it is appropriate to refer to them as having hearing loss or being **hard of hearing. Deaf** is also acceptable but is typically reserved for those persons whose hearing loss is severe. *Deafness* is commonly thought of as a complete loss of hearing, but even those with profound hearing loss retain some amount of residual hearing, making true deafness—that is, the inability to hear at all—extremely rare. *Deaf* with a capital *D* denotes a member of the **Deaf community.** Those individuals whose hearing loss is severe but who do not identify with the Deaf community use the term *deaf* with a lowercase *d*.

PREVALENCE AND INCIDENCE ●

The reported prevalence of hearing loss among children varies significantly, depending on the criteria used to identify the loss. Some reports include only profound loss, whereas others include all types of hearing loss, even minimal and temporary losses. The rates also vary according to the age group of children studied. Historically, statistics showed only 1 or 2 children per 1,000 as born with significant hearing loss. However, universal newborn screening programs are identifying more children as exhibiting significant loss at birth, indicating that children have been previously underidentified. The early hearing detection and intervention (EDHI) program found 5 to 6 infants per 1,000 children as born with hearing loss (Centers for Disease Control and Prevention, 2001). This apparent discrepancy is most likely due to previous classification of hearing loss as acquired when it was actually congenital.

Although relatively few school-age children exhibit severe or profound permanent hearing loss—estimated at about 1 to 2% of students — a surprisingly large number of students exhibit hearing loss that is serious enough to impact their educational achievement. Estimates from research conducted in the last 2 decades suggest that about 15% of schoolchildren have a hearing loss that is educationally significant (Niskar, Kieszak, Holmes, Esteban, et al., 1998). The term *educationally significant* refers to a hearing loss that is serious enough to impact a child's ability to perform well educationally. About one-third of these students also exhibit additional disabilities, which increases their educational risk (Laurent Clerk National Deaf Education Center, 2007). Currently in American schools, about 72,000 students between the ages of 6 and 21 receive specific educational services solely for hearing loss or deafness (U.S. Department of Education, 2006).

There are several reasons for the high rates of hearing loss among schoolchildren. First, these prevalence estimates include cases of acquired hearing loss attributable to middle-ear infections; current estimates suggest that 41% of children experience ongoing middle-ear infections throughout childhood (Auinger, Lanphear, Kalkwarf, & Mansour, 2003), which typically result in intermittent mild-to-moderate hearing loss. Second, the hearing apparatus is a delicate yet complex set of structures that can be negatively impacted through a host of causes. Prevalence estimates include cases of congenital hearing loss resulting from prenatal genetic influences (i.e., heredity, genetic syndromes), prenatal or perinatal injuries (e.g., birth trauma, fetal alcohol exposure), and peri- or postnatal illnesses (e.g., meningitis, measles). Identification methods are constantly improving so that hearing loss resulting from these many causes can be more readily identified.

IMPACT

Given the integrative relationships among hearing, speech, language, and communication, hearing loss in children varies considerably in how much it impacts these areas of development. In many ways, the impact on communication is the major handicapping influence of hearing loss. If communication is not affected, hearing loss may have little or no impact on a child's life and should not be seen as a disability. This is true, for instance, of children who are born congenitally deaf, are reared to speak American Sign Language (ASL) as their first language, and have a community in which to use this native language. On the other hand, if communication ability is compromised and children with hearing loss do not develop a native language in a timely manner, hearing loss may significantly affect a child's life, including the ability to develop relationships with parents and peers, to succeed academically, and to be involved with extracurricular activities. In such cases, hearing loss may exert a handicapping influence on broad areas of development.

What is particularly important in determining the impact of hearing loss is how a family responds to the loss and when the loss is identified. If hearing loss is identified early and the child's family responds proactively and intensively, the hearing loss may have little if any adverse impact on the child's life, even if the loss is severe. Consider Ashley, the 9-year-old girl with severe hearing loss who is featured on the accompanying CD-ROM. Because of early intervention, the effects of her hearing loss on her life at home and at school are minimal, if not nonexistent. On the other hand, if a hearing loss is not identified and a family is not able to respond proactively, the impact on the child's life can be profound, even if the hearing loss is mild or moderate.

Integration into the Community

When a significant hearing loss is identified early in a child's life, preferably at birth through newborn hearing screening, parents must make a series of important decisions about their child's identity and place in the community; they must choose a communication mode and orientation. *Communication mode* refers to how the child will communicate—the two common alternatives being speech and sign language. *Orientation* refers to whether the child with hearing loss will be a member of the oral community or the Deaf community. These decisions are not easy for the family of a newborn but are potentially the most important they will make.

More than 80% of children with hearing loss are born to parents with normal hearing. A study conducted by the Gallaudet Research Institute (2006) of 37,352 hard-of-hearing children ranging in age from 1 to 18 years showed that for 28,498 of the children, both parents were hearing; less than 4% of the children had two deaf or hard-of-hearing parents. Not surprisingly, then, many parents of children with hearing loss do not link their families with the Deaf community because they themselves are part of the hearing society. Of children and youth who are deaf or hard of hearing, only 26% have family members who regularly sign; 69% have family members who do not sign (Gallaudet Research Institute, 2001). Parents with normal hearing often focus on integrating their children into the mainstream oral community. Many of these children learn to listen and speak with the use of assistive technology such as hearing aids, and they require considerable intervention to meet the goal of integration.

On the other hand, some parents whose children are identified as deaf or profoundly hard of hearing may choose to support their children's entry into the Deaf community. This is most likely for children with hearing loss who are born to parents already in the Deaf community, which views deafness as central to its identity. Membership in the Deaf community is contingent on many factors. First, it is a choice to align oneself with the Deaf community; the choice is typically influenced by family identity and shared experiences and ideas. Second, there must be a common language or communication mode, usually ASL. Membership in the community implies an appreciation of the history, folklore, and traditions of the community and an active role in the group's activities.

The Deaf Community

The identity of the Deaf community is centered on shared attitudes and a common language, which in the United States is American Sign Language (ASL). The Deaf community does not reside in its own geographical space but is a social community based on a shared set of beliefs. The members of the Deaf community are as diverse as those belonging to the larger society and have formed a community for many of the same reasons—primarily, the desire for the companionship of others with similar psychological and social needs (Scheetz, 2001).

A common belief of the Deaf community is that deafness is an attribute rather than a deficiency, in contrast to the perspective of the more mainstream society, in which deafness is seen as a disability that should be corrected/treated (Scheetz, 2001). For the Deaf community, deafness is akin to left-handedness. Being unable to hear need not present any disadvantage to a person, just as being left-handed need not be disabling.

The Deaf community of the United States has many of the same cultural materials that other communities have:

- Deaf magazines, such as *Deaf Life*
- Deaf newspapers, such as *SIGNews*
- Deaf schools, such as the Atlanta Area School for the Deaf
- Deaf universities, such as Gallaudet University
- Deaf recreational clubs, such as Seattle's Greater Seattle Club for the Deaf
- Deaf sports organizations, such as the American Deaf Volleyball Association
- Deaf theatrical groups, such as Cleveland's Signstage Theatre
- Deaf churches, such as the Calvary Baptist Deaf Church in Auburn, Washington
- Deaf film festivals, such as Amsterdam's International Deaf Film Festival

Parents who are not part of the Deaf community but whose children are deaf must consider this reality carefully and decide whether they can see their

DISCUSSION POINT:
Consider the case of Mesha in Case Study 13.1, whose parents are deaf. Identify specific ways in which Mesha's socialization and education will be influenced by her parents' membership in the Deaf community.

children as members of the Deaf community. Do they want their children to develop ASL as a native language and align themselves with that community? Or will they raise their children to be truly bilingual and bicultural, fully integrated into the Deaf community but functioning equally well in the larger society? Is this possible? An alternative is to raise their children as hearing children, whose hearing loss will be corrected or treated through medical means and other intervention.

Communication Development

Critical to the healthy development of a child with hearing loss are early identification and intervention—preferably before 6 months of age (Yoshinaga-Itano, Sedey, Coulter, & Mehl, 1998). Consequently, most states have initiated infant assessment programs to identify children with hearing loss at birth. However, while the age of children being identified with significant congenital hearing loss is shifting to the first few months of life, nationally many children who fail the initial hearing screening are lost to follow-up (Centers for Disease Control, 2001).

> **DISCUSSION POINT:**
>
> What are some explanations for the difficulty in identifying hearing problems in infants and toddlers?

When early identification does not occur or when intervention efforts are either fragmented or ineffective in communication development (whether oral or manual), hearing loss will likely result in delayed receptive and expressive speech and language development. These delays may range from mild to profound and are likely to have further deleterious impact on the child's cognitive development, academic achievement, self-concept, and social-emotional well-being (Yoshinaga-Itano, 2003). In turn, any or all of these are likely to have a negative impact on vocational choices and the child's long-term occupational achievements. The relationship between the severity of hearing loss and psychosocial and educational concerns is depicted in Table 13.1.

The speech and language delay associated with hearing loss can include difficulties in (1) vocabulary (semantics), (2) grammar (syntax), (3) communicative intent and interaction style (pragmatics), and (4) speech intelligibility (phonology). In the area of vocabulary, children with hearing loss typically learn concrete words like *red, car, four,* and *push* since they can be matched to an object or action. However, function words like *an* or *the* and abstract concepts such as *think* or *earlier* are very difficult for these children to grasp. Additionally, words or phrases with multiple or subtle meanings can be confusing (see Figure 13.1), because these tend to require a well-developed vocabulary. In the area of grammar, the use of grammatical morphemes—such as the past tense *-ed,* the plural *-s,* the possessive *'s,* and the present progressive *-ing*—all may be delayed in development. These markers tend to be particularly difficult to hear in spoken language; they are not stressed in a word and/or occur at the end of a word, which is spoken with less intensity and loudness. Consequently, children with hearing loss may not understand or use common structures that broaden and enhance word use and grammatical development.

In the area of pragmatics, certain aspects of conversation are difficult for children with hearing loss. They may miss out on subtle aspects of communication in group settings and have difficulties following the use of figurative language, such as idioms and humor. Delays in language development can also impact a child's ability to negotiate with peers, initiate communicative acts with others, and navigate the structured turn-taking of conversations.

TABLE 13.1 The degree of hearing loss and possible impacts

Degree of Hearing Loss in dB HL	Potential Impact		
	Speech and Language	Education	Social-Emotional Adjustment
Normal hearing, −10 to +15	In the presence of background noise, may have difficulty discriminating speech	None	None
Minimal, 16 to 25	May have difficulty detecting faint and distant speech, listening in a noisy room, and detecting word-sound distinctions (e.g., verb tenses, plural forms, possessives, etc.)	May miss 10% of classroom instruction; may appear inattentive or uninterested; may be more fatigued because of increased listening effort	If missing fast pace or subtleties of peer conversation, may act awkward or uninterested or respond inappropriately; may behave immaturely
Mild, 26 to 40	Depending on degree of loss, may miss 25–50% of speech signal, including many consonants necessary for intelligibility; language development and articulation affected	May appear to daydream or listen only when interested; likely to be more fatigued or irritable	May impact self-concept and cause confusion as speech is increasingly unclear; may feel stress and uneasiness and perceive a lack of ability to succeed
Moderate, 41 to 55	Without amplification will miss 75% or more of speech signal; likely to have delayed syntax, limited vocabulary, imperfect speech production, and voice quality issues	Will have difficulty with receptive and expressive language, reading, spelling, and other school concepts; will miss most of classroom instruction presented orally	Will lack socialization with peers, leading to isolation and loneliness; may be judged/judge self as incompetent learner
Moderately severe, 56 to 70	Will miss up to 100% of speech signal; will have marked difficulty in both one-on-one and group conversations; will show delayed language and syntax and reduced voice quality and speech intelligibility; may be 75% unintelligible in speech	Will not be able to keep up with oral instruction and will fall behind academically, probably in all subjects	Will have difficulty with social behaviors; may experience a sense of frustration and rejection; poor self-concept
Severe, 71 to 90, and profound, 91+	Without amplification may not develop speech and/or language; if acquired condition, may lose preexisting skills	Without intervention, will not be able to participate in typical academic setting	Without spoken or manual language, will not be able to communicate with others, leading to severe isolation and possible social and emotional problems
Unilateral loss (mild or worse)	May have difficulty hearing faint or distant speech, localizing sounds, and understanding speech in poor listening conditions	May miss important oral instructions or descriptions (particularly in noise), leading to incomplete concept development or misunderstanding	May be more distractible, frustrated, dependent; less attentive and less confident

Source: Based on Flexer (1994).

Finally, phonology is often impacted when a child exhibits moderate to more severe hearing loss. If a child cannot adequately hear the sounds of speech, the natural development of accurate production of those sounds does not occur (Ling, 2001), affecting both vowels and consonants. For children with significant hearing loss, as many as 80% of spoken words may be unintelligible (Tye-Murray, 2000). Other aspects of speech production are also affected—resonance

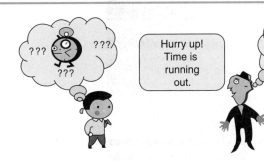

FIGURE 13.1

An illustration of comprehension difficulties due to figurative language.

characteristics, causing hyponasality; fluency charac-teristics, resulting in slow speaking rate; and prosodic characteristics, producing a monotonic and arhythmic speech (Tye-Murray, 2000).

Academic achievement for children with hearing loss is challenging on many levels, particularly read-ing and mathematical concepts (Allen, 1986; Berg, 2001; Bess, Dodd-Murphy, & Parker, 1998). As children progress through school, the gaps between children with typical hearing and those with hearing loss tend to widen, particularly when appropriate and intensive early intervention is not in place. Without appropriate management, children with bilateral mild to moderate hearing loss achieve, on average, one to four grade levels less than their peers with normal hearing (American Speech-Language Hearing Association [ASHA], 2008b). A unilateral hearing loss causes similar academic concerns.

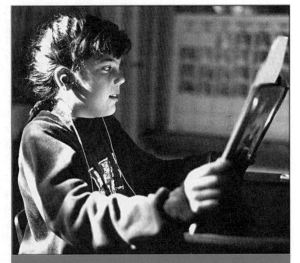

Without proactive intervention, children who have a severe to profound hearing loss often do not achieve reading and writing skills beyond a third-grade level.

HOW IS PEDIATRIC HEARING LOSS CLASSIFIED?

Hearing loss in children and adolescents is typically classified according to its etiology, its manifestation and impact, and its severity.

ETIOLOGY

Hearing loss results from many different causes. In characterizing the etiology of hearing loss, experts identify the genetic or environmental cause, the age of onset, and the type of loss.

Genetic or Environmental Cause

Genetic and environmental factors that can result in hearing loss are numerous, although in many cases the specific cause is unknown (ASHA, 2008b). The high-risk register identifies conditions present in infants that signal an elevated risk of hearing loss (see Figure 13.2).

When congenital loss is present, about 50% of the cases result from genetic causes, in which hearing loss is transmitted from parents to their offspring. With *autosomal dominant hearing loss,* one parent has a hearing loss and is a carrier

FIGURE 13.2

The high-risk register: Indicators of elevated risk of hearing loss in infancy.

- Family history of congenital hearing loss
- Congenital infection linked to hearing loss (e.g., herpes, rubella)
- Craniofacial anomaly affecting the ear
- Low birth weight
- Ototoxic medications
- Bacterial meningitis and other infectious diseases associated with hearing loss (e.g., measles)
- Low Apgar scores at birth
- Mechanical ventilation for 10 days or longer
- Presence of syndrome associated with hearing loss (e.g., Down syndrome)
- Head trauma during or soon after birth

Sources: Based on Joint Committee on Infant Hearing (1991); Martin (1994).

of a dominant gene for hearing loss, which is passed on to the child (ASHA, 2008b). The child then has a 50% chance of having a genetic-linked hearing loss. With *autosomal recessive hearing loss,* both parents carry a recessive trait for hearing loss, but neither exhibits hearing loss. Their offspring has a 25% chance of congenital hearing loss, which might be unexpected by the parents.

Children can also experience congenital hearing loss due to infection, injury, or illness in the prenatal, perinatal, or 28-day postnatal period. Possible prenatal causes include maternal diabetes, cytomegalovirus, rubella, herpes, syphilis, and toxoplasmosis. Perinatal causes include anoxia (i.e., lack of oxygen to the brain), head trauma, and hyperbilirubinemia (i.e., excessive bile pigments in the blood). Further, in the first 28 days after birth, children who receive ototoxic medications for any reason may experience damage to the ear. Unfortunately, this is a side effect of some medicines for which the alternative, including death, is clearly worse than loss of hearing. In addition, some children are born with specific physical deformities, like malformation of the outer or middle ear, or with syndromes such as Down syndrome that make hearing loss probable.

Beyond these physical or biological causes, the environment can occasionally induce a child's hearing loss. Although less common than biologically based loss, exposure to noise in the environment can result in a noise-induced hearing loss, which can range from mild to profound. Noise exposure from ventilation systems and other medical equipment in the neonatal intensive care unit (NICU) can cause permanent hearing loss in children who stay in the NICU for a long period of time. Sudden exposure to loud noise, such as a gunshot close to the ear, can also permanently damage the ear, as can barotrauma, a sudden change in air pressure.

DISCUSSION POINT:
Compare and contrast the causes of hearing loss for the two children described in Case Study 13.1.

Age of Onset

The age of onset for hearing loss is typically differentiated into developmental or acquired. Developmental loss is present at birth; acquired loss occurs sometime after birth. Experts also differentiate between prelingual and postlingual loss, with prelingual loss occurring before language is acquired and postlingual loss occurring after language is acquired. There is no consistent age that separates prelingual from postlingual loss. However, the more time a child has had to develop language and speech through oral means before a hearing loss occurs, the more likely it is that oral communication can be conserved.

SPOTLIGHT ON LITERACY

Reading Achievement in Children and Adolescents with Hearing Loss

Reading provides a child with an alternate form of communication and access to the world, which is particularly beneficial in children with hearing loss who may experience difficulty accessing spoken language. The importance of literacy for children with hearing loss goes well beyond access; reading provides children with an alternate avenue to improve language, vocabulary, spelling, and many other important academic skills. Yet, high school children with hearing loss historically have achieved reading comprehension test scores that correspond to a fourth-grade reading level (Traxler, 2000). This is not surprising considering that deaf adults, when surveyed about their early reading experiences, often indicate that they did not like reading (Schleper, 1995). Parents of children with hearing loss report that they are less likely to read to their children as a result of feeling that the vocabulary and concepts in storybooks are too difficult (Gioia, 2001).

Promoting early parent-child book reading and increasing children's willingness to persist in language and literacy exchanges are practical approaches to improving reading outcomes. However, parent-child storybook reading can present some potential challenges for children with hearing loss. Early in life, children who are learning spoken language may have limited world language experience if they are not immersed in the language of their parents. This lack of language knowledge may make it difficult for some children to comprehend the subtleties of storybook language, known as *decontextualized literate language features*. Conversely, children who learn to communicate early through sign language may struggle with the features of written English. Kaderavek and Pakulski (2007) identify motivating and effective ways of promoting language and literacy. Some practical solutions include (1) arranging seating to maximize child's ability to access information (visual or auditory), (2) gaining child's focus of attention (line of regard), (3) drawing attention to main points and pausing for child to absorb information, (4) choosing books with manipulative features, and (5) creating books about the child or his interests.

Literacy issues continue through school age. Children with hearing loss often cannot keep up with the expectations of reading, which include listening, attending, and responding to teacher questioning. Further, the books that appeal to school-age children often contain language that is well beyond the child's ability, and school-age children would consider books written at an appropriate language level to be babyish. Strategies that may enhance reading in school-age children with hearing loss include the following: (1) enlist the child to read a simple book to a younger "book buddy," which motivates the older child to read a language-appropriate text; (2) maintain interest by monitoring "language load" and rewording age-appropriate books (when given text is too difficult); and (3) role-play or read aloud with support (a concept known as Reader's Theatre).

Type of Loss

Type of loss identifies the auditory structures that are affected. In considering the pathway of sound from the outer ear to the brain, we must differentiate between two sets of mechanisms that transport the sound. The outer ear and middle ear are considered *conductive* mechanisms, whereas the cochlea and auditory nerve are considered *sensorineural* mechanisms. Three types of loss are possible, based on the extent to which these mechanisms are involved:

1. **Conductive hearing loss** is caused by damage to the outer or middle ear, with the inner ear and cochlea intact.

2. **Sensorineural hearing loss** is caused by damage to the cochlea or the auditory nerve, with the outer and middle ear intact.

3. **Mixed hearing loss** is caused by damage to both the conductive and sensorineural mechanisms.

In classifying the hearing loss of a given individual, experts consider all these sources of information—cause of loss, age of onset, and type of loss. Consider Ashley from the companion CD-ROM. Ashley is a 9-year-old girl with a moderate to severe hearing loss. She has a congenital (prelingual) mixed loss; the sensorineural component resulted from an unknown cause, whereas the conductive aspect resulted from chronic middle-ear infections.

MANIFESTATION

Hearing loss is also classified according to the aspects of audition that are impacted—that is, how the disorder is manifested. Some children with hearing loss experience loss of hearing acuity, referring to the precision of hearing at different levels of loudness. Loss of hearing acuity can range from slight to profound in one or both ears; it results in sounds being softer or less audible. You can experience the impact of such a loss by turning down the radio until it is only slightly audible or by putting cotton in your ears. The individual with a loss of hearing acuity strains to hear what others can hear without straining.

More problematic than a loss in acuity is a decrease in auditory comprehension of spoken language and speech perception, which can accompany hearing loss. Whereas several technologies, such as hearing aids, can increase sound intensity (volume) to make up for a decrease in acuity, a loss of speech perception is more difficult to manage. A child who experiences loss of acuity can turn up the television temporarily or use a hearing aid when conversing with friends. When a loss of auditory comprehension and speech perception occurs, as it may with sensorineural loss, a child must compensate in many ways, such as paying attention to visual cues or requesting written notes.

SEVERITY

Hearing loss is also classified according to its severity, using the decibel (dB) system. **Decibels,** which are the standard unit of sound intensity, represent the differences in loudness available to human hearing, from the threshold of sound at 0 dB (the drop of a pin) to the threshold of pain between 120 dB and 140 dB (a fire alarm close to your ear). The prevailing approach to hearing loss is to identify the **threshold,** or earliest point, at which a person can begin to hear—that is, the *threshold of hearing.* For normal hearing, this threshold is between −10 and +15 dB. The threshold of hearing becomes higher as hearing loss becomes more severe:

- 16 to 25 dB: Minimal hearing loss
- 26 to 40 dB: Mild hearing loss
- 41 to 55 dB: Moderate hearing loss
- 56 to 70 dB: Moderately severe hearing loss
- 71 to 90 dB: Severe hearing loss
- 91 dB or higher: Profound hearing loss

Estimates from the Gallaudet Research Institute (2008) show that hearing loss among children and youth runs the full range of severity. Recent data on children from birth through 18 years who are considered deaf or hard of hearing show these rates of occurrence:

- 19% with minimal hearing loss
- 13% with mild hearing loss
- 14% with moderate hearing loss

- 12% with moderately severe hearing loss
- 14% with severe hearing loss
- 28% with profound hearing loss

Typically, hearing loss is not described in percentages of loss, even though you may occasionally see references such as "Joey has a 15% hearing loss in the right ear." Experts caution against using percentiles to describe hearing loss, because the decibel system is not amenable to this type of interpretation. The decibel system is a logarithmic system in which the relationship between units is not linear, and the scale increases exponentially. Thus, the difference between 15 dB and 30 dB is not the same as the difference between 70 dB and 85 dB in magnitude; as the decibel level increases, the difference between decibels increases exponentially. Because percentage rankings imply an equal difference between units, they do not do a good job of characterizing hearing loss. To say that Henry has a 15% hearing loss and Tisha has a 40% hearing loss is basically meaningless, given the logarithmic nature of decibels.

Hearing level in decibels is plotted on a graph called an *audiogram,* as shown in Figure 13.3. The *y*-axis denotes decibels and loudness perception for the range of –10 dB to 120 dB, which is the normal range of human hearing from just audible to extremely loud. The threshold of hearing is plotted on the *x*-axis in hertz (Hz) along the frequency range of human hearing, from very low (125 Hz) to very high (8,000 Hz). The audiogram presented in Figure 13.3 shows where different speech sounds are located perceptually for the dimensions of pitch (i.e., frequency) and loudness.

The severity of hearing loss can vary across the frequency range. For example, a child with bilateral hearing damage from noise exposure may have normal hearing (threshold between –10 dB and 15 dB) for all the frequencies except 4,000 Hz and 8,000 Hz, at which the threshold is 40 dB, indicating a high-frequency hearing loss. A child with persistent bilateral middle-ear infections may have depressed hearing thresholds (about 30 dB to 40 dB) across all frequencies from 125 Hz to 8,000 Hz.

It is important to note that the level of severity in decibels does not necessarily correspond to the severity of impairment. A slight hearing loss does not imply a slight problem, nor does a profound hearing loss indicate a complete loss of sound. In fact, the severity of a loss does not necessarily correspond with its manifestation. We must differentiate between the concepts of *loss,* which is an objective term used to describe hearing status, and *disability,* which is a subjective term describing the impact of the loss on a person's life. Someone with a mild hearing loss may have a significant disability, whereas someone with a severe loss may have virtually no disability.

> **DISCUSSION POINT:**
> To understand the difference between hearing loss and hearing disability, compare and contrast the ways in which a mild hearing loss might affect the owner of a pesticide company versus a 911 dispatcher.

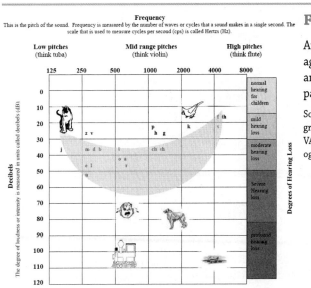

FIGURE 13.3

Audiogram depicting average range of speech energy and levels of hearing impairment in dB HL.

Source: From "Teaching Audiogram" by A. S. Mehr, n.d., Reston, VA: American Academy of Audiology. Reprinted with permission.

WHAT ARE THE DEFINING CHARACTERISTICS OF PREVALENT TYPES OF PEDIATRIC HEARING LOSS?

The outer and middle ear make up the conductive hearing mechanism—that is, they conduct, or deliver, the sound to the inner ear. Thus, damage to the outer or middle ear results in a conductive hearing disorder. The inner ear is the sensory system where the actual "sense" of hearing is located, and the auditory nerve represents the neural portion. Together, the inner ear, or cochlea, and the auditory nerve make up the sensorineural hearing mechanism. Damage to either of these systems is collectively termed *sensorineural hearing loss.* A mixed hearing loss occurs if both conductive and sensorineural loss occurs simultaneously.

Identifying a child's hearing loss as conductive, sensorineural, or mixed is one of the most prevalent ways of classifying pediatric hearing loss. Here we consider the defining characteristics of each type of loss, as well as common causes and risk factors.

CONDUCTIVE HEARING LOSS

Defining Characteristics

When sound is not conducted efficiently through the outer or middle ear, the result is an attenuation, or reduction, of the sound heard. This attenuation of sound is the defining characteristic of a conductive hearing loss. You can readily experience a temporary conductive hearing loss by putting your index fingers into your ears (not too far, please!). A conversation in the near distance can still be heard, but the loudness of it is reduced.

Children who have a conductive hearing loss, whether it is temporary or persistent, experience this attenuation of loudness. When a conductive hearing loss is present, children often report that their ears feel plugged or full. This sense of fullness makes sounds around a person appear softer but exaggerates the sense of loudness of the individual's own voice or the noise of chewing crunchy foods. You can try yet another simulation by plugging your ears while eating some chips or other crunchy foods. The reason your voice seems so loud is because of **bone conduction,** which is the transmittal of sound vibrations along the bones of the skull.

Conductive hearing loss generally causes a slight to moderate loss of hearing in one or both ears. The impact is not severe, because some sounds still travel to the auditory processing system of the brain via bone conduction. As long as the cochlea is functioning, it will carry some sound information to the brain. However, the sound's loudness is attenuated, and thus some auditory information may be lost. Conductive hearing loss is typically amenable to medical or surgical intervention and therefore is often a temporary loss if it is identified and treated.

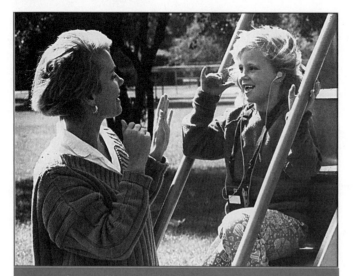

Hearing loss and hearing disability are two different concepts. A child with a profound hearing loss may have no disability, given high-quality exposure to a language system.

Causes and Risk Factors

Children frequently experience conductive hearing loss, which in many cases can be reversed. Cerumen (i.e., ear wax) blockage is a common cause. Because it is unwise to clean the ear canal with cotton swabs and because many children have narrow ear canals, wax buildup can occur frequently and block sound transmission. Foreign objects inappropriately put into ear canals or inflammation of the ear canal (e.g., swimmer's ear) can also block the transmission of sounds to cause conductive hearing loss.

In addition, malformations of the outer and middle ear can cause conductive hearing loss. Sometimes children are born with a malformed or absent external auditory canal or a congenital blockage of the ear canal, so there is no opening through which sound waves can travel. And some types of oral-facial anomalies result in underdeveloped or missing ossicles (malleus, incus, or stapes), so they do not work together to transmit sound waves through the middle ear.

The most common cause of conductive hearing loss in children is middle-ear dysfunction caused by **otitis media,** which results from a viral or bacterial infection of the middle-ear space. Some estimates indicate that at least 70% of children experience otitis media at least once and more than 40% will experience repeated otitis media (Auinger et al., 2003), which may be an underestimation since some ear infections have no symptoms. Typically, otitis media progresses in the following way: First, the child has an infectious organism in the pharyngeal area, which makes its way into the middle-ear space through the eustachian tube, usually via a sneeze or a nose-blow (Martin, 1994). Second, a eustachian-tube dysfunction results in a buildup of negative pressure behind the eardrum. Third, fluid builds up in the middle-ear space, which may or may not be infected. Here, pus can accumulate, and the mucosal lining of the middle-ear cavity can swell. Fourth, the fluid and pressure eventually perforate the tympanic membrane. Most young children do not show outward signs until the problem has developed into a fluid-filled middle ear or a perforated tympanic membrane, both of which cause significant hearing loss.

With intervention, this progression of events can be halted. For instance, the bacterial infection can be brought under control with antibiotics. Also, pressure-equalizing (PE) tubes can be inserted through the eardrum to equalize the pressure building up in the inflamed middle ear and to release any fluids. Careful monitoring of infection and skilled intervention to decrease the impact on hearing and communication are critical to the well-being of children.

Otitis media is common among children because of several factors. First, from a biological standpoint, the angle and short length of the eustachian tube in young children make it easier for organisms to enter and move through the tube. With age, the tube takes on more of an S-shape, but in children it is relatively straight and short. Second, from an environmental standpoint, some allergens, such as cigarette smoke, seem to make children more susceptible to otitis media (Martin, 1994). Third, some evidence points to group child care as possibly posing a significant risk factor (Auinger et al., 2003).

Young children who attend early child care programs do experience greater rates of otitis media than do children who are cared for at home. Estimates show that children under the age of 2 who attend daycare are three times more likely to have a history of otitis media than are children not attending daycare. With the number of single-parent households on the rise, as well as the number of households in which both parents work outside the home, more children are attending child care programs today; current statistics show that more than 50% of young children are cared for outside the home. However, it is not care

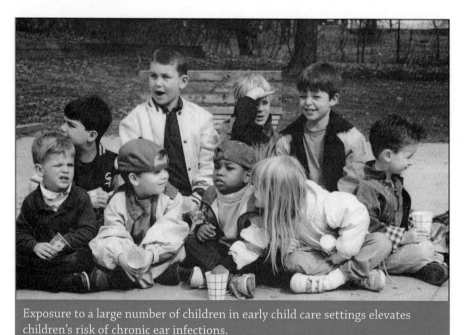

Exposure to a large number of children in early child care settings elevates children's risk of chronic ear infections.

outside the home that seems to be the defining variable; rather, it is the number of children with whom a given child interacts. Thus, children who attend large-population child care centers face greater risk of otitis media than do children attending centers with fewer children (Auinger et al., 2003).

SENSORINEURAL HEARING LOSS

Defining Characteristics

Sensorineural hearing loss is the most common type of hearing loss; it results from damage to the cochlea or the auditory nerve that travels from the cochlea to the brain. The presence of a sensorineural hearing loss can cause a slight to profound loss of hearing in one or both ears. Even though sensorineural disorders are thought of as a decrease in overall loudness, they are also associated with a decrease in speech perception and a decreased ability to distinguish speech from background noise. Thus, not only is loudness affected, but also the clarity of what is heard. Some children also experience ringing in the ears (i.e., tinnitus) and reduced tolerance of loud sounds. Sensorineural loss can be treated effectively with amplification or other types of intervention, but hearing cannot usually be restored.

Causes and Risk Factors

Most often, sensorineural hearing loss is present at birth as a congenital hearing loss. The most influential factors include maternal health during pregnancy, the birth process, the child's health at birth, hereditary factors, exposure to medications that are toxic to the ear, and disease. The following present the greatest risk:

1. Serious illness, drug use, or other problems of the mother during pregnancy
2. In utero infections, including CMV, herpes, toxoplasmosis, syphilis, and rubella

FOCUS ON TECHNOLOGY

Bilateral Cochlear Implantation

There is an exciting technology that is changing the educational trajectory for children with hearing loss—the cochlear implant. The U.S. Food and Drug Administration (FDA) first approved cochlear implant devices for children in 1990; today FDA guidelines provide approval for children at 12 months of age, and some children are being implanted as early as 6 months of age if need can be demonstrated. More than 10,000 children have received cochlear implants worldwide. A growing body of research has demonstrated that children who receive cochlear implants when they are very young make substantial gains in acquiring age-appropriate listening and language skills, and they are often on track by the time they enter kindergarten.

A cochlear implant is a computerized device that allows people with severe to profound sensorineural hearing loss to detect sound; the device works by directly stimulating the auditory (eighth) nerve with electrical signals. The stimulation bypasses damaged hair cells of the cochlea. The device consists of an external portion that sits behind the ear and houses the *microphone, speech processor,* and *transmitter* and the internal parts, including the *receiver* and *electrodes.* The microphone picks up the sound and sends it to the speech processor, a computerized device that digitizes and analyzes the sound. The transmitter and receiver convert the coded speech signals to electrical signals, which are sent to the electrodes. An array of electrodes that are surgically implanted in the cochlea stimulate the fibers of the auditory nerve so that sounds can be perceived despite damaged sensory cells in the ear. The website of the cochlear implant manufacturer MED-EL provides useful demonstrations of how these devices work: www.medel.com.ar/ENG/US/10_Understanding_CI/20_Understanding_the_CI/050_how_ci_works.asp#].

3. Complicated birth process or poor infant health, including hyperbilirubinemia, oxygen deprivation, low birth weight, or trauma

4. Family history of permanent childhood hearing loss

5. Noise exposure, including exposure to mechanical ventilation

6. Syndrome associated with hearing loss or craniofacial anomaly

7. Recurrent or persistent otitis media with effusion (i.e., fluid) for at least 3 months (Martin & Greer Clark, 2002)

Data from the Gallaudet Research Institute's annual survey of deaf and hard-of-hearing children and youth provide useful information about the leading causes of sensorineural hearing loss, ranging in severity from minimal to profound. The 2006–2007 survey interviewed over 37,000 deaf and hard-of-hearing children and youth, ranging in age from birth to young adulthood. For 57% of the children, the cause of hearing loss was unknown; among the remaining 49%, the leading causes of deafness and hearing loss included these:

- Genetics and heredity (23% of children surveyed)
- Pregnancy related (10%)
- Postbirth disease or injury (12%)

MIXED HEARING LOSS

When both conductive and sensorineural loss exist, the loss is termed *mixed.* For example, a child with a congenital sensorineural hearing loss may also acquire a conductive hearing loss from a bout of chronic otitis media or because of cerumen buildup. Thus, a mixed hearing loss typically includes a permanent reduction of sound (the sensorineural component) as well as additional temporary loss of hearing from the conductive component.

DISCUSSION POINT:
What are some possible causes of a mixed hearing loss?

HOW IS PEDIATRIC HEARING LOSS IDENTIFIED? ●

Assessment for hearing loss in pediatric populations requires a multitiered approach, as illustrated in Figure 13.4, to include both identification and ongoing monitoring. Identification of a hearing loss often begins with a routine screening, such as an infant hearing screening conducted in the hospital immediately after birth. Once a hearing loss is identified, ongoing monitoring is essential to track changes over time and to monitor the effects of specific interventions.

THE ASSESSMENT PROCESS

Referral

Early diagnosis of hearing impairment (EDHI) programs are present in most states; their goal is to detect hearing loss at birth, while the infant is still in the hospital. Infants who do not pass EDHI screenings are referred by their pediatricians to an audiologist for follow-up testing.

In the toddler and preschool years, children who exhibit developmental delays in communication, who have a hereditary predisposition to hearing loss, or who develop diseases or disorders that impact the auditory mechanism should be referred for a hearing screening or evaluation. Typically, the referral is made by the pediatrician or speech-language pathologist. Additionally, children with risk factors for hearing loss should receive regular audiological monitoring. If no specific risk factors are present, children are typically evaluated for hearing acuity in kindergarten, first through third grades, and then again in seventh and eleventh grades.

Screening

Screening generally falls into two categories, depending on the child's age. Infant hearing screenings, also called *newborn hearing screenings,* are completed at birth and involve specialized testing that is typically completed before a newborn leaves the hospital. Older children are screened using conventional methods, involving an audiometer, headphones, and tones presented to both ears. If a

FIGURE 13.4

The assessment process.

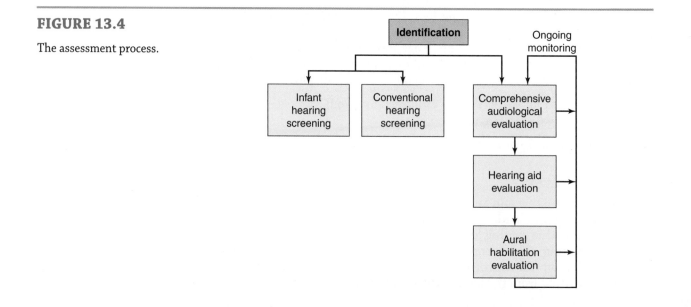

child does not pass a screening, a comprehensive audiological evaluation is scheduled. Depending on the suspected cause of loss (e.g., birth anomaly or disease), medical evaluation may also be warranted.

Infant Screening. Infant screening includes objective tests that do not require a response from the infant. There are two commonly used measures, each of which is administered relatively quickly while the infant sleeps, causing little or no discomfort. **Otoacoustic emissions** (OAEs) are a measure of cochlear function (specifically, the functioning of the outer hair cells) and are considered a good indicator of hearing acuity. **Evoked auditory potentials** (EAPs) measure the electrical response of the auditory system to a sound stimulus. Audiologists or trained personnel under their supervision provide infant screenings.

Conventional Hearing Screening. Conventional screenings require a child to respond when a soft tone is heard. Any screening that requires a child's response is called *behavioral testing.* Soft-level tones are introduced into each ear using an audiometer at three test frequencies, typically 1,000, 2,000 and 4,000 Hz. The examiner determines the child's ability to detect each frequency in each ear at the threshold of 20 dB. The examiner may allow younger children to respond in the form of a play activity (e.g., dropping a block into a box) or by raising their hand. Speech-language pathologists, audiologists, and other supervised, trained personnel provide conventional hearing screenings for children 3 years and older, but only audiologists can screen younger children. Children who fail to respond to a tone at any frequency in either ear are considered to have failed the screening and need to be rescreened within 2 weeks or referred for a comprehensive audiological evaluation (Martin & Greer Clark, 2002).

Comprehensive Audiological Evaluation

A comprehensive audiological evaluation assesses the type and degree (i.e., severity) of hearing loss, speech discrimination and auditory perception abilities in quiet and in noisy conditions, and any other concerns (e.g., loudness tolerance level). The evaluation also provides information about the cause of any loss. When a comprehensive evaluation indicates a significant hearing loss, a hearing aid evaluation is often conducted if the family so chooses. The hearing aid evaluation involves assessment for and fitting of amplification or other assistive technology. The major tools of the evaluation include (1) case history and interview, (2) other interviews and observation, (3) otoscopic examination, (4) audiometry, and (5) objective measures. Pediatric audiologists also assess related family and child needs—such as social or emotional concerns, educational problems, and speech/language functioning—to inform their assessment and to determine the need for referral to other professionals.

Case History and Interview. As a first step in the comprehensive audiological evaluation, the parent or primary caregiver completes a case history form and a case interview with the clinician. The case history and interview are important in uncovering further concerns or behaviors related to the auditory problems. Combined, the case history and interview help the clinician determine the primary reason for referral, family background, health and developmental history, communication history, and other important concerns.

Other Interviews and Observation. Interviews are inexpensive and useful ways to obtain parental input about a child's auditory and communicative behaviors and to gather input from other professionals who work with the child, such as a speech-language pathologist, a special or general educator, or an early interventionist. Observations can be used to understand a child's strengths and needs in many different contexts, including the clinic, home, classroom, and various community settings.

A variety of tools are available to the pediatric audiologist. One of these instruments, Auditory Behavior in Everyday Life (ABEL; Purdy, Moran, Chard, & Hodgson, 2002), is shown in Figure 13.5. This brief questionnaire, completed by parents, provides useful information concerning children's auditory behaviors in everyday activities with family members and peers.

The audiologist is likely to supplement interview data with direct observations of the child's listening behaviors. For instance, after administration of parent and teacher questionnaires, a school-based audiologist would observe the following in the child's classroom:

- Listening demands in the classroom and curriculum
- Teacher and student speaking behaviors
- Level of noise in classroom

For the student being assessed, the audiologist would document oral and aural behaviors (e.g., responses to the teacher, asking questions) as well as social-communicative behaviors (e.g., turn-taking with peers, voice use).

Otoscopic Examination.   An otoscope is a lighted magnifying device used to evaluate the structures of the outer and middle ear. With this instrument, the audiologist can inspect the external auditory canal and the tympanic membrane. The purpose of the **otoscopic examination** is to detect any abnormalities in these structures and to ensure a clear external auditory canal prior to testing. The otoscopic examination is an important tool for studying the characteristics of the tympanic membrane; it will reveal whether there is negative pressure behind the membrane (the membrane would be retracted), whether the middle ear is inflamed (the membrane would appear red), and whether there is fluid in the middle-ear chamber (the line of fluid might be discernible through the transparent membrane).

Audiometry.   **Audiometry,** also called *pure-tone testing,* provides objective information about hearing acuity. Audiometric testing is a behavioral measure, because it relies on a child's cooperation and participation. Typically, children repeat words and respond to tones (e.g., by pushing a button or raising a hand). When preschool or older children are tested, toys and visual displays are used to reinforce responses. This is called *play audiometry,* since the child is engaged in what appears to be a game. For example, a child might be taught to put colorful pegs in a peg board each time a sound is heard. While the child enjoys the game, the audiologist is able to gain valuable auditory information from the child's responses.

Audiometric testing is completed in a specialized test room or a sound-treated booth that is designed to minimize interference from background noise. The audiometer produces pure-tone sounds in a range of frequencies (from 125 Hz to 8,000 Hz) and a range of intensities from soft to loud (−10 dB to 110 dB). The sounds, or pure tones, can be delivered through a variety of transducers, including earphones placed over the ears or into the ear canals, loudspeakers, or a small vibratory device placed on the mastoid bone behind the ear. When the pure-tone sounds are delivered through earphones or loudspeakers, air conduction of

FIGURE 13.5

Auditory Behavior in Everyday Life (ABEL) Parent Questionnaire

by S. C. Purdy, C. A. Moran, L. L. Chard, S.-A. Hodgson

Child's name: _____ Completed by:_____ Date: _____

Instructions: We would like to know how you feel about your child's auditory development. Please circle the number beside each item that best describes your child's behavior during the past week.

0 Never   1 Hardly ever   2 Occasionally   3 About half the time
4 Frequently   5 Almost always   6 Always

1. Initiates spoken conversations with familiar people.	0	1	2	3	4	5	6
2. Says a person's name to gain their attention.	0	1	2	3	4	5	6
3. Says "please" or "thank you" without being reminded.	0	1	2	3	4	5	6
4. Responds verbally to greeting from familiar people.	0	1	2	3	4	5	6
5. Initiates spoken conversations with unfamiliar people.	0	1	2	3	4	5	6
6. Takes turns in conversations.	0	1	2	3	4	5	6
7. Answers telephone appropriately.	0	1	2	3	4	5	6
8. Responds to own name spoken in the same room.	0	1	2	3	4	5	6
9. Talks using a normal voice level.	0	1	2	3	4	5	6
10. Asks for help in situations where it is needed.	0	1	2	3	4	5	6
11. Makes inappropriate vocal noises.	0	1	2	3	4	5	6
12. Shows interest in spoken conversations around him/her.	0	1	2	3	4	5	6
13. Responds verbally to greeting from unfamiliar person(s).	0	1	2	3	4	5	6
14. Says the names of siblings, family members, classmates.	0	1	2	3	4	5	6
15. Responds to a door bell or knock.	0	1	2	3	4	5	6
16. Will whisper a personal message.	0	1	2	3	4	5	6
17. Quietens activity when asked to.	0	1	2	3	4	5	6
18. Asks about sounds heard around him/her (e.g., planes, trucks, animals).	0	1	2	3	4	5	6
19. Knows when making loud sounds (e.g., slamming doors, stomping feet).	0	1	2	3	4	5	6
20. Ignores telephone ringing.	0	1	2	3	4	5	6
21. Plays cooperatively in a small group without adult supervision.	0	1	2	3	4	5	6
22. Sings.	0	1	2	3	4	5	6
23. Knows when hearing aids are not working.	0	1	2	3	4	5	6
24. Experiments with newly discovered sounds.	0	1	2	3	4	5	6

Source: From "A Parent Questionnaire to Evaluate Children's Auditory Behavior in Everyday Life (ABEL)" by S. C. Purdy, D. R. Farringon, C. A. Moran, L. L. Chard, and S. Hodgson, 2002, *American Journal of Audiology, 11,* pp. 72–82. Copyright 2002 by ASHA. Reprinted with permission.

sounds is being tested. **Air conduction** is the way most sounds are delivered to the cochlea and auditory pathway; the sound waves pass along the auditory canal and then, as mechanical energy, through the middle-ear space. Air-conduction testing provides information about hearing acuity, particularly the functioning of the outer and middle ear. Air-conduction testing is illustrated in part A of Figure 13.6.

Pure-tone sounds can also be delivered directly to the inner ear by transmitting sound vibrations across the mastoid bone. In this case, the audiologist places vibratory devices that look like headphones against the bones right behind the ears (see part B in Figure 13.6). This form of testing is called *bone conduction;* it provides information on the functioning of the cochlea and auditory nerve. The audiologist can then compare results from the bone-conduction and the air-conduction testing to help determine the type of hearing loss. For instance, an individual may exhibit a significant hearing loss at low frequencies with air-conduction testing but not with bone-conduction testing, suggesting that the cochlea and auditory nerve are functioning but the outer- and middle-ear pathways are not.

As described earlier, the audiologist plots hearing acuity on a graph called an *audiogram.* You may recall that the softest level at which a person can detect a pure-tone sound is called a *threshold,* and it is measured in decibels from –10 dB to 120 dB hearing level (HL). Unlike other units of measurement, 0 dB HL does not represent an absence of sound but rather the threshold of hearing. The audiologist measures an individual's threshold of hearing on a range of frequencies between 250 Hz and 8,000 Hz. As shown in Figure 13.7, the audiogram maps hearing for the frequency range (perceived as pitch) from very low (250 Hz) to very high (8,000 Hz) and the intensity range (perceived as loudness) from very soft (–10 dB HL) to very loud (110 dB HL). A person's hearing acuity, or threshold, is recorded for each frequency. This audiogram also shows several sounds with which most readers are familiar (e.g., a leaf falling, a phone ringing) and the frequency intensity levels for some speech sounds (e.g., M, O).

Sample audiograms illustrating the three types of hearing loss—conductive, sensorineural, and mixed—are shown in Figure 13.8. The shaded portion of the audiogram represents the average region for speech sound energy. When a child's hearing is below the shaded region, many key speech sounds will not be naturally audible. On the first audiogram (A), showing a conductive hearing loss, note the normal bone conduction thresholds (representing the functioning of the cochlea and the auditory nerve) and the diminished air-conduction thresholds

FIGURE 13.6

Air (A) and bone (B) conduction pathways.

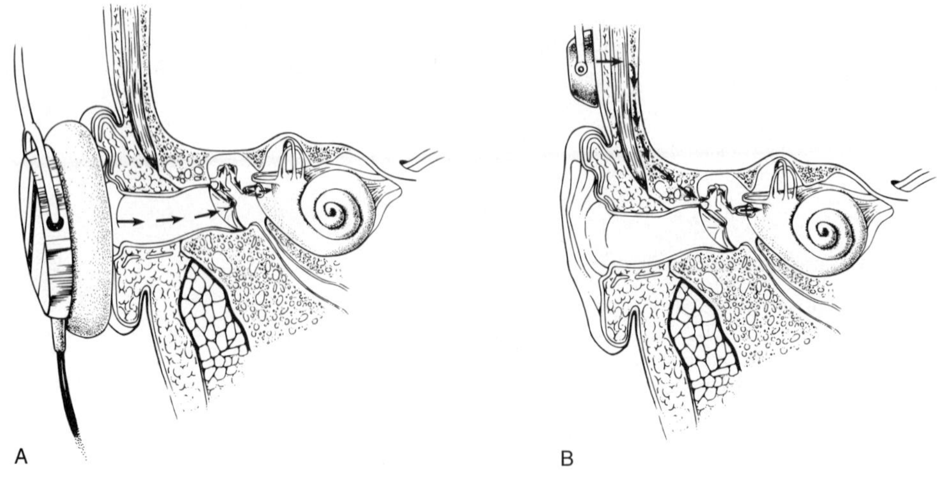

A   B

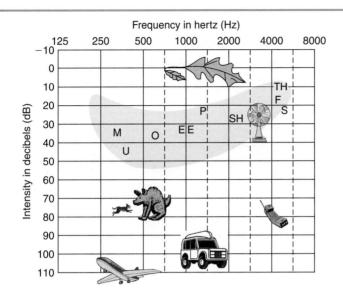

FIGURE 13.7

Deciphering an audiogram.

Source: From "Understanding Your Audiogram" by A. S. Mehr, 2005, Reston, VA: American Academy of Audiology. Retrieved January 25, 2008, from www.audiology.org/ aboutaudiology/consumered/ guides/audiogram.htm. Reprinted with permission.

(representing an abnormality in the outer or middle ear). The difference between these two thresholds is called the *air-bone gap.* The hearing loss represented on this audiogram would be typical of cerumen blockage, otitis media, or a congenital closure of the external auditory canal.

In the second audiogram (B), showing a sensorineural hearing loss, there is no air-bone gap, but there is a decrease in hearing threshold when tested by both air and bone conduction. Loss is more severe at higher frequencies. This audiogram might be seen with a genetic disorder, long-term use of ototoxic medications, or auditory nerve damage.

A mixed hearing loss, as shown in the third audiogram (C), occurs when both sensorineural and conductive problems are present. Consequently, both air- and bone-conduction thresholds are diminished and an air-bone gap is present. The air-bone gap occurs because air-conduction testing detects both the conductive and sensorineural components of the mixed loss, whereas bone-conduction testing detects only the sensory component.

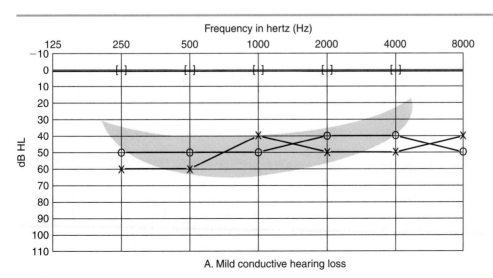

A. Mild conductive hearing loss

FIGURE 13.8

Pure-tone audiograms illustrating three types of hearing loss.

Continued

FIGURE 13.8

Continued.

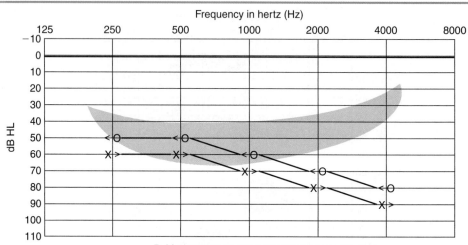

B. Moderate to severe sensorineural hearing loss

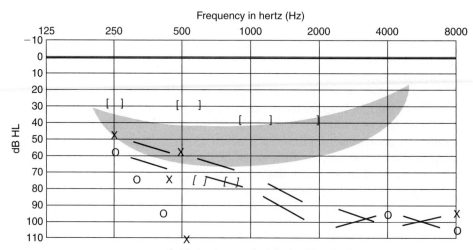

C. Moderate to profound mixed hearing loss

Audiometric Symbols

	Right ear	**Left ear**
Air conduction	O	X
Bone conduction	<	>
	[	]
Unaided Aided	Soundfield	

An audiologist uses speech audiometry as a companion to pure-tone testing to study an individual's hearing responses to speech. In this case, an audiometer delivers a speech signal via a microphone, either live speech or a recording. A child's ability to discriminate words in the presence of background noise or other adverse listening conditions can also be evaluated. It is important to understand that hearing acuity and speech perception may not be directly related. For example, a child may have poor speech perception even when hearing loss is minimal. Conversely, many children with profound hearing loss have good speech perception when the speech signal is audible through hearing aids or a cochlear implant.

Objective Measures. The audiologist can use a set of objective measures to evaluate middle-ear function, auditory acuity, and the integrity of the auditory system. Objective tests require expensive equipment and extensive training, but they can be completed on infants and children of all ages and do not require a child to respond. In fact, the infant or child is typically asleep during testing.

- *Immittance.* **Immittance** describes the acoustic flow of energy through the middle-ear space; *admittance* is the forward flow of energy, and *impedance* is the oppositional energy against the flow. These two forces are tested by studying the vibratory movements of the tympanic membrane. Thus, immittance testing evaluates middle-ear function. The audiologist uses several different tools, including **tympanometry,** which examines tympanic membrane movement, or vibration, and graphs the results on a tympanogram. Children with conductive hearing loss—perhaps from wax blockage, otitis media, or perforated eardrums—will have abnormal tympanograms. When a sensorineural hearing loss is present, the tympanogram should be normal.

- *Otoacoustic emissions.* Otoacoustic emissions (OAEs) are a relatively new form of objective testing; they provide an inexpensive, noninvasive, and relatively quick screening or diagnostic tool. The audiologist introduces a series of tones into the ear canal, using insert-style earphones (earbuds), and records the responses of the auditory system. These responses are called *otoacoustic emissions.* The sensory cells of the cochlea produce an audible by-product, like an echo, in response to sounds; these can be detected and recorded in the ear canal. The audiologist studies OAEs for children who have no evidence of middle-ear dysfunction, which would interfere with the delivery of the sound stimulus to the cochlea. When the cochlea is impaired, the OAEs are abnormal or absent.

- *Evoked auditory potentials.* Evoked auditory potentials (EAPs) are another type of effective, objective test. EAPs test the auditory nervous system's electrical response to sound stimulation. Although EAPs do not directly assess hearing acuity, the results provide information about the integrity of the auditory pathway. The audiologist measures EAPs by delivering tones or clicks to the ears through headphones. Electrodes attached to the head then record electrical activity in the brain as a result of the auditory stimuli. The audiologist graphs the results to study the integrity of the auditory pathway.

Hearing Aid Evaluation

An audiologist who identifies a hearing loss in a child works with the child and the child's family to determine the most appropriate avenue for habilitation. For children with permanent hearing loss and a family desiring an oral orientation, a **hearing aid** will likely be considered. Hearing-aid evaluations are used to fit and monitor the use of hearing aids, cochlear implants, and other assistive listening devices. The hearing-aid assessment uses several important approaches, including probe microphone measurement and electroacoustic evaluation.

Probe Microphone Measurement. **Probe microphone measurement,** or real ear testing, is an objective, computerized method of measuring hearing-aid function in a child's ear. The audiologist places a small probe in the ear canal, along with the hearing aid. A computer generates a series of sounds and measures the output of the hearing aid near the tympanic membrane. Probe micro-

DISCUSSION POINT:
What problems might arise for a child who is over- or underamplified?

phone measures consider the individual characteristics of the ear canal and the hearing loss.

Sophisticated hearing-aid programs are available that consider age, hearing loss, and type of hearing aid and that prescribe an appropriate amount of amplification. Comparing the hearing-aid output with the computer-generated prescription provides information about whether the hearing aid is meeting the prescribed target. If it is not, changes can be made on the hearing aid, and the effects will be immediately observed. Probe microphone measurement is a critical step in ensuring that children are not over- or underamplified.

Electroacoustic Evaluation.   Electroacoustic testing electronically verifies the sound properties of a hearing aid. Audiologists use electroacoustic evaluation to choose an appropriate hearing aid for a child and verify that the hearing aid is working properly. Testing is completed in a specially designed box that eliminates outside noise and interfaces with a computer capable of generating and measuring a wide range of sounds. The audiologist studies three key features of the hearing aid:

- *Gain:* amount of amplification
- *Output:* intensity of sound the hearing aid can produce at full volume
- *Frequency response:* the pitch range amplified by the hearing aid

Electroacoustic evaluation is a quick, easy way to determine whether an aid is working properly.

THE IMPORTANCE OF ACCURATE DIAGNOSIS

Hearing loss is an invisible disorder; there is typically no outward physical sign that a problem exists. This complicates the identification and treatment of hearing loss among children of all ages, as the case studies of Ashley in the Companion CD-ROM and Mesha in Case Study 13.1 illustrate. Too often, children's hearing loss is not diagnosed until after it has exerted a deleterious impact on communication development.

Among this nation's schoolchildren, the number who have unidentified hearing loss is significant (ASHA, 2002b). Implementation of newborn hearing screening programs is a necessary and important step to reduce that rate among infants. Among older children, including those of preschool or elementary age, screening programs can fail to identify those who are experiencing ongoing conductive and sensorineural loss, particularly in group screening programs in which audiometers can easily become uncalibrated and where noise levels interfere with test results. It is important that educators and other professionals who work with children remain vigilant in detecting signs of hearing loss in children.

As important as it is to identify children with hearing loss, professionals must also take care not to mistake other conditions for hearing loss. The misdiagnosis of a hearing loss is certainly possible, given the difficulty of ensuring that children's responses to audiometric tasks truly represent auditory performance. Children might respond inconsistently, attempt to fake a loss, or simply not cooperate in hearing screening or assessment. These possibilities underscore the importance of a comprehensive test battery that includes reliability checks and objective measures. A misdiagnosis would lead to inappropriate treatment, and it could damage the cochlear sensory cells if overamplification is provided. In addition, it is possible that a child could be mistakenly diagnosed as having a

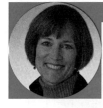

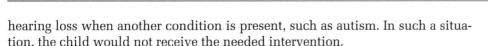

hearing loss when another condition is present, such as autism. In such a situation, the child would not receive the needed intervention.

HOW IS PEDIATRIC HEARING LOSS TREATED?

COMMUNICATION CHOICES

The overarching goal of all interventions for pediatric hearing loss is the development of healthy, socially and emotionally balanced individuals who are able to integrate fully into society and lead productive lives. Achieving this goal often is dependent on the extent to which these children can form meaningful, sensitive relationships. And that capability relates to their own sense of identity and the way they relate to the world around them (Scheetz, 2001). Consideration of self-concept, or identity, is particularly relevant in discussions of children who are deaf or hard of hearing, for the parents of these children will need to choose whether to embrace the Deaf community or the mainstream oral community. Even though the Deaf community functions within the larger mainstream oral community, the general approach to life may differ significantly for members of this community.

To understand the importance of parental orientation, we must understand that children are not *taught* speech and language. Rather, they learn the language in which they are immersed through incidental learning and exposure. Children with significant prelingual hearing loss whose parents use oral language will not develop speech and language spontaneously. In fact, to develop speech and language orally, these children will need significant and intensive amounts of

DISCUSSION POINT:
For two parents who are hard of hearing and users of American Sign Language, what would be some pros and cons of raising their hearing infant to use ASL versus spoken language?

intervention, the extent of which will be strongly influenced by the age of identification and treatment. Children who are treated early with hearing aids or cochlear implantation are more likely to take advantage of auditory neuroplasticity (e.g., Sharma, Tobey, Dorman, Bharadwaj, et al., 2004; Werker & Tess, 2005) and developmental synchrony (Robbins, Koch, Osberger, & Zimmerman-Philips, 2004), which may result in development of speech and language skills commensurate with their peers (Yoshinaga-Itano, et al., 1998). On the other hand, children who are deaf or hard of hearing (and even those with normal hearing) who are raised in a home using a manual language (e.g., American Sign Language) will learn to communicate in that language as effortlessly as a hearing child reared in a home with spoken language, assuming the parent is fluent in sign language.

For children born with a significant hearing loss, families need to make several very important decisions regarding communication choices. For some families, the choice will be to maximize their children's hearing so they can learn to speak and listen. Other families may choose to communicate primarily through sign language, focusing on building their children's competence in a manual system. But families are not limited to these two choices; there is a wide continuum from which to choose, as shown in Figure 13.9. Many families will not choose a strict orientation (i.e., ASL or spoken English) but will use a combination of approaches called *total communication,* employing a variety of techniques to support the speech, language, and hearing of their children. Of the children who are hard of hearing or deaf, 36% use both speech and sign language, whereas 52% use only speech and 11% use only sign language (Gallaudet Research Institute, 2006).

FIGURE 13.9

A continuum of communication choices.

American Sign Language (ASL)	A mixture of language features representing manual and/or spoken languages with various syntactical structures from ASL and English						Spoken English
	Pidgin signed English (PSE)	Manually coded English	Seeing Essential English and Signing Exact English	Cued speech	Aural/oral	Auditory-verbal	
Manual	Manual	Manual or combined	Manual or combined	Combined	Oral, visual, and auditory cues	Oral and auditory cues	Oral
Distinct grammatical language	Mixture of syntax features from ASL & English	ASL signs produced using English syntax	English words signed, may include word endings	Phonemically based, uses physical gestures to enhance speech reading	Spoken English learned with residual hearing; supplemented with visual cues	Spoken English learned using residual hearing	Distinct grammatical language

Source: From "Auditory-Verbal Therapy for Children with Hearing Loss" by M. Harrison, June 1999, presented at Listening to Learn: Partnering Families and Professionals to Teach Children with Hearing Loss, Celebrate the Power Conference, Department of Special Education, Eastern Michigan University, Ypsilanti, MI. Adapted with permission.

Nearly 50% of the children who are deaf or hard of hearing attend regular schools with hearing children, receiving their education in the mainstream education setting. The other half attend school in a self-contained program for children with hearing loss and other disabilities or a residential school or center.

AMPLIFICATION AND LISTENING DEVICES

Many children with mild to severe hearing loss are fitted with amplification devices; data from the Gallaudet Research Institute (2006) show that 59% of students and youth with hearing loss use hearing aids for instructional purposes; 12% have cochlear implants. Amplification devices include hearing aids and other assistive listening devices, as well as surgically placed cochlear implants. None of these devices restore hearing, but they do make sounds accessible to a child's auditory system.

> **DISCUSSION POINT:**
> In what ways might the daily regimen of caring for hearing aids impact a child's life at home and at school?

Hearing Aids

Hearing aids are available in many styles and electronic configurations. Children are typically fitted with behind-the-ear hearing aids (BTEs) rather than the in-the-ear aids that adults prefer for their small size and cosmetic appeal. BTEs are coupled to the ear with an earmold that fits into the outer portion of the ear and attaches to the aid with a connecting tube. Earmolds are custom-made of silicone or similar materials for each child. The earmolds, tubing, and hearing aid all help to shape the sound as it enters the ear. BTEs offer several distinct advantages for children: They are sturdy, and the earmold is more flexible and damage resistant than an in-the-ear aid. BTEs also have longer battery life (2–3 weeks) and can accommodate more options, because they are relatively large; they can be fitted with tamper-resistant battery doors and volume controls, as well as specialized components that couple with other assistive listening devices.

Hearing aids have improved greatly in recent years because of technological advances. Historically, hearing-aid users complained of volume control issues and poor speech perception in noise. These were legitimate complaints of the older analog models, which could amplify sound but were not well configured to an individual's specific type of hearing loss. New innovations, including digital processing and multiple-microphone technology, help to maximize hearing in many difficult listening conditions.

Assistive Listening Devices

Many devices can be used in lieu of hearing aids or in conjunction with personal amplification. Assistive listening devices (ALDs) are designed to improve a person's ability to hear in difficult listening situations, such as background noise or distance, both of which are common conditions in classrooms. Sometimes ALDs are used to enhance the amplification of personal hearing aids; at other times, ALDs are used instead of hearing aids.

The most common ALD used by children is an **FM system,** which is a personal amplification system that can be used independently or with hearing aids. FM systems are used both in noisy situations and with distant speakers or signals. FM technology relies on radio waves to send a signal from the speaker's microphone/transmitter to the listener's device (the receiver). The receiver can be an ear-level device or a desktop speaker. In a classroom, a child might be provided a personal FM system to amplify the teacher's voice during instruction.

A similar type of system is the soundfield system, which is a type of public address system. Soundfield amplification distributes enhanced sound across an entire room, again using wireless FM microphones. In this case, the sound-field surrounds the classroom space. These wireless listening systems are often beneficial not only to the child with hearing loss, but also to all the children in the classroom. However, this system is susceptible to interference from other electronic equipment, such as cellular phones.

Cochlear Implants

A **cochlear implant** is a surgically placed device that provides direct electrical stimulation to the auditory nerve; it is appropriate for children who have severe to profound sensorineural hearing loss. The cochlear implant delivers sound directly to the auditory nerve via an array of electrodes that are surgically implanted in the turns of the cochlea. The implant relies on an external microphone, a speech-processing device, and a transmitter to deliver the sound signals to the internal device. Cochlear implants require extensive testing prior to approval for surgery; factors considered include a child's overall health, chronological age, hearing age, severity of hearing loss, speech perception, spoken language skill, and family expectations and support.

Cochlear implants restore access to sound as soon as they are activated. However, hearing sensitivity alone does not ensure understanding of speech and language. Early implantation and long-term intervention to support speech and language development can maximize the benefit. Outcome studies are just emerging, since cochlear implants are a relatively new option for young children; the results are impressive (Svirsky, 2003; Tomblin, Barker, Spencer, Zhang, et al., 2005). Other implantable devices are in various stages of use or investigation, including middle-ear and brain-stem devices.

AURAL HABILITATION

Hearing loss among children and adolescents requires individualized intervention, called **aural habilitation,** to achieve fluent communication in a manual or oral modality. Audiologists and speech-language pathologists must carefully design treatment strategies that account for differences in hearing ability and learning style and must work with classroom teachers to ensure carryover into the child's learning environment. Aural habilitation typically involves the following set of activities:

- Reception and comprehension of language
- Speech and voice production
- Auditory training
- Speech reading and visual cues
- Communication strategies
- Education and counseling
- Family/caregiver participation
- Follow-up service (ASHA, 1997)

Three general best-practice principles are commonly used for all children learning to use oral language: ensuring an appropriate listening environment, maximizing audition, and supporting listening development.

Ensuring an Appropriate Listening Environment

Children with hearing loss require listening environments that are sensitive to their hearing needs. An appropriate listening environment requires that auditory distractions be minimized—turning off an unwatched television, decreasing radio volume, and running a dishwasher at night (rather than during the day) all help to alleviate background noise at home. School classrooms may also have sources of unnecessary sounds that add to the overall background noise, and modifications should be made. Typical and inexpensive solutions include placing carpet or rugs on the floor; putting cut tennis balls on the bottoms of chairs (if they are sitting on hard floors); hanging window treatments; and placing absorbent materials on the walls, such as tapestries, banners, and even egg cartons. FM technology should also be considered.

Maximizing Audition

Maximizing audition for a child with hearing loss is imperative but is often overlooked as an essential aspect of habilitation. Digital hearing aids, FM and soundfield systems, and even cochlear implants are beneficial but must be appropriately fitted, programmed, and properly maintained. Maximizing audition involves more than simply using good equipment; it requires attention to the details of audition.

A pediatric audiologist begins the process with state-of-the-art fitting methods, utilizing every decibel of hearing available to a child and continually striving for improvement. Once the potential for maximum audition is in place, children's hearing devices must be checked on a daily basis. Each day, parents should check the instruments with a listening *stethoset* (a device used to listen to another person's hearing instrument); they should visually inspect for damage, moisture buildup, or wax blockage; and they should perform a battery check. This check is best done each evening, since battery energy can store up temporarily overnight and provide inaccurate results in the morning. As children grow older, they can take on both the visual inspection and the battery check.

Further, adults who interact with children with hearing loss should enhance the acoustic signal to provide more audible cues during interactions. This is known as *acoustic highlighting* and includes a variety of techniques:

- A slower rate
- Nearness to the listener
- Increased pitch and rhythm
- Increased repetition and redundancy
- Shorter sentences
- Emphasis on key words
- Emphasis on unstressed function words (i.e., pronouns, articles, verb tense markers, prepositions)
- Emphasis on end of sentence (Simser, 1995)

Supporting Listening Development

Aural habilitation typically features a range of activities to improve auditory detection, discrimination, identification, and comprehension (see Figure 13.10). A clinician supports a child's development of listening skills by gradually increasing the auditory demands of tasks and providing the amount of support needed for the child to be successful. The clinician might give visual cues (e.g., pictures or gestures) or use a technique called *auditory sandwiching*. An auditory sandwich involves saying the word, signing or providing a visual cue, and then saying

FIGURE 13.10

A hierarchy of listening development.

Detection	• Noise and nonspeech sounds
	• Speech sounds with reinforcement
	• Speech sounds without reinforcement
	• Response to own name
Discrimination	• Two or more items differing in suprasegmental (i.e., pitch, stress) features
	• Linguistic ("moo" vs. "go," "car" vs. "pencil")
	• Nonlinguistic (joyful voice vs. angry voice, male voice vs. female voice, child voice vs. adult voice)
Identification	• Three or more items differing in segmental features
	• Single-syllable words varying in vowel and consonant content
	• Words in which vowel is constant and consonant varies in manner, place, and voicing
	• Two or more elements varied in a phrase
Comprehension	• Familiar phrases
	• Simple and complex directions
	• Sequence of directions and events in a story
	• Conversation with cues (e.g., picture context or familiar story)
	• Connected discourse
	• Different settings (in quiet, then noise)
	• Onomatopoeic words

Source: From "Learning Through Listening: A Hierarchy" by C. Edwards and W. Estabrooks, 1994, in W. Estabrooks (Ed.), *Auditory-Verbal Therapy for Parents and Professionals* (p. 58), Washington, DC: Alexander Graham Bell Association for the Deaf. Copyright 1994 by Alexander Graham Bell Association for the Deaf. Adapted with permission.

the word again (e.g., say "apple," sign apple, say "apple"). The clinician is coupling visual cues with auditory cues and over time will reduce the visual cues.

INTERVENTION PRINCIPLES

Infants, Toddlers, and Preschoolers

When first identified with hearing loss, infants and young children have different intervention needs from those of older children. Because they are learning language, treatment focuses on facilitating natural developmental sequences and promoting acquisition of functional communication. The guiding principles for providing aural habilitation to infants, toddlers, and preschoolers are consistent with the principles of other forms of intervention for children of this age, including early intervention, parental involvement, naturalistic environments, social interaction, and functional outcomes.

Early Intervention.   Early intervention is the single most important factor in determining long-term achievement for children with hearing loss. Implementing intervention before 6 months of age is optimal. Even though clinicians do not provide conventional therapy for an infant, they do provide hearing aids or other listening devices and guide parents' use of natural and developmentally appropriate interactions to encourage communication development.

Parental Involvement.   Parents who understand natural developmental sequences and use that information to creatively expose their children to language and learning opportunities are the most important change agent in children's developmental achievements. Parents also monitor services to ensure carryover and coordination among professionals; they are the advocates and the negotiators on whom their children depend.

Naturalistic Environments.   Intervention for children with hearing loss is most effective when it engages them in those environments in which they must use their skills. Naturalistic environments include the home and the classroom. And although children may be seen for intervention in therapy contexts, the room should be child friendly, with activities centered on the floor or on child-sized furniture. Working across multiple environments also provides valuable information about the child's ability to generalize skills from one environment to the next, and multiple exposure to key concepts in multiple environments reinforces the child's experiences and learning.

Social Interaction.   Generally, children are social by nature. Communication facilitates social interaction, and in turn, social interaction creates opportunities for communication development. Supporting the development of children with hearing loss within authentic social interactions is considered an essential best practice. It is not uncommon that a child and one or both parents learn sign language but that other family members and friends do not, leaving the child unable to communicate effectively and independently with other family and friends, thus inhibiting social engagement and interaction. A clinician works closely with the child's family to enhance the child's opportunity and potential for socially embedded communication experiences.

Functional Outcomes.   The average age of identification of children with congenital hearing loss ranges from birth to 2 years. If a 2-year-old child has little or no language, frustration and related behavioral problems are likely. Thus, it is imperative that intervention focus on developing the child's capacity for functional communication and provide the child a means to communicate in everyday contexts, whether with words, signs, or gestures. As communication skills improve, functional communication targets become more sophisticated but no less important.

School-Age Children

School-age children diagnosed with an acquired hearing loss or an undetected congenital loss have established audition, speech, and language skills. Although their communication skills may be delayed or disordered, school-age children with hearing loss have a foundation from which to begin intervention. However, increasing levels of academic complexity and social sophistication continually challenge these children; frequently, they find themselves interested in activities and experiences that relate to their peers, but they lack the communication skills to effectively participate. Professionals and families must be mindful of the intervention principles that guide service provision to school-age children: an effective means of communication, self-advocacy, and literacy.

An Effective Means of Communication.   Children with severe to profound hearing loss often struggle with communication, and some fail to develop a fluent and effective means of communicating with people across different environments. Instead, they may flounder between inadequate oral and sign language skills. By the time a child reaches school age, an effective means of communication must be established.

If a child is an inadequate oral communicator, parents must consider enhancing communication with sign language or seek ways to improve audition such as cochlear implantation. A child who is taught sign language must have the support of family (and friends to the extent possible), or the child must be given other opportunities (e.g., cochlear implant) to maximize hearing and improve oral communication skills. Further, families should foster the development of relationships with peers who share the same language (e.g., ASL) if children are not naturally involved in activities or experiences with other children with whom they can communicate.

Self-Advocacy.   Children with hearing loss often have special needs with respect to communication, particularly outside the home. They may need to request clarification, assistance, or special consideration. In class, students may require that instructions be repeated or written down, or they may need the assistance of an interpreter. Participation in a sporting event may require assistance with technology to enable the athlete to hear the coach from a distance. In a restaurant or noisy cafeteria, students may benefit from moving to a small table away from the kitchen. Children who are able and willing to seek support and assistance develop into confident adults who can have their needs met through effective communication.

Literacy.   Literacy includes more than reading and writing; it also includes literate thought, or the ability to think critically and reflectively and to use language to solve problems and reason (Paul, 1998). Literate thought, as well as reading and writing, requires the acquisition of a solid language foundation (whether oral or manual) at the earliest age possible; literacy skills will enhance and extend this early foundation (Paul, 1998). Because children with hearing loss too often exhibit weaknesses in their language base, literacy is often compromised. School-age children must be given consistent and intensive supports to achieve literacy and literate thought. Audiologists, speech-language pathologists, reading specialists, and special educators must work together.

WHAT IS AUDITORY PROCESSING DISORDER, AND HOW IS IT IDENTIFIED AND TREATED? ●

An auditory processing disorder (APD) is a type of hearing loss that adversely affects an individual's processing, or interpretation, of auditory messages. An individual with APD has problems in one or more of the following aspects of auditory processing:

1. Sound localization and lateralization with both ears
2. Auditory discrimination (i.e., hearing the differences between different sounds)
3. Recognition of patterns of sound

4. Differentiation of the temporal aspects of sound

5. Reduced auditory performance when the message is incomplete or when competing acoustic signals are present (ASHA, 1996; Schow, Seikel, Chermak, & Berent, 2000)

Auditory processing disorders are not typically accompanied by a loss of hearing acuity. Rather, these reflect difficulty processing specific elements of the auditory signal, such as timing or patterns.

Terms used to describe auditory processing disorders in children include *central auditory processing disorder* (CAPD), *central deafness, auditory perception deficit,* and *auditory comprehension disorder.* The terms *auditory processing disorder* and *central auditory processing disorder* indicate that the disorder is in the auditory center of the brain, not in the peripheral auditory system that includes the ear and the auditory nerve. Thus, the problem lies in deciphering a message as opposed to hearing it.

DEFINING CHARACTERISTICS

APD is a neurological problem in which a child has difficulty interpreting and processing auditory information, even though hearing acuity is intact. Thus, the child exhibits no apparent problems with the outer-, middle-, or inner-ear functions or structures; the problem resides in the areas of the brain that process auditory information. Although the child may have some subtle auditory difficulties, the processing of auditory information tends to be particularly degraded in the presence of background noise or other distractions (Martin & Greer Clark, 2002). Children with auditory processing problems exhibit academic and communicative difficulties, including inability to follow complex verbal directions, poor performance on verbally instructed tasks, spelling and reading deficits, and inability to engage in classroom discussion. Some of the most common indicators of APD include the following:

- Behaves as if a hearing loss is present although it is not
- Shows problems following complex, multistep directions
- Exhibits difficulties with reading and spelling performance
- Reveals degraded listening and audition in noisy environments or with competing auditory stimuli
- Appears to seek out visual cues from the environment (e.g., from other children)
- Has a history of fluctuating hearing loss, including middle-ear infections
- Has difficulty staying on task, finishing assignments, and working independently (Bellis, 1996)

Although children with auditory processing disorders exhibit many of the negative impacts experienced by children with more general hearing loss, there are numerous differences. Since auditory processing disorders do not cause a loss of hearing acuity, children with APD typically demonstrate little difficulty with speech production. However, their vocabulary development, pragmatics, listening, and academic achievement may be affected. In addition, amplification through hearing aids is not an option for children with APD, as the child's auditory difficulties are not related to hearing acuity.

CAUSES AND RISK FACTORS

Scientists do not fully understand the underlying processes of the auditory processing mechanisms or the ways they malfunction to result in communication disorders. Consequently, the specific cause of APD is often unknown. In children, APD is sometimes associated with other disorders, including dyslexia, attention deficit disorder, autism spectrum disorder, specific language impairment, and developmental delay (National Institute for Deafness and Other Communication Disorders, 2003).

ASSESSMENT

DISCUSSION POINT:
A comprehensive auditory processing assessment should include a speech and language evaluation. What might the speech and language evaluation uncover that would not be discovered in an assessment by only an audiologist?

The brain's auditory processing centers form a complex system. There is currently no gold standard for identifying the presence of an auditory processing disorder, although an audiologist does have a set of tools to study auditory processing capabilities. Because these often involve asking the individual to listen carefully and respond behaviorally to auditory stimuli for a long period of time in a soundproof booth, auditory processing assessment is not recommended for children under 7 years of age (Bellis, 1996). The assessment tasks examine sensitivity to the temporal ordering of sounds, the ability to listen to sounds when they are degraded or have other sounds competing, and the ability to listen to different stimuli in both ears simultaneously. The audiologist also uses observation and interview to determine how the child functions in different listening environments, such as the classroom. Typically, additional professionals are involved with auditory processing evaluation such as special educators, speech-language pathologists, and neuropsychologists.

TREATMENT APPROACHES

Currently, treatment for APD focuses on reducing the symptoms of the disorder. The most common symptoms cluster into four areas of concern: behavior, such as problems listening and attending; literacy, such as problems with phonological awareness, reading, and spelling; linguistic ability, such as vocabulary and pragmatics; and organization, such as difficulties with planning responses and tasks (Bellis, 1996).

Audiologists work directly with teachers and speech-language pathologists to provide treatment that involves three main approaches: environmental modification, remediation activities, and compensatory strategies (Bellis, 1996). Environmental modification changes the learning environment so that it provides highly redundant and better-quality auditory information. Common techniques include notetakers, frequent checks for clarification, assistive listening devices, and preferential seating. Remediation activities focus on alleviating the disorder by improving auditory processing abilities. The clinician engages the child in structured activities designed to stimulate various aspects of the auditory processing system, such as training in the temporal organization of sounds. Compensatory strategies teach the child to be a proactive listener and communicator and to use strategies that improve both roles. The child is helped to learn when communication breakdowns occur and to implement approaches that resolve them.

CASE ANALYSIS

Review the case of Andy on the Companion Website at www.pearsonhighered.com/justice2e. Reflect on how his communication skills may affect his social experience at school.

CHAPTER SUMMARY

Hearing loss is a complex problem that has the potential to dramatically impact children's lives. Children's communication skills and academic achievement influence their identity and course in life. Deafness in particular is unique, because it involves a separate community with its own language and values for those who choose to embrace it.

Hearing loss covers a broad spectrum of problems. The loss may be temporary, permanent, or fluctuating. It can vary in degree from slight to profound, and it can affect one or both ears. The loss can affect hearing acuity, comprehension, and speech perception, all of which influence development of functional communication and cognition.

Parents, teachers, physicians, or other professionals may make the initial referral for a hearing loss. Screening tests are often used to establish the underlying problem. Depending on the nature of the problem, an audiologist develops a comprehensive test battery. Audiometry and immittance are used to determine the type and degree of hearing loss. Audiologists use a separate, four-factored test battery for children with auditory processing problems. If a hearing loss exists, parents are counseled regarding communication options. If families choose to have their child use spoken language, the audiologist determines the need for amplification and assesses aural habilitation needs. An aural habilitation evaluation requires an interdisciplinary team to evaluate speech, language, cognition, and other factors such as social-emotional concerns.

Once an intervention plan is developed, the clinician initiates therapy and works with other professionals to maximize the child's communicative success. Aural habilitation includes targets for development/remediation and strategies to achieve those targets and may take place across contexts. Intervention principles are geared toward the individual child and family. With early and appropriate identification and intervention, children can learn to listen and speak.

KEY TERMS

air conduction, p. 448
audiometry, p. 446
auditory processing disorders,
    p. 428
aural habilitation, p. 456
bone conduction, p. 440
cochlear implant, p. 456
conductive hearing loss, p. 437
congenital hearing loss, p. 429
deaf/Deaf, p. 430
Deaf community, p. 430

decibels, p. 338
evoked auditory potentials,
    p. 445
FM system, p. 455
hard of hearing, p. 430
hearing aid, p. 451
hearing loss, p. 427
immittance, p. 451
mixed hearing loss, p. 437
otitis media, p. 441
otoacoustic emissions, p. 445

otoscopic examination, p. 446
postlingual hearing loss,
    p. 429
prelingual hearing loss,
    p. 429
probe microphone
    measurement, p. 451
sensorineural hearing loss,
    p. 437
threshold, p. 438
tympanometry, p. 451

ON THE WEB

Check out the Companion Website at www .pearsonhighered.com/justice2e. On it you will find:

- suggested readings
- reflection questions

- a self-study quiz
- links to additional online resources, including current technologies in communication sciences and disorders

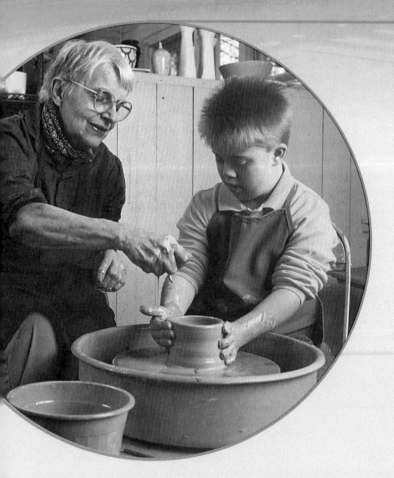

HEARING LOSS IN ADULTS

L. A. Pakulski

FOCUS QUESTIONS

This chapter answers the following questions:

1. What is hearing loss in adults?

2. How is adult hearing loss classified?

3. What are the defining characteristics of prevalent types of adult hearing loss?

4. How is adult hearing loss identified?

5. How is adult hearing loss treated?

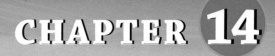
INTRODUCTION

Mr. Jones picks up the telephone, listens for a moment, and asks, "You're trying to save the nation?" "No, sir," the voice responds, "I said I'm trying to get some information!" Mr. Jones hangs up in frustration, still not understanding what the call was all about. This brief snippet provides a glimpse into the life of an adult with a moderate hearing loss. Mr. Jones is not aware of the loss, nor are any of his family members or friends, although his wife occasionally wonders if her husband is losing his hearing. Consequently, even though Mr. Jones experiences daily difficulties in his communication with others, he has yet to receive any assistance. His condition remains undiscovered.

As Mr. Jones's experiences illustrate, hearing loss in adults is called an *invisible disability* because there are often no outward signs of diminished hearing. And because hearing loss in adults often emerges gradually with age, the symptoms of hearing loss may be mistaken for other conditions, such as cognitive decline or psychological issues like irritability or depression. Nonetheless, untreated hearing loss among adults can have detrimental effects on an individual's social-emotional, psychological, and physical well-being (e.g., Dalton, Cruikshanks, Klein, Klein, et al., 2003; Jerger, 2007; Kirkwood, 1999). Beyond the personal cost, untreated or mismanaged hearing loss costs the U.S. economy billions of dollars annually. However, these costs need not occur; hearing loss can be treated through a wide array of technologies and interventions.

More than 31 million Americans have hearing loss, representing about 10% of the population (Kochkin, 2008). Estimates also show that well over one-fourth of the adult population will experience a hearing loss sometime in their lifetime (Cruikshanks et al., 1998). In fact, it is nearly guaranteed that individuals who are fortunate enough to live a long life will experience a significant decline in hearing; epidemiological studies show that 90% of persons over age 80 have hearing loss (Cruikshanks et al., 1998). Thus, it is not surprising that hearing loss ranks third among common health complaints of older adults, with only hypertension and arthritis ranking higher (Bance, 2007).

In the next decade, the number of adults living with hearing loss will increase substantially, as 1 in 6 of the "rockin' and rollin' baby boomers" have a hearing problem (Kochkin, 2008). Fortunately, these individuals will have numerous technologies and interventions available to help compensate for their hearing loss. However, less than 24% of those who might benefit from intervention receive services; estimates suggest that more than "23 million Americans do not use hearing aids to compensate for their hearing loss" (Kochkin, 2008).

Adults often resist seeking intervention for hearing loss for several reasons: (1) a perception that the hearing loss is not severe enough, (2) concerns about the costs associated with treatment, and (3) negative images associated with hearing aids (Erler & Garstecki, 2002; Kirkwood, 1999). Additionally, because hearing screenings occur rarely during routine medical visits (Newman & Sandridge, 2004), physicians on the front line miss important opportunities to identify hearing loss among their patients and to refer them for proactive interventions. Fortunately, when appropriate intervention does occur, adults can learn to live well with hearing loss with little or no negative impact on daily life (e.g., Backenroth & Ahlner, 2000; Bridges & Bentler, 1998; Lewis et al., 2003).

This chapter considers hearing loss among the adult population. Although adults between the ages of 21 and 65 experience hearing loss, the elderly comprise the largest percentage of the affected population. This chapter reintroduces and builds on many concepts introduced in Chapter 13. Consequently, you are encouraged to study these two chapters in the order in which they occur in this text.   ●●●

WHAT IS ADULT HEARING LOSS? ●

DEFINITION

DISCUSSION POINT:
Consider Kristina and Mr. Johnson in Case Study 14.1. To what extent does each of these individuals exhibit a hearing handicap in addition to a hearing loss?

Hearing loss is a "deviation or change for the worse in either auditory structure or auditory function" that differs significantly from normal (ASHA, 1981, p. 293). When this deviation impacts a person negatively, it is considered a hearing handicap or a hearing impairment, suggesting the disadvantage to an individual's daily living routines, including communication (ASHA, 1981).

A hearing loss results from change in the outer, middle, or inner ear or the auditory nerve to the brain. When the disorder affects the outer or middle ear, it is a conductive disorder. Sensorineural loss results from outer or inner hair cell damage in the cochlea or damage to the auditory nerve, which travels from the cochlea to the brain (Killion & Niquette, 2000). Among adults, sensorineural hearing loss is most common; it is the cochlea and the auditory nerve that are most readily affected by aging, noise exposure, illness, disease, and injury. Recall from Chapter 13 that among children, conductive hearing loss is most prevalent because of the high rates of middle-ear infections in early childhood. Among adults, conductive problems occur relatively infrequently.

Cochlear damage results in a loss of sensitivity to sound, or a decrease in hearing acuity. Consequently, a person experiences difficulty hearing soft sounds (e.g., a bird chirping) and understanding soft speech (e.g., a spouse speaking from another room). The change in hearing sensitivity also affects people's perception of loud sounds. Specifically, they may experience a reduced tolerance for loud sounds, termed *recruitment*. **Recruitment** makes it difficult for a person with hearing loss to tolerate common loud sounds, such as the increase in volume of a typical television commercial or a crying baby. Many adults with hearing loss also experience another auditory phenomenon called *tinnitus*. **Tinnitus** is described as a ringing, roaring, buzzing, or hissing sound in one or both ears. It may be occasional or frequent, intermittent or continuous. Tinnitus may be a result of damage to the ears (e.g., excessive noise exposure), or it may be related to high blood pressure, stress, fatigue, excessive caffeine, or other physical concerns.

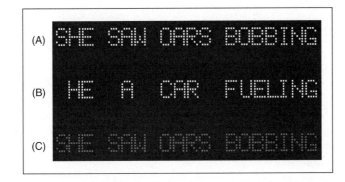

A visual analogy of normal hearing, loss of clarity, and loss of acuity.

FIGURE 14.1

Note: Imagine an electronic sign in which each lightbulb has its own wire that delivers the electrical current. Each bulb represents an inner hair cell, and each wire represents a neuron. When a bulb is out, it can be because of the bulb itself (inner hair cell damage) or a cut wire (neuron damage).

A: All lights are lit normally; thus all components are functioning properly.

B: Approximately 35% of the bulbs are burned out, leading to interpretation of the original message as "HE A CAR FUELING." This illustrates a loss of clarity. If additional damage occurs, it may be impossible to interpret any of the message, even if the remaining bulbs are very bright.

C: The lights are all working, but they are quite dim. This corresponds to a loss of acuity due to outer hair cell damage. The message may be difficult to read, but amplification can make up for the loss of sensitivity.

Source: From "What Can the Pure-Tone Audiogram Tell Us About a Patient's SNR Loss?" by M. C. Killion and P. A. Niquette, 2000, *Hearing Journal, 53,* pp. 46–53. Copyright 2000 by Lippincott Williams & Wilkins. Adapted with permission.

Damage to the cochlea can also result in a decrease in clarity of speech perception, especially in noise. Such a decrease is different from a decrease in audibility or acuity, as shown in Figure 14.1. Hearing loss and loss of speech clarity due to inner hair cell damage are termed **signal-to-noise ratio (SNR) loss.** SNR loss is a relatively new concept that explains why some people complain that they can hear just fine if people wouldn't mumble or if there wasn't so much background noise. This type of loss is based on the relationship of a signal (e.g., the voice of a friend in the room) to the noise in the environment (e.g., a fan and a television). In general, signals become more difficult to discern as noise levels increase, a concept referred to as the *signal-to-noise ratio.* However, individuals with SNR loss experience difficulty even when the signal-to-noise ratio is relatively low. They require a greater signal intensity than other people.

Although rare, sensorineural hearing loss can also result from damage to the eighth cranial nerve, the auditory nerve, referred to as *neural loss.* Loss of or damage to neurons along the auditory pathway causes a loss of hearing acuity and a loss of clarity.

In defining adult sensorineural hearing loss, it is important to consider the impact of the loss on both hearing acuity and hearing clarity. Even though the symptoms often co-occur, the loss of clarity is actually independent of hearing acuity (Killion & Niquette, 2000). Loss of hearing acuity can be readily improved by amplifying sound, as with a hearing aid. On the other hand, loss of clarity due to inner hair cell or neural damage results in a reduction in or degradation of the flow of auditory information to the brain (Killion & Niquette, 2000). This cannot be remedied with amplification alone but requires an improved signal-to-noise ratio. The presence of either recruitment or SNR loss is a particularly important consideration in choosing the appropriate amplification device to

DISCUSSION POINT:
SNR loss causes a reduction in clarity, especially in noise. How does this differ from a loss of acuity?

CASE STUDY 14.1   Hearing Loss in Early and Later Adulthood

KRISTINA, age 22, is a single mother of an 8-month-old daughter. Kristina has a hearing loss that was first identified when she was in high school. She tried hearing aids briefly at that time but was not satisfied and discontinued use. Recently, she started taking college courses and working part-time at a convenience store. Her hearing loss interferes with her ability to hear her daughter, understand her instructors in the classroom, and communicate with customers. Kristina shared her concerns with her physician, who recommended a hearing evaluation.

Kristina saw a student intern at the university, who conducted a comprehensive hearing evaluation. The results showed a moderately severe high-frequency sensorineural hearing loss in both ears. An aural rehabilitation assessment was also completed and found that Kristina is an adequate speech/lip-reader. Based on self-perception surveys, it appears that Kristina has a perception of significant handicap related to her hearing loss. A conversational observation, completed with her mother as communication partner, revealed many communication breakdowns, inadequate use of repair strategies, inappropriate topic shifts, and an imbalance in conversational turn-taking.

Audiometric and aural rehabilitation findings were explained to Kristina. The intern recommended that she reconsider hearing aids and undergo a hearing aid assessment and trial program with digital amplification that can be programmed to match her current hearing loss contour. An aural rehabilitation program was also suggested to counter the negative consequences of Kristina's untreated hearing loss.

Internet research

1 What laws protect the rights of employees with hearing loss? What changes might her employer have to make to accommodate Kristina's loss?

2 What sources of funding are available for lower-income persons to cover the cost of hearing aids? How much does a digital hearing aid typically cost?

Brainstorm and discussion

1 In what ways will amplification impact Kristina's communication with her daughter?

2 What are some possible explanations for Kristina's limited use of hearing aids in the past? Why might she be more likely to use amplification now?

● ● ●

MR. JOHNSON is a 68-year-old man with sensorineural hearing loss. Mr. Johnson served in the military and was also exposed to industrial noise through his occupation. It is likely that both noise exposure and aging factors (presbycusis) contributed to his diminished hearing. Fortunately for Mr. Johnson, he does not experience tinnitus, which is common among adults with his hearing history.

Like many adults, Mr. Johnson first noticed problems with his hearing when his wife would complain that he did not hear her. He reported that he could "get by" for a long time. When considering how he got by, Mr. Johnson remembers that his quality of life was affected. He would sometimes feign understanding; other times he would have to walk across the house to be in the same location as the person talking with him. He learned to rely heavily on lip-reading. Eventually, Mr. Johnson realized that he was missing too much and sought intervention.

Mr. Johnson's hearing loss causes him to have problems hearing softer sounds of speech; he also has difficulty with hearing clarity. He was fitted with bilateral behind-the-ear hearing aids. With his hearing aids, Mr. Johnson reports that he can hear much better in most listening situations, and his quality of life in general has improved dramatically. In noisy situations, such as busy restaurants, Mr. Johnson still has some difficulty.

Mr. Johnson's treatment plan included three elements: counseling, fitting and maintenance of the amplification devices, and aural rehabilitation. Since insurance companies and other third-party payers do not cover these services, Mr. Johnson had to make a decision about budgeting for and purchasing hearing aids and the associated services. After becoming a hearing-aid user and seeking the appropriate treatment, Mr. Johnson realizes that the benefits far outweigh the costs.

Internet research

1 If a person such as Mr. Johnson experiences work-related hearing loss, what recourse does he have from his employer?

2 What can be done to prevent hearing loss in the workplace? From aging?

3 If third-party payers do not cover hearing aids and related services and a client cannot afford them, what other possible funding sources or options are available?

Brainstorm and discussion

1 What are some activities that Mr. Johnson and his family could practice to promote better communication?

2 What are some approaches Mr. Johnson's wife might use to support his pursuit of intervention?

ensure that sounds are perceived as clearly and comfortably as possible in both quiet and noisy conditions.

Social-Emotional, Psychological, and Physical Impact

Hearing loss goes undetected or untreated in more than 75% of adults with hearing loss (Newman & Sandridge, 2004). When left untreated, hearing loss—particularly the sensorineural variety, which impacts hearing acuity and clarity—can have devastating effects on an individual's social-emotional and psychological well-being, physical health, lifestyle, and educational and vocational choices. Sometimes, people are aware of a hearing loss and make changes in their lifestyles rather than admit the loss and seek intervention; others are unaware of their loss, and it goes undetected by medical professionals and family members, too. Regardless, hearing loss can impact life in many ways. Consider Jorges, an elderly grandfather who decides to quit attending family functions because "no one is interested in what an old man has to say," and he's tired of sitting alone at gatherings with no one to talk to. In reality, after years of increasingly difficult communication because of his poor hearing ability, Jorges's family has stopped taking the time to converse with him in group settings. Contrast Jorges's experience with that of Mr. Johnson on the Companion CD-ROM. Mr. Johnson's hearing loss from noise exposure has little effect on his life because of his use of hearing aids and participation in habilitation programs.

What is particularly striking about hearing loss in the adult population is that its effects can be significant even when the hearing loss is minimal, as with a unilateral loss or a mild bilateral loss (Newman, Hug, Jacobson, & Sandridge, 1997). In a major survey commissioned by the National Council on Aging (NCOA), researchers found that people who do not appropriately manage their hearing loss report significantly higher rates of these problems:

- Depression (e.g., fatigue, insomnia, thinking a lot about death)
- Anger and frustration (likely to get annoyed and irritated easily)

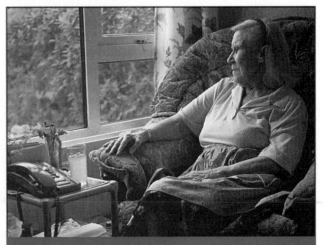
Significant others may limit their conversations with family members with hearing loss, given the challenges of communicating effectively.

- Paranoia (believing they are blamed for something that is not their fault)
- Denial of the severity and extent of hearing-related problems
- Feelings of loss of control
- Pretending to understand others when they do not
- Violating the rules of communication (e.g., interrupting a speaker or inappropriately shifting topics; Kirkwood, 1999)

DISCUSSION POINT:
Many individuals seek treatment for hearing loss when the problem reaches a crisis stage. What example of a crisis might propel an adult to seek treatment for a hearing loss?

Unmanaged hearing loss directly impacts interpersonal relationships with family members, coworkers, and friends. Adults with untreated hearing loss and their spouses suffer in both their social and their family roles and report more negativity and arguments in their relationships, often leading to crises (Armero, 2001; Chia, Wang, Rochtchina, Cumming, et al., 2007; Dalton et al., 2003).

However, untreated hearing loss results in significant lifestyle limitations that go far beyond socialization. This is particularly true for individuals who have had ongoing hearing loss since early childhood that has been untreated or treated with fragmented approaches. The reading abilities and educational outcomes of adults who have congenital hearing loss are staggeringly low; studies show the average reading ability at a fourth-grade level (Gallaudet University Center for Assessment and Demographic Study, 1998). Labor force participation is also lower for people with hearing loss (Mohr et al., 2000), and they show less involvement in community activities, such as volunteering. Hearing loss also influences retirement decisions; more people with hearing loss retire early (i.e., between the ages of 51 and 61) than do their typical hearing peers (Mohr et al., 2000). And more retired people with hearing loss report that poor health led to their retirement.

DISCUSSION POINT:
If the impact of hearing loss is so far reaching, why is there such a stigma attached to hearing loss and hearing-aid use?

Estimates suggest that untreated hearing loss costs the U.S. economy billions of dollars in lost productivity and medical care. People with hearing loss in the workforce earn only about 50 to 70% of the income of their hearing peers, reducing their earnings by up to $500,000 in a lifetime (Mohr et al., 2000). The costs of economic-induced hearing loss are also considerable, specifically **noise-induced hearing loss** caused by exposure to occupational noise. As the second most common cause of sensorineural hearing loss among adults, noise-induced hearing loss costs the American economy greatly in unemployment and disability benefits (Daniell, Fulton-Kehoe, Smith-Weller, & Franklin, 1998).

TERMINOLOGY

As introduced in Chapter 13, the term *hearing loss* is objective and refers specifically to a decrease in hearing acuity or clarity as a malfunction of the hearing mechanisms. The terms *handicap, disability,* and *impairment* reference the impact of hearing loss on an individual's daily living activities.

Hearing loss that occurs as a result of aging is called **presbycusis.** The noise-induced hearing loss just discussed is acquired from exposure to noise, often through occupational conditions (e.g., machinery operation) or recreational activities (e.g., gun use). *Nerve loss* is a term often used incorrectly to describe sensorineural hearing loss, which *can* be caused by neuron damage but is far more often the result of damage to the hair cells of the cochlea.

PREVALENCE AND INCIDENCE

Hearing loss is the third most prevalent chronic condition in the older population (Bance, 2007). Approximately 10% of the population, or 31 million Americans, have hearing loss, and this number is expected to increase significantly over the

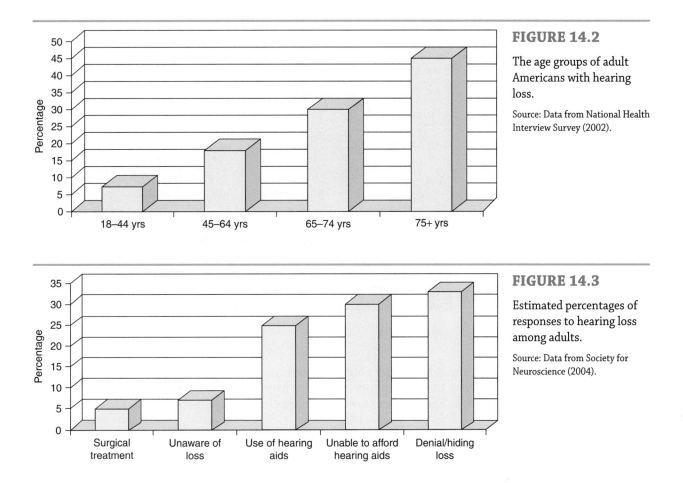

FIGURE 14.2

The age groups of adult Americans with hearing loss.

Source: Data from National Health Interview Survey (2002).

FIGURE 14.3

Estimated percentages of responses to hearing loss among adults.

Source: Data from Society for Neuroscience (2004).

next decades, particularly for people of advanced age (Kochkin, 2008). The incidence of acquired hearing loss increases dramatically with age, as shown in Figure 14.2. In contrast to the number of persons exhibiting hearing loss, the number of adults receiving treatment or intervention for it is much lower, estimated at about 25% of adults with hearing loss, as shown in Figure 14.3.

HOW IS ADULT HEARING LOSS CLASSIFIED? ●

Hearing loss in the adult population is classified in terms of etiology, manifestation, and severity.

ETIOLOGY

Identifying the cause of adult hearing loss is a common way to classify the different types of loss. Etiology identifies the area of the auditory pathway or brain that is affected (e.g., outer ear, middle ear, cochlea, auditory nerve). A conductive loss places the site of breakdown in the outer or middle ear. A sensorineural loss occurs from a breakdown either of the outer or inner hair cells of the cochlea or of the auditory nerve.

As discussed in Chapter 13, hearing loss can be congenital or acquired. Among the adult population with hearing loss, most often the loss is acquired

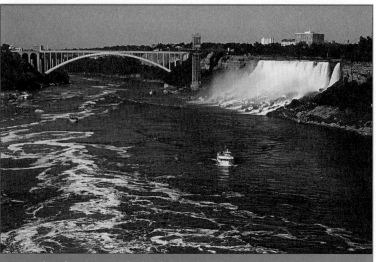

From the observation decks the roar of Niagara Falls is about 80 dB
and thus would be inaudible to persons with profound hearing loss.

sometime during the course of adulthood, either from a sudden event, such as
a tumor of the auditory nerve, or from a gradual process, such as illness or
disease. The most common causes include the following:

- Head trauma
- Barotrauma (excessive change in atmospheric pressure that cannot be
  matched by ear pressure changes)
- Tumor (e.g., acoustic neuroma, a tumor on the auditory nerve)
- Ototoxic drugs
- Infection/disease (e.g., Meniere's disease)
- Illness
- Noise exposure/damage
- Aging

The last two are the most prevalent causes of adult acquired hearing loss.

MANIFESTATION

Hearing loss is also classified according to the aspects of audition that are
affected, or the ways the disorder is manifested. This approach considers
whether the loss impacts acuity and audibility of sounds alone or whether comprehension of spoken language and speech perception (i.e., clarity) are affected
as well. A change in hearing acuity is the most commonly recognized manifestation of hearing loss; a decrease in hearing acuity results in sounds being softer
or less audible, a symptom familiar to many whose grandparents may have
asked them to "speak a little louder." More problematic, however, is an SNR
loss, resulting in a decrease in comprehension of spoken language and speech
clarity. With an SNR loss, the speech signal itself is compromised and
degraded. Whereas sound intensity (i.e., volume) can be increased to make up
for a decrease in acuity, a loss of clarity is more complicated to treat. Commonly

FIGURE 14.4

Commonly reported problems of adults with hearing loss and of their significant others.

Problems of adults with hearing loss

- Environmental challenges
  - Sounds in background noise
  - Conversations in the dark or poor lighting
  - Sounds at a distance or in another room
  - Speech or music in the automobile
  - Large group situations
  - Rooms with poor acoustics
  - Conversations outdoors (particularly in noisy places or on windy days)
  - Telephone and cellular phone conversations
  - Voices on television, radio, or film

- Speaker challenges
  - Conversations with multiple speakers
  - Unfamiliar speaker or a foreign accent
  - Unfamiliar topic (e.g., medical explanation)
  - Speaker who looks away or provides poor facial cues (e.g., covering face with veil, beard, or hand)
  - Speaking without getting attention of listener
  - Misinterpreting listener's failure to understand

- Listener challenges
  - Isolation
  - Trying to concentrate, even when fatigued
  - Loss of spontaneity and/or intimacy

Problems of significant others

- Speaking challenges
  - Remembering to get listener's attention, speak clearly, and face the listener
  - Reducing conversational frequency/duration

- Interpersonal challenges
  - Not being able to determine when listener understands
  - Variability in listener's ability to understand
  - Finding creative ways to make listener understand
  - Having to repeat a lot
  - Responding when listener doesn't understand another speaker
  - Failure of listener to pay attention
  - Attempting to get listener to understand in emergency situations
  - Minimizing frustration
  - Being patient, even when fatigued
  - Having to act as an interpreter
  - Not being able to enjoy certain activities (e.g., traveling, theater)
  - Isolation imposed by significant other
  - Loss of spontaneity and/or intimacy

- Other challenges
  - Television or radio volume too loud

Source: From *Living with Hearing Loss Workbook* by S. Trychin, 2002, Erie, PA: Author. Copyright 2002 by S. Trychin. Adapted with permission.

experienced problems resulting from loss of both acuity and clarity are provided in Figure 14.4.

SEVERITY

The severity of hearing loss ranges from mild to profound and is typically defined using decibels (dB):

- −10 dB to 15 dB: Normal hearing
- 16–25 dB: Slight loss
- 26–40 dB: Mild loss
- 41–55 dB: Moderate loss
- 56–70 dB: Moderately severe loss
- 71–90 dB: Severe loss
- > 91 dB: Profound loss

These numbers indicate the decibel level at which an individual is able to detect sound. Thus, an individual with normal hearing detects sounds when they are between −10 dB and 15 dB. By contrast, a person who does not detect sounds until they are at about 30 dB has a mild loss.

DISCUSSION POINT: Consider the cases of Kristina and Mr. Johnson in Case Study 14.1. Identify the cause of hearing loss for each of these individuals. Which causes could have been prevented?

Literacy Issues among Adults with Hearing Loss

As mentioned in Chapter 13, many high school students with hearing loss do not progress beyond a fourth-grade reading level. This trend can continue into adulthood, with many adults with serious and persistent hearing loss exhibiting inadequate reading and writing skills to perform well in the twenty-first century workplace. Learning to read and write effectively as an adult is a daunting task, particularly when a person does not hear and communicates using American Sign Language.

Fortunately, there are specialized programs available to support the reading and writing development of adults with hearing loss. The Program for Deaf Adults (PDA) at LaGuardia Community College is one such example. For more than 30 years, PDA has offered specialized higher-education opportunities for deaf adults and offers courses on basic academic skills (reading, writing, and math), as well as American Sign Language, Drivers Education, Computing, and Telecommunication Skills.

It might be helpful to consider the decibel levels of various environmental sounds (Van Bergeijk, Pierce, & David, 1960):

- 10 dB: Rustle of leaves
- 20 dB: Whisper at 20 feet
- 30 dB: Quiet street with no traffic
- 40 dB: Night noises in a city
- 50 dB: A car engine 10 feet away
- 60 dB: The interior of a department store
- 70 dB: Busy traffic on a city street
- 80 dB: Niagara Falls

Using these reference points, consider the experiences of a person with a mild or moderate hearing loss. In everyday living, numerous sensory experiences would be missed, and conversations with friends and family members would likely be impaired unless some communication enhancements are used.

WHAT ARE THE DEFINING CHARACTERISTICS OF PREVALENT TYPES OF HEARING LOSS? ●

CONDUCTIVE HEARING LOSS

Defining Characteristics

Conductive hearing loss is less common among adults than it is among children. As described in Chapter 13, this type of hearing loss occurs when sound is not conducted efficiently through the outer and/or middle ear, resulting in an attenuation of the sound. Conductive hearing loss results in a sense of fullness or plugged ears and generally causes a slight to moderate loss of hearing in one or both ears. It is typically amenable to medical or surgical intervention and therefore is often a temporary loss.

Causes and Risk Factors

A common cause of conductive loss in adulthood is cerumen blockage, particularly due to the use of cotton swabs. Even though many people use cotton swabs to keep their ears clean, their use is actually detrimental. The human ear produces cerumen as a protective agent to keep objects out of the ear canal and to keep it lubricated and healthy. When swabs are pushed into the ear, they serve as a plunger, removing some wax while pushing other wax deep into the ear canal. When significant wax builds up, sound transmission is blocked. Wax pushed into the ear canal near the tympanic membrane can become hard and stiff and difficult to remove, necessitating its removal by an audiologist. Attempting to remove cerumen that is deep in the ear canal makes the tympanic membrane vulnerable to rupture.

Foreign objects inappropriately put into the ear canals or inflammation of the ear canal can also block the transmission of sound, causing conductive hearing loss. One elderly woman who suffered from Alzheimer's disease mistakenly placed her hearing aid battery in her ear canal rather than in the hearing aid. It was not discovered for several months, by which time it had turned into a serious infection and had to be removed surgically.

Adults also experience otitis media, although it occurs far less frequently than it does with children because of structural changes in the ear mechanism (e.g., the lengthening and curving of the eustachian tube) and an improved immune system, which allows adults to resist chronic infections. Adults who have allergies, sinus-related problems, and a childhood history of chronic otitis media are at greatest risk for adult bouts of otitis media. As with children, otitis media needs to be treated thoroughly and well to minimize its impact on the middle-ear structures and hearing acuity.

Damage to the outer- and middle-ear structures can also cause conductive hearing loss. For example, individuals who suffer head trauma in an automobile accident may experience perforation of the eardrum or disarticulation (i.e., dislocation) of the ossicles. Sometimes trauma is self-induced, as it was with a college student who fell asleep and jammed her pencil into her ear, perforating the tympanic membrane. Accidents like this are very painful but can be repaired surgically in most cases. *Myringoplasty* is a medical intervention in which tissue is grafted onto the tympanic membrane to repair perforations. However, with clean tears, the membrane can often heal itself.

Another cause of adult-onset conductive hearing loss is **otosclerosis,** a condition in which abnormal bone growth develops around the ossicles (especially the stapes). That bone growth impedes the movement of the stapes, compromising the transmission of sound energy along the ossicular chain to the footplate of the stapes, which transmits energy to the cochlea through the oval window. The bone growth can also invade the inner ear. Otosclerosis is relatively common, affecting approximately 1 of 100 adults in the United States, with the incidence in women approximately twice that in men (Martin & Greer Clark, 2002). There is a strong genetic link in the risk for this disease, and it seems to be aggravated by hormonal changes in pregnancy or menopause. Although otosclerosis can be treated surgically—often through a *stapedectomy,* in which the diseased bone is replaced with a prosthesis—a significant, long-term conductive hearing loss is common.

SENSORINEURAL HEARING LOSS

Defining Characteristics

Sensorineural hearing loss is the most common type of hearing loss in adulthood, resulting most often from damage to the outer or inner hair cells of the cochlea. Whereas outer hair cell damage often results in difficulty with hearing acuity, inner hair cell damage results in a more complicated problem—SNR loss. SNR loss, which also occurs with auditory nerve damage, results in both a decrease in acuity and a loss of clarity, especially in noise. Depending on the location of damage, people may experience recruitment and/or tinnitus as well. Sensorineural loss can be treated effectively with amplification or other types of intervention, but hearing cannot usually be restored.

Causes and Risk Factors

There are many causes of sensorineural hearing loss, the most frequent being presbycusis and noise exposure. Presbycusis is a degeneration of the inner ear and other auditory structures as a result of the normal aging process. It is a progressive loss that begins in early adulthood but may not be noticeable until the fifth or sixth decade of life. Figure 14.5 illustrates expected hearing levels by decade, considering only aging factors. Presbycusic losses result in a decrease in the high-frequency range and may be accompanied by SNR loss, tinnitus, and recruitment; these losses are more prevalent and severe in men. Some individuals are genetically predisposed to presbycusis and may be more susceptible to these changes. Thus, a parent with age-related hearing loss increases the risk of a son or daughter having age-related hearing loss (Gates, Couropmitree, & Myers, 1999). Other risk factors include disease or illness (e.g., diabetes), cardiac problems and high blood pressure, noise exposure, and certain medications.

Noise-induced hearing loss results from exposure to damaging levels of noise. This exposure can be in the form of industrial or construction noise, music, gunfire, or other sounds greater than 85 dB. Some common activities with very high noise levels include taking an aerobics class (78–106 dB), playing in an orchestra (87–98 dB), running a power mower (107 dB), spending time in a club or a bar (110 dB), listening to stereo headphones (110 dB), or attending a rock concert (130 dB; Wilson & Herbstein, 2003). A single exposure to noises at these levels may not be enough to result in permanent damage, because the hair cells of the cochlea are able to self-repair within a relatively short period of time. If you have had a temporary hearing loss due to a loud noise (e.g., a rock concert), you have experienced this self-repair. However,

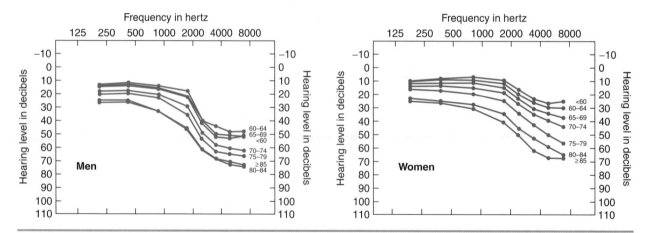

FIGURE 14.5   Expected hearing level decreases for aging men and women.

Source: From *Geriatric Audiology* by B. E. Weinstein, 2000, New York: Thieme. Copyright 2000 by Thieme. Reprinted with permission.

with ongoing exposure, the self-repair mechanisms of the cochlea become overwhelmed or unable to compensate, as several well-known musicians (e.g., The Who's Pete Townsend) have learned the hard way. The alarming rates of noise-induced hearing loss due to occupational conditions have resulted in numerous hearing conservation programs in American industries with high noise levels, such as mining, lawn care, the airline industry, machine-repair shops, and construction. An estimated 30 million Americans experience excessive noise in their workplace, and efforts are under way to enhance hearing screening and protection.

Like presbycusis, noise-induced hearing loss appears to have a strong genetic link. Animal studies indicate that the gene that influences presbycusic loss can also influence susceptibility to noise-induced hearing loss (Tremblay & Cunningham, 2002). Other influencing factors include (1) the intensity of the noise, (2) the length of exposure, (3) the use of hearing protection, (4) the recovery time between exposures, and (5) other forms of damage to the cochlea. Table 14.1 illustrates the relationship between intensity level and hours of safe exposure.

Ototoxicity is another common cause of inner-ear damage and sensorineural hearing loss. An ototoxic drug is one that negatively affects the hearing mechanism, such as certain antibiotics (e.g., streptomycin and neomycin), aspirin (salicylates) in large quantities, diuretics (e.g., Lasix), and chemotherapy drugs (e.g., cisplatin). Damage may be temporary, but it is more often permanent, particularly when the medication is used for a long period of time at high dosages. Drugs that are known to be ototoxic are often administered because of their life-saving effects. For instance, the drug quinine is used to prevent malaria, although it has a clear ototoxic effect. For people who travel frequently to malarial regions, the impact on hearing may be an unfortunate but necessary trade-off for protection from the potentially life-threatening disease. Occasionally, a substitute, nonototoxic drug can be given when testing indicates signs of damage to the outer hair cells, which are particularly susceptible to ototoxic agents. When ototoxic drugs are used, hearing should be carefully monitored.

> **DISCUSSION POINT:**
> Mr. Johnson, described in Case Study 14.1, has a noise-induced hearing loss, which is preventable. What might a prevention program for noise-induced hearing loss look like?

TABLE 14.1	The relationship between the intensity level of noise and the hours of safe exposure	
	Hours of Safe Exposure	
Noise Level (dB)	**Without Hearing Protection**	**With 15 dB Hearing Protection**
90	8	Unlimited
95	4	Unlimited
100	2	Unlimited
105	1	8
110	½	4
115	¼	2
120	0	1
125 or greater	0	0

Source: Data from Occupational Safety and Health Administration (OSHA) (1992).

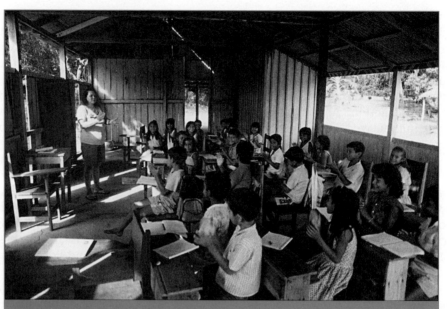

Antimalarial treatment can cause hearing loss, but it can also save one's life by preventing malaria.

Many diseases and infections can also cause sensorineural hearing loss, including Meniere's disease and labyrinthitis, cerebral-vascular disease, diabetes, tuberculosis, kidney disease, autoimmune diseases, and HIV and other sexually transmitted diseases, including herpes. **Meniere's disease** and **labyrinthitis** affect the labyrinth of the inner ear in both the vestibular and cochlear mechanisms. The vestibule of the inner ear controls balance functions, whereas the cochlea mediates hearing. When both the vestibule and the cochlea are damaged, as occurs in these two disorders, the symptoms include hearing loss, vertigo (i.e., dizziness), and tinnitus. Labyrinthitis is a short-term infection that is treated medically; Meniere's disease is a long-term disorder caused by an overproduction or underabsorption of endolymph, a fluid that circulates in the inner ear, resulting in a progressive hearing loss. Between 3 and 5 million cases are present in the United States (American Academy of Otolaryngology—Head and Neck Surgery, 2004). Meniere's disease typically strikes between 20 and 50 years of age, affecting men and women equally.

An additional illness that can result in sensorineural hearing loss is meningitis, which is also one of the leading causes of acquired postnatal hearing loss, accounting for about 6% of cases (Gallaudet Research Institute, 2001). Meningitis is an inflammation of the meninges, a layer of tissues that encase the brain. Meningitis occurs from both viral and bacterial agents; it is not spread by casual contact but through close or prolonged physical contact between two people. Those who care for people with bacterial meningitis must take special care, including antibiotic treatment, not to contract the illness themselves. Symptoms include a rapid-onset high fever, vomiting, extreme weakness, spots on the body, and painful, achy joints.

Finally, tumors, particularly along the auditory nerve, can cause sensorineural hearing loss, primarily because of the space they occupy. Described as *acoustic neuromas,* tumors can be hard to identify and are usually noticed first by a decrease in hearing in one ear, followed by a feeling of fullness or pressure. Surgical removal of the tumor can result in a complete loss of hearing and facial paralysis. Although surgeons try hard to preserve hearing in the removal of acoustic neuromas, their immediate goal is always to remove the tumor and preserve the patient's life. The most efficient route to removal is through the ear directly, which can damage much of the ear and result in a significant unilateral loss.

MIXED HEARING LOSS

Defining Characteristics, Causes, and Risk Factors

When people with a sensorineural hearing loss experience a bout of otitis media or a buildup of cerumen, the concomitant loss is termed a *mixed hearing loss.* It is a combination of a permanent reduction of sound (i.e., the sensorineural component) and a temporary loss of hearing from a conductive component.

HOW IS HEARING LOSS IDENTIFIED? ●

THE ASSESSMENT PROCESS

Assessment of hearing loss in adults can be initiated with an audiometric screening, but it more often begins with a complete hearing evaluation. Generally, assessment tools fall into three categories: (1) observation and self-assessment, (2) conventional audiometry, and (3) objective measurement. Screenings can include questionnaires completed by the individual or a significant other and observations about communication in various environments/situations. Screenings also include measurement of auditory system response to sounds through conventional audiometry or objective measures (e.g., otoacoustic emissions).

A comprehensive audiometric test battery is described in Chapter 13; it includes conventional audiometry as well as objective measures, such as otoacoustic emissions (OAEs) and evoked auditory potentials (EAPs). Adults and their significant others can also provide substantial information through self-assessment instruments. Assessment should determine hearing acuity (or degree of loss), the type of loss (e.g., outer versus inner hair cell damage) and likely cause, and speech perception ability in quiet and noise (e.g., presence of SNR loss). If there are specific medical concerns, such as acoustic neuroma or otosclerosis, testing of auditory system integrity (e.g., EAP, OAEs) should also be completed.

Once a hearing loss is diagnosed, assessment for hearing aids should follow, as described in Chapter 13:

- Conventional audiometry in a sound-treated room to determine functional improvement in the aided condition for tones and for speech perception
- Electroacoustic testing
- Probe microphone or real-ear assessment

SPOTLIGHT ON TECHNOLOGY

Telecommunications

People communicate in many ways, including during face-to-face conversations and over the telephone; we also communicate through electronic media and receive important alerting or warning sounds. While hearing aids are useful in face-to-face communication, other forms of communication sometimes require additional assistive listening devices to maximize a person's reception. Communicating on the telephone is one particularly difficult situation for many people with hearing loss, with or without hearing aids. A device known as a *telecoil* is built into the hearing aid and can provide an audible signal to the listener. Other options include special telephone amplifiers that replace the telephone handset, that attach to the phone between the handset and the phone (in-line amplifiers), or that attach to the handset (portable amplifiers). Each of these amplifiers can be used with or without a hearing aid.

For those who cannot understand voices over the telephone, even with amplification, there are other options such as the Voice Carry Over (VCO) or "read and talk" telephones. Used with the telephone relay service, VCO allows a person to talk directly to the other party while an operator translates what the other party says into print that is displayed on a small LCD screen. Other telecommunications options for people who experience difficulty understanding speech over the telephone include e-mail, instant messaging, TTYs, and two-way pagers.

The audiologist also conducts an aural habilitation assessment to develop a comprehensive and appropriate intervention plan. That assessment includes careful evaluation of the following:

- The individual's background, including health status, stage of life, and audiological expectations
- Identification of audiological concerns
- Conversational skills, including appropriateness of topic shifts or balance of turn-taking
- Use and effectiveness of communication strategies, such as lip-reading, using gestures, and asking for clarification
- Status of any current assistive technologies, including hearing aids or cochlear implants
- Degree and areas of perceived handicap, such as problems communicating with spouse or in public forums
- Educational/vocational goals and challenges
- Specific lifestyle concerns, such as family issues, hobbies, and recreational activities

DISCUSSION POINT:
Consider the case of Mr. Johnson in Case Study 14.1. To what extent would auditory rehabilitation be useful for him? What might it entail?

THE IMPORTANCE OF ACCURATE DIAGNOSIS

Hearing loss among adults often has no outward signs. Since it frequently has a gradual onset, the affected person may not be aware that a problem exists or may be unaware of its severity. Nevertheless, the negative consequences of untreated or mismanaged hearing loss can be devastating and far reaching, impacting general well-being, lifestyle, interpersonal relationships, and economic livelihood. The importance of accurate diagnosis is underscored by the improved quality of life for those who obtain appropriate intervention. Specifically, hearing-aid use, and to a lesser extent aural rehabilitation, results in improved personal well-being, enhanced interpersonal relationships, higher productivity, and greater success (Backenroth & Ahlner, 2000; Hawkins, 2005; Jerger, 2007; Lewis et al., 2003). However, an inaccurate diagnosis can lead to inappropriate hearing aid fitting, which can lead to additional loss of hearing if the hearing aid's output is too intense for the individual's hearing level.

DISCUSSION POINT:
Consider some possible explanations for a misdiagnosis of a hearing loss when hearing is, in fact, intact.

HOW IS HEARING LOSS TREATED?

Research shows that the human auditory system, including the brain systems that support audition, remains plastic throughout life, suggesting that the auditory system can be retrained in its functions (Fallon, Irvine, & Shepherd, 2008; Tremblay, 2003). The most effective treatment approach for adult hearing loss is an individualized and comprehensive plan that combines counseling, fitting of amplification devices, and aural rehabilitation (Montgomery & Houston, 2000; Tye-Murray, 2004). Counseling enables an individual to learn how to live life with a hearing loss and not permit it to become a handicap. Counseling also helps family and friends cope with the loss. Amplification devices provide a means to improve hearing acuity and, to some extent, hearing clarity. And aural rehabilitation provides an opportunity to learn compensatory approaches to contend with the hearing loss and a chance to help the auditory system relearn and improve some of its lost or impaired functions.

Despite the known benefits of such an approach, services are too often limited to basic counseling and hearing-aid orientation (Pakulski & Hinkle, 2003; Schow, Balsara, Smedley, & Whitcomb, 1993). Many professionals, particularly those working in private practice and hospital programs, indicate that this gap in service provision is due, at least in part, to the fact that most third-party payers do not reimburse for hearing aids or adult aural rehabilitation services (Pakulski & Hinkle, 2003; Prendergrast & Kelley, 2002). Other explanations include client perceptions that problems are not severe enough to warrant such services, professional concerns about cost-effectiveness and time constraints, and the costs of rehabilitation.

DISCUSSION POINT:
Advocates such as ASHA and the American Academy of Audiology (AAA) continually lobby insurance companies and Congress to cover the cost of hearing-aid services for adults. Why do you think there is resistance to covering these important services?

LIMITATIONS OF CURRENT APPROACHES

Considering the high cost of untreated hearing loss, as well as the stigma attached to both hearing loss and hearing-aid use (Erler & Garstecki, 2002), professionals must continually seek creative ways to make comprehensive services accessible to clients, increase client satisfaction with those services, and reach more individuals in need of such services. Less than one-quarter of all adults with hearing loss get hearing aids, and far fewer participate in aural rehabilitation. It is not surprising, then, that 40% of hearing-aid users report dissatisfaction with their hearing aids (Kochkin, 2002), and more than 15% of people completely reject them following a trial period (Kochkin, 2002; Strom, 2001).

A recent survey of the experiences of 651 hearing-aid recipients examined the types of information and services they received from their audiologists (Stika, Ross, & Cuevas, 2002). Most of the recipients received information focused on aspects of the hearing aid:

- Audiogram results (78%)
- Reasons for the specific hearing-aid selection (79%)
- Care of the hearing aid (79%)

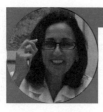

SPOTLIGHT ON RESEARCH AND PRACTICE

NAME: RANDA MANSOUR-SHOUSHER, AuD, CCC-A

PROFESSION/TITLE
Doctor of Clinical Audiology/Clinical Audiologist
Northwest Ohio Hearing Clinic

A DAY AT WORK

Every day is different. Usually my schedule is packed with patients who need simple hearing testing of pre- and post-op audiograms. Engs/VNGs and OAEs are in the mix along with hearing aid fittings and tinnitus patients who are constantly coming in for rechecks on their specific treatment/adjustment to the tinnitus. In between, I will order supplies, including hearing aids; return phone calls; respond to e-mails; pay bills; and write reports. In the mix of that, I teach our AuD student and allow undergraduates time to observe and lecture the medical students or residents.

HOW INTEREST STARTED

I grew up in a medical household. My father was a pediatrician who always told us that medicine was the best field for a career. He was very devoted and committed to his patients and never had hobbies other than medicine and his family. I knew that I didn't want the lifestyle of a physician and balance it with a family without being stressed. Audiology is a good mix that allows me to sleep at night without worrying that the phone will ring in the middle of the night and take me away from home.

PRACTICE INTEREST

My practice interest lies in the area of tinnitus and the comparison between those patients who are using hearing aids and tinnitus treatment devices and those who are just using tinnitus devices.

MOST EXCITING PROFESSIONAL ACCOMPLISHMENTS

I am a first-generation Palestinian and have a desire to help the refugees in the West Bank of Palestine. With the situation and war status, there are many who are exposed to bombing and extreme noise, causing hearing loss. I am currently working on obtaining hearing aids and equipment to send overseas to help the less-fortunate individuals.

FUTURE TRENDS

The next item that I would like to see improvements with is hearing aids that adapt with ease to telephone usage with better Bluetooth capabilities. Along with that, the modifications of BAHA hearing aids to true digital technology.

- Care of the hearing-aid battery (67%)
- Hygiene for the hearing aid and earmold (60%)

However, the survey showed that other types of information were neglected. Only 21% of the audiologists involved spouses or other family members in discussions of strategies for coping with hearing loss, only 19% of hearing-aid recipients received information about consumer resources and self-help groups for persons with hearing loss, only 17% received information about strategies to improve communication, and only 13% received information about communication strategies for dealing with hearing loss at work (Stika, Ross, & Cuevas, 2002).

Thus, although most professionals provide counseling and **hearing-aid orientation,** the scope and focus of those services may not be sufficient. Counseling that focuses on a client's cognitive and emotional response to the hearing loss promotes appropriate expectations for hearing-aid use and for living well with hearing loss (Hallberg, Hallberg, & Kramer, 2008). In addition, there

DISCUSSION POINT:
What might counseling focus on for Kristina, whose case is described in Case Study 14.1? How important is it that she be provided with counseling as well as amplification?

are remarkable benefits in interpersonal relationships when the significant others and family members of individuals with hearing loss are included in counseling (Armero, 2001).

Further, the fitting of amplification devices is often limited to hearing-aid orientation and evaluation of the instrument. However, many hearing-aid users benefit from extended training in use of hearing aids in various situations and settings and in coupling their devices with other forms of technology (e.g., cellular phones or sound systems in theaters). And even short-term training in aural rehabilitation provides benefit to adults with hearing loss and their significant others (Hawkins, 2005). However, many do not receive aural rehabilitation, because they do not seek treatment for hearing loss in general or they do not understand the potential of rehabilitating the auditory system.

AMPLIFICATION AND ASSISTIVE LISTENING DEVICES

Hearing Aids and FM Systems

For most adults who seek treatment for hearing loss, hearing aids are the intervention of choice to improve access to auditory information and increase communication effectiveness (Weinstein, 2000). Modern technology provides many solutions, depending on the etiology, severity, and manifestations of the hearing loss. Hearing aids are available with a wide range of processing abilities, ranging from analog to completely digital. Hearing instruments for adults also vary in size and cosmetic appeal, as illustrated in Figure 14.6. Although most hearing instruments are custom fitted, there are disposable devices that can be used for emergency situations, such as when a hearing aid is being repaired. Consequently, prices range from a few hundred dollars to several thousand dollars. Such a wide array of possibilities can be overwhelming for the consumer without the proper assistance and support of professionals.

Individuals whose hearing loss is caused by damage to the outer hair cells of the cochlea or who have a long-term conductive hearing loss have many choices in instrumentation, since their primary concern is a loss of sensitivity and hearing acuity. When the hearing loss is related to inner hair cell damage or neural damage, resulting in SNR loss, there are two problems to solve: acuity and clarity. The acuity can be remedied quite well with appropriate hearing aids, but the remaining SNR loss cannot be solved with amplification alone (Killion & Christensen, 1998; Killion & Niquette, 2000). Especially if it is moderate to severe or profound, an SNR loss requires an improvement in the signal-to-noise ratio in order to improve the clarity of speech in noise.

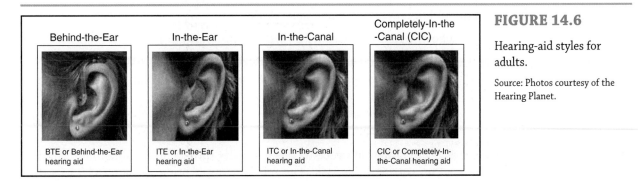

Behind-the-Ear	In-the-Ear	In-the-Canal	Completely-In-the -Canal (CIC)
BTE or Behind-the-Ear hearing aid	ITE or In-the-Ear hearing aid	ITC or In-the-Canal hearing aid	CIC or Completely-In-the-Canal hearing aid

FIGURE 14.6

Hearing-aid styles for adults.

Source: Photos courtesy of the Hearing Planet.

Technological advances have provided several methods of improving SNR for adults. Some adults couple their hearing aids to FM systems that require a speaker to use a small wireless transmitter/microphone, which sends the speech signal to a compact FM receiver. This technology provides remarkable improvement in the SNR of listening situations. For meetings or small groups, FM transmitters are available in the form of a conference microphone, which can be placed in the center of a table. However, this equipment is not suitable for all situations, such as group settings with multiple speakers or with people moving around.

An alternative to FM systems is hearing-aid microphone technology. Directional microphones have long been used on hearing aids to focus reception on the pathway directly in front of the instrument. An omnidirectional microphone detects sounds all around the instrument. A good directional microphone improves the SNR sufficiently for a mild to moderate loss of clarity, but individuals whose SNR loss is more severe require an array of microphones (i.e., multiple microphone technology) to compensate for their loss of clarity (Killion & Niquette, 2000).

Assistive Listening Devices

Assistive listening devices (ALDs) include a variety of technologies—telephone amplifiers, strobe-light doorbells, amplified or lighted fire alarms, and vibrating alarm clocks. All of these provide important options for safety, lifestyle, and vocational choices. Nonetheless, ALDs are not widely used, primarily because of cost. Hearing aids are a significant purchase, and many users believe that the hearing aids alone should handle most situations. Consequently, situation-specific ALDs, which may be helpful, are considered an unnecessary luxury. Awareness of these devices and their availability are other factors. Many audiologists do not dispense ALDs.

DISCUSSION POINT:

People do not typically wear hearing aids to bed at night. What circumstances might arise while someone is asleep that would call for the use of ALDs?

Cochlear Implants and Other Implantable Devices

Recent years have seen dramatic scientific advances in the restoration of hearing following a sensorineural loss. Individuals with severe and profound loss now have access to surgically implantable devices, including cochlear implants and middle-ear and brain-stem implants, which are designed to restore function to damaged areas of the auditory system. A cochlear implant involves placing a device in the cochlea and using an external sound processor (see Figure 14.7) to capture sounds from the environment. Such implants are widely used but may be controversial for some adults.

Not all adults with significant hearing loss are candidates for cochlear implants. Those who desire implantation must go through an extensive evaluation to determine their candidacy. Adults considered optimal candidates for implantation have these characteristics:

- Postlingual deafness with severe to profound loss
- Marginal or no speech-perception benefit from hearing aids
- Good health with no physical abnormalities that will compromise implantation
- Access to optimal education and habilitation services following implementation (National Institutes of Health [NIH], 1995)

The implantation procedure is generally quite safe, although any surgical procedure carries some risk. The rate of complication is about 5%, less than

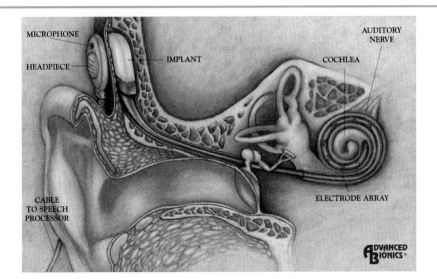

FIGURE 14.7

Anatomy of the cochlear implant.

Source: Photo courtesy of Clarion.

other implantation procedures (e.g., placement of a defibrillator; NIH, 1995). Major complications that are possible, albeit rare, include failure of the device, migration of the device from the site of original placement, and facial palsy resulting from surgical damage to the facial nerve.

Since cochlear implants restore access to sound, adults who have used their sense of hearing to listen and speak prior to their loss can receive great benefit. However, the sound, or sensations, received via the cochlear implant are markedly different from the acoustical sounds to which most listeners are accustomed. Consequently, adults require aural rehabilitation to learn to listen again and to interpret the information provided by the cochlear implant.

AURAL REHABILITATION

Living Well with Hearing Loss

There are a multitude of treatment strategies that can be used to meet the unique needs of adults with hearing loss. All strategies are aimed at preventing hearing loss from diminishing the quality of life, particularly for individuals whose hearing loss has gone undetected or untreated. When hearing loss interferes with perception of self-worth and ability to function appropriately in daily life, a diminished sense of personal well-being negatively affects interpersonal relationships, resulting in concomitant problems such as loss of intimacy and strained interactions. Individual counseling focuses on issues of self-perception, understanding hearing loss and its manifestations, and learning how to live well with hearing loss. Some of the strategies addressed in counseling are presented in Figure 14.8.

Group counseling is a useful tool to examine **communication breakdowns** and the ways they affect relationships. People converse dozens of times each day with family, friends, colleagues, service providers, and even strangers. And conversation occurs in every imaginable situation and listening environment, many of which are not conducive to good communication. For instance, people may say hello as they pass in a stairwell and then continue the conversation as one climbs up and the other down. For people with hearing loss, these daily conversations on the run can be impossible to manage and often produce misunderstandings or hurt feelings. Imagine that

DISCUSSION POINT:
Communication breakdowns occur for everyone at some time. What are some strategies you use to repair breakdowns during communicative interactions?

FIGURE 14.8

Strategies for living well with hearing loss.

Environment
• Optimize visual cues with good lighting.
• Reduce extraneous background noise (e.g., television in the background).
• Minimize distance between speaker and listener (e.g., don't try to converse in different rooms).
• Determine best location for listening in important settings.

Communication style
• Take responsibility for communication needs (e.g., request that TV be turned off during conversation).
• Ask for assistance when needed (e.g., Will you please look at me when you speak?).
• Do not bluff.
• Be patient.
• Take interest in the speaker and concentrate on the conversation.

Expectations
• Be realistic. Hearing aids do not restore hearing; they make sounds accessible.
• Some listening situations are difficult for everyone, including those with good hearing.
• Relearning to listen takes time. Think of it as retraining the brain now that the ears can hear.
• Seek professional help when problems arise.
• Use hearing aids consistently, every day, not just for special occasions.

Jill has a hearing loss and passes her neighbor in a busy grocery store. Without stopping to chat, Jill mindlessly asks, "How are you?" Her neighbor, having just found out that her mother is gravely ill, replies, "Not great—it's been a difficult week for us." But Jill hears only "great" and replies, "Glad to hear it."

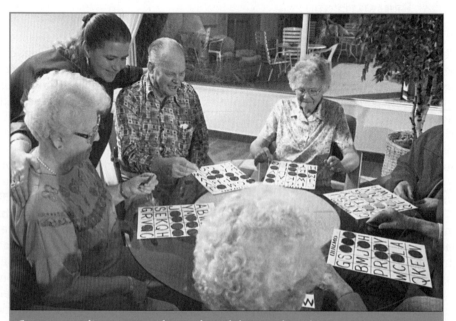

Group counseling can provide people with hearing loss the opportunity to identify and discuss reasons for communication breakdowns.

Goals of Aural Rehabilitation

The overarching goal of aural rehabilitation is to improve the fluency and effectiveness of communication, which is key to quality of life. Specific targets include (1) evaluating communication partners' roles in conversation, (2) determining whether social rules are broken (e.g., with inappropriate topic shifts), and (3) teaching strategies to facilitate communication and repair breakdowns effectively. Such strategies can incorporate a variety of methods—for example, improving use of visual cues or building listening and attention skills. Some communication training strategies are listed in Figure 14.9.

FIGURE 14.9

Communication training strategies.

Strategies for significant others

- Do not talk too loudly or abnormally slowly; speak naturally and distinctly
- Rephrase rather than repeat
- Get a person's attention before starting conversation and emphasize the subject or idea you are speaking about
- Do not try to speak from another room or from a distance
- Follow rules of conversation (e.g., turn taking, shared ideas, etc.)

Strategies for listeners with hearing loss

Keys to good listening

- Practice paying attention
- Be assertive; admit the presence of hearing loss and explain how others can be helpful
- Do not try to get every word; concentrate on the thread and spirit of the message
- Manipulate the environment to facilitate communication
- Be prepared; review topics or be familiar with concepts before attending a listening event (e.g., movie)

Using visual cues to enhance listening

- Practice interpreting gestures and facial expressions and pay attention to these cues during conversation
- Observe situational cues
- Consider linguistic constraints
- Practice and use visual recognition of sounds (speech and/or lip-reading)

Preventing communication breakdowns

- Follow rules of conversation
- Choose topics of importance and interest to conversational partners
- Take turns; make sure one person does not do all the talking
- Change topics in an orderly fashion
- Do not bluff or disregard missed information
- Be specific when requesting clarification
- Stay focused and attentive; choose appropriate moment to get clarification if something is missed
- Be prepared for difficult situations (e.g., communicating in the car or at a large gathering)

Repairing communication breakdowns

- Request clarification or missed information thoughtfully (e.g., be specific about what was not clear)
- Ask for repetition of entire message, a specific aspect, key word, or unclear content
- Choose a repair strategy and implement it at an appropriate moment
- Be patient and appreciative of partner's efforts

Source: Information on communication breakdowns based on Tye-Murray (2004).

As a function of improving communication, rehabilitation focuses on maintaining (or restoring) an individual's lifestyle and vocation. Age, stage of life, and lifestyle will all strongly influence a treatment approach. For example, a corporate executive will need to listen effectively in a variety of settings and may require ALDs (e.g., conference microphone/FM system) or hearing aids interfacing with a cellular telephone. A retired homemaker who lives alone might benefit from safety/alerting devices, as well as ways to communicate with people outside the home (e.g., amplified telephone or e-mail). Maintaining lifestyle and vocation is also addressed along with protecting hearing from further loss.

Building Treatment Plans

Following diagnosis of hearing loss and evaluation for any treatable medical causes (e.g., otitis media), a hearing-aid evaluation and aural rehabilitation assessment are completed to develop an effective treatment plan. A hearing-aid fitting includes counseling regarding expectations as well as orientation to device operation and use. A hearing-aid trial period (typically 30 days) is initiated, during which time additional hearing-aid evaluations are completed to ensure that the instrument is providing appropriate amplification.

When the appropriateness of the fitting is confirmed, the aural rehabilitation program is initiated, which takes into account a wide range of concerns related to individual needs. Depending on the severity, length, and type of loss, clients' rehabilitation needs will vary from minimal to extensive. One program incorporates five areas of rehabilitation, using the acronym *FACES:*

- **F**amily/significant other participation
- **A**uditory skill building
- **C**onversation strategies
- **E**ducation and counseling
- **S**peech reading and visual cues (Schow, 2001; Weinstein, 2000)

The participation of family/significant others refers to the ongoing commitment and involvement of family members in the rehabilitation process. Family members should receive training in how to change their communication styles to enhance the audibility of their speech, how to address communication-related relationship issues, and how to support the individual with hearing loss in use of amplification devices.

Auditory skill building concerns the ability of the person with hearing loss to relearn how to listen. For cochlear implant users, auditory skill building may need to start with basic sound detection (e.g., whether the radio is on or off), discrimination (e.g., attending to the stress or length of an utterance), and identification (e.g., identifying a spoken phrase). Individuals who receive implants soon after the loss of hearing and whose language skills were good prior to the loss will likely progress well through this rehabilitation process. For new hearing-aid users, problems are often situational—listening in noise or comprehending spoken language from a distance. Consequently, auditory skill building may focus on use of instrumentation or accommodations to improve the audibility of sounds (e.g., interfacing with a telephone at work or using an FM system at church or in the theater).

Conversational strategies address issues related to maintaining conversational fluency—facilitating conversation and repairing communication breakdowns. Examples of both facilitative and repair strategies are provided in Figure 14.10.

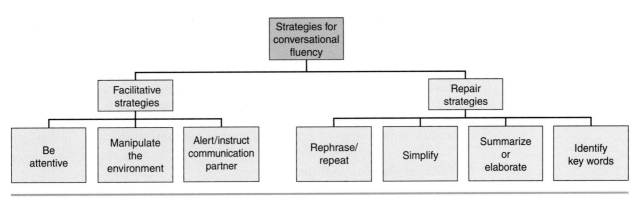

Strategies for maintaining conversational fluency.

FIGURE 14.10

Teaching these strategies through example and practice is effective and may involve group therapy so that individuals can apply specific strategies in interactions with others. For example, Karen might ask Susan, "Did you borrow my yellow cardigan last week?" Susan might hear something about borrow but not understand the message. If she says, "What?" or "I didn't hear you," Karen will have to repeat the entire phrase. Instead, Susan should determine which key words she understood and then simplify her request: "I didn't get that. You asked if I borrowed what?"

In turn, Karen can learn strategies for giving clearer messages. She can use repetition and simpler phrasing: "My sweater, did you borrow my sweater?" Thus, analyzing a conversation provides invaluable information that can be used to discuss and train communication partners in the elements of shared conversation with persons with hearing loss. Through practice and attention to what is heard and not heard, miscommunication and frustration are less likely, and individuals with hearing loss can improve their communication participation and their fluency.

Also important are education and counseling at the time of hearing-aid fitting; this can significantly reduce the self-perception of a hearing handicap (Hallberg et al., 2008; Hawkins, 2005), a perception that often leads to rejection of hearing aids or high rates of infrequent use and dissatisfaction (Armero, 2001). Other important aspects that should be addressed include these:

- Function, use, and maintenance of hearing aids/related devices
- An understanding of hearing loss and the impact on communication
- Realistic expectations of instrumentation
- Social, emotional, and psychological underpinnings of hearing loss

Despite the known benefits of counseling, many professionals have received little training in counseling and psychology (Armero, 2001) and have difficulty with the emotions of personal and relationship counseling. Nonetheless, significant others share in the handicapping effect of hearing loss, experiencing a reduced quality of life, embarrassment in public communication situations, and social withdrawal (Armero, 2001; Preminger, 2003). The impact of hearing loss is considerable and extends far beyond the client.

A treatment plan should also include speech and lip-reading and other visual cues, which are useful tools in interpreting messages. Given minimal instruction, people can learn to read sounds and words as they are formed and use this skill to help fill in missing parts of conversation in difficult listening situations. However, some subtle auditory cues that provide information about emotion or meaning may not be audible, even with hearing aids, or may not be accessible to speech reading. For example, a wife may question her husband with hearing loss: "You're going to wear *that*?" with heavy emphasis on the final word. Her husband would miss the subtle auditory cue, but if he was able to detect nonverbal cues like facial expression, he could still determine that his wife was not thrilled with his selection. Aural rehabilitation provides an individual with a range of tools for effective communication.

Early Identification and Intervention

Early identification is just as important for adults with hearing loss as it is for children. Adult-onset hearing loss typically manifests itself as a gradual decrease in hearing acuity, often in the higher frequencies, as well as a possible loss of clarity. Consequently, people first notice that they do not seem to understand as well as they used to or they miss some sounds. Yet the auditory system still functions, and individuals learn to make do with the hearing they have, sometimes relying on visual or other cues to help decipher messages. When prompted by a family member or a physician to get a hearing assessment or a hearing aid, the common response is that the problem is not "that bad." This situation is complicated by the fact that only about 16% of senior citizens receive a hearing screening as part of their routine physical (Kochkin, 2002).

As people experience a gradual decrease in auditory acuity and clarity, they become increasingly accustomed to a more quiet world. The auditory system is relied on less and less, especially as individuals make significant changes in lifestyle to avoid difficult situations. Much like a muscle that is not exerted for a long period of time, the auditory system becomes unaccustomed to deciphering speech or managing noise. People who avoid hearing aids and treatment for many years often find it difficult, if not impossible, to adjust to amplification. However, early identification of adult hearing loss, combined with appropriate amplification, allows the auditory system to maintain function and continue its auditory capability. Timely intervention maximizes the chance of maintaining good listening skills.

Healthy People 2010, an initiative of the U.S. Department of Health and Human Services (USDHHS), focuses on health promotion for the American people and seeks to increase the number of referrals primary care physicians make for hearing evaluations. *Healthy People 2010* recommends frequent hearing screenings for anyone over age 50 (USDHHS, 2000). Physicians can identify individuals who should receive audiological screenings by asking a few pointed questions that focus on whether hearing difficulties are impacting life.

One quick, easy, and free tool is the Hearing Handicap Inventory for the Elderly—Screening Version (Ventry & Weinstein, 1982), which provides 10 questions a physician or other professional can ask to determine whether a hearing loss exists. Examples of questions include these:

- Does a hearing problem cause you to attend religious services less often than you would like?
- Does a hearing problem cause you to have arguments with family members?
- Does a hearing problem cause you difficulty when listening to the TV or radio?

The items on the inventory identify ways in which a person's life might be impacted by a hearing loss. Scores can range from 0 to 40; a score of 10 or higher warrants a referral for an audiological evaluation. Tools like this, which can be administered in minutes, are important in increasing the identification of hearing loss among the adult population and improving access to services.

> **CASE ANALYSIS**
>
> Study the case of Emily (Case Study 9 on the Companion Website at www.pearsonhighered.com/justice2e). Reflect on how her hearing loss may impact her quality of life.

● CHAPTER SUMMARY

At this time, about 10% of the population experiences hearing loss. However, the incidence of hearing loss is expected to increase dramatically as baby boomers reach advanced age after years of loud music in addition to work-related and environmental noise exposure. Considering the incredible advances in technology, the likelihood of successful rehabilitation is greater than ever. Yet research continues to show that, as a whole, people with hearing loss are reluctant to seek treatment. In fact, fewer than 25% of those with significant hearing loss use hearing aids. Failure to seek initial treatment stems from financial concerns as well as denial of the severity and extent of the problem.

Many individuals who do seek treatment have mediocre success, because they delay intervention until the problem reaches alarming severity, and they fail to participate in comprehensive aural rehabilitation programs. Professionals report that the gap in service provision can be attributed to their inability to convince potential clients of the benefits of aural rehabilitation, coupled with a lack of third-party reimbursement.

Research consistently shows that individuals with hearing loss who do not seek treatment (especially those who function in the hearing world and then experience a deterioration in their hearing) suffer significant reductions in quality of life. In fact, the cost of untreated or mismanaged hearing loss is enormous on both the personal and societal levels.

Audiologists and speech-language pathologists have the tools to provide intervention to those who seek it. Amplification and other assistive devices, coupled with comprehensive aural rehabilitation programs, are highly effective in improving access to auditory information as well as countering the negative impact of hearing loss. Professionals are challenged to reach potential clients early and convince them to avail themselves of services.

● KEY TERMS

communication breakdowns, p. 485
hearing-aid orientation, p. 482
labyrinthitis, p. 478
Meniere's disease, p. 478

noise-induced hearing loss, p. 470
otosclerosis, p. 475
ototoxicity, p. 477
presbycusis, p. 470

recruitment, p. 466
signal-to-noise ratio (SNR) loss, p. 467
tinnitus, p. 466

● ON THE WEB

Check out the Companion Website at www.pearsonhighered.com/justice2e. On it you will find:

- suggested readings
- reflection questions

- a self-study quiz
- links to additional online resources, including current technologies in communication sciences and disorders

FEEDING AND SWALLOWING DISORDERS

Cynthia O'Donoghue
Mary C. Tarbell
Laura M. Justice

FOCUS QUESTIONS

This chapter answers the following questions:

1. What are feeding and swallowing disorders?

2. What are the defining characteristics of pediatric feeding and swallowing disorders?

3. How are pediatric feeding and swallowing disorders identified and treated?

4. What are the defining characteristics of adult dysphagia?

5. How is adult dysphagia identified and treated?

INTRODUCTION

Like all other species, humans must eat and drink to develop and maintain themselves physically, cognitively, and psychologically. Drinking and eating is also a typical component of most social activities that we enjoy—birthday parties, holiday dinners, even popcorn at the movies. Yet, for some children and adults, the ability to eat and drink efficiently and safely is compromised due to disease or injury.

Individuals with disruptions in their swallowing ability may find eating to be a burden, or they may be limited in what foods or liquids they can safely consume such that meals are no longer pleasurable. This impairment in the ability to swallow is known as **dysphagia,** which is a type of **feeding disorder,** because the individual with dysphagia can no longer eat safely. Dysphagia occurs across the age spectrum for a variety of reasons due to developmental, neurological, or structural problems that alter the normal swallowing process.

Speech-language pathologists (SLPs) are the professionals who evaluate and treat this disorder (ASHA, 2002c). To many students beginning their studies in Communication Sciences and Disorders, the role of evaluating and treating clients with swallowing disorders is a new concept. However, speech-language pathologists have been involved with management of dysphagia and feeding disorders for some time. The premier textbook *Evaluation and Treatment of Swallowing Disorders* was published in the early 1980s (Logemann, 1983), and many SLPs were already actively engaged in the management of persons with swallowing impairments. Recognizing these additional clinical responsibilities for many practicing therapists, ASHA has expanded the Scope of Practice for Speech-Language Pathology to include swallowing disorders and in 1987 provided an initial policy statement titled "Knowledge and Skills Needed by Speech-Language Pathologists Providing Services to Dysphagic Patients/ Clients" (ASHA, 2002c). Dysphagia and feeding management for children and adults is now a major component of the SLP's daily professional responsibilities in many settings, including hospitals, rehabilitation centers, nursing homes, outpatient clinics, and even public schools. In fact, dysphagia services now constitute more than 50% of the SLP's clinical caseload in medical settings (ASHA, 2002d).

SLPs who specialize in feeding and swallowing disorders in children or dysphagia in adults will play a direct role in assessment and treatment. They will conduct a comprehensive assessment of structures and functions involved with feeding and swallowing abilities and, if these are impaired, will provide treatment to strengthen the oral-motor system and build the individual's capacity for safe feeding and swallowing. The **oral-motor system** refers to the physical structures and neuromuscular functions involved with both eating and speaking. The SLP focuses on improving **oral-motor functions** (i.e., the strength and coordination of the articulators), **oral-motor muscular tone** (i.e., the tension and posture of the articulators), and **oral-motor sensation** (i.e., the sensitivity to taste, movement, and textures; Creskoff & Haas, 1999). Simultaneously, the therapist will investigate and implement strategies to help the individual drink and eat safely to the extent this is possible.

Providing clinical services to persons with dysphagia requires specialized skills and knowledge given that mismanagement of this disorder may have life-threatening consequences. Individuals with dysphagia are at risk for choking and blocking the airway, aspirating foods into their lungs, pneumonia, and potentially death. Although these risks present challenges, improving one's ability to eat safely and pleasurably can be especially rewarding. ●●●

WHAT ARE FEEDING AND SWALLOWING DISORDERS? ●

PEDIATRIC FEEDING DISORDERS

The American Psychiatric Association (APA; 1994) defines a *feeding disorder* as a child's "persistent failure to eat adequately" for a period of at least 1 month, which results in a significant loss of weight or a failure to gain weight (p. 98). Feeding disorders among children most often manifest themselves in the first year of life, often as part of a broader medical or developmental condition, such as cleft palate; however, feeding disorders can occur in apparent isolation and with no clear cause. In addition to the failure to eat adequately, the child with a feeding disorder usually demonstrates one or more of the following:

- Unsafe or inefficient swallowing patterns
- Growth delay affecting height and/or weight
- Lack of tolerance of food textures and tastes
- Poor appetite regulation

Mild and transient feeding problems are common in young children; 25 to 35% of parents report that their young children have feeding issues (Linscheid, 1992). These temporary feeding problems may emerge at certain developmental points, such as the transition to solid foods, but they usually resolve easily with no negative effect on the developing child (Black, Cureton, & Berenson-Howard, 1999). More serious and persistent feeding problems are less common; their prevalence is difficult to estimate. As many as 10% of young children experience malnutrition, although it is not clear how many of these cases are due to feeding and swallowing disorders (Kessler, 1999). Of children admitted to the hospital for failure to gain adequate weight, about half are due to feeding disturbances (APA, 1994).

Feeding disorders become more prevalent in the context of specific risk factors. For instance, about 8% of all babies born in the United States have a very low birth weight—308,470 babies in the year 2000 (Maternal and Child Health Bureau, 2002). These and other conditions described later greatly elevate the likelihood of feeding or swallowing disorders in young children (Black et al., 1999; Satter, 1999).

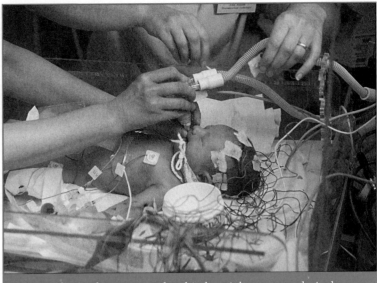

Infants who are born at very low birth weights are at relatively greater risk of developing feeding problems.

Conditions that cause frailty in infants are increasing in their prevalence, such as being born at low birth weight. In the last decade, the likelihood that very-low-birth-weight infants would survive to leave the hospital increased 10%, from 74% to 84% (Lemons et al., 2001). From the very start of their lives, many of these children exhibit significant impairments of feeding and require the earliest of interventions while in the **neonatal intensive care unit** (NICU). Not only do these children's fragile medical states complicate the feeding process, but the NICU treatments themselves can directly interfere with the development of pleasurable oral experiences—for example, the use of nasogastric feeding tubes for high-calorie nutritional support and ventilators to provide oxygen, as described in Table 15.1.

In addition, children served in the NICU may have limited exposure to foods and thus may have missed out on the opportunity to progress normally and/or safely in the early stages of feeding development, learn feeding routines, and to experience different tastes and textures. These children may have an inability to manipulate food safely in their mouths and may have increased aversion to foods because of their lack of experience. This may increase the likelihood that these children will demonstrate food refusal, inappropriate meal time behaviors, and/or inefficient ingestion.

> **DISCUSSION POINT:**
> What conditions can you think of that cause frailty in young children? Of these, which would you expect to increase a child's risk for feeding or swallowing problems?

DYSPHAGIA

A *swallowing disorder,* or dysphagia, occurs when an individual exhibits an unsafe or inefficient swallowing pattern that undermines the eating/drinking process. These can occur at any time of the human life span but are most common among infants and the elderly. Swallowing, also called **deglutition,** is the complex neuromuscular act of moving substances from the oral cavity to the esophagus. The substance being moved is generically called the *bolus.*

Swallowing safely is often taken for granted. However, it is important to recognize that only a slim margin of error separates the pathway for breathing (i.e., the airway) from the pathway of the bolus. Unsafe swallowing can be a

Procedure	Purpose	Description
Enteral (tube) feeding	• Provides a temporary means to improve the child's nutrition and growth when at least 80% of nutritional needs cannot be met orally and weight loss or no gain occurs for 3 months • Used for prematurity, lack of weight gain, gastrointestinal dysfunctions, severe diarrhea, coma, feeding refusal, failure to thrive	• Nasogastric tube passed through nose and esophagus for short-term feeding (>3 months) • Gastrostomy tube surgically placed directly into the stomach for long-term feeding (3 months) • Jejunostomy tube surgically placed into the jejunum, or small intestine, also for long-term feeding
Tracheostomy	• Provides an alternative airway when the airway is blocked by congenital or acquired airway obstruction • Also used to provide oxygen supplements for cardiopulmonary disease or an infant unable to breathe adequately because of prematurity or trauma and requiring a ventilator.	• An incision made into the trachea, or airway • A tracheostomy tube placed into the incision to provide an airway that bypasses the oral/nasal cavity
Ventilation	• Provides an alternative or supplementary source of oxygen when a child cannot breathe because of an immature respiratory system or an injury or impairment of the respiratory system (e.g., chronic lung disease) • Supplemental oxygen needed by nearly one-fourth of very-low-birth-weight children up to 9 months after birth	• Mechanical ventilation attached to child via a tracheostomy tube

TABLE 15.1   Common neonatal intensive care procedures that can impact feeding and swallowing development

Sources: Based on Kedesdy and Budd (1998); Lemons, Bauer, Oh, et al. (2001); Schauster and Dwyer (1996).

life-or-death matter, as poor management and coordination of swallowing increases a child's or adult's risk of penetration or aspiration of food or liquid into the laryngeal area, which serves as the gateway to and the protector of the lungs (see Figure 15.1). With **penetration,** food or liquid enters the larynx, which can cause choking and respiratory distress. With **aspiration,** the food or liquid passes through the larynx and into the lungs, which can interfere with the exchange of air in the lungs and cause asphyxiation or a pulmonary infection, such as pneumonia. To more properly understand what happens when swallowing goes wrong, we provide in the next section a review of the phases of the normal swallow, discussed previously in Chapter 3.

FIGURE 15.1

An infant's laryngeal area, depicting pathways for nutrition and respiration.

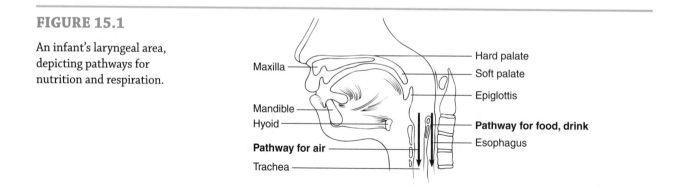

CASE STUDY 15.1	Feeding and Swallowing Disorders

LILY is a 2-year-old girl living in Omaha, Nebraska. She was born with the umbilical cord tightly wrapped around her neck, resulting in brain damage from lack of oxygen during the birthing process that led to cerebral palsy and oral motor dysfunction. At birth, Lily could not coordinate a suck-swallow-breathe pattern and demonstrated frequent choking and gagging. A modified barium swallow study at 2 weeks revealed aspiration during bottle feeding and poor coordination of the tongue during sucking. Lily had a gastrostomy tube placed at 3 weeks to provide nutrition. Now, on her second birthday, her parents would like to begin feeding her orally. Lily uses a wheelchair for mobility and positioning and has no functional use of her hands. Cognitively, Lily is delayed but appears to understand some family members' names.

Internet research

1 How common is it for children to be born with the umbilical cord wrapped around their neck?

2 What kind of community resources are available in Omaha, Nebraska, for Lily's family?

3 How prevalent is cerebral palsy due to perinatal birth trauma?

Brainstorm and discussion

1 How do you think Lily's feeding and swallowing difficulties affect her family?

2 Given that Lily has been on a feeding tube for 2 years, why would her parents want to pursue oral intake at this time?

3 What other aspects of Lily's life might be affected by her dependence on a gastrostomy tube for nutrition?

● ● ●

SYLVIA ANDERSON is a 78-year-old female who currently lives at Pleasant Valley Nursing Home. Sylvia has Alzheimer's dementia, diagnosed approximately 11 years ago. She also has a history of hypertension, diabetes, bilateral hip replacements, osteoarthritis, and intermittent unexplained bronchitis. Sylvia has resided at Pleasant Valley for 2 years, and although she needs supervision for her safety, she is ambulatory with a cane and completes her daily dressing, bathing, and feeding with minimal to moderate assistance.

Recently, the nursing assistants have noted that Sylvia is not finishing her meals and that midway through her meal, she has a gurgly voice quality with excessive throat clearing. Three days ago, Sylvia had a severe coughing episode while eating fried chicken. The nursing staff consulted the only speech-language pathologist in the facility to evaluate Sylvia for possible dysphagia. He completed a clinical bedside examination of swallowing and found Sylvia pleasant, cooperative, and able to follow short instructions, although cognitive impairments were evident. Assessment findings suggested that Sylvia has a pharyngeal phase swallowing

problem, and an instrumental assessment at the local hospital is scheduled.

Internet research

1 What is the prevalence of Alzheimer's dementia in the United States?

2 What is the percentage of nursing home residents over 65 years of age suspected to have dysphagia?

3 Find a website that provides information on Alzheimer's disease and support for clients and their families. What kinds of supports are most prevalent?

Brainstorm and discussion

1 Transporting Sylvia to the local hospital for an instrumental examination of dysphagia is costly. Is this cost justifiable?

2 How will Sylvia's cognitive decline and dementia diagnosis affect treatment of dysphagia?

THE NORMAL SWALLOW

Swallowing is so natural that we do it approximately 580 times daily without even thinking about it (Logemann, 1998). Even though we do not consciously think about how to swallow, there are specific physiological components of a normal swallow that occur in a series of unfolding stages. These swallowing stages, also called *phases,* include the oral preparatory phase, the oral phase, the pharyngeal phase, and the esophageal phase. Each of these is essential for safely and efficiently moving food and drink from the oral cavity through the pharynx (i.e., throat) and into the esophagus toward the intestines. The four phases of swallowing must work seamlessly and efficiently to keep food and drink from taking possibly dangerous routes.

The Oral Preparatory Phase

The role of the oral preparatory phase is to prepare the substance to be swallowed for swallowing. This phase starts as the food or liquid enters the mouth, and it includes containing the material in the oral cavity by closing the lips and then manipulating and preparing the food or liquid into a cohesive ball, or bolus. As food enters the oral cavity, saliva production increases to assist in bolus formation. Also, the soft palate lowers toward the tongue to contain the bolus and prohibit the flow of ingested material into the pharyngeal region until the bolus is adequately prepared. Chewing, or *mastication,* occurs as the lips, tongue, teeth, mandible, and cheeks work cooperatively to grind the food into a manageable texture to swallow. Even with liquids, a bolus is formed that assists in controlling the flow of the liquid.

The time to complete the oral preparatory phase is variable, depending on the substance eaten. Oral preparation for liquids (e.g., tea, milkshake) is more rapid than for foods requiring mastication (e.g., potato chips, popcorn). Throughout the oral preparatory phase, respiration continues with inhalation and exhalation through the nose.

The Oral Phase

The role of the oral phase is to move the bolus to the rear of the oral cavity and prepare it for propulsion down the throat. The oral phase begins as the tongue propels the bolus to the back of the mouth. This "stripping action" is accomplished as the tongue presses upward against the hard palate. This tongue movement, coupled with tension in the cheeks created by the *buccal muscles,* creates a pressure that pushes the bolus backward toward the pharynx. You can experience this by chewing a cracker. Notice that once the cracker is prepared into a ball in the oral preparatory phase, you move it back into the throat by pushing the tongue against the roof of the mouth. The oral phase typically is completed within 1 to 1.5 seconds (Logemann, 1998). In this phase, the individual still maintains a normal respiratory pattern, breathing through the nose.

The Pharyngeal Phase

The role of the pharyngeal phase is to propel the bolus downward through the throat to the entrance of the esophagus. The pharyngeal phase begins when the bolus reaches the posterior portion of the oral cavity, specifically the *anterior faucial pillars.* These pillars comprise a band of muscular tissue that extends from both sides of the palate to the tongue. The muscle forms a sphincter that contracts to initiate the pharyngeal phase of the swallow.

The pharyngeal phase is complex, with many important physiological occurrences happening simultaneously and quickly. At the start of this phase, the **pharyngeal swallow reflex** is triggered; the posterior pharyngeal wall and the back of the tongue move toward one another to create a pressure that, in conjunction with the squeezing pharyngeal muscles, moves the bolus downward through the pharynx toward the entrance to the esophagus. The *cricopharyngeus muscle,* also called the *upper esophageal sphincter,* is the juncture between the pharynx and the esophagus. It opens to allow passage of the bolus into the esophagus.

The pharyngeal phase is important; at this point, the bolus can potentially enter the laryngeal pathway to the lungs or the nasal cavity, prohibiting breathing. However, there are multiple protective mechanisms in place within the pharyngeal phase to prevent either from happening. First, the soft palate elevates to form a barrier between the pharynx and the nasal cavity; this keeps the bolus from flowing upward into the nasal area. Second, the larynx moves forward and higher in the neck, making the risk of material entering the airway less probable. Third, the epiglottis folds downward to form a cover over the larynx. Fourth, both the false and true vocal folds approximate (i.e., come together) to close and prevent ingested materials from entering the larynx, or airway.

If for some reason material does go the wrong way, a reflexive cough occurs to propel the material back out. The **reflexive cough** is a protective reflex in which exhaled air is forced upward through the vocal folds to expel any foreign matter. In addition, during the pharyngeal phase of a normal swallow, respiration experiences a brief halt, called an **apneic moment.** This short period of halted breathing further minimizes the risk of material entering the airway. In all, this stage lasts about 1 second from the time the pharyngeal swallow reflex is triggered until the bolus passes into the esophagus.

> **DISCUSSION POINT:**
> During which swallowing phase is Sylvia's (Case Study 15.1) swallowing difficulty appearing to occur? In your own words, describe what happens in this phase of swallow.

The Esophageal Phase

The esophageal phase moves the bolus through the esophagus into the stomach. This process starts as the bolus passes through the upper esophageal sphincter (UES). The bolus is propelled through the esophagus by an involuntary wave, or contraction. It then passes through the lower esophageal sphincter (LES) into the stomach. The esophageal phase ranges from about 8 to 20 seconds for adults. Age influences the variation in duration, with esophageal movement slowing as we age—referred to as a decrease in *esophageal motility* (DeVault, 2002). In summary, the normal swallowing process is a complex yet innate ability, as presented in Figure 15.2.

THE DISORDERED SWALLOW: DYSPHAGIA

Dysphagia is a condition in which an individual exhibits difficulty in at least one of the phases of the swallow, causing swallowing to be inefficient or unsafe. When swallowing is inefficient, it does not provide adequate nutrition. For instance, individuals may spend so much time in the oral preparatory phase that they are fatigued and unable to consume enough food to meet their nutritional needs.

When swallowing is unsafe, individuals are at risk of penetration or aspiration because of poor coordination or management of the bolus as it moves through the swallowing phases. Of particular concern is when silent aspiration occurs, as there is no sign—such as choking, coughing, or speaking with a wet or gurgly voice—to suggest that aspiration is occurring. For instance, an infant

FIGURE 15.2

Bolus movement during a normal swallow.

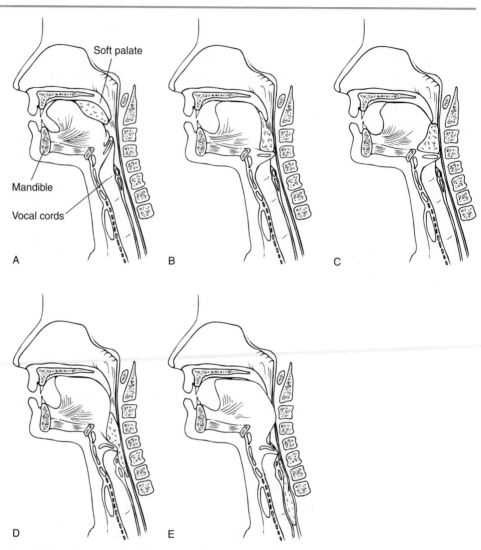

Lateral view of swallow, beginning with initiation of swallow by tongue (A); the triggering of the pharyngeal swallow (B); the bolus in the valleculae area (C); the tongue base retraction against the pharyngeal wall (D); the bolus in the cervical esophagus (E).

may have severe pharyngeal phase dysphagia characterized by excessive aspiration but may exhibit no outward signs that aspiration is occurring. In such instances, only a direct examination of the infant's pharyngeal area during swallowing, made possible through a technique called *videofluoroscopy,* will identify the infant's aspiration. Both penetration and aspiration present hazards: Penetration can result in choking, causing a loss of oxygen to the brain and leading to brain damage or death, and aspiration can result in pneumonia and pulmonary damage.

Individuals with dysphagia may be unable to intake certain food consistencies safely and must, as a result, have their diets altered. With such diet changes, individuals frequently have difficulty maintaining their hydration and nutrition. If the situation persists, these individuals need to be fed through an alternative means, such as an **enteral feeding tube,** which directs a liquid formula to the stomach and is typically placed through the nose (i.e., nasogastric tube) or directly into the stomach (i.e., gastrostomy tube). The liquid formula provides for nutritional maintenance, and water can also be given to keep persons hydrated.

A Symptom, Not a Disease

Dysphagia is not a disease but rather is a symptom that results from an underlying etiology, or cause. Swallowing problems can result from neurological injuries; progressive disease processes; head and neck cancers; or even the medical treatments prescribed to combat a disease, such as radiation to treat laryngeal cancer. Dysphagia among young children often results from medical complications associated with low birth weight, prematurity, or presence of developmental disabilities like cleft palate.

WHAT ARE THE DEFINING CHARACTERISTICS OF PEDIATRIC FEEDING AND SWALLOWING DISORDERS? ●

Pediatric feeding and swallowing disorders may be characterized by such symptoms as a refusal to eat, eating nonnutritive substances, and rigidity in eating. A summary of prevalent behaviors that characterize various types of feeding and swallowing disorders is presented in Table 15.2.

Regardless of what specific behaviors are demonstrated, it is important to identify how, exactly, the child's feeding and swallowing behaviors differ from the norm. Normal feeding and swallowing are safe, efficient, and organized. Consequently, a disorder of feeding/swallowing typically features one or more of these characteristics:

1. Feeding and/or swallowing is unsafe.
2. Feeding and/or swallowing is inadequate.
3. Feeding and/or swallowing is inappropriate.

UNSAFE FEEDING AND SWALLOWING

Defining Characteristics

At birth, an infant must skillfully implement a coordinated pattern of suckling, swallowing, and breathing. This coordination is not always perfect in young infants, but minor deviations do not usually pose a risk (Arvedson & Rogers, 1997). Some children, however, cannot negotiate the suck-swallow-breathe pattern, and feeding and swallowing become unsafe. Feeding and swallowing are unsafe when they pose a risk of penetration or aspiration of the bolus into the airway.

Unsafe swallowing (dysphagia) typically results from the dysfunction of or damage to a child's oral-motor system or an inappropriate eating rate, either too fast or too slow. Swallowing dysfunction can affect planning, timing, coordination, organization, and sensation. Consider, for instance, children who have cardiac or pulmonary issues who may breathe too rapidly to coordinate a suck-swallow-breathe pattern. When liquid is pulled into the oral cavity but allowed to linger, it can create a pool in the *valleculae,* the space created when the epiglottis folds down to cover the trachea during swallowing. If milk pools there, it can easily spill over into the airway before or after a swallow has been triggered, putting the child at risk for aspiration.

TABLE 15.2   Behaviors characteristic of pediatric feeding and swallowing disorders

Behavior	Description
Food refusal	• Resistance to eating and/or drinking that cannot be attributed to a lack of food or a medical condition
Food selectivity	• Severely self-restricted diet based on resistance to certain types, textures, or volumes of food available • May range from mild ("picky eating") to extreme (e.g., refusal to eat all but one color of food)
Rumination	• Persistent regurgitation and reingestion of food for a period of 1 month or longer • Voluntary (self-induced), pleasurable, usually involving small portions, and not associated with nausea
Vomiting	• Persistent voluntary or involuntary expulsion of a typically large volume of food or drink • Associated with nausea, distress, and acute weight loss
Pica	• Ingestion of nonnutritive substances for 1 month or longer (e.g., clay, soil, insects, animal droppings, paint, pebbles, leaves, hair)
Limited food intake	• Inadequate eating and nutritional intake, perhaps due to passivity, lack of interest or appetite, or excessive selectivity
Excessive food intake	• Persistent overintake of food • May result from an insatiable appetite (hyperphagia)
Oral-motor hypersensitivity	• Excessive sensitivity of the oral-motor structures (e.g., teeth, lips, cheeks, tongue) or functions (e.g., swallowing too soon, gagging)
Oral-motor hyposensitivity	• Inadequate sensitivity of the oral-motor structures (e.g., teeth, lips, cheeks, tongue) or functions (e.g., inability to trigger swallow or detect drooling)
Chewing problems	• Inability to adequately chew or a prolonged chewing of food due to poor coordination, limited muscle control, or structural problems
Sucking or swallowing problems	• Weak or ineffective suck or swallow, including delayed trigger of swallow and inadequate timing of suck-swallow coordination
Delays in self-feeding and self-drinking	• Slow acquisition of skills in independently transporting food or liquid for eating and drinking • May stem from motor control difficulties, behavioral difficulties, or cognitive delays
Disruptive behaviors	• Inappropriate or excessive show of tantrums, screaming, kicking, hitting, biting, throwing food, playing with food, talking, and other aggressive behaviors during mealtime • Most often associated with food refusal
Pace of intake	• Inappropriately slow or fast rate of oral intake during mealtime

Sources: Based on American Psychiatric Association (1994); Babbitt, Hoch, and Coe (1994); Ginsberg (1988); Kedesdy and Budd (1998).

DISCUSSION POINT:
A physician may prescribe an NPO status due to concerns about swallowing safety. How does NPO status affect an individual's quality of life?

Children who are very unsafe in their swallowing may receive a physician's order of NPO, which loosely means "nothing per oral." Children who are NPO cannot ingest anything through their mouths and will receive a supplemental feeding tube.

Causes and Risk Factors

Dysphagia frequently accompanies a number of syndromes, particularly those that feature low muscle tone (*hypotonia*), delayed motor development, and physical deformities affecting the oral-motor area (Arvedson & Rogers, 1997). For instance, children with Down syndrome may exhibit hypotonia, contributing to a weak suck, which can result in a swallowing impairment. **Cerebral palsy** (CP), a neuromuscular disorder that affects about 1 in 1,000 children, also presents a significant risk factor for dysphagia (Kuban & Leviton, 1994). CP can result from a variety of causes, including a lack of oxygen to the infant's brain (i.e., anoxia) during birth. During the first year of life, 57% of children with CP have problems with sucking, 38% have problems with swallowing, and 33% exhibit failure to thrive (FTT) or malnutrition (Reilly, Skuse, & Poblete, 1996). Over time, these problems can become more severe as the child's nutritional needs increase. Children with CP may require supplemental nutrition if they are unable to develop the oral-motor skills needed for oral feeding.

Other conditions in which dysphagia is seen at elevated rates include significant anomalies of the physical structures required for swallowing, including the hard and soft palate, tongue, lips, tonsils, and pharynx; chronic or recurrent respiratory problems, including pneumonia; and cardiopulmonary diseases that cause fatigue during feeding and rapid breathing. Cleft lip or palate is an example of a physical impairment that can affect safe feeding. Children with this condition have an opening, or cleft, in their lip and/or palate. Children with *cleft lip* may be unable to create a strong enough seal around the nipple to efficiently excise the formula or breast milk. Children with **cleft palate** require help achieving a good oral seal, as the hole in the palate creates a loss of pressure during sucking and can result in formula, breast milk, or solid foods entering the nasal cavity. Surgical repair of clefts typically does not occur until after 12 months of age. Thus, during the first year of life, children may require either an adapted nipple or an alternative feeding method for safe and efficient feeding.

INADEQUATE FEEDING AND SWALLOWING

Inadequate feeding and swallowing refers to cases in which the child is unable to achieve the nutrition needed for healthy growth and development. Inadequate nutrition occurs for four primary reasons: inefficiency, overselectivity, refusal, or feeding delay.

Defining Characteristics

Inefficiency.   Children who are inefficient at feeding and swallowing are unable to meet their caloric and nutritional needs, because the process is not productive. During feeding, inefficient feeders may fatigue too easily, become breathless, or show disinterest or a lack of persistence. They may be inattentive and frequently off task. These characteristics can contribute to undernutrition and growth delays (Kedesdy & Budd, 1998) as the child's inefficiency does not keep pace with nutritional needs.

Overselectivity.   Some children eat too little because of moderate to extreme **overselectivity.** Children with overselective eating patterns are restrictive in the taste, type, texture, or volume of food they will eat (Kedesdy & Budd, 1998). Taste/type restrictions involve rejection of all members of a particular food group because of taste or type—all vegetables or all green foods, for example. Texture restrictions involve resistance to particular textures; the child may eat only one texture, such as liquids. Volume restrictions tend to involve a refusal to eat large portions and can, in the extreme, involve total resistance to eating.

Rigidity in eating is not uncommon in children; about one-third of parents report that their children are picky or finicky eaters (Reau, Senturia, Lebailly, & Christoffel, 1996). Pickiness is a problem when it creates significant stress for the

DISCUSSION POINT:
Think about your own eating likes and dislikes. Make a list of foods you refuse to eat. Are there patterns to your dislikes in terms of specific food groups, appearances, or textures?

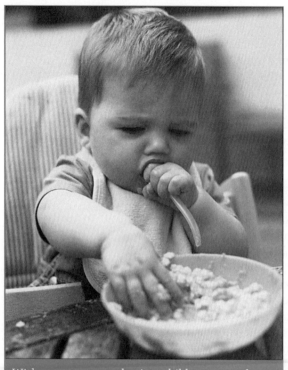

With extreme overselection, children may refuse to eat any food that is not a particular texture or color.

family and when it provides a diet that is inadequate in nutrients and calories. For instance, Kedesdy and Budd (1998) describe a 2-year-old child who ate only formula from a bottle, cookies, and sweet dry cereal. One author of this chapter worked with a child who ate only chicken nuggets from a fast-food restaurant. You can imagine the stress on family dynamics as well as the implications for children's growth.

Refusal.   Some cases of pediatric undernutrition result from a complete refusal to eat (Kedesdy & Budd, 1998). Although most young children will periodically resist foods (Young & Drewett, 2000), an ongoing refusal to eat is a serious matter that can occur for several reasons. First, the child may have a physical or medical issue that has not been resolved. For example, a child may have poor appetite regulation because of constipation—refusing food on days when stooling has not occurred. Constipation has a significant impact on oral intake, because food is not moving through the intestines, resulting in disrupted appetite and hunger.

Second, a child may have gastrointestinal distress, such as reflux. With **reflux,** gastric acid is regurgitated into the esophagus and even the pharynx, resulting in a burning of the esophagus and throat. As many as 40% of infants regurgitate once daily (Orenstein, 1994). When regurgitation is more frequent, significant problems with feeding may occur, including food aversion, loss of appetite, and malnutrition. Because reflux is so painful, children may attempt to avoid eating or may eat only small amounts at one time. Some infants have silent reflux, which produces no visible regurgitation, and hence, no treatment is pursued. Without treatment, a child may resist eating or may seriously limit intake (Krebs, 1999). The extent to which a child experiences symptoms of gastrointestinal distress—vomiting, diarrhea, and constipation—is strongly associated with refusal to eat and mealtime struggles (Johnson & Harris, 2004).

Third, a child may experience a traumatic event that results in resistance to eating, described as **conditioned dysphagia.** Some children resist eating after experiences with severe choking, ingestion of poison, or severe allergic reactions (Kedesdy & Budd, 1998).

Feeding Delay.   Because of developmental delays, illnesses, or trauma, some children experience delayed development of feeding skills. These children are slow to meet major milestones, such as the transition from a bottle to a cup or the emergence of finger feeding. However, major milestones correspond to increasing nutritional needs, such as the transition to table foods, which provides greater nutritional variety to support growth and development. Thus, when children do not transition, their delays may contribute to insufficient feeding.

Causes and Risk Factors

Insufficient feeding occurs for many reasons, including trauma, abuse, accidents, illnesses, developmental disabilities, oral-motor dysfunction, and the like. Several of the more prevalent causes of pediatric feeding disorders that are related to inadequate feeding include low birth weight, prematurity, and prenatal drug exposure.

Children who are born exceptionally small—that is, infants born with low or very **low birth weight** (LBW or VLBW)—are at great risk of feeding and swallowing disorders and of failing to achieve adequate nutrition on their own (MacDorman, Minino, Strobino, & Guyer, 2002). Poor postnatal growth in these babies is very common, affecting 99% of infants who weigh less than 1,000 grams (about 2.2 pounds) at birth (Lemons et al., 2001).

Prematurity.   **Prematurity** occurs when a child is born at or before 37 weeks of gestation. In the year 2000, nearly 12 in 100 births were preterm, and very preterm births (< 32 weeks of gestation) comprised almost 2 in 100 births (MacDorman et al., 2002). Children who are born preterm face many challenges, including feeding and swallowing with a neurologically immature system, and have many systems that are immature, especially the digestive and respiratory systems. Thus, preterm infants have a diminished ability to coordinate the suck-swallow-breathe pattern, which compromises safe and efficient swallowing (Kedesdy & Budd, 1998).

Prenatal Drug Exposure.   Prenatal exposure to alcohol, tobacco, cocaine, heroin, and other toxic substances has been linked to prematurity and low birth weight, as well as to longer-term growth failure and depressed neurological functioning, any one of which can impede a young child's feeding development and swallowing skills (Frank & Wong, 1999). Alcohol consumption by pregnant mothers can result in fetal alcohol syndrome (FAS), alcohol-related birth defects (ARBD), or alcohol-related neurodevelopmental disorder (ARND). Current best estimates of prevalence of these three alcohol-related disorders suggest that about 10 in 1,000 infants are affected (May & Gossage, 2001), and symptoms include an increased likelihood of problems with feeding. Prenatal exposure to opiates, such as heroin, increases suckling problems in infants, which in turn impede feeding and nutrition. In addition, maternal drug use can impede the feeding connection between caregiver and child (Frank & Wong, 1999). The development of feeding skills and achievement of coordinated behavioral routines within a stable and structured caregiving context is a critical variable in preventing feeding disturbances (Yoos, Kitzman, & Cole, 1999).

Diet Restrictions.   Some children are placed on strict or modified diets in response to diabetes, phenylketonuria, and other metabolic disorders (Kedesdy & Budd, 1998). Diabetes is a disorder in which the body does not produce enough insulin. Nearly 2 in 1,000 children are affected by insulin-dependent diabetes (American Diabetes Association, 1996) and face carefully controlled diets, in addition to insulin injections and blood testing. The challenges of such strict diets—for example, not being allowed to snack and eating meals different from those of other children—can result in feeding issues and a resistance to eating (Kedesdy & Budd, 1998).

Similar challenges are associated with **phenylketonuria** (PKU), a metabolic disorder characterized by a deficient liver enzyme and elevated levels of the amino acid phenylaline (National Institutes of Health, 2000). PKU affects about 1 in 15,000 infants born in the United States, although the prevalence is much higher in other countries in which PKU screening is not common. PKU management is essential to preventing the growth deficiencies and mental retardation that frequently result from the buildup of unmetabolized amino acids. However,

DISCUSSION POINT:
Expectant mothers are screened for PKU prior to giving birth to prepare for early interventions if needed. What other kinds of developmental disabilities or metabolic problems are screened for during pregnancy?

because of strict dietary management, children with PKU may have poor appetite, food aversions, and serious anxieties about eating (Kedesdy & Budd, 1998).

INAPPROPRIATE FEEDING AND SWALLOWING

Defining Characteristics

Children who exhibit inappropriate feeding behaviors demonstrate undesirable and disruptive behaviors during mealtimes. If the inappropriate behaviors are significant, the children's growth and development may be compromised as successful feeding is disrupted, turning mealtime interactions into serious and stressful struggles between caregivers and children. Inappropriate feeding behaviors include screaming, spitting, throwing, hitting, and other similar actions (Kedesdy & Budd, 1998). Some children may drop food on the floor, let food fall out of their mouths, or eat very, very slowly, resulting in never-ending mealtimes. In contrast, some children may eat excessively fast—as many as 20 bites of food per minute (Kedesdy & Budd, 1998). Eating too slowly can cause nutritional deficiencies, whereas eating too fast can cause choking or aspiration. Some children may wholly resist letting any food touch their faces or mouths, as discussed previously.

Causes and Risk Factors

About one-third of feeding disorders in young children result from nonorganic causes (Budd et al., 1992). Feeding difficulties can stem from behaviors and attributes of the caregiver or the child that become complexly intertwined in the feeding process. During the first year of a child's life, parents and children develop a feeding relationship that has immediate and long-term consequences. Many parent behaviors can undermine or impair the feeding relationship:

- Being overactive and overstimulating
- Being underactive, passive, and unengaged
- Being rigid, directive, and demanding
- Being chaotic, disorganized, and frenzied
- Being overly concerned, anxious, and fearful (Satter, 1999)

Such behaviors may be more prevalent in caregivers who are poor, depressed, drug-dependent, socially isolated, stressed, or undereducated about nutrition (Yoos et al., 1999).

HOW ARE PEDIATRIC FEEDING AND SWALLOWING DISORDERS IDENTIFIED AND TREATED? ●

EARLY IDENTIFICATION AND REFERRAL

The timely identification of pediatric feeding and swallowing disorders is critical so that immediate intervention can sustain the child's health and nutrition. Typically, newborns stay in the hospital for 48 to 72 hours when there are no complications, and longer when complications are evident or when the child is underweight or premature. Nurses, parents, and physicians are usually well aware when feeding is not progressing well, because the newborn's weight and feeding behaviors are monitored frequently. Interventions are then readily available, ranging from consultation with a breast-feeding specialist to surgical intervention.

SPOTLIGHT ON LITERACY

Prematurity and Reading Difficulties

Prematurity occurs when a child is born at or before 37 weeks of gestation, and it occurs fairly commonly in the United States. About 12% of infants are preterm, and 2% are very preterm (born prior to 32 weeks of gestation). As discussed in this chapter, preterm infants face increased risks for a range of adverse developmental events during infancy, including problems with feeding and swallowing. Recent research has begun to consider more closely some of the long-term challenges preterm infants may face as they grow older. These include difficulties with oral language development, including vocabulary and grammar skills in the early elementary grades (e.g., Jennische & Sedin, 2001). Given the strong interrelationships between oral language abilities and reading development, it is not surprising that preterm infants also show an increased risk for reading problems. Many preterms will show diffuse difficulties in reading skills in the elementary grades, and these are typically most profound for those children born very prematurely (gestational age < 28 weeks, e.g., Grunau, Whitfield, & Davis, 2002). Problems in reading achievement are often accompanied by significant difficulties with writing including handwriting legibility (Feder, Majnemer, Bourbonnais, Platt, et al., 2005). Such findings show that many children who are born prematurely will require long-term supports to achieve their fullest potential, not only in early developmental functions such as feeding and swallowing but also over the long-term in literacy specifically and academically more generally.

Speech-language pathologists (SLPs) who work with the neonatal population on feeding and swallowing issues can play an important role in helping parents of these infants begin to build literacy foundations early in children's lives in an effort to prevent reading difficulties from emerging. As a very simple approach, SLPs can provide parents of premature infants with storybooks and encourage them to read these books to their neonates even while they are in the NICU. The speech-language pathologist can help parents think about the important role that they will play in helping their children become readers and writers in the not-so-distant future.

However, many children do not immediately demonstrate overt feeding disorders. In those cases, it is usually the parent or the pediatrician who identifies a feeding or swallowing difficulty. During the first year of life, children's height and weight are carefully monitored to reveal any deviation or faltering. During routine well-child visits, pediatricians and nurses ask parents to report on feeding and nutrition. Should the parent report any anomaly—excessive feeding time, poor weight gain, rigid eating behaviors, discomfort during feeding—the pediatrician will problem-solve with the parent to prevent early problems from persisting and becoming more serious. Common caregiver concerns about infants under 6 months of age who are bottle- or breast-fed include arching the back, crying, and turning away from the nipple. Then, around 6 months, some children do not transition well from liquids to solids.

Pediatricians and parents must be extremely vigilant during this period of time. A survey at the Montreal Children's Hospital Failure to Thrive and Feeding Disorders Clinic found that the mean age of onset of pediatric feeding problems was 3 months and the mean onset age of failure to thrive or poor growth was about 9 months. Unfortunately, the mean referral age by the pediatrician to the feeding clinic was 19 months. These results indicate that feeding problems emerge much earlier than referral typically occurs. And when feeding problems persist, problematic secondary behaviors can emerge (Ramsay, Gisel, & Boutry, 1993).

> **DISCUSSION POINT:**
> Ask members of your family what you were like as a young eater. Were you finicky or selective? What foods did you like and dislike? Did these preferences change over time?

COMPREHENSIVE ASSESSMENT

The speech-language pathologist will conduct a comprehensive assessment that includes a case history, a physical feeding/swallowing evaluation, and observation of mealtime interactions.

Case History

A careful and detailed history is central to assessing children with feeding and swallowing difficulties. The case history gathers information on the child's and family's eating and feeding experiences to explore possible problems, study changes in behaviors over time, and document specific manifestations of the disorder.

Of particular importance is the child's feeding history. A parental report on the length of meals, the quality of intake, and the child's progression from breast/bottle to purees and solids helps the specialist identify where any breakdowns might have occurred. A history of formulas used and volumes tolerated gives the specialist helpful information regarding potential referral to other professionals, such as an allergist or endocrinologist.

Physical Feeding and Swallowing Evaluation

Following the case history, the specialist completes a careful evaluation of the structures and functions of the child's oral-motor mechanism. This includes observation of the lips, tongue, jaw, teeth, and hard and soft palates. The structural examination studies the physical nature of these structures, whereas the functional examination assesses how they work together during eating and swallowing. The specialist examines the structures and functions at rest (when not being used for feeding or swallowing) and during feeding. The specialist is likely to first watch the child's oral-motor mechanisms during play and other everyday activities and as the child eats and drinks various substances—thin liquids (water), thickened liquids (milkshake), purees (applesauce), and solids (crackers).

During the functional examination, the specialist ascertains both the safety and the efficiency of feeding and swallowing, as well as the quality of intake. The specialist studies how the child handles substances of various textures and looks for any inability to move food, difficulty breaking down foods, extensive chewing, excessive drooling, swallowing whole foods without chewing, and easy fatigue (Creskoff & Haas, 1999). The specialist also looks for behaviors such as coughing, choking, changes in facial color, vocal stridor, a wet or gurgly voice quality, vomiting, or increased or decreased heart rate. Figure 15.3 lists major signs of oral-motor dysfunction, any one of which may suggest unsafe or insufficient feeding or swallowing.

If any of these signs are seen, the feeding specialist will likely refer the child for a **modified barium swallow** (MBS) study, also called a *video swallow study* (VSS). This is conducted by the speech-language pathologist working closely with a radiologist and is one of the only ways to look directly at the structures and functions as swallowing occurs.

TREATMENT GOALS IN PEDIATRIC FEEDING AND SWALLOWING

The immediate and foremost goals of pediatric feeding and swallowing treatment are to ensure that nutritional needs are met for healthy growth and development and that feeding and swallowing do not endanger a child's life. In some cases, this means providing alternative or supplemental nutrition via tube feeding. Once those immediate goals are achieved, specialists focus on improving a child's own ability to meet his or her nutritional needs and to see eating as a psychologically pleasant experience. The specialist may need to increase specific desirable behaviors and skills, such as accepting solid foods, while decreasing undesirable behaviors and skills, such as gagging when chewing. Both physiological and psychological aspects of feeding and swallowing are targeted.

FIGURE 15.3

Signs to watch for during the oral-motor examination for feeding and swallowing problems.

Oral Motor Structures

- Excessive drooling
- Forward thrust of tongue
- Asymmetry of one or more oral or facial features
- Tongue protrusion or low mobility
- Deviation of tongue to left or right
- Enlarged tonsils
- Abnormal height or width of palatal arch
- Weakness of tongue, lips, or jaw
- Abnormal color of pharynx (back of oral cavity)
- Clefting of palate

Oral Motor Functions

- excessive drooling or saliva
- food falls out of mouth
- unable to form food into bolus
- residual food after swallowing
- difficulty pursing lips for such
- easy fatigue
- extended chewing
- slow chewing
- inadequate chewing
- inability to move food around
- pocking food or drink in cheeks
- spitting out food
- vomiting or regurgitating before, during, or after feeding from oral or nasal cavity
- couching or choking
- resisting food
- resisting touch or pressure to oral structures
- crying during eating or drinking
- gurgly or wet voice quality after feeding
- gagging

Sources: Creskoff & Haas, 1999; Shipley & McAfee (1998).

Physiology of Feeding and Swallowing

Physiological targets emphasize the organic and neurodevelopmental aspects of eating and drinking, such as muscle tone, articulator movement and coordination, oral-motor sensitivity, and body posture. For swallowing disorders, treatment focuses on improving the coordination of the swallow to achieve efficiency and safety. Interventions typically feature a hierarchical continuum of training targets, each of which is a small, discreet, and easily attainable behavior or skill. These short-term goals begin at the child's present skill level and progress toward independent eating, which is typically the long-term goal (Kedesdy & Budd, 1998).

Psychology of Feeding and Swallowing

Psychological targets emphasize the behavioral aspects of eating and drinking, such as accepting certain food types or textures, decreasing resistance and

SPOTLIGHT ON TECHNOLOGY

The Modified Barium Swallow Study (MBS)

A modified barium swallow study (MBS) uses videofluoroscopy to follow a substance as it enters an individual's mouth through the oral, pharyngeal, and esophageal phases to see whether aspiration or penetration is occurring. Other names for this procedure include *videofluoroscopic swallow study* (VFSS) or *video swallow study* (VSS). The MBS couples fluoroscopy, a radiographic imaging technique, with videotaping to create, in essence, a moving picture of the swallow as it is executed. Speech-language pathologists conduct the MBS by having clients ingest a variety of food consistencies and using videofluoroscopy to watch the functioning of the swallow. MBS is sometimes called a *cookie study,* because the client chews and swallows a variety of different foods, often including a cookie. A radiopaque contrast material, such as barium, is mixed with the foods for visualization. When conducting the MBS, the client is administered liquids and foods in graduated and controlled trials to ascertain swallowing competency. Generally, the procedure flows in the following steps:

1. A baseline picture of structures, including the posterior portion of the mouth, the soft palate, the pharynx, the larynx, and the upper esophageal sphincter

2. Administration and observation of liquids and foods in the following order:
   a. Thin liquids (e.g., apple juice)
   b. Thick liquids if indicated (e.g., tomato juice or apricot nectar)
   c. Purees (e.g., applesauce)
   d. Mechanical soft items (e.g., Rice Krispies)
   e. Regular foods (e.g., graham cracker)
   f. Pills

3. Study of different compensatory strategies to assess their impact on swallowing efficiency and safety while different textures are ingested (e.g., a chin tuck, leaning, or a head turn)

---

fussiness when eating, following a consistent meal schedule, and the like. For children who receive nutrition supplementally or alternatively, goals correspond to a gradual reduction in tube feedings. Therapists usually utilize behavioral principles to deliver treatment, such as shaping, conditioning and reinforcement, and systematic desensitization (Kedesdy & Budd, 1998).

With *shaping,* the therapist moves a child incrementally toward a desired goal. For instance, if a long-term goal is to increase a child's consumption of foods that have texture, the therapist will gradually shape the child's experiences with textured foods—from touching a new texture to the lips without gagging to eating a variety of textured foods during a single mealtime. With *conditioning and reinforcement,* a child learns to associate a stimulus with a particular outcome, such as receiving a preferred food for eating a nonpreferred food. Social approval from a parent ("That was great! I am very proud of you!") is one form of positive reinforcement that then might be paired with the new behavior to increase its frequency. With *systematic desensitization,* the therapist trains a child to accept an aversive sensory experience (e.g., eating a new texture) by breaking it down into small steps and showing the child that each step is safe and possible.

Alternative and Supplemental Feeding

Children who are unable to meet their own nutritional needs orally and whose growth is faltering require an alternative solution. Children who are candidates for supplemental or alternative nutrition are those (1) who cannot meet 80% of their caloric needs orally, (2) who have not gained weight or who have continuously lost weight for 3 months, (3) whose weight and height ratio is below the 5th percentile, or (4) whose feeding time is greater than 5 to 6 hours daily (Smith & Pederson, 1990).

The most common solution is *enteral,* or tube, feeding, in which liquid nutrition is delivered through a tube. In some cases, the tube feeding is supplemental, providing supportive therapy in combination with oral intake (Smith & Pederson, 1990). For instance, a child with cerebral palsy might be able to meet some but not all nutritional needs orally, in which case tube feeding is supplemental. In other cases, tube feeding might be the sole avenue for a child's nutrition, as in the case of a child with very low birth weight or one who is very premature.

For short-term treatment, a **nasogastric tube** is used, which is passed through the nasal cavity and into the esophagus. No surgery is required, and the tube should not impact communication, although it may interfere with breathing and cause throat irritation. For longer-term treatment, a *gastrostomy tube* or a *jejunostomy tube* is placed surgically into the stomach or small intestine. Nutritional support is then delivered either intermittently or continuously. With intermittent feeding, nutrition is provided four to eight times daily to mimic the timing of normal feeding, whereas with continuous feeding, nutrition is provided nonstop. For children requiring enteral feeding, a team of professionals works closely with the families to determine the best approach.

When children receive alternative nutritional support, therapists work to ensure that the caregiver-child feeding relationship also receives special support; it is a special context in which the overall relationship develops, as well as important communicative abilities. In addition, therapists and parents must promote children's oral abilities even when these are not being used for feeding. Children who receive no nutrition orally may become orally hypersensitive or aversive to touch around their mouths, creating significant problems for parents and therapists once these children are more medically stable and ready to eat.

WHAT ARE THE DEFINING CHARACTERISTICS OF ADULT DYSPHAGIA? ●

The defining characteristics of adult dysphagia typically relate to (1) the phase of swallow affected, (2) the underlying pathology or cause, and (3) the severity of the disorder.

PHASE AFFECTED

Dysphagia can be characterized by the phase affected to identify the site at which the swallowing system breaks down. The speech-language pathologist is primarily concerned with disorders in the oral preparatory, oral, and pharyngeal phases, also called *oral-pharyngeal dysphagia*. **Gastroenterologists,** internists, radiologists, and other professionals study and treat *esophageal dysphagia,* resulting from impairments of the esophageal phase of swallowing. Characteristics of difficulties in the oral and pharyngeal phases are summarized here.

Oral Preparatory Phase

Breakdowns in the oral preparatory phase occur when the structures and functions of the lips, tongue, cheeks, and mandible do not function as they should. Some disorders that may result in an oral preparatory dysphagia include stroke, Parkinson's disease, and head and neck cancers. Characteristics of oral preparatory phase dysphagia include the following:

1. Decreased lip closure, resulting in problems intaking foods or liquids from an eating utensil, straw, or cup and allowing food materials to leak from the mouth

2. Problems controlling the ingested materials, such that food or liquid falls in the space between the teeth and gums (i.e., the **sulci**)

3. Difficulty biting or chewing, thus hindering the formation of a bolus

4. Inefficient oral preparation due to reduced range of motion of the tongue and/or weakness of the tongue, requiring increased time to prepare the bolus for swallowing

5. Impaired sensitivity of the tongue, lips, and other oral structures that hinders food positioning and management

Oral Phase

In the oral phase, the formed bolus moves posteriorly in the mouth toward the pharynx to trigger the swallow. Oral phase dysphagia occurs with strokes, progressive neurological diseases such as ALS, and even tooth loss. Characteristics of oral phase dysphagia include these:

1. Difficulty moving the bolus to the pharynx, resulting in food or liquid residuals remaining in the mouth (typically in the sulci or adhering to the hard palate)

2. Inability to adequately control the bolus flow, such that some materials spill into the pharyngeal region prematurely

3. Delayed initiation of the bolus movement, increasing the transit time from the oral to the pharyngeal phase

Pharyngeal Phase

Breakdowns in the pharyngeal phase occur when the pharyngeal structures do not function as they should to move the bolus through the pharynx to the entrance of the esophagus. The pharyngeal phase directs the prepared bolus through the pharynx into the esophagus, while simultaneously making physiological adjustments to protect the airway. This phase is critical because the greatest threat is that of materials entering the airway. Unlike the oral preparatory and oral phases, which are more readily observable at the bedside, pharyngeal phase difficulties are not readily transparent. Pharyngeal phase dysphagia occurs with neurological disorders, and with head and neck cancers. Characteristics of pharyngeal stage dysphagia include the following:

1. Incomplete palatal elevation to seal off the nose from the pharynx, allowing foods or liquids into the nasal cavity (i.e., **nasal reflux**)

2. Delayed initiation of the pharyngeal swallow reflex, allowing materials to move deeper into the pharynx or larynx, thus increasing the risk of aspiration

3. Diminished tongue and pharyngeal muscle force to move the bolus through the pharynx, resulting in materials "hanging" in the throat

4. Reduced laryngeal elevation and closure, making the airway more prone to entering materials (i.e., aspiration)

5. Inadequate opening of the cricopharyngeus muscle (i.e., the upper esophageal sphincter), hindering the movement of the bolus into the esophagus and enabling the retention of food residuals within the pharynx

UNDERLYING PATHOLOGY OR CAUSE

Dysphagia is a secondary disorder, meaning that it results from another primary cause. The most common causes of dysphagia are neurological damage due to a stroke, a brain injury, or a disease (e.g., Parkinson's disease), and laryngeal damage due to radiation, surgical removal of the larynx (laryngectomy), or trauma. Figure 15.4 lists acquired conditions that commonly result in oropharyngeal dysphagia. Speech-language pathologists usually manage dysphagia cases stemming from brain injury, progressive neurological diseases, and head and neck cancer treatments.

Brain Injury

Stroke.   Stroke is a leading cause of disability and even death among adults. The percentage of those developing dysphagia following stroke is relatively high—50% or even higher (Mann, Hankey, & Cameron, 1999; Martino, Pron, & Diamant, 2000). A stroke results from an interruption in the blood supply to the brain, robbing the brain tissue of required oxygen and nutrients. As a result, brain tissue is damaged. After a stroke, individuals are prone to oropharyngeal dysphagia, which increases

> **DISCUSSION POINT:**
> What symptoms might be present providing evidence of an individual's difficulty in the oral phase of swallowing?

FIGURE 15.4

Acquired conditions frequently resulting in oropharyngeal dysphagia.

Traumatic brain injury
  Closed-head injury
  Open-head injury

Single stroke
  Lower brain-stem stroke
  High brain-stem stroke
  Cerebral cortex stroke (left and/or right hemispheres)

Multiple strokes

Head and neck cancer

Spinal cord injury

Surgical trauma (e.g., removal of brain-stem tumor)

Poliomyelitis

Guillain-Barre disease

Cerebral palsy

Riley-Day syndrome

Multiple sclerosis

Huntington's disease

Dementia

Parkinson's disease

Wilson's disease

Infectious disease (e.g., meningitis, Lyme disease)

Sources: Based on Buchholz and Robbins (1997); Logemann (1998).

the risk of malnutrition, aspiration, and pneumonia. As many as 55% of stroke patients aspirate, increasing their risk of developing pneumonia (Ding & Logemann, 2000). Estimates suggest that approximately one-third of stroke patients die from pneumonia caused by aspiration (Odderson, Keaton, & McKenna, 1995).

Traumatic Brain Injury.   Traumatic brain injuries (TBIs) are caused by car accidents, falls, and physical acts of violence and often result in diffuse brain damage. Dysphagia is a common complication of TBI (Morgan & Mackey, 1999), with one-fourth to three-fourths of individuals with TBI exhibiting dysphagia (Mackey, Morgan, & Bernstein, 1999; Schurr, Ebner, Maser, Sperling, et al., 1999). Even at the lower estimate, dysphagia is a common concern. The dysphagia commonly seen with TBI includes a significant delay in the pharyngeal swallow reflex, diminished pharyngeal constriction, and oral-motor compromises (Lazarus & Logemann, 1987). In addition, the frequent disturbance in cognitive functioning, such as low level of arousal and attention, can make swallowing further unsafe or inefficient.

Progressive Neurological Disease

Progressive neurological diseases are disorders of the nervous system producing discoordination and weakness of motor skills as well as decreased sensory abilities. These disorders are called *progressive,* because the neurological problems and resulting symptoms become more disabling over time as the disease follows its course.

Parkinson's Disease.   Parkinson's disease (PD) is a progressive neurological disease characterized by gradual depletion of the neurotransmitter dopamine, which hinders functioning of the basal ganglia. This alteration produces a movement disorder characterized by tremors, difficulty initiating movements, and a slow and rigid motion. As the disease progresses, it can also result in cognitive deterioration similar to that of dementia, with confusion and agitation.

Swallowing disorders in PD are common, impacting somewhere between 50 and 92% of individuals (Nilsson, Ekberg, Olsson, & Hindfelt, 1996; Stroudley & Walsh, 1991). This variability in estimates likely results from the fact that many PD clients are unaware of or fail to report dysphagia (Bird, Woodward, Gibson, Phyland, et al., 1994). Dysphagia in PD affects the oral, pharyngeal, and esophageal phases of the swallow, with common difficulties including drooling, abnormalities in bolus preparation and transport, delayed triggering of the swallow reflex, residual materials in the pharynx, aspiration, and diminished esophageal motility.

Amyotrophic Lateral Sclerosis.   Amyotrophic lateral sclerosis (ALS) is more commonly recognized as Lou Gehrig's disease. ALS is a rapidly progressing motor-neuron disease resulting in severe deterioration of the muscles and motoric systems of the body, including the muscles for respiration. Although individuals with ALS experience significant physical deterioration, their cognitive abilities remain intact. Dysphagia is prevalent in ALS because of the disruptions in respiratory, phonatory, and articulatory functions. All persons with ALS experience oropharyngeal dysphagia at some point in the disease process. Swallowing dysfunction typically starts in the oral phase and progresses to the pharyngeal stage. Dysphagia may be one of the first symptoms of ALS, leading individuals to seek medical treatment based on changes in their swallowing ability and weight loss (Logemann, 1998).

DISCUSSION POINT:

In what ways does presence of a swallowing disorder influence the quality of life for persons with progressive neurological disease?

Dementia.   *Dementia* is a global term referring to alterations in cognitive skills. It has numerous etiologies, including Alzheimer's, dementia from multiple strokes, or progressive diseases such as Parkinson's disease or Huntington's chorea. One of the most common causes of dementia is Alzheimer's disease (AD), which is a progressive deterioration in mental capacity and later affects both sensory and motor functions. The incidence of dysphagia in AD is relatively low in the early disease stages. However, as AD progresses to moderate and severe levels of impairment, dysphagia is seen in more than one-fourth of individuals (Chouinard, 2000; Kalia, 2003). Oropharyngeal deficits include the inability to recognize foods as something to eat, resulting from a more general condition of *agnosia,* in which individuals do not recognize things for what they are; difficulty in bolus preparation and transit, often due to apraxia; delayed initiation of the pharyngeal swallow reflex; and poor pharyngeal constriction. The mental decline in these individuals places them at greater risk of aspiration and pneumonia (Wada et al., 2001).

Head and Neck Cancer Treatments

Cancerous growths of the mouth, pharynx, and larynx are currently treated with surgery, radiation, and possibly chemotherapy. Dysphagia is often present prior to medical treatment for these cancers, but it frequently becomes more severe immediately following these interventions, which are necessary for survival. The impact of head and neck cancers on swallowing function relates directly to the type, size, and location of the growth (Colangelo, Logemann, & Rademaker, 2000; Pauloski et al., 2000) and the extent of surgical intervention and radiation therapy. Head and neck cancers often result in oral or pharyngeal stage dysphagia, which can be readily managed for many individuals.

Surgical Management.   Since a malignant cancer is potentially life-threatening, removal of the diseased tissue or structures is necessary. When components of swallowing are either partially or totally removed, as occurs in *glossectomy* (tongue removal) or *laryngectomy* (larynx removal), changes in swallowing function are probable.

In some cases a tracheotomy is required, either temporarily or permanently. This surgical procedure places a tube through the neck directly into the trachea (see Figure 15.5) to maintain the airway and to allow for pulmonary hygiene. The tracheostomy tube affects swallowing performance by altering the normal airflow through the nose or oral cavities and vocal folds; air is now inhaled and exhaled through the tube. Physiological changes in the laryngeal muscles also hinder the swallowing process.

Radiation Therapy. Radiation is often used in addition to surgical management. Radiation treatment itself reduces saliva production (known as *xerostomia*) and also results in edema (water retention in tissues), tooth decay, and pain. All of these factors negatively influence swallowing capability.

Chemotherapy. In certain situations, chemotherapy is part of the treatment regimen for head and

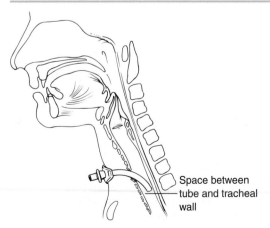

Space between tube and tracheal wall

FIGURE 15.5

Tracheostomy tube placement.

neck cancers. The side effects of chemotherapy—such as nausea, vomiting, and fatigue—can lead to swallowing concerns, particularly adequate intake to achieve good nutritional status. Fortunately, advances in chemotherapy medications mean they are producing fewer unpleasant side effects.

SEVERITY

The severity of dysphagia can range from mild to severe. The Penetration-Aspiration Scale (Rosenbek et al., 1996) provides one way to approximate severity, using an 8-point scale to describe the degree of airway protection during the swallow. A score of 1 indicates that no material enters the airway, whereas a score of 8 indicates that material is aspirated and the individual shows no effort to cough and no gag reflex. A patient with a score of 8 would be at very high risk for aspiration.

The New Zealand Index for Multidisciplinary Evaluation of Swallowing (NZIMES; Huckabee, 2004) provides a comprehensive rating of an individual's swallowing status from the oral phase to the esophageal phase, assessing performance on a variety of indicators (e.g., positioning of bolus in oral phase) and using a scale of 0 (no impairment) to 4 (profound impairment). The NZIMES identifies mild to profound impairments in each function and structure involved in safe swallowing (Huckabee, 2004).

A mild impairment of swallowing includes some difficulties with oral preparation and pharyngeal functioning but overall good mastication and safe, independent feeding and swallowing. A moderate impairment indicates some dangers of aspiration and penetration into the airway. Those may result from such difficulties as problems clearing a spoon of a bolus because of lingual and labial uncoordination or weakness, problems clearing the mouth when creating the bolus, problems masticating solid foods, and a slow trigger of swallow. A severe impairment indicates a serious risk of aspiration and penetration, and a profound impairment indicates that a person is unable to safely swallow, thus requiring an alternative means of nutrition.

HOW IS ADULT DYSPHAGIA IDENTIFIED AND TREATED? ●

The speech-language pathologist is typically the key professional responsible for evaluating clients with suspected dysphagia. This assessment process includes a clinical swallowing examination and, when indicated, an instrumental dysphagia evaluation using MBS.

CLINICAL SWALLOWING EXAMINATION

Upon referral, the speech-language pathologist will often conduct a clinical swallowing examination, also referred to as a **bedside swallow examination,** because it typically occurs at a client's bedside. In this procedure, SLPs do the following:

1. Review current and past medical records
2. Complete a comprehensive client interview to learn medical, social, and family history, with particular attention to the history of the swallowing problem (e.g., When did the problem start? What foods are most troublesome?)

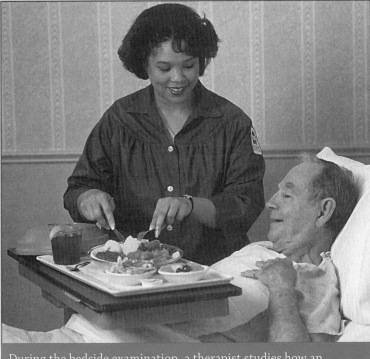

During the bedside examination, a therapist studies how an individual takes in food and drink and considers the safety and efficiency of swallowing.

3. Conduct a thorough oral mechanism examination of the mouth and throat to determine structural and functional adequacy for swallowing

4. Attempt trial feedings or observe the client during a meal

5. Make feeding recommendations if appropriate

6. Refer the client for instrumental assessment of swallowing if indicated

7. Refer the client to other professionals for any specialized testing that is needed

A sample report used in a typical swallowing examination is presented in Figure 15.6. If the clinical swallowing examination cannot clearly determine the nature of the swallowing problem, an instrumental assessment of dysphagia, typically an MBS, is required to study the swallowing phases more thoroughly. This assessment uses radiography and other instrumentation and should be used only when it is necessary for further diagnosis. These five indicators suggest the need for instrumentation to quantify swallowing problems (ASHA, 2004c):

1. Clinical bedside findings are inconsistent with reported signs and symptoms of dysphagia.

2. Instrumentation is needed to assist in determining the medical diagnosis.

3. Dysphagia diagnosis or the safety and efficiency of the swallow require confirmation.

4. Nutritional or pulmonary compromises are present, and oropharyngeal dysphagia is suspected as a contributing factor.

5. Specific swallowing information is required to design and implement a treatment plan.

FIGURE 15.6

An outline of a clinical swallowing examination and report.

CLINICAL SWALLOW EXAMINATION

Client:
Date of Birth:
Date of Exam:
Diagnosis:
Referral Source:
Client Identification Number:

History. This section includes all relevant past medical, social, and family history, as well as current medical diagnoses, procedures and results, medications, and allergies. Specific interview questions include these:

- What is your chief complaint and the nature of the problem?
- How long has this been a problem?
- Do you experience this problem more at certain times of day? (e.g., better at breakfast and worse at dinner?)
- Are there certain food textures (e.g., liquids, soft foods) that make the problem better or worse?
- When you experience swallowing problems, what happens?
- Have you found things that make you swallow better?
- Have you had a change in weight? If so, how much and over what time span?

Oral Mechanism Exam. This section includes observation of oral structures at rest and in use. Rate, strength, and direction of the movements of structures used in articulation, phonation, and resonance are noted. If a tracheostomy tube is present, the type, size, and duration of tube placement are determined.

Feeding Trials. This section reports observations of swallowing performance for various consistencies. Optimally, this includes liquids, purees, soft foods, foods requiring much chewing, and pills. Problems across the phases of the swallow are identified. In addition, techniques to compensate for or improve swallowing performance are attempted, and benefits, if present, are noted. If the client is not taking foods or liquids by mouth, this is noted, and the type of feeding tube, current formula, and feeding schedule are listed.

Clinical Impressions. This section summarizes findings on the presence of dysphagia, its severity, specific swallowing deficits, and prognosis for improvement.

Recommendations. This portion outlines the recommendations for oral intake, optimal diet, and safety strategies. Referrals for instrumental assessment or professional services are indicated. If therapy is indicated, an intervention plan is suggested that includes the frequency and duration of treatment, measurable goals, and specific treatment techniques.

Signature of speech-language pathologist
Credentials
State license number

CC: Others receiving a copy of this report

When instrumental evaluation is required, the SLP initiates the referral process through the appropriate physician. Most instrumental procedures require a physician's prescription if they are to be paid for by the insurance company. SLPs are typically responsible for actually conducting the instrumental dysphagia examination, but they work closely with other professionals, especially radiologists, in carrying out and interpreting the assessment.

INSTRUMENTAL DYSPHAGIA EXAMINATION

Evaluation of swallowing problems using technology, or instrumentation, typically provides a more objective and quantifiable measure of swallowing functions, including the safety of those functions, than the bedside examination. Commonly used instrumentation includes fiberoptic endoscopic evaluation, ultrasonography, and videofluoroscopy.

Fiberoptic Endoscopic Examination

The **fiberoptic endoscopic examination of swallowing,** commonly referred to as *FEES,* provides direct visualization of the swallowing mechanism. A fiberoptic endoscope, a flexible tube containing a small camera, is passed through the nose and into the pharynx, yielding a real-time picture of swallowing, both before and after the swallow. However, pharyngeal movement during the swallow makes imaging impossible during the actual swallow itself. FEES is videotaped so that replay of the test is possible, and it has no radiation exposure. Complications can include nasal laceration, hemorrhaging, or allergic reaction to topical anesthetics.

Ultrasonography

Ultrasonography, or ultrasound, is the same technology long used to visualize a fetus in the mother's womb. In dysphagia evaluation, ultrasound uses high-frequency sound waves to create a black-and-white picture of the structures targeted. A transducer, placed either at the chin or at the thyroid area at the front of the neck, generates sound waves to create the image. Ultrasound is most beneficial in oral phase evaluation; pharyngeal phase assessment with ultrasound is poor. Ultrasound is without known risk and is noninvasive. Further, it is portable, so it can be used at bedside.

Videofluoroscopy

Videofluoroscopy, or MBS (see Spotlight on Technology: The Modified Barium Swallow Study [MBS]), is the most commonly used instrumentation for swallowing evaluation and is the gold standard in most cases. Although this procedure yields information on all phases of the swallow, there are certain drawbacks. The MBS uses radiation, so client exposure must be considered and minimized. Further, the MBS is not readily portable in most environments, so client transport and positioning needs should be considered. Finally, MBS is an expensive procedure that requires highly specialized instruments and skilled professionals. Not all facilities are equipped with both.

TREATING DYSPHAGIA

Following assessment, the speech-language pathologist often provides direct treatment to remediate oropharyngeal dysphagia using two types of rehabilitation strategies: compensatory and restorative approaches.

Compensatory Approaches

Compensatory techniques are strategies that compensate for a specific problem in order to make swallowing safe and efficient. For example, for clients who experience oral leakage of foods or who pack food in the cheeks, the speech-language pathologist might place a mirror in front of them during meals so that they can monitor and correct this problem. Or the SLP might help clients with left facial weakness place food on the stronger right side of their mouths during the oral preparatory phase. Postural techniques are used quite commonly; for instance, the chin-down posture, in which the individual touches the chin to the front of the neck while swallowing, is helpful for reducing aspiration of thin liquids (Logemann et al., 2008).

In addition to modifications in the way individuals take in food, SLPs use diet modifications as a compensatory approach. This typically involves changing the viscocity of foods. For example, if chewing is difficult for a client, meals can be customized to use chopped rather than whole meats. Or if an individual is at risk for aspirating thin liquids like water or juice, a thickening agent can be added, based on the premise that thickened liquids can be managed more readily in the swallowing process. Additional compensatory techniques are listed in Figure 15.7. A recent large-scale study contrasted three compensatory

---

FIGURE 15.7

Compensatory strategies.

- *Diet modifications*
  Change the consistency of foods and drinks
  Change the temperature of foods and drinks

- *Altered positioning during swallowing*
  Have client tuck chin in (chin tuck)
  Place client on side
  Have client turn head to the left or right side

- *Intake modifications*
  Alternate solids and liquids
  Encourage extra swallows per bite
  Change food placement in the mouth
  Alter bite size

- *Meal set-up/environment*
  Minimize distractions
  Monitor tray placement
  Use adaptive feeding equipment, such as high-rimmed bowls, feeding utensils, nonslide
  placemats to secure plates, cups that control the rate of liquid flow
  Have staff monitor and assist

- *Prosthetic devices or appliances*

---

techniques for eliminating aspiration among adults with dysphagia secondary to Parkinson's disease or dementia (Logemann et al., 2008): use of a chin-down posture while swallowing, use of liquids thickened to a nectar consistency, and use of liquids thickened to a honey consistency. The use of MBS for each of the three techniques showed that honey-thickened liquid was most effective for eliminating aspiration of thin liquids, followed by nectar-thickened liquid and then the chin-down posture. However, no single technique had total success: 53% of the adults aspirated with the honey-thickened consistency, 63% with nectar-thickened, and 68% with the chin-down posture.

Restorative Techniques

Restorative techniques are intended to improve or restore swallow function. Examples include oral and pharyngeal exercises and biofeedback. For an individual with a delayed swallow reflex, the therapist might use thermal stimulation to improve the sensitivity of the oral area and the timeliness of the swallow reflex. In the case of a weak swallow, the therapist might train the client to use an effortful swallow in the pharyngeal phase to help propel the bolus downward without leaving residue behind. However, this requires considerable muscular effort and an ability to follow directions, so it might not be suitable for some clients with language impairment, cognitive decline, or muscular fatigue (Logemann, 1998). Figure 15.8 lists these and other commonly used restorative treatments.

NUTRITION AND DIETARY CONSIDERATIONS

The importance of nutritional health to an individual with dysphagia cannot be overestimated. Because dysphagia results from an underlying disease, individuals must achieve adequate nutrition to promote healing of and recovery from the

FIGURE 15.8

Restorative strategies.

- *Thermal stimulation:* The therapist rubs a cold laryngeal mirror on the faucial pillars to improve the timeliness of the swallow reflex.

- *Effortful swallow:* The client tries to swallow hard using the swallowing muscles.

- *Mendelsohn maneuver:* The client learns to catch the swallow during elevation of the larynx, increasing the duration of the upper esophageal opening.

- *Supraglottic swallow:* In this multistep maneuver clients hold their breath before swallowing, then swallow, and finally cough to improve the closure of the airway.

- *Oral motor exercise:* The client completes exercises of the swallowing structures to improve strength and efficiency.

- *Electromyography (EMG):* This biofeedback approach enhances awareness and self-monitoring of performance.

underlying disease. For example, persons recovering from neurological injuries such as stroke or traumatic brain injury have greater nutritional needs than they did prior to their illness. Unfortunately, however, swallowing dysfunction places them at a higher risk of malnutrition and dehydration. A speech-language pathologist works closely with a registered dietitian to assess diet and adjust recommendations to meet nutritional demands; typical diet levels are presented in Figure 15.9.

Despite dietary modifications and compensatory strategies, some individuals are unable to meet their nutritional requirements orally. In these cases, alternative

FIGURE 15.9

Typical diet levels.

- *NPO (non per os):* This level indicates that no liquids or foods are to be consumed orally. These clients require intravenous or tube feedings to maintain their nutritional needs.

- *Thin liquids:* This level allows thin liquids such as juices and water. It also includes foods that melt to a liquid consistency, such as gelatins.

- *Thickened liquids:* This level allows liquids that are more viscous, such as tomato juice or nectars. If clients are unable to tolerate thin liquids, commercial thickening agents are added to achieve the required thickness.

- *Puree:* These items have well-blended, smooth consistencies that require relatively little oral preparation (e.g., applesauce or pudding).

- *Mechanical soft:* These foods require oral preparation but are soft, so that chewing demands are limited. Examples include soft cooked vegetables, canned fruits, and moist, tender meats that are sometimes ground or finely chopped.

- *Soft:* This level includes most foods except those that are difficult to manage orally, such as peanuts, raw apples, and hard candy.

- *Regular:* This is an unrestricted level that allows all foods.

- *Medications:* Many dysphagia clients experience difficulties swallowing needed medications. In these cases medications can be given in liquid form or crushed, if not contraindicated.

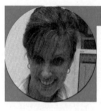

SPOTLIGHT ON RESEARCH AND PRACTICE

NAME: LORI M. BURKHEAD, PH.D., CCC-SLP

PROFESSION/TITLE
Assistant Professor and Lead Speech Pathologist, Medical College of Georgia, Department of Otolaryngology

PROFESSIONAL RESPONSIBILITIES
Evaluation and treatment of dysphagia, clinical research, teaching.

A DAY AT WORK
A typical day contains a combination of patient care and data collection. I also provide formal lectures and didactic mentoring to residents in otolaryngology, medical students, and fellow speech-language pathologists in the community.

HOW INTERESTS IN COMMUNICATION SCIENCES AND DISORDERS BEGAN
I was originally an elementary education major. I took a required course entitled "Speech Pathology for the Classroom Teacher" taught by a dynamic professor, Dr. Bryce Evans. He invited me to observe in the on-campus clinic. I sat behind a one-way mirror with a woman watching her husband struggle to communicate. She explained that, as a former attorney, language was his strength. She looked me in the eye and said, "Honey, if you go into this field and help people like my husband, your life will mean something." I changed my major that day. As I worked with adults with communication disorders, I realized that more than half also had dysphagia. Many patients and families expressed that dysphagia impacted their health and quality of life as much if not more than the communication disorder. My patients' goals dictated that dysphagia therapy took the forefront in our sessions. Recognizing the need for more widespread education in our field regarding dysphagia as well as the need for more focused and methodologically based treatments, I pursued a Ph.D. to expand my opportunities for teaching and research.

CURRENT RESEARCH AND PRACTICE INTERESTS
Developing more effective and efficient methods for evaluation and treatment of dysphagia.

MOST EXCITING/INTERESTING PROFESSIONAL ACCOMPLISHMENT IN CSD
One of my most memorable moments was a phone call from a patient who tearfully expressed gratitude for being able to eat Thanksgiving dinner with his family. For the year and a half prior to that, he had been feeding-tube dependent following a stroke and frequently expectorated into a cup, as he was unable to safely swallow even saliva. After 8 weeks of aggressive therapy, he enjoyed Thanksgiving dinner without difficulty or fear. When days get long and demands are high, those moments motivate me to stay the course.

nutritional means, such as a feeding tube, are necessary to supplement intake by mouth; it is not unusual for dysphagia clients to receive both oral intake and tube feedings. The same types used with pediatric populations, as discussed previously in this chapter—including nasogastric and gastostomy tubes—are used for adults. The type of tube is determined by a client's physician, who considers the nature of the dysphagia, the individual's clinical profile, and the anticipated duration of tube placement.

CASE ANALYSIS

Study the case of Joseph on the Companion Website at www.pearsonhighered.com/justice2e (Case Study 10). Reflect on how his swallowing disorder affects his quality of life.

CHAPTER SUMMARY

A *pediatric feeding disorder* refers to a persistent failure to eat adequately for a period of 1 month or longer. Children with feeding disorders may experience growth delay, lack of tolerance of food textures and tastes, poor appetite regulation, or rigid eating patterns. A swallowing disorder, or dysphagia, is a type of feeding disorder in which safe and efficient swallowing is compromised; dysphagia occurs most commonly in very young children or older adults. Prematurity, low birth weight, and developmental disability are common causes of dysphagia among young children; for adults, dysphagia is usually associated with a brain injury, such as that resulting from stroke or from neurological disease or injury.

Pediatric feeding and swallowing disorders are typically characterized as to whether feeding or swallowing is unsafe, inadequate, or inappropriate. Unsafe feeding/swallowing occurs when there is dysfunction or damage to a child's oral-motor system or the child uses an inappropriate eating rate, either too fast or too slow. Inadequate feeding/swallowing occurs when the child is unable to achieve the nutrition needed for healthy growth and development, perhaps because feeding/swallowing is inefficient or the child is overselective in what he or she eats. Inappropriate feeding/swallowing occurs when the child growth and development is compromised due to undesirable and disruptive behaviors during mealtimes.

Adult dysphagia is typically characterized by the phase of the swallow affected, the etiology of the swallowing impairment, and its severity. Oral preparatory and oral phase dysphagia typically occur due to problems with preparing the bolus for transport or initiating movement of the bolus to the pharynx. Pharyngeal phase dysphagia involves an impairment of the movement of the bolus through the pharynx toward the esophagus. In terms of etiology, dysphagia typically occurs due to brain injury or neurological disease, including dementia, Parkinson's disease, and ALS. Severity can range from mild to severe.

Assessment of pediatric feeding and swallowing disorders emphasizes early identification and referral to promote healthy growth and development in young children. When treatment is required, behavioral approaches commonly include conditioning, reinforcement, shaping, and desensitization. For very young children, including those in the NICU, ongoing oral-motor stimulation and communicative supports are vital. For some children, supplemental or alternative feeding is needed, including enteral feeding systems.

The evaluation of adult dysphagia includes a clinical swallowing or bedside examination and, when indicated, instrumental assessment using fiberoptic endoscopy, ultrasonography, or videofluoroscopy (MBS).

Treatment plans incorporate both compensatory and restorative interventions to optimize current performance and future recovery. Strategies implemented should be evidence based and measurable in terms of client progress. The rehabilitation plan must be sensitive to the client's quality of life and ethnocultural background.

KEY TERMS

apneic moment, p. 499
aspiration, p. 496
bedside swallow examination,
    p. 516
cleft palate, p. 503
cerebral palsy, p. 503
conditioned dysphagia, p. 504
deglutition, p. 495
dysphagia, p. 493
enteral feeding tube, p. 500

feeding disorder, p. 493
fiberoptic endoscopic examination, p. 518
gastroenterologist, p. 511
low birth weight, p. 505
modified barium swallow, p. 508
nasal reflux, p. 512
nasogastric tube, p. 511
neonatal intensive care unit
    (NICU), p. 495

oral-motor function, p. 494
oral-motor system, p. 493
oral-motor muscular tone,
    p. 494
oral-motor sensation, p. 494
overselectivity, p. 503
penetration, p. 496
pharyngeal swallow reflex,
    p. 499
phenylketonuria (PKU), p. 505

prematurity, p. 505
reflexive cough, p. 499

reflux, p. 504
sulci, p. 512

ultrasonography, p. 519
videofluoroscopy, p. 519

● ON THE WEB

Check out the Companion Website at www
.pearsonhighered.com/justice2e! On it you will find:

• suggested readings
• reflection questions

• a self-study quiz
• links to additional online resources, including current technologies in communication sciences and disorders

REFERENCES

Aaron, P. G., Joshi, M., & Williams, K. A. (1999). Not all reading disabilities are alike. *Journal of Learning Disabilities, 32,* 120–137.

AAC TechConnect. (2008). Device assistant. Retrieved March 13, 2008, from www.aactechconnect.com/da.cfm.

Abbs, J. H., Gracco, V. L., & Cole, K. J. (1984). Control of multi-movement coordination: Sensorimotor mechanisms in speech motor programming. *Journal of Motor Behavior, 16*(2), 195–231.

Abitol, J. (1995). *Atlas of laser voice surgery.* San Diego, CA: Singular.

Acharya, K., & Msall, M. E. (2008). The spectrum of cognitive-adaptive developmental disorders in intellectual disability. In P. Accardo (Ed.), *Neurodevelopmental disabilities in infancy and childhood, volume II: The spectrum of neurodevelopmental disabilities* (3d ed., pp. 241–259). Baltimore, MD: Paul H. Brookes.

Adams, M. J., Foorman, B., Lundberg, I., & Beeler, D. (1998). *Phonemic awareness in young children.* Baltimore, MD: Paul H. Brookes.

Adams, S. G. (1997). Hypokinetic dysarthria in Parkinson's disease. In M. R. McNeil (Ed.), *Clinical management of sensorimotor speech disorders* (pp. 261–285). New York: Thieme.

Adams, S. G., Page, A. D., & Jog, M. S. (2002). Summary feedback schedules and speech motor learning in Parkinson's disease. *Journal of Medical Speech-Language Pathology, 10,* 215–220.

Adamson, L. B., & Chance, S. E. (1998). Coordinating attention to people, objects, and language. In A. M. Wetherby, S. F. Warren, & J. Reichle (Eds.), *Transitions in prelinguistic communication.* Baltimore, MD: Paul H. Brookes.

Addy, D. A., Golinkoff, R. M., Sootsman, J. L., Pence, K., Pulverman, R., Salkind, S., & Hirsch-Pasek, K. (2003, June). *Understanding /ing/: Sensitivity to grammatical morphemes precedes their production.* Paper presented at the Jean Piaget Society. Chicago, IL.

Agency for Healthcare and Quality. (2004). *Literacy and health outcomes: Summary.* [Evidence Report.] Washington, DC: U.S. Department of Health and Human Services, Agency for Healthcare Research and Quality.

Alant, E. (2007, August). Training and intervention in South Africa. *The ASHA Leader.*

Alcock, K. J., Passingham, R. E., Watkins, K. E., & Vargha-Kadem, F. (2000). Oral dyspraxia in inherited speech and language impairment and acquired dysphasia. *Brain and Language, 75,* 17–33.

Allen, T. E. (1986). Patterns of academic achievement among hearing impaired students: 1974 and 1983. In A. N. Schildroth & M. A. Karchmer (Eds.), *Deaf children in America* (pp. 161–202). San Diego, CA: College-Hill Press.

Ambrose, N. G., Cox, N., & Yairi, E. (1997). The genetic basis of persistence and recovery in stuttering. *Journal of Speech, Language, and Hearing Research, 40,* 567–580.

Ambrose, N. G., & Yairi, E. (1999). Normative disfluency data for early childhood stuttering. *Journal of Speech, Language, and Hearing Research, 42,* 895–909.

Ambrose, N. G., & Yairi, E. (2002). The Tudor study: Data and ethics. *American Journal of Speech-Language Pathology, 11,* 190–203.

Ambrose, N. G., Yairi, E., & Cox, N. (1993). Genetic aspects of early childhood stuttering. *Journal of Speech and Hearing Research, 36,* 701–706.

American Academy of Otolaryngology—Head and Neck Surgery. (2004). *Meniere's disease.* Retrieved February 11, 2004, from www.entnet.org/healthinfo/balance/meniere.cfm.

American Association on Mental Retardation. (2002). *Mental retardation: Definition, classification, and systems of supports* (10th ed.). Washington, DC: Author.

American Diabetes Association. (1996). *National diabetes fact sheet.* Washington, DC: Author.

American Psychiatric Association. (1994). *Diagnostic and statistical manual of mental disorders* (4th ed.). Washington, DC: Author.

American Speech-Language-Hearing Association. (1981). On the definition of hearing handicap. *ASHA, 23,* 293–297.

American Speech-Language-Hearing Association. (1993). Definitions of communication disorders and variations. *AHSA, 35*(Suppl. 10), 40–41.

American Speech-Language-Hearing Association. (1996). Central auditory processing: Current status of research and implications for clinical practice. *American Journal of Audiology, 5,* 41–54.

American Speech-Language-Hearing Association. (1997). *Preferred practice patterns for the profession of audiology* (pp. 43–46). Rockville, MD: Author.

American Speech-Language-Hearing Association. (1998). *National outcomes measurement system.* Rockville, MD: Author.

American Speech-Language-Hearing Association. (1999). *Terminology pertaining to fluency and fluency disorders: Guidelines* [Guidelines]. Available from www.asha.org/policy.

American Speech-Language-Hearing Association. (2000a). Asking your audiologist about preventing and identifying hearing loss through audiologic screening and audiology services. *Audiology Information Series, 1,* 1–4.

American Speech-Language-Hearing Association (2000b). Clinical indicators for instrumental assessment of dysphagia (guidelines). *ASHA Desk Reference, 3,* 225–233.

American Speech-Language-Hearing Association. (2001). *Roles and responsibilities of speech-language pathologists with respect to reading and writing in children and adolescents (guidelines).* Rockville, MD: Author.

American Speech-Language-Hearing Association. (2002a). Augmentative and alternative communication knowledge and skills for service delivery. ASHA Supplement, *22,* 97–106.

American Speech-Language Hearing Association. (2002b). *Guidelines for audiology service provision in and for schools.* Rockville, MD: Author.

American Speech-Language-Hearing Association. (2002c, April 16). Roles of speech-language pathologists in swallowing and feeding disorders: Position statement. *ASHA Leader,* 7(Suppl. 22), 73.

American Speech-Language-Hearing Association. (2002d, October 8). SLPs in health care settings: Survey results. *ASHA Leader, 7,* 8.

American Speech-Language-Hearing Association. (2002e). 2002 *Omnibus survey salary report: Annual salaries.* Rockville, MD: Author.

American Speech-Language-Hearing Association. (2004b). Knowledge and skills needed by speech-language pathologists performing videofluoroscopic swallowing studies. *ASHA Suppl. 24.*

American Speech-Language-Hearing Association. (2004b). *Roles and responsibilities of speech-language pathologists with respect to augmentative and alternative communication: Technical report.* Retrieved from www.asha.org/policy.

American Speech-Language-Hearing Association. (2004a). *Scope of practice in audiology.* Rockville, MD:Author.

American Speech-Language-Hearing Association. (2005a). *(Central) Auditory processions disorders* [Technical Report]. Retrieved from www.asha.org/policy.

American Speech-Language-Hearing Association. (2005b). Membership and certification handbook of the American Speech-Hearing Association, for speech-language pathology (effective January 1, 2005). Rockville, MD: Author. Retrieved February 15, 2008, from www.asha.org/about/membership-certification/handbooks/slp/slp_standards.htm.

American Speech-Language-Hearing Association. (2005c). *Roles and responsibilities of speech-language pathologists with respect to augmentative alternative communication: Position statement.* Retrieved from www.asha.org/policy.

American Speech-Language-Hearing Association. (2006). *2006 Schools Survey.* Rockville, MD: Author.

American Speech-Language-Hearing Association. (2007a). *Scope of practice in speech-language pathology.* Rockville, MD: Author.

American Speech-Language-Hearing Association. (2007b). *The 2007 audiology standards.* Rockville, MD: Author. Retrieved February 15, 2008, from www.asha.org/about/membership-certification/certification/au_standards_new.htm.

American Speech-Language-Hearing Association. (2008a). *Back to school: Language and learning.* Retrieved from www.asha.org/about/news/tipsheets/language_and_learning.htm.

American Speech-Language Hearing Association. (2008b). Effects of hearing loss on development. Retrieved January 23, 2008, from www.asha.org/public/hearing/disorders/effects.htm.

Anderson, K. (1989). *Screening instrument for targeting educational risk (SIFTER).* Austin, TX: Pro-Ed.

Anderson, K. (2001). *Early listening function: Discovery tool for parents and caregivers of infants and toddlers.* Retrieved October 1, 2003, from www.phonak.com/index.cfm?article_id=7281.

Anderson, K., & Matkin, N. (1996). *Screening instrument for targeting educational risk in preschool children (age 3–kindergarten) (Preschool SIFTER).* Tampa, FL: Educational Audiology Association.

Anderson, K., & Smaldino, J. (1998). *Listening inventory for education: An efficacy tool.* Tampa, FL: Educational Audiology Association.

Anderson, K., & Smaldino, J. (2001). *Children's home inventory for listening difficulties (CHILD).* Retrieved October 1, 2003, from www.phonak.com/index.cfm?article_id=7281.

Anderson, T. K., & Felsenfeld, S. (2003). A thematic analysis of late recovery from stuttering. *American Journal of Speech-Language Pathology, 12,* 243–253.

Andrews, G., Morris-Yates, A., Howie, P., & Martin, N. (1991). Genetic factors in stuttering confirmed. *Archives of General Psychiatry, 48,* 1034–1035.

Andrews, M. L., & Summers, A. C. (2002). *Voice treatment for children and adolescents* (2d ed.). San Diego, CA: Singular Publishing.

Anglin, J. M. (1993). Vocabulary development: A morphological analysis. *Monographs of the Society for Research in Child Development, 58,* 1–186.

Aram, D. M. (1988). Language sequelae of unilateral brain lesion in children. In F. Plum (Ed.), *Language, communication and the brain* (pp. 171–198). New York: Raven Press.

Aram, D. M., & Biron, S. (2004). Intervention programs among low SES Israeli preschoolers: The benefits of joint storybook reading and joint writing to early literacy. *Early Childhood Research Quarterly, 19,* 588–610.

Aram, D. M., Morris, R., & Hall, N. E. (1993). Clinical and research congruence in identifying children with specific language impairment. *Journal of Speech and Hearing Research, 36,* 580–591.

Armero, O. (2001). Effects of denied hearing impairment on the significant other. *Hearing Journal, 54,* 44–47.

Armson, J., Kiefte, M., Mason, J., & DeCroos, D. (2006). The effect of SpeechEasy on stuttering frequency in laboratory conditions. *Journal of Fluency Disorders, 31,* 137–152.

Arndt, J., & Healey, E. C. (2001). Concomitant disorders in school-age children who stutter. *Language, Speech, and Hearing Services in Schools, 32,* 68–78.

Aronson, A. E. (1990). *Clinical voice disorders: An interdisciplinary approach.* New York: Thieme, Inc.

Arvedson, J. C., & Rogers, B. T. (1993). Pediatric swallowing and feeding disorders. *Journal of Medical Speech Language Pathology, 1,* 203–221.

Arvedson, J. C., & Rogers, B. T. (1997). Swallowing and feeding in the pediatric patient. In A. L. Perlman & K. S. Schulze-Delrieu (Eds.), *Deglutition and its disorders* (pp. 419–448). San Diego: Singular Publishing.

Assistive Technology Funding & Systems Change Project. (1999). *Medicaire, managed care, and AAC devices.* Washington, DC: United Cerebral Palsy Association.

August, D., & Hakuta, K. (Eds.). (1997). *Improving schooling for language-minority children.* Washington, DC: National Academy Press.

Auinger, P., Lanphear, B. P., Kalkwarf, H. J., & Mansour, M. E. (2003). Trends in otitis media among children in the United States. *Pediatrics, 112*(3), 514–520.

Ausetermann Hula, S. N., Robin, D. A., Maas, E., Ballard, K. J., & Schmidt, R. A. (2008). Effects of feedback frequency and timing on acquisition, retention, and transfer of speech skills in acquired apraxia of speech. *Journal of Speech, Language, and Hearing Research, 5,* 1088–1113.

Autism Society of America. (2000). *Advocate, 33*(1), 3.

Avent, J. R. (1997). Group treatment in aphasia using cooperative learning methods. *Journal of Medical Speech-Language Pathology, 5*(1), 9–26.

Avent, J. R. (2004). Group treatment for aphasia using cooperative learning principles. *Topics in Language Disorders, 24*(2), 118–124.

Awan, S. N., & Mueller, P. B. (1996). Speaking fundamental frequency characteristics of white, African American, and Hispanic kindergarteners. *Journal of Speech and Hearing Research, 39,* 573–577.

Babbitt, R. L., Hoch, T. A., & Coe, D. A. (1994). Behavioral feeding disorders. In D. N. Tuchman & R. S. Walter (Eds.), *Disorders of feeding and swallowing in infants and children* (pp. 77–95). San Diego, CA: Singular.

Backenroth, G. A., & Ahlner, B. H. (2000). Quality of life of hearing-impaired persons who have participated in audiological rehabilitation counselling. *International Journal for the Advancement of Counselling, 22,* 225–240.

Baddeley, A. D., & Longman, D. J. A. (1978). The influence of length and frequency of training session on the rate of learning to type. *Ergonomics, 21,* 627–635.

Badian, N. (2005). Does a visual-orthographic deficit contribute to reading disability? *Annals of Dyslexia, 55,* 28–52.

Baker, C. (2000). *A parents' and teacher's guide to bilingualism* (2d ed.). Tonawanda, NY: Multilingual Matters.

Balandin, S. (2002). Message from the president. *The ISAAC Bulletin, 67*(2), 2.

Balasubramanian, V., & Max, L. (2004). Crosses apraxia of speech: A case report. *Brain and Cognition, 55,* 240–246.

Ballard, K. J. (2001). Response generalization in apraxia of speech treatments: Taking another look. *Journal of Communication Disorders, 34,* 3–20.

Ballard, K. J., Granier, J. P., & Robin, D. A. (2000). Understanding the nature of apraxia of speech: Theory, analysis, and treatment. *Aphasiology, 14*(10), 969–995.

Ballard, K. J., Maas, E., & Robin, D. A. (2007). Treating control of voicing in apraxia of speech with variable practice. *Aphasiology, 21*(12), 1195–1217.

Ball, L. J., Beukelman, D. R., & Pattee, G. L. (2004). Acceptance of augmentative and alternative communication technology by persons with amyotrophic lateral sclerosis. *Augmentative & Alternative Communication 20(2),* 113–122.

Bance, M. (2007). Hearing and aging. *Canadian Medical Association Journal, 176,* 925–928.

Bankson, N., & Bernthal, J. (1990). *Quick screen of phonology.* Chicago, IL: Riverside Press.

Barlow, J. (2001). Case study: Optimality theory and the assessment and treatment of phonological disorders. *Language, Speech, and Hearing Services in Schools, 32,* 242–256.

Barlow, S. (1999). *Handbook of clinical speech physiology.* San Diego, CA: Singular.

Bartlett, C., Flax, J., Logue, M., Vieland, V. J., Tallal, P., & Brzustowica, L. M. (2002). A major susceptibility locus for specific language impairment is located on 13q21. *American Journal of Human Genetics, 71,* 45–55.

Bashir, A. S., Conte, B., & Heerde, S. M. (1998). Language and school success: Collaborative challenges and choices. In D. D. Merritt & B. Culatta (Eds.), *Language intervention in the classroom* (pp. 1–36). San Diego, CA: Singular Publishing.

Basso, A., Marangolo, P., Piras, F., & Galluzzi, C. (2001). Acquisition of new "words" in normal subjects: A suggestion for the treatment of anomia. *Brain and Language, 77,* 45–59.

Battle, D. (2002). Communication disorders in a multicultural society. In D. E. Battle (Ed.), *Communication disorders in multicultural populations* (pp. 3–32). Woburn, MA: Butterworth-Heinemann.

Bauman-Waengler, J. (2004). *Articulatory and phonological impairments: A clinical focus* (2d ed.). Boston: Allyn & Bacon.

Bavelier, D., & Neville, H. J. (2002). Cross-modal plasticity: Where and how? *Nature Reviews: Neuroscience, 3,* 443–452.

Bayles, K. A., & Kim, E. S. (2003). Improving functioning of individuals with Alzheimer's disease: Emergence of behavioral interventions. *Journal of Communication Disorders, 36*(5), 327–343.

Bayles, K. A., & Tomoeda, C. K. (1993). *Arizona battery for communication disorders of dementia.* Tucson, AZ: Canyonlands Publishing, Inc.

Bayles, K. A., & Tomoeda, C. K. (1995). *The ABCs of dementia* (2d ed.). Tuscon, AZ: Canyonlands Publishing, Inc.

Bays, C. L. (2001). Quality of life of stroke survivors: A research synthesis. *Journal of Neuroscience Nursing, 33,* 310–322.

Bear, D. R., Invernizzi, M., Templeton, S., & Johnston, F. (2008). *Words their way: Word study for phonics, vocabulary, and spelling instruction* (4th ed.). Upper Saddle River, NJ: Pearson Education, Inc.

Beck, I. L., McKeown, M. G., & Kucan, L. (2002). *Bringing words to life.* New York: Guilford.

Beitchman, J., Hood, J., Rochon, J., Peterson, M., Mantini, T., & Majumdar, S. (1989). Empirical classification of speech/language impairment in children I. Identification of speech/language categories. *Journal of the American Academy of Child and Adolescent Psychiatry, 28,* 112–117.

Bellis, T. (1996). *Assessment and management of central auditory processing disorders in the educational setting: From science to practice.* San Diego, CA: Singular.

Benjamin, B., & Croxson, G. (1987). Vocal nodules in children. *Annals of Otology, Rhinology, and Laryngology, 96,* 530–533.

Bereiter, C., & Engelman, S. (1966). *Teaching disadvantaged children in the preschool.* Englewood Cliffs, NJ: Prentice-Hall.

Bergbom-Engberg, E., & Haljamae, H. (1989). Assessment of patients' experience of discomforts during respirator therapy. *Critical Care Medicine, 17,* 1068–1071.

Berg, F. (2001). Educational management of children who are hearing impaired. In R. H. Hull (Ed.), *Aural rehabilitation: Serving children and adults* (pp. 169–185). Canada: Singular.

Bernhardt, B., & Stoel-Gammon, C. (1994). Non-linear phonology: Introduction and clinical application. *Journal of Speech, Language, and Hearing Research, 37,* 123–143.

Berninger, V. W., Abbot, R. D., Jones, J., Wolf, B. J., Gould, L., Anderson-Youngstrom, M., Shimada, S., & Apel, K. (2006). Early development of language by hand: Composing, reading, listening, and speaking connections; three letter-writing modes; and fast mapping in spelling. *Developmental Neuropsychology, 29,* 61–92.

Bernstein Ratner, N. (1997). Stuttering: A psycholinguistic perspective. In R. Curlee & G. Siegel (Eds.), *Nature and treatment of stuttering: New directions* (2d ed., pp. 97–127). Boston: Allyn & Bacon.

Bernthal, J. E., & Bankson N. W. (2004). *Articulation and phonological disorders* (5th ed.). Boston: Allyn & Bacon.

Bess, F. H., Dodd-Murphy, J., & Parker, R. A. (1998). Children with minimal sensorineural hearing loss: Prevalence, educational performance, and functional status. *Ear and Hearing, 19,* 339–354.

Best, W., Herbert, R., Hickin, J., Osborne, F., & Howard, D. (2002). Phonological and orthographic facilitation of word-retrieval in aphasia: Immediate and delayed effects. *Aphasiology, 16,* 151–168.

Beukelman, D. R., & Ansel, B. M. (1995). Research priorities in augmentative communication. *Augmentative and Alternative Communication, 11,* 131–134.

Beukelman, D. R., & Mirenda, P. (1998). *Augmentative and alternative communication: Management of severe communication disorders in children and adults.* Baltimore: Paul H. Brookes.

Beukelman, D. R., & Mirenda, P. (2005). *Augmentative and alternative communication: Supporting children and adults with complex communication needs* (3d ed.). Baltimore, MD: Brookes.

Beukelman, D. R., & Yorkston, K. M. (1991). Traumatic brain injury changes the way we live. In D. R. Beukelman & K. M. Yorkston (Eds.), *Communication disorders following traumatic brain injury: Management of cognitive, language, and motor impairments* (pp. 1–14). Austin, TX: Pro-Ed.

Bhatnagar, S. C. (2007). *Neuroscience for the study of communicative disorders* (3d ed.). Baltimore, MD: Lippincott, Williams, & Wilkins.

Bhatnagar, S. C., & Andy, O. J. (1995). *Neuroscience for the study of communicative disorders.* Baltimore, MD: Williams & Wilkins.

Bickerston, D. (1995). *Language and human behavior.* Seattle, WA: University of Washington Press.

Birks, J. (2006). Cholinesterase inhibitors for Alzheimer's disease. *Cochrane Database of Systematic Reviews, 25*(1): CD005593.

Bishop, D. V., & Edmundson, A. (1987). Language-impaired 4-year-olds: Distinguishing transient from persistent impairment. *Journal of Speech and Hearing Disorders, 52,* 156–173.

Black, M. M., Cureton, P. L., & Berenson-Howard, J. (1999). Behavior problems in feeding: Individual, family, and cultural influences. In D. B. Kessler & P. Dawson (Eds.), *Failure to thrive and pediatric undernutrition: A transdisciplinary approach* (pp. 151–172). Baltimore, MD: Paul H. Brookes.

Blackstone, S. (1999). Communication partners. *Augmentative Communication News, 12*(1–2), 1–16.

Blackstone, S. W., & Hunt Berg, M. (2003). *Social networks: A communication inventory for individuals with complex communication needs and their communication partners.* Monterey, CA.: Augmentative Communication, Inc.

Blissymbolic Communication International. (2008). Retrieved March 13, 2008, from www.blissymbolics.org/.

Blitzer, A., & Brin, M. F. (1992). The dystonic larynx. *The Journal of Voice, 6,* 294–297.

Blomgren, M., Roy, N., Callister, T., & Merrill, R. M. (2005). Intensive stuttering modification therapy: A multidimensional assessment of treatment outcomes. *Journal of Speech, Language, and Hearing Research, 48,* 509–523.

Blonsky, E., Logemann J., & Boshes, B. (1975). Comparison of speech and swallowing function in patients with tremor disorders and in normal geriatric patients: A cine fluorographic study. *Journal of Gerontology, 30,* 299–305.

Blood, G. W. (1994). Efficacy of a computer-assisted voice treatment protocol. *American Journal of Speech-Language Pathology, 3,* 57–66.

Blood, G. W. (1995). POWER: Relapse management with adolescents who stutter. *Language, Speech, and Hearing Services in Schools, 26,* 169–179.

Blood, G. W., Blood, I. M., Bennett, S., Simpson, K. C., & Susman, E. J. (1994). Subjective anxiety measurements and cortisol responses in adults who stutter. *Journal of Speech and Hearing Research, 37,* 760–768.

Blood, G. W., Thomas, E. A., Ridenour, J. S., Qualls, C. D., & Hammer, C. S. (2002). Job stress in speech-language pathologists working in rural, suburban, and urban schools: Social support and frequency of interactions. *Contemporary Issues in Communication Sciences and Disorders, 29,* 132–140.

Bobrick, B. (1995). *Knotted tongues: Stuttering in history and the quest for a cure.* New York: Simon & Schuster.

Bollinger, R. L., Musson, N. D., & Holland, A. L. (1993). A study of group communication intervention with chronically aphasic persons. *Aphasiology, 7,* 301–313.

Bondy, A., & Frost, L. (1994). The picture exchange communication system. *Focus on Autistic Behavior, 9,* 1–19.

Bondy, A., & Frost, L. (1995). Educational approaches in preschool: Behavior techniques in a public school setting. In E. Shopler & G. Mesibov (Eds.), *Learning and cognition in autism* (pp. 311–333). New York: Plenum.

Borden, G. J., Harris, K. S., & Raphael, L. J. (1994). *Speech science primer: Physiology, acoustics, and perception of speech* (3d ed.). Baltimore: Williams & Wilkins.

Bortfeld, H., Rathbun, K., Morgan, J., & Golinkoff, R. (2003). What's in a name? Highly familiar items anchor infants' segmentation of fluent speech. In B. Beachley, A. Brown, & F. Conlin (Eds.), *BUCLD 27: Proceedings of the 27th Annual Boston University Conference on Language Development.* Somerville, MA: Cascadilla Press.

Botting, N., Faragher, B., Simkin, Z., Knox, E., & Conti-Ramsden, G. (2001). Predicting pathways of specific language impairment: What predicts good and poor outcome? *Journal of Child Psychology and Psychiatry, 42,* 1013–1020.

Boudreau, D. (2002). Literacy skills in children and adolescents with Down syndrome. *Reading and Writing: An Interdisciplinary Journal, 15,* 497–525.

Boudreau, D. M., & Hedberg, N. L. (1999). A comparison of early literacy skills in children with specific language impairment and their typically developing peers. *American Journal of Speech-Language Pathology, 8,* 249–260.

Bourgeois, M. S., & Hickey, E. M. (2007). Dementia. In D. R. Beukelman, K. L. Garrett, & K. M. Yorkston (Eds.), *Augmentative communication strategies for adults with acute or chronic medical conditions* (pp. 243–285). Baltimore, MD: Brookes.

Boyer, L., & Mainzer, R. W. (2003). Who's teaching students with disabilities? A profile of characteristics, licensure status, and feelings of preparedness. *Teaching Exceptional Children, 35*(6), 8–11.

Brackenbury, T., & Fey, M. E. (2003). Quick incidental learning in 4-year-olds: Identification and generalization. *Journal of Speech, Language, and Hearing Research, 46,* 313–327.

Brainard, M. S., & Doupe, A. J. (2000). Auditory feedback in learning and maintenance of vocal behavior. *Nature Reviews: Neuroscience, 1,* 31–40.

Bray, M. A., Kehle, T. J., Lawless, K. A., & Theodore, L. A. (2003). The relationship of self-efficacy and depression to stuttering. *American Journal of Speech-Language Pathology, 12,* 425–431.

Brice, A. (1992). The Adolescent Pragmatics Screening Scale: A comparison of language-impaired students, bilingual/Hispanic students, and regular education students. *Howard Journal of Communications, 4,* 143–156.

Brice, A. (2002). *The Hispanic child: Speech, language, culture and education.* Boston: Allyn & Bacon.

Brin, M. F., Fahn, S., Blitzer, A., Ramig, L. O., & Stewart, C. (1992). Movement disorders of the larynx. In A. Blitzer, M. F. Brin, C. T. Sasaki, S. Fahn, & K. S. Harris (Eds.), *Neurological disorders of the larynx.* New York: Thieme Medical.

Brodnitz, F. S. (1998). *Keep your voice healthy* (2d ed.). Austin, TX: Pro-Ed.

Broen, P. A., & Moller, K. T. (1993). Early phonological development and the child with cleft palate. In K. T. Mollerr & C. D. Starr (Eds.), *Cleft palate: Interdisciplinary issues and treatment* (pp. 219–249). Austin, TX: Pro-Ed.

Brookshire, R. H. (2003). *Introduction to neurogenic communication disorders* (6th ed.). St. Louis, MO: Mosby.

Brown, I. (2007). What is meant by intellectual and developmental disability? In I. Brown and M. Percy (Eds.), *A comprehensive guide to intellectual and developmental disabilities* (pp. 3–15). Baltimore, MD: Paul H. Brookes.

Brown, R. (1973). *A first language: The early stages.* Cambridge: Harvard University Press.

Bruck, M. (1990). Word recognition skills of adults with childhood diagnoses of dyslexia. *Developmental Psychology, 26,* 439–454.

Bruechert, L., Lai, Q., & Shea, C. H. (2003). Reduced knowledge of results frequency enhances error detection. *Research Quarterly for Exercise and Sport, 74*(4), 467–472.

Bruns, J., Hauser, W. A. (2003). The epidemiology of traumatic brain injury: A review. *Epilepsia, 44*(Suppl. 10), 2–10.

Bryan, K. L. (1989). *The right hemisphere language battery.* Leicester, GB: Far Communications.

Buchholz, D. W., & Robbins, J. (1997). Neurological diseases affecting oropharyngeal swallowing. In A. L. Perlman & K. Schulze-Delrieu (Eds.), *Deglutition and its disorders* (pp. 319–342). San Diego, CA: Singular.

Bunton, K. (2005). Patterns of lung volume use during extemporaneous speech task in persons with Parkinson disease. *Journal of Communication Disorders, 38,* 331–348.

Busch, C. (1994, October). How is a treatment plan for an aphasic person reviewed in terms of Medicare policy and guidelines? *Neurophysiology and neurogenic speech and language disorders special interest Division 2 newsletter* (pp. 14–17). Rockville, MD: American Speech-Language-Hearing Association.

Cahill, L. M., Turner, A. B., Stabler, P. A., Addis, P. E., Theodoros, D. G., & Murdoch, B. E. (2004). An evaluation of continuous positive airway pressure (CPAP) therapy in the treatment of hypernasality following traumatic brain injury: A report of three cases. *Journal of Head Trauma Rehabilitation, 19*(3), 241–253.

Cain, K., Oakhill, J., Barnes, M., & Bryant, P. (2001). Comprehension skill, inference making ability and their relation to knowledge. *Memory & Cognition, 29,* 850–859.

Camarota, S. (2001). *Immigrants in the United States—2000.* Washington, DC: Center for Immigration Studies. Retrieved February 12, 2008, from http://cis.org/articles/2001/back101.pdf.

Campbell, T. F. (1999). Functional treatment outcomes in young children with motor speech disorders. In N A. J. Caruso & E. A. Strand (Eds.), *Clinical management of motor speech disorders in children* (pp. 385–396). New York: Thieme.

Cann, C. I., Rothman, K. J., & Fried, M. P. (1996). The epidemiology of the laryngeal cancer. In M. P. Fried (Ed.), *The larynx: A multidisciplinary approach* (pp. 425–436). St. Louis, MO: Mosby.

Cannito, M. P., Burch, A. R., Watts, C., Rappold, P. W., Hood, S. B., & Sherrard, K. (1997). Disfluency in spasmodic dysphonia: A multivariate analysis. *Journal of Speech, Language, and Hearing Research, 40,* 627–641.

Cao, Y., Vikingstad, E. M., George, K. P., Johnson, A. F., & Welch, K. M. (1999). Cortical language activation in stroke patients recovering from aphasia with functional MRI. *Stroke, 30,* 2331–2340.

Capone, G. T., Roizen, N. J., & Rogers, P. T. (2008). Down syndrome. In P. J. Accardo (Ed.), *Neurodevelopmental disabilities in infancy and childhood: Volume II, the spectrum of neurodevelopmental disabilities* (2d ed., pp. 285–308). Baltimore, MD: Paul H. Brookes.

Carding, P. N., Roulstone, S., Northstone, K., & ALSPAC Study Team. (2006). The prevalence of childhood dysphonia: A cross-sectional study. *Journal of Voice, 20,* 623–630.

Carey, S., & Bartlett, E. (1978). Acquiring a single new word. *Papers and Reports on Child Language Development, 15,* 17–29.

Carta, J., Greenwood, C., Walker., D., Kaminski, R., Good, R., et al. (2002). Individual Growth and Development Indicators (IGDIs): Assessment that guides intervention for young children. In M. Ostrosky & E. Horn (Eds.), *Assessment: Gathering meaningful information.* Longmont, CO: Sopris West.

Case, J. L. (1996). *Clinical management of voice disorders* (3d ed.). Austin, TX: Pro-Ed.

Case, J. L. (2002). *Clinical management of voice disorders* (4th ed.). Austin, TX: Pro-Ed.

Cassar, M., & Treiman, R. (2004). Developmental variations in spelling: Comparing typical and poor spellers. In C. A. Stone, F. R. Silliman, B. J. Ehren, & K. Apel (Eds.), *Handbook of language and literacy: Development and disorders* (pp. 627–643). New York: Guilford Press.

Cassar, M., Treiman, R., Moats, L., Pollo, T. C., & Kessler, B. (2005). How do the spellings of children with dyslexia compare with those of nondyslexic children? *Reading and Writing, 18,* 27–49.

Catts, H., Adolf, S., Hogan, T., & Ellis Weismer, S. (2005). Are specific language impairment and dyslexia distinct disorders? *Journal of Speech, Language, and Hearing Research, 48,* 1378–1396.

Catts, H. W., Adolf, S. M., & Ellis Weismer, S. (2006). Language deficits in poor comprehenders: A case for the simple view of reading. *Journal of Speech, Language, and Hearing Research, 49,* 278–293.

Catts, H. W., Fey, M. E., Zhang, X., & Tomblin, J. (2001b). Language deficits in poor comprehenders: A case for the simple view of reading. *Journal of Speech, Language, and Hearing Research, 49,* 278–293.

Catts, H. W., Fey, M. E., Zhang, X., & Tomblin, J. B. (2001a). Estimating the risk of future reading difficulties in kindergarten children: A research-based model and its clinical implications. *Language, Speech, and Hearing Services in Schools, 32,* 38–50.

Catts, H. W., Fey, M. E., Tomblin, J. B., & Zhang, X. (2002). Longitudinal investigation of reading outcomes in children with language impairment. *Journal of Speech, Language, and Hearing Research, 45,* 1142–1157.

Catts, H. W., Hogan, T. P., & Adlof, S. M. (2005). Developmental changes in reading and reading disabilities. In H. W. Catts & A. G. Kahmi (Eds.), *Connections between language and reading disabilities.* Mahwah, NJ: Erlbaum.

Catts, H. W., & Kahmi, A. G. (2005). Classification of reading disabilities. In H. W. Catts and A. G. Kahmi (Eds.), *Language and reading disabilities* (2d ed., pp. 50–71). Boston, MA: Allyn & Bacon.

Centers for Disease Control and Prevention. (2005). *Preventing lead poisoning in young children.* Atlanta: Author.

Centers for Disease Control and Prevention Early Hearing Detection Intervention (EHDI). (2001). *Health communication and follow-through related to early identification of deafness and hearing loss in newborns.* Retrieved September 25, 2003, from www.cdc.gov.ncbddd/ehdi/ehdi.htm.

Center for the Voice. (2004). *Professions at risk for voice disorders.* Retrieved October 1, 2004, from www.nyee.edu/cfv-professions.hmtl#about.

Chall, J. S. (1996). *Stages of reading development.* Fort Worth, TX: Harcourt Brace & Company.

Champlin, C. A. (2000). Hearing science. In R. B. Gillam, T. P. Marquardt, & F. N. Martin (Eds.), *Communication sciences and disorders: From science to clinical practice.* San Diego: Singular.

Chaney, C. (1998). Preschool language and metalinguistic skills are links to reading success. *Applied Psycholinguistics, 19,* 433–466.

Chapman, K. L., Hardin-Jones, M., & Halter, K. A. (2003). The relationship between early speech and later speech and language performance for children with cleft lip and palate. *Clinical Linguistics and Phonetics, 17,* 173–197.

Chapman, R. S., Seung, H. K., Schwartz, S. E., & Kay-Raining Bird, E. (1998). Language skills of children and adolescents with Down syndrome: II. Production deficits. *Journal of Speech, Language, and Hearing Research, 41,* 861–873.

Cheang, H. S., & Pell, M. D. (2007). An acoustic investigation of Parkinsonian speech in linguistic and emotional contexts. *Journal of Neurolinguistics, 20,* 221–241.

Chermak, G. D., & Musiek, F. E. (1997). *Central auditory processing disorders: New perspectives.* San Diego, CA: Singular Publishing Group.

Cherney, L., Halper, A., Holland, A., & Cole, R. (2008). Computerized script training for aphasia: Preliminary results. *American Journal of Speech-Language Pathology, 17,* 19–34.

Chia, E., Wang, J., Rochtchina, E., Cumming, R., Newall, P., & Mitchell, P. (2007). Hearing impairment and health-related quality of life: The Blue Mountains Hearing Study. *Ear & Hearing, 28,* 187–195.

Chouinard, J. (2000). Dysphagia in Alzheimer's disease: A review. *The Journal of Nutrition Health and Aging, 4,* 214–217.

Christensen, J., Trovato, M. K., Saolorio, C., Brandys, E., Morozova, O., et al. (2008). Traumatic brain injury. In P. Accardo (Ed.), *Neurodevelopmental disabilities in infancy and childhood, volume I: Neurodevelopmental diagnosis and treatment* (3d ed., pp. 615–637). Baltimore, MD: Paul H. Brookes.

Churchill, J., Hodson, B., Jones, B., & Novak, R. (1988). Phonological systems of speech-disordered clients with positive/negative histories of otitis media. *Language, Speech, and Hearing Services in Schools, 19,* 100–106.

Clark, H. M. (2003). Neuromuscular treatments for speech and swallowing: A tutorial. *American Journal of Speech-Language Pathology, 12,* 400–415.

Clark, H. M., Stierwalt, J. A. G., & Robin, D. A. (2000). Motor speech disorders. In J. B. Tomblin, H. L. Morris, & D. C. Spriestersbach (Eds.), *Diagnosis in speech-language pathology* (Chapter 12). San Diego: Singular.

Cleave, P. L., & Fey, M. E. (1997). Two approaches to the facilitation of grammar in children with language impairments: Rationale and description. *American Journal of Speech-Language Pathology, 6,* 22–32.

Colangelo, L. A., Logmann, J. A., & Rademaker, A. W. (2000). Tumor size and pretreatment speech and swallowing in patients with resectable tumors. *Archives of Otolaryngology—Head and Neck Surgery, 122,* 653–661.

Coleman, T. J., & McCabe-Smith, L. (2000). Key Terms and concepts. In T. Coleman (Ed.), *Clinical management of communication disorders in culturally diverse children* (pp. 3–12). Boston, MA: Allyn & Bacon.

Conti-Ramsden, G., & Jones, M. (1997). Verb use in specific language impairment. *Journal of Speech, Language, and Hearing Research, 40,* 1298–1413.

Conture, E. G. (1990). *Stuttering* (2d ed.). Upper Saddle River, NJ: Prentice Hall.

Cook, S. (2001). *Handbook of multiple sclerosis* (3d ed.). NY: Informa Healthcare.

Cooper, W. E., & Klouda, G. V. (1987). Intonation in aphasic and right-hemisphere-damaged patients. In J. H. Ryalls (Ed.), *Phonetic approaches to speech production in aphasia and related disorders.* (chapter 12, pp. 59–77). Boston, MA: Little, Brown and Company.

Costa, D., & Kroll, R. (2000). Stuttering: An update for physicians. *Canadian Medical Association Journal, 1621,* 1849–1855.

Council for Exceptional Children. (2001). *CEC knowledge and skill base for all beginning special education teachers of students in individualized general curriculums.* Washington, DC: Author.

Coyne, M. D., Kame'enui, E., & Carnine, D. (2007). *Effective teaching strategies that accommodate diverse learners.* Boston: Allyn & Bacon.

Craig, A., Hancock, K., Tran, Y., Craig, M., & Peters, K. (2002). Epidemiology of stuttering in the community across the entire life span. *Journal of Speech, Language, and Hearing Research, 45,* 1097–1105.

Creskoff, N., & Haas, A. (1999). Oral-motor skills and swallowing. In D. B. Kessler & P. Dawson (Eds.), *Failure to thrive and pediatric undernutrition: A transdisciplinary approach* (pp. 309–318). Baltimore, MD: Paul H. Brookes.

Cruikshanks, K. J., Wiley, T. L., Tweed, T. S., Klein, B. E. K., Klein, R., Mares-Perlman, J. A., & Nondahl, D. M. (1998). Prevalence of hearing loss in older adults in Beaver Dam,

Wisconsin: The epidemiology of hearing loss study. *American Journal of Epidemiology, 148,* 879–886.

Curenton, S., & Justice, L. M. (2004). Low-income preschoolers' use of decontextualized discourse: Literate language features in spoken narratives. *Language, Speech, and Hearing Services in Schools, 35,* 240–253.

Curlee, R. F., & Yairi, E. (1997). Early intervention with early childhood stuttering: A critical examination of the data. *American Journal of Speech-Language Pathology, 6*(2), 8–18.

Curtis, H., & Barnes, S. (1989). *Biology* (5th ed.). New York: Worth.

Curtis, M. E. (2005). The role of vocabulary instruction in adult basic education. In J. Comings, B. Garner, & C. Smith (Eds.), *Review of adult learning and literacy: Connecting research, policy, and practice* (pp. 43–70). New York: Routledge.

Dalton, D., Cruickshanks, K., Klein, B., Klein, R., Wiley, T., & Nondahl, D. (2003). The impact of hearing loss on quality of life in older adults. *Gerontologist, 43,* 61–68.

Daly, D. A., Simon, C. A., & BurnettStolnack, M. (1995). Helping adolescents who stutter focus on fluency. *Language, Speech, and Hearing Services in Schools, 26,* 162–168.

Damasio, A. (1981). The nature of aphasia: Signs and syndromes. In M. T. Sarno (Ed.), *Acquired aphasia* (pp. 51–65). New York: Academic Press.

Damasio, A. R. (1995). *Descartes' error: Emotion, reason, and the human brain.* New York: Quill.

Damasio, H. (2001). Neural basis of language disorders. In R. Chapey (Ed.), *Language intervention strategies in aphasia and related neurogenic communication disorders* (pp. 18–36). Baltimore, MD: Lippincott, Williams & Wilkins.

Damico, J. S. (1991). Clinical discourse analysis: A functional approach to language assessment. In C. S. Simon, *Communication skills and classroom success.* Eau Claire, WI: Thinking Publications.

Daniell, W. E., Fulton-Kehoe, D., Smith-Wellerr, T., & Franklin, G. M. (1998). Occupational hearing loss in Washington state, 1984–1991. Morbidity and associated costs. *American Journal of Industrial Medicine, 33,* 529–536.

Darley, F. L., Aronson, A. E., & Brown, J. R. (1969). Clusters of deviant speech dimension in the dysarthrias. *Journal of Speech and Hearing Research, 12,* 462–496.

Davis, B. L. (2005). Clinical diagnosis of developmental speech disorders. In A. Kamhi & K. Pollack (Eds.), *Phonological disorders in children* (pp. 3–22). Baltimore, MD: Paul H. Brookes.

Davis, B. L., Jakielski, K. J., & Marquardt, T. P. (1998). Developmental apraxia of speech: Determiners of differential diagnosis. *Clinical Linguistics & Phonetics, 12*(11), 25–45.

Davis, L. F. (1982). Respiration and phonation in cerebral palsy: A developmental model. *Seminars in Speech and Language, 8,* 101–106.

DeFeo, A. B., & Schaefer, C. M. (1983). Bilateral facial paralysis in a preschool child: Oral-facial and articulatory characteristics (a case study). In W. R. Berry (Ed.), *Clinical dysarthia* (pp. 165–186). San Diego, CA: College Hill Press.

DeVault, K. R. (2002). Presbyesophagus: A reappraisal. *Current Gastroenterology Reports, 4,* 193–199.

Diamond, P. T., Gale, S. D., & Denkhaus, H. K. (2001). Head injuries in skiers: An analysis of injury severity and outcome. *Brain Injury, 15,* 429–434.

DiMeo, J. H., Merritt, D. D., & Culatta, B. (1998). Collaborative partnerships and decision making. In D. D. Merritt &

B. Culatta (Eds.), *Language intervention in the classroom.* (pp. 37–98). San Diego, CA: Singular Publishing.

Ding, R., & Logemann, J. A. (2000). Pneumonia in stroke patients: A retrospective study. *Dysphagia, 15,* 51–57.

Dodd, B., Gillon, G., Oerlemans, M., Russell, T., Syrmis, M., & Wilson, H. (1995). Phonological disorder and the acquisition of literacy. In B. Dodd (Ed.), *Differential diagnosis and treatment of children with speech disorder* (pp. 125–146). London: Whurr.

Dollaghan, C., & Campbell, T. (1998). Nonword repetition and child language impairment. *Journal of Speech, Language, and Hearing Research, 41,* 1136–1146.

Dowden, P. A. (1999). Augmentative and alternative communication for children with motor speech disorders. In A. J. Caruso & E. A. Strand (Eds.), *Clinical management of motor speech disorders in children* (pp. 345–383). San Diego, CA: Singular.

Dowden, P., & Cook, A. M. (2002). Choosing effective selection techniques for beginning communications. In J. Reichle, D. R. Beukelman, & J. C. Light (Eds.), *Exemplary practices for beginning communicators: Implications for AAC* (pp. 395–431). Baltimore, MD: Brookes Publishing.

Dronkers, N. F. (1996). A new brain region for coordinating speech articulation. *Nature, 384,* 159–161.

Drumwright, A. (1971). *The Denver Articulation Examination.* Denver, CO: Ladoca Project and Publishing Foundation.

Duff, M. C., Proctor, A., & Yairi, E. (2004). Prevalence of voice disorders in African American and European American Preschoolers. *Journal of Voice, 18,* 348–353.

Duffy, J. R. (1995). *Motor speech disorders: Substrates, differential diagnosis, and management.* St. Louis, MO: Mosby.

Duffy, J. R. (2005). *Motor speech disorders: Substrates, differential diagnosis, and management* (2d ed.). St. Louis, MO: Elsevier Mosby.

Duffy, J. R. (2006). Apraxia of speech in degenerative neurologic disease. *Aphasiology, 20*(6), 511–527.

Dworkin, J. P., Marunick, M. T., & Krouse, J. H. (2004). Velopharyngeal dysfunction: Speech characteristics, variable etiologies, evaluation techniques, and differential treatments. *Language, Speech, and Hearing Services in Schools, 35,* 333–352.

Eadie, T. L., Yorkston, K. M., Klasner, E. R., Dudgeon, B. J., Deitz, J. C., Baylor, C. R., Miller, R. M., & Amtmann, D. (2006). Measuring communicative participation: A review of self-report instruments in speech-language pathology. *American Journal of Speech-Language Pathology, 15,* 307–320.

Edwards, C., & Estabrooks, W. (1994). Learning through listening: A hierarchy. In W. Estabrooks (Ed.), *Auditory-verbal therapy for parents and professionals.* Washington, DC: Alexander Graham Bell Association for the Deaf.

Ehlers, S., & Gillberg, C. (1993). The epidemiology of Asperger syndrome: A total population study. *Journal of Child Psychology and Psychiatry, 34,* 1327–1350.

Ehri, L. C. (2005). Learning to read words: Theory, findings, and issues. *Scientific Studies of Reading, 9,* 167–188.

Einarsdóttir, J., & Ingham, R. (2005). Have disfluency-type measures contributed to the understanding and treatment of developmental stuttering? *American Journal of Speech-Language Pathology, 14,* 260–273.

Ekwall, E. E., & Shanker, J. L. (1985). *Teaching reading in the elementary school.* Columbus, OH: Charles E. Merrill.

Elbert, M. (1997). From articulation to phonology: The challenge of change. In B. W. Hodson & M. L. Edwards (Eds.),

Perspectives in applied phonology (pp. 43–60). Gaithersburg, MD: Aspen Publishers.

Ellis Weismer, S., Murray-Branch, J., & Miller, J. F. (1994). A prospective longitudinal study of language development in late talkers. *Journal of Speech and Hearing Research, 37,* 852–867.

Ellis Weismer, S., & Robertson, S. (2006). Focused stimulation approach to language intervention. In R. McCauley and M. Fey (Eds.), *Treatment of language disorders in children.* Baltimore, MD: Paul H. Brookes.

Elman, R. J., & Bernstein-Ellis, E. (1995). What is functional? *American Journal of Speech-Language Pathology, 4,* 115–117.

Erard, M. (2007). *Um: Slips, stumbles, and verbal blunders, and what they mean.* New York: Random House.

Erler, S. F., & Garstecki, D. C. (2002). Hearing loss- and hearing aid-related stigma: Perceptions of women with age-normal hearing. *American Journal of Audiology, 11,* 83–91.

Ertmer, D. (2004). How well can children recognize speech features in spectograms? Comparisons by age and hearing status. *Journal of Speech, Language, and Hearing Research, 47,* 484–495.

Ezell, H. K., & Goldstein, H. (1991). Observational learning of comprehension monitoring skills in children who exhibit mental retardation. *Journal of Speech and Hearing Research, 34,* 141–154.

Ezrati-Vinacour, R., Platzky, R., & Yairi, E. (2001). The young child's awareness of stuttering-like disfluency. *Journal of Speech, Language, and Hearing Research, 44,* 368–380.

Fager, S. K., Doyle, M., & Karantounis, R. (2007). Traumatic brain injury. In D. R. Beukelman, K. L. Garrett, & K. M. Yorkston (Eds.), *Augmentative communication strategies for adults with acute or chronic medical conditions* (pp. 131–162). Baltimore, MD: Brookes.

Fallion, J., Irvine, D., & Shepherd, R. (2008). Cochlear implants and brain plasticity. *Hearing Research, 238,* 110–117.

Feder, K. P., Majnemer, A., Bourbonnais, D., Platt, R., Blayney, M., & Synnes, A. (2005). Handwriting performance in preterm children compared with term peers at age 6 to 7 years. *Developmental Medicine and Child Neurology, 47,* 163–170.

Felsenfeld, S., McGue, M., & Broen, P. A. (1995). Familial aggregation of phonological disorders: Results from a 28-year follow-up. *Journal of Speech and Hearing Research, 38,* 1901–1107.

Felsenfeld, S., & Plomin, R. (1997). Epidemiological and offspring analyses of developmental speech disorders using data from the Colorado Adoption Project. *Journal of Speech, Language, and Hearing Research, 40,* 778–791.

Fenson, L., Pethick, S., Renda, C., Cox, J. L., Dale, P. S., & Reznick, J. S. (2000). Short-form versions of the MacArthur Communicative Development Inventories. *Applied Psycholinguistics, 21,* 96–116.

Fey, M. (1986). *Language intervention with young children.* Boston, MA: College-Hill.

Fey, M. E., Long, S. H., & Finestack, L. M. (2003). Ten principles of grammar facilitation to children with specific language impairments. *American Journal of Speech-Language Pathology, 12,* 3–15.

Finn, P. (1996). Establishing the validity of recovery from stuttering without formal treatment. *Journal of Speech and Hearing Research, 39,* 1171–1181.

Fisher, K. V., Scherer, R. C., Guo, C. G., & Owen, A. S. (1996). Longitudinal phonatory characteristics after Botulinum toxin type A injection. *Journal of Speech and Hearing Research, 39,* 968–980.

Fitch-West, J., & Sands, E. S. (1987). *Bedside evaluation screening test.* Rockville, MD: Aspen.

Flax, J., Realpe-Bonilla, T., Hirsch, L. S., Brzustowic, L. M., Bartlett, C., & Tallal, P. (2003). Specific language impairment: Co-occurrence in families. *Journal of Speech, Language, and Hearing Research, 46,* 530–543.

Fletcher, J. (2003, December). *Validity of alternative approaches to the identification of LD: Operationalizing unexpected underachievement.* Presentation to the National Research Center on Learning Disabilities. Retrieved June 1, 2008, from www.nrcld.org/symposium2003/fletcher/fletcher2.html.

Fletcher, J. M., Shaywitz, S. E., Shankweiler, D. P., Katz, L., Liberman, I. Y., Stuebing, K. K., et al. (1994). Cognitive profiles of reading disability: Comparisons of discrepancy and low achievement definitions. *Journal of Educational Psychology, 86,* 6–23.

Flexer, C. (1994). *Facilitating hearing and listening in young children.* San Diego, CA: Singular.

Flynn, F. C., Benson, D. F., & Ardila, A. (1999). Anatomy of the insula: Functional and clinical correlates. *Aphasiology, 13,* 55–78.

Folkins, J. W. (1985). Issues in speech motor control and their relation to the speech of individuals with cleft palate. *Cleft Palate Journal, 22*(2), 106–122.

Folkins, J. W., & Bleile, K. M. (1990). Taxonomies in biology, phonetics, phonology, and speech motor control. *Journal of Speech and Hearing Disorders, 55,* 596–611.

Folkins, J. W., Moon, J. B., Luschei, E. S., Robin, D. A., Tye-Murray, N., & Moll, K. L. (1995). What can nonspeech tasks tell us about speech motor disabilities? *Journal of Phonetics, 23,* 139–147.

Folstein, M. F., Folstein, S. E., & McHugh, P. R. (1975). "Mini-mental state": A practical method for grading the mental state of patients for the clinician. *Journal of Psychological Research, 12,* 189–198.

Fombonne, E. (2003). Epidemiological surveys of autism and other pervasive developmental disorders: An update. *Journal of Autism and Developmental Disorders, 33,* 365–382.

Ford, C. N. (1996). Thyroplasty: Indications, techniques, and outcome. In M. P. Fried (Ed.), *The larynx: A multidisciplinary approach* (2d ed., pp. 243–252). Baltimore, MD: Mosby.

Ford, J., & Milosky, L. (2008). Inference generation during discourse and its relation to social competence: An online investigation of children with and without language impairment. *Journal of Speech, Language, and Hearing Research, 51,* 367–380.

Forrest, K., & Weismer, G. (1995). Dynamic aspects of lower lip movement in Parkinsonian and neurologically normal geriatric speakers' production of stress. *Journal of Speech and Hearing Research, 38,* 260–272.

Foundas, A., Bollich, A., Corey, D., Hurley, M., & Heilman, K. (2001). Anomalous anatomy of speech-language areas in adults with persistent developmental stuttering. *Neurology, 57,* 207–215.

Fowler, A., & Swainson, B. (2004). Relationships of naming skills to reading, memory, and receptive vocabulary: Evidence for imprecise phonological representations of words by poor readers. *Annals of Dyslexia, 54,* 247–280.

Fox, C. M., Morrison, C. E., Ramig, L. O., & Sapir, S. (2002). Current perspectives on the Lee Silverman Voice Treatment (LSVT) for individuals with idiopathic Parkinson disease. *American Journal of Speech-Language Pathology, 11,* 111–123.

Fox, C. M., & Ramig, L. O. (1997). Vocal sound pressure level and self-perception of speech and voice of men and women with idiopathic Parkinson disease. *American Journal of Speech-Language Pathology, 6,* 85–94.

Francis, D. J., Fletcher, J. M., Catts, H. W., & Tomblin, J. B. (2005). Dimensions affecting the assessment of reading comprehension. In S. A. Stahl & S. G. Paris (Eds.), *Children's reading comprehension and assessment* (pp. 369–394). Mahwah, NJ: Erlbaum.

Franic, D. M., & Bothe, A. (2008). Psychometric evaluation of condition-specific instruments used to assess health-related quality of life, attitudes, and related constructs in stuttering. *American Journal of Speech-Language Pathology, 17,* 60–80.

Frank, D. A., & Wong, F. (1999). Effects of prenatal exposures to alcohol, tobacco, and other drugs. In D. B. Kessler & P. Dawson (Eds.), *Failure to thrive and pediatric undernutrition: A transdisciplinary approach* (pp. 275–280). Baltimore, MD: Paul H. Brookes.

Frankenburg, W., Dodds, J., Archer, P., Bresnick, B., Maschka, P., Edelman, N., & Shapiro, H. (1990). *Denver II: Screening manual.* Denver, CO: Denver Developmental Materials.

Frattali, C. M., Thompson, C. M., Holland, A. L., Wohl, C. V., & Ferketic, M. M. (1995). *The American Speech-Language-Hearing Association functional assessment of communication skills for adults (ASHA FACS).* Rockville, MD: ASHA.

Freedman, S. E., Maas, E., Caligiuri, M. P., Wulf, G., & Robin, D. A. (2007). Internal vs. external: Oral-motor-performance as a function of attentional focus. *Journal of Speech, Language, and Hearing Research, 50*(1), 131–136.

Fried, M. P., & Lauretano, A. M. (1996). Conservation surgery for glottic carcinoma. In M. P. Fried (Ed.), *The larynx: A multidisciplinary approach* (2d ed., pp. 519–523). Baltimore, MD: Mosby.

Frost, L., & Bondy, A. S. (1994). *PECS: The picture exchange communication system training manual.* Cherry Hill, NJ: Pyramic Educational Consultants.

Fucci, D., & Luss, N. J. (1999). *Fundamentals of speech science.* Boston, MA: Allyn & Bacon.

Fuchs, D., & Fuchs, L. S. (2005). Responsiveness-to-intervention: A blueprint for practitioners, policymakers, and parents. *Teaching Exceptional Children,* September–October, 57–61.

Fuchs, L. S., & Fuchs, D. (2007). The role of assessment in the three-tier approach to reading instruction. In D. Haager, J. Klingner, & S. Vaughn (Eds.), *Evidence-based reading practices for response to intervention* (pp. 29–44). Baltimore, MD: Paul H. Brookes.

Fudala, J., & Reynolds, W. (2000). *Arizona Articulation Proficiency Scale* (3d ed.). Los Angeles, CA: Western Psychological Services.

Fujiki, M., Brinton, B., Morgan, M., & Hart, C. H. (1999). Withdrawn and sociable behavior of children with language impairment. *Language, Speech, and Hearing Services in Schools, 30,* 183–195.

Fujiki, M., Brinton, B., & Todd, C. M. (1996). Social skills in children with specific language impairment. *Language, Speech, and Hearing Services in Schools, 27,* 195–201.

Fuller, D. R., Lloyd, L. L., & Stratton, M. M. (1997). Aided AAC symbols. In L. L. Lloyd, D. R. Fuller, & H. H. Arvidson (Eds.), *Augmentative and alternative communication: A handbook of principles and practices* (pp. 48–79). Needham Heights, MA: Allyn & Bacon.

Functional MRI Research Center. (2008). The future role of functional MRI in medical applications. NY: Functional MRI Research Center, Columbia University. Retrieved February 18, 2008, from www.fmri.org/fmri.htm.

Gallaudet Research Institute. (2001). *Regional and national summary report of data from the 1999–2000 annual survey of deaf and hard of hearing children and youth.* Washington, DC: Gallaudet University.

Gallaudet Research Institute. (2006). *Regional and national summary report of data from the 2006–2007 annual survey of deaf and hard of hearing children and youth.* Washington, DC: Gallaudet University.

Gallaudet University Center for Assessment and Demographic Study. (1998). 30 years of annual surveys of deaf and hard-of-hearing children and youth: A glance over the decades. *American Annals of the Deaf, 142,* 72–76.

Ganske, K. (2000). *Word journeys: Assessment-guided phonics, spelling, and vocabulary instruction.* NY: Guilford.

Gates, G. A., Couropmitree, N. M., & Myers, R. H. (1999). Genetic associations in age-related hearing thresholds. *Archives of Otolaryngology—Head and Neck Surgery, 125,* 654–659.

Genesee, F., Paradis, J., & Crago, M. B. (2004). *Dual language development and disorders: A handbook on bilingualism and second language learning.* Baltimore: Brookes.

Gerring, J. P., Brady, K. D., Chen, A., Vasa, R., Grados, M., Bradeen-Roche, K. J., et al. (1998). Premorbid prevalence of ADHA and development of secondary ADHA after closed head injury. *Journal of the American Academy of Child and Adolescent Psychiatry, 37,* 647–654.

Gertner, Y., Fisher, C., & Eisengart, J. (2006). Abstract knowledge of word order in early sentence comprehension. *Psychological Science, 17,* 684–691.

Gierut, J. (1989). Maximal opposition approach to phonological treatment. *Journal of Speech and Hearing Disorders, 54,* 9–19.

Gierut, J. (2005). Phonological intervention: The how or the what? In A. Kamhi & K. Pollack (Eds.), *Phonological disorders in children: Clinical decision making in assessment and intervention* (pp. 201–211). Baltimore, MD: Paul H. Brookes.

Gierut, J. A. (1998). Treatment efficacy: Functional phonological disorders in children. *Journal of Speech, Language, and Hearing Research, 41,* S85–S100.

Gierut, J. A. (2007). Phonological complexity and language learnability. *American Journal of Speech-Language Pathology, 16,* 6–17.

Gierut, J. A., Morrisette, M. L., Hughes, M. T., & Rowland, S. (1996). Phonological treatment efficacy and developmental norms. *Language, Speech, and Hearing Services in Schools, 27,* 215–230.

Gillam, R. (1999). Computer-assisted language intervention using Fast Forward®: Theoretical and empirical considerations for decision-making. *Language, Speech, and Hearing Services in Schools, 3,* 363–370.

Gillam, R., Loeb, D. F., Hoffman, L., Bohman, T., Champlin, C., et al. (2008). The efficacy for Fast ForWard language intervention in school-age children with language impairment:

A randomized controlled trial. *Journal of Speech, Language, and Hearing Research, 51,* 97–119.

Gillis, R. J. (1996). *Traumatic brain injury rehabilitation for speech-language pathologists.* Boston: Butterworth-Heinemann.

Gillon, G. (2000). The efficacy of phonological awareness intervention for children with spoken language impairment. *Language, Speech, and Hearing Services in Schools, 31,* 126–141.

Gillon, G. T. (2002). Follow-up study investigating the benefits of phonological awareness intervention for children with spoken language impairment. *International Journal of Language and Communication Disorders, 37,* 381–400.

Gillon, G. (2004). *Phonological awareness. From research to practice.* New York: Guilford Press.

Ginsberg, A. J. (1988). Feeding disorders in the developmental disabled population. In D. C. Russo & J. H. Kedesdy (Eds.), *Behavioral medicine with the developmentally disabled* (pp. 21–41). New York: Plenum.

Gioia, B. (2001). The emergent language and literacy experiences of three deaf preschoolers. *International Journal of Disability, Development and Education, 48,* 411–428.

Girolametto, L., Pearce, P. S., & Weitzman, E. (1996). Interactive focused stimulation for toddlers with expressive vocabulary delays. *Journal of Speech and Hearing Research, 39,* 1274–1283.

Girolametto, L., Weitzman, E., & Greenberg, J. (2000). *Teacher interaction and language rating scale.* Toronto, ON: The Hanen Centre.

Girolametto, L., Wiigs, M., Smyth, R., Weitzman, E., & Pearce, P. (2001). Children with history of expressive vocabulary delay: Outcomes at 5 years of age. *American Journal of Speech-Language Pathology, 10,* 358–369.

Giuffrida, C. G., Shea, J. B., & Fairbrother, J. T. (2002). Differential transfer benefits of increased practice for constant, blocked, and serial practice schedules. *Journal of Motor Behavior, 34,* 353–365.

Goffman, L., Gerken, L., & Lucchesi, J. (2007). Relations between segmental and motor variability in prosodically complex nonword sequences. *Journal of Speech, Language, and Hearing Research, 50,* 444–458.

Goldberg, S. (1993). *Clinical intervention: A philosophy and methodology for clinical practice.* New York: Merrill.

Goldman, R. M., & Fristoe, M. (2000). *Goldman-Fristoe Test of Articulation-2.* Circle Pines, MN: American Guidance Service.

Goldman, S. L., Hargrave, J., Hillman, R. E., Holmberg, E., & Gress, C. (1996). Stress, anxiety, somatic complaints, and voice use in women with vocal nodules: Preliminary finds. *American Journal of Speech-Language Pathology, 5,* 44–54.

Golinkoff, R. M., & Hirsch-Pasek, K. (1999). *How babies talk: The magic and mystery of language in the first three years of life.* New York: Dutton.

Gomi, H., Honda, M., Ito, T., & Murano, E. Z. (2002). Compensatory articulation during bilabial fricative production by regulating muscle stiffness. *Journal of Phonetics, 30,* 261–279.

Goodglass, H., & Kaplan, E. (1983). *The assessment of aphasia and related disorders* (2d ed.). Philadelphia, PA: Lea & Febriger.

Goodman, R., & Yude, C. (1996). IQ and its predictors in childhood hemiplegia. *Developmental Medicine and Child Neurology, 38,* 881–890.

Gough, P. B., & Tunmer, W. E. (1986). Decoding, reading, and reading disability. *Remedial and Special Education, 7,* 6–10.

Gottwald, S. R., & Starkweather, C. W. (1995). Fluency intervention for preschoolers and their families in the public schools. *Language, Speech, and Hearing Services in Schools, 26,* 117–126.

Gray, H. *Anatomy of the human body.* Philadelphia: Lea & Febiger, 1918; Bartleby.com, 2000. Retrieved from www.bartleby.com/107/. [Online Edition].

Gray, S., Plante, E., Vance, R., & Henrichson, M. (1999). The diagnostic accuracy of four vocabulary tests administered to preschool-age children. *Language, Speech, and Hearing Services in Schools, 30,* 196–206.

Gresham, F. M., & Elliot, S. N. (1990). *Social skills rating system.* Circle Pines, MN: AGS.

Grice, H. P. (1975). Logic and conversation. In P. Cole and J. Morgan (Eds.), *Syntax and semantics: Speech acts* (vol. 3). New York: Academic Press.

Grigorenko, E. (2005). A conservative meta-analysis of linkage and linkage-association studies. *Scientific Studies of Reading, 9,* 285–316.

Gruber, F. A. (1999). Probability estimates and paths to consonant normalization in children with speech delay. *Journal of Speech, Language, and Hearing Research, 42,* 448–459.

Grunau, R. V., Whitfield, M. F., & Davis, C. D. (2002). Pattern of learning disabilities in children with extremely low birth weight and broadly average intelligence. *Archives of Pediatrics & Adolescent Medicine, 156,* 615–620.

Grunwell, P. (1987). *Clinical phonology* (2d ed.). Baltimore: Williams & Wilkins.

Grunwell, P. (1997). Natural phonology. In M. Ball & R. Kent (Eds.), *The new phonologies: Developments in clinical linguistics.* San Diego, CA: Singular Publishing Group, Inc.

Guenther, F. H. (2006). Cortical interactions underlying the production of speech sounds. *Journal of Communication Disorders, 39,* 350–356.

Guenther, F. H., Hampson, M., & Johnson, D. (1998). A theoretical investigation of reference frames for the planning of speech movements. *Psychological Review, 105,* 611–633.

Guitar, B. (1998). *Stuttering: An integrated approach to its nature and treatment* (2d ed.). Baltimore: Lippincott Williams & Wilkins.

Guitar, B. (2005). *Stuttering: An integrated approach to its nature and treatment* (3d ed.). New York: Lippincott Williams & Wilkins.

Guralnick, M. J. (1997). *The effectiveness of early intervention.* Baltimore, MD: Paul H. Brookes.

Gutiérrez-Clellen, V. F., & Peña, E. (2001). Dynamic assessment of diverse children: A tutorial. *Language, Speech, and Hearing Services in Schools, 32,* 212–224.

Haelsig, P. C., & Madison, C. L. (1986). A study of phonological processes exhibited by 3-, 4-, and 5-year-old children. *Language, Speech, and Hearing Services in Schools, 17,* 107–144.

Hagen, C. (1981). Language disorders secondary to closed head injury. *Topics in Language Disorders, 1,* 73–87.

Hagen, C. (1998). *Rehabilitation of the head injured adult: Comprehensive physical management* (3d ed.). Downey, CA: Association of the Ranchos Los Amigos Hospital, Inc.

Hagen, M. C., & Pardo, J. V. (2002). PET studies of somatosensory processing of light touch. *Behavioral Brain Research, 135,* 133–140.

Hall, J. W., & Mueller, H. G. (1997). *Audiologists' desk reference: Volume I*. San Diego, CA: Singular Publishing Group.

Hall, K. D., Amir, O., & Yairi, E. (1999). A longitudinal investigation of speaking rate in preschool children who stutter. *Journal of Speech, Language, and Hearing Research, 42,* 1367–1377.

Hall, P. K. (2007a). Familial and genetic factors: Co-occurring associations or possible contributions to the etiology? In P. K. Hall, L. S. Jordan, & D. A. Robin (Eds.), *Developmental apraxia of speech, theory and clinical practice* (2d ed., pp. 165–189). Austin, TX: Pro-Ed.

Hall, P. K. (2007b). Neurological and psychological factors in children with DAS. In P. K. Hall, L. S. Jordan, & D. A. Robin (Eds.), *Developmental apraxia of speech theory and clinical practice* (2d ed., pp. 123–163). Austin, TX: Pro-Ed.

Hall, P. K., Jordan, L. S., & Robin, D. A. (2007). *Developmental apraxia of speech: Theory and clinical practice* (2d ed.). Austin, TX: Pro-Ed.

Hallberg, L., Hallberg, U., & Kramer, S. (2008). Self-reported hearing difficulties, communication strategies, and psychological general well-being (quality of life) in patients with acquired hearing loss. *Disability and Rehabilitation, 30,* 203–212.

Halliday, M. A. K. (1975). *Learning how to mean: Explorations in the development of language development*. London: Edward Arnold.

Halliday, M. A. K. (1977). *Exploration in the functions of language*. New York: Elsevier North-Holland.

Halliday, M. A. K. (1978). *Language as a social semiotic: The social interpretation of language and meaning*. Baltimore, MD: University Park Press.

Halper, A., Cherney, L. R., & Burn, M. S. (1996). *Clinical management of right hemisphere dysfunction* (2d ed.). Rockville, MD: Aspen.

Hanks, R. A., Wood, D. L., Millis, S., Harrison-Felix, C., Pierce, C. A., Rosenthal, M., et al. (2003). Violent traumatic brain injury: Occurrence, patient characteristics, and risk factors from the Traumatic Brain Injury Model Systems Project. *Archives of Physical Medicine and Rehabilitation, 84,* 249–254.

Hardin-Jones, M., Chapman, K. L., & Schulte, J. (2003). The impact of cleft type on early vocal development in babies with cleft palate. *Cleft Palate-Craniofacial Journal, 40,* 453–459.

Hardin-Jones, M., Chapman, K., & Scherer, N. J. (2006, June 13). Early intervention in children with cleft palate. *The ASHA Leader, 11*(8), 8–9, 32.

Hardy, J. C. (1983). *Cerebral palsy*. Englewood Cliffs, NJ: Prentice-Hall.

Harris, V., Onslow, M., Packman, A., Harrison, E., & Menzies, R. (2002). An experimental investigation of the impact of the Lidcombe Program on early stuttering. *Journal of Fluency Disorders, 27,* 203–214.

Harrison, P., Kaufman, A., Kaufman, N., Bruinicks, R., Rynders, J., Ilmore, S., Sparrow, C., & Cicchetti, D. (1990). *Early screening profiles*. Circle Pines, MN: American Guidance Service.

Hart, B., & Risley, T. R. (1995). *Meaningful differences in the everyday experience of young American children*. Baltimore, MD: Paul H. Brookes.

Hartman-Maeir, A., Soroker, N., Oman, S. D., & Katz, N. (2003). Awareness of disabilities in stroke rehabilitation: A clinical trial. *Disability and Rehabilitation, 25*(1), 35–44.

Harvey, P. L. (1996). *Behavioral management of the performing voice*. In M. P. Fried (Ed.), *The larynx: A multidisciplinary approach* (2d ed., pp. 253–269). Baltimore, MD: Mosby.

Hawke, J. L., Wadsworth, S. J., & DeFries, J. C. (2006). Genetic influences on reading difficulties in boys and girls: The Colorado Twin Study. *Dyslexia, 12,* 21–29.

Hawking, S. (2003). *My experience with ALS*. Retrieved from www.hawking.org.u/diable/disable.html.

Hawkins, D. (2005). Effectiveness of counseling-based adult aural rehabilitation programs: A systematic review of the evidence. *Journal of the American Academy of Audiology, 16,* 485–493.

Heath, S. M., & Hogben, J. H. (2004). Cost effective prediction of reading disabilities. *Journal of Speech, Language, and Hearing Research, 47,* 751–765.

Heflin, L. J., & Simpson, R. L. (1998). Interventions for children and youth with autism: Prudent choices in a world of exaggerated claims and empty promises. Part 1: Intervention and treatment option review. *Focus on Autism and Other Developmental Disabilities, 13,* 194–211.

Heilman, K. M. (2004). Intentional neglect. *Frontiers in Bioscience, 9,* 694–705.

Helm-Estabrooks, N., & Albert, M. L. (1991). *Manual of aphasia therapy*. Austin, TX: Pro-Ed.

Helm-Estabrooks, N., & Holtz, G. (1991). *Brief test of head injury*. Chicago: Riverside.

Herrington-Hall, B., Lee, L., Stemple, J., Niemi, K., & McHone, M. (1988). Description of laryngeal pathologists by age, sex, and occupation in a treatment seeking sample. *Journal of Speech and Hearing Disorders, 53,* 57–65.

Herzberg, T. S., Stough, L. M., & Clark, C. (2004). Teaching and assessing the appropriateness of uncontracted braille. *Journal of Visual Impairment and Blindness, 98,* 773–779.

Hetzroni, O. E. (2004). AAC and literacy. *Disability and Rehabilitation, 26,* 1305–1312.

Heward, W. L. (2003). *Exceptional children: An introduction to special education* (7th ed.). Upper Saddle River, NJ: Merrill Prentice-Hall.

Hillenbrand, J., Cleveland, R. A., & Erikson, R. L. (1994). Acoustic correlates of breathy vocal quality. *Journal of Speech and Hearing Research, 37,* 769–778.

Hillis, A. E., Work, M., Barker, P. B., Jacobs, M. A., Breese, E. L., & Maurer, K. (2004). Re-examining the brain regions crucial for orchestrating speech articulation. *Brain, 127,* 1479–1487.

Hixon, T. J., Hawley, J. L., & Wilson, K. J. (1982). An around-the-house device for the clinical determination of respiratory driving pressure: A note on making simple even simpler. *Journal of Speech and Hearing Disorders, 47,* 413–415.

Hodson, B. (1997). Disordered phonologies: What have we learned about assessment and treatment? In B. W. Hodson & M. L. Edwards (Eds.), *Perspectives in applied phonology* (pp. 197–224). Gaithersburg, MD: Aspen Publishers.

Hodson, B. W., & Paden, E. P. (1991). *Targeting intelligible speech* (2d ed.). Austin, TX: Pro-Ed.

Hoff, E. (2003). The specificity of environmental influence: Socioeconomic status affects early vocabulary development via maternal speech. *Child Development, 74,* 1368–1378.

Hoff-Ginsberg, E. (1997). *Language development*. Pacific Grove, CA: Brooks Cole Publishing.

Hogan, T. P., Catts, H. W., & Little, T. D. (2005). The relationship between phonological awareness and reading: Implications for the assessment of phonological awareness. *Language, Speech, and Hearing Services in Schools, 36,* 285–293.

Holmberg, E., Hillman, R., Hammarberg, B., Södersten, M., & Doyle, P. (2001). Efficacy of a behaviorally based voice therapy protocol for vocal nodules. *Journal of Voice, 15,* 395–412.

Hooper, C. (2004). Treatment of voice disorders in children. *Language, Speech, and Hearing Services in Schools, 35,* 320–326.

Hoover, W. A., & Gough, P. B. (1990). The simple view of reading. *Reading and Writing: An Interdisciplinary Journal, 2,* 127–160.

Huckabee, M. (2004). *New Zealand Index for Multidisciplinary Evaluation of Swallowing.* Christchurch, NZ: University of Canterbury.

Hughes, D., McGillivray, L., & Schmidek, M. (1997). *Guide to narrative language: Procedures for assessment.* Eau Claire, WI: Thinking Publications.

Hymes, D. (2001). On communicative competence. In A. Duranti (Ed.), *Linguistic anthropology: A reader* (pp. 53–73). Boston: Blackwell Publishing.

Individuals with Disabilities Education Act. (2004). P. L. 108–446.

Individuals with Disabilities Education Act Data. (2006). *Annual report tables* Retrieved from www.ideadata.org/ AnnualTables.asp.

Ingham, J. C. (2003). Evidence-based treatment of stuttering. I. Definition and application. *Journal of Fluency Disorders, 28,* 197–207.

Ingham, R. J., Finn, P., & Bothe, A. K. (2005). "Roadblocks" revisited: Neural change, stuttering treatment, and recovery from stuttering. *Journal of Fluency Disorders, 30,* 91–107.

International Phonetic Association. (1996). *International phonetic alphabet.* London: Author.

Invernizzi, M., Justice, L. M., Landrum, T., & Booker, K. (2004). Early literacy screening in kindergarten: Widespread implementation in Virginia. *Journal of Literacy Research, 36,* 479–500.

Invernizzi, M., Meier, J., & Sullivan, A. (2004). *Phonological awareness and literacy screening—PreK.* Charlottesville, VA: University of Virginia.

Iverson, G. L., Gaetz, M., Lovell, M. R., & Collins, M. W. (2004). Cumulative effects of concussion in amateur athletes. *Brain Injury, 18*(5), 433–443.

Iverson, J. M., & Thal, D. J. (1998). Communicative transitions: There's more to the hand than meets the eye. In A. M. Wetherby, S. F. Warren, & J. Reichle (Eds.), *Transitions to prelinguistic communication* (pp. 59–86). Baltimore, MD: Paul H. Brookes.

Jacobsen, B., Johnson, A., Grywalski, C., Silbergleit, A., Jacobson, G., et al. (1997). The Voice Handicap Index: Development and validation. *American Journal of Speech-Language Pathology, 6,* 66–70.

Jennett, B., & Teasdale, G. (1981). *Management of head injuries.* Philadelphia: F. A. Davis.

Jennische, M., & Sedin, G. (2001). Linguistic skills at 6½ years of age in children who required neonatal intensive care in 1986–1989. *Acta Paediatricia, 90,* 199–212.

Jerger, J. (2007). Do hearing aids really improve quality of life? *Journal of American Academy of Audiology, 18,* 97.

Johnson, C. J. (2007). Prevalence of speech and language disorders in children. In *Canadian Language and Literacy Research Network, Encyclopedia of language and literacy development* (pp. 1–10). London, ON: Author. Retrieved February 24, 2008, from www.literacyencyclopedia.ca/pdfs/ topic.php?topId=24.

Johnson, C. J., Beitchman, J. H., Young, A., Escobar, M., Atkinson, L., Wilson, B., et al. (1999). Fourteen-year follow-up of children with and without speech-language impairments: Speech/language stability and outcomes. *Journal of Speech, Language, and Hearing Research, 42,* 744–760.

Johnson, R., & Harris, G. (2004). A preliminary study of the predictors of feeding problems in late infancy. *Journal of Reproductive and Infant Psychology, 22,* 183–188.

Joint Committee on Infant Hearing. (1991). Joint Committee on Hearing 1990 position statement. *ASHA, 3*(Suppl. 5), 3–6.

Jones, K. C., Peach, R. K., & Schneck, M. J. (2003). Must the insula be damaged in apraxia of speech? Poster presented at the Clinical Aphasiology Conference, Orca's Island, WA.

Jones, M., Onslow, M., Harrison, E., & Packman, A. (2000). Treating stuttering in young children: Predicting treatment time in the Lidcombe Program. *Journal of Speech, Language, and Hearing Research, 43,* 1440–1450.

Juel, C. (1988). Learning to read and write: A longitudinal study of 54 children from first through fourth grades. *Journal of Educational Psychology, 80,* 437–447.

Justice, L. M. (2006). Evidence-based practice, response-to-intervention, and prevention of reading difficulties. *Language, Speech, and Hearing Services in Schools, 37,* 1–14.

Justice, L. M., Bowles, R., & Skibbe, L. (2006). Measuring preschool attainment of print concepts: A study of typical and at-risk 3- to 5-year-old children. *Language, Speech, and Hearing Services in Schools, 37,* 1–12.

Justice, L. M., & Ezell, H. K. (1999). Vygotskian theory and its application to language assessment: An overview for speech-language pathologists. *Contemporary Issues in Communication Science and Disorders, 26,* 111–118.

Justice, L. M., & Ezell, H. K. (2000). Stimulating children's print and word awareness through home-based parent intervention. *American Journal of Speech-Language Pathology, 9,* 257–269.

Justice, L. M., & Ezell, H. K. (2001). Descriptive analysis of written language awareness in children from low income households. *Communication Disorders Quarterly, 22,* 123–134.

Justice, L. M., & Ezell, H. K. (2001). Written language awareness in preschool children from low-income households: A descriptive analysis. *Communication Disorders Quarterly, 22,* 123–134.

Justice, L. M., & Ezell, H. K. (2002). *The syntax handbook.* Eau Claire, WI: Thinking Publications.

Justice, L. M., & Ezell, H. K. (2004). Print referencing: An emergent literacy enhancement technique and its clinical applications. *Language, Speech, and Hearing Services in Schools, 35,* 185–193.

Justice, L. M., & Fey, M. (2004). Evidence-based practices in schools: Integrating craft and theory with science and data. *ASHA Leader, 4–5,* 30–32.

Justice, L. M., Invernizzi, M. A., & Meier, J. D. (2002). Designing and implementing an early literacy screening protocol: Suggestions for the speech-language pathologist. *Language, Speech, and Hearing Services in Schools, 33,* 84–101.

Justice, L. M., & Kaderavek, J. (2004). Embedded-explicit emergent literacy I: Background and description of approach. *Language, Speech, and Hearing Services in Schools, 35,* 201–211.

Justice, L. M., Meier, J., & Walpole, S. (2005). Learning new words from storybooks: Findings from an intervention with at-risk kindergarteners. *Language, Speech, and Hearing Services in Schools, 36,* 17–32.

Justice, L. M., & Pullen, P. (2003). Promising interventions for promoting emergent literacy skills: Three evidence-based approaches. *Topics in Early Childhood Special Education, 23,* 99–113.

Justice, L. M., Pullen, P. C., & Pence, K. (2008). Influence of verbal and nonverbal references to print on preschoolers' visual attention to print during storybook reading. *Developmental Psychology, 44,* 855–866.

Justice, L. M., & Schuele, M. (2003). Phonological awareness: Description, assessment, and intervention. In J. Bernthal and N. Bankson (Eds.). *Articulation and phonological disorders* (5th ed., pp. 376–406). New York: Allyn & Bacon.

Justice, L. M., Sofka, A., & McGinty, A. (2007). Targets, techniques, and treatment contexts in emergent literacy intervention. *Seminars in Speech and Hearing 28,* 14–24.

Kaderavek, J., & Justice, L. M. (2002). Shared storybook reading as an intervention context: Practices and potential pitfalls. *American Journal of Speech-Language Pathology, 11,* 395–406.

Kaderavek, J., & Justice, L. M. (2004). Embedded-explicit emergent literacy II: Goal selection and implementation in the early childhood classroom. *Language, Speech, and Hearing Services in Schools, 25,* 212–228.

Kaderavek, J. N., & Pakulski, L. A. (2007). Mother-child storybook interactions: Literacy orientation of preschools with hearing impairment. *Journal of Early Childhood Literacy, 7,* 49–72.

Kagan, A., Black, S., Duchan, J., Simmons-Mackie, N., & Square, P. (2001). Training volunteers as communication partners using "Supported Conversation for Adults with Aphasia" (SCA): A controlled trial. *Journal of Speech, Language, and Hearing Research, 44,* 624–639.

Kalia, M. (2003). Dysphagia and aspiration pneumonia in patients with Alzheimer's disease. *Metabolism, 52,* 36–38.

Kalinowski, J., Armson, J., Roland-Mieszkowski, M., Stuart, A., & Gracco, V. L. (1993). Effects of alterations in auditory feedback and speech rate on stuttering frequency. *Language and Speech, 36,* 1–16.

Kalinowski, J., Stuart, A., & Armson, J. (1996). Perceptions of stutterers and nonstutterers during speaking and nonspeaking situations. *American Journal of Speech-Language Pathology, 5,* 61–66.

Kalmanson, B., & Seligman, S. (1992). Family-provider relationships: The basis of all interventions. *Infants and Young Children, 4,* 46–52.

Kandel, E. R., Schwartz, J. H., & Jessell, T. M. (2001). *Principles of neural science* (4th ed.). New York: McGraw-Hill.

Karmody, C. S. (1996). The history of laryngology. In M. P. Fried (Ed.), *The larynx: A multidisciplinary approach* (2d ed., pp. 3–14). Baltimore, MD: Mosby.

Kart, C. S., & Kinney, J. M. (2001). *The realities of aging: An introduction to gerontology* (6th ed.). Boston: Allyn & Bacon.

Kashinath, S., Woods, J., & Goldstein, H. (2006). Enhanced generalized teaching strategy use in daily routines by parents of children with autism. *Journal of Speech, Language, and Hearing Research, 49,* 466–485.

Katz, J. (Ed.). (1994). *Handbook of clinical audiology* (4th ed.). Baltimore, MD: Williams & Wilkins.

Katz, W. F., Bharadwaj, S. V., & Carstens, B. (1999). Electromagnetic articulography treatment for an adult with Broca's aphasia and apraxia of speech. *Journal of Speech, Language, and Hearing Research, 42,* 1355–1366.

Katzir, T., Kim, Y., Wolf, M., O'Brien, B., Kennedy, B., Lovett, M., & Morris, R. (2006). Reading fluency: The whole is more than its parts. *Annals of Dyslexia, 56,* 51–82.

Kaufman, A. S., & Kaufman, N. L. (1990). *Kaufman Brief Intelligence Test.* Circle Pines, MN: American Guidance Service.

Kaut, K. P., DePompei, R., Kerr, J., & Congeni, J. (2003). Reports of head injury and symptom knowledge among college athletes: Implications for assessment and intervention. *Clinical Journal of Sports Medicine, 13*(4), 213–221.

Kedesky, J. H., & Budd, K. S. (1998). *Childhood feeding disorders.* Baltimore, MD: Paul H. Brookes.

Keenan, J. S., & Brassell, E. G. (1975). *Aphasia language performance scales.* Murfreesboro, TN: Pinnacle Press.

Keller, H. (1933). *Helen Keller in Scotland: A personal record by herself* (J. Love, Ed.). London: Methuen & Co.

Kenneally, S. M., Bruck, G. E., Frank, E. M., & Nalty, L. (1998). Language intervention after three years of isolation: A case study of a feral child. *Education and Training in Mental Retardation and Developmental Disabilities, 33,* 13–23.

Kent, R. D. (1994). *Reference manual for communicative sciences and disorders: Speech and language.* Austin, TX: Pro-Ed.

Kent, R. D. (1997). *The speech sciences.* San Diego, CA: Singular.

Kent, R. D., Adams, S. G., & Turner, G. S. (1996). Models of speech production. In N. J. Lass (Ed.), *Principles of experimental phonetics* (pp. 3–45). St. Louis, MO: Mosby.

Kent, R. D., Kent J. F., Duffy, J. R., Thomas, J. E., Weismer, G., & Stuntebeck, S. (2000). Ataxic dysarthria. *Journal of Speech, Language, and Hearing Research, 43,* 1275–1289.

Kent, R. D., & Rosenbek, J. C. (1983). Acoustic patterns of apraxia speech. *Journal of Speech and Hearing Research, 26,* 231–249.

Kertesz, A. (1982). *Western aphasia battery.* New York: Grune & Stratton.

Kesey, K. (1973). *One flew over the cuckoo's nest.* New York: Viking Press.

Kessler, D. B. (1999). Failure to thrive and pediatric undernutrition: Historical and theoretical context. In D. B. Kessler & P. Dawson (Eds.), *Failure to thrive and pediatric undernutrition: A transdisciplinary approach* (pp. 3–18). Baltimore, MD: Paul H. Brookes.

Khalifa, N., & von Knorring, A. (2003). Prevalence of tic disorder and Tourette syndrome in a Swedish school population. *Developmental Medicine and Child Neurology, 23,* 315–319.

Khan, L. M. (2002). The sixth view: Assessing preschoolers' articulation and phonology from the trenches. *American Journal of Speech-Language Pathology, 11,* 250–254.

Kiliç, M., Okur, E., Yildirim, I., & Güzelsoy, S. (2004). The prevalence of vocal fold nodules in school age children. *International Journal of Pediatric Otorhinolaryngology, 68,* 409–412.

Killion, M. C., & Christensen, L. (1998). The case of the missing dots: AI and SNR loss. *The Hearing Journal, 51*(5), 32–47.

Killion, M. C., & Niquette, P. A. (2000). What can the pure-tone audiogram tell us about a patient's SNR loss? *Hearing Journal, 53,* 46–53.

Kintsch, W. (2004). The construction-integration model of text comprehension and its implications. In R. B. Ruddell & N. J. Unrau (Eds.), *Theoretical models and processes of reading*

(5th ed., pp. 1270–1328). Newark, DE: International Reading Association.

Kirkwood, D. (1999). Major survey documents negative impact of untreated hearing loss on quality of life. *Hearing Journal, 52,* 32–40.

Klapp, S. T. (2003), Reaction time analysis of two types of motor preparation for speech articulation: Action as a sequence of chunks. *Journal of Motor Behavior, 35,* 135–150.

Klein, E. S. (1996). Phonological/traditional approaches to artic-ulation therapy: A retrospective group comparison. *Language, Speech, and Hearing Services in Schools, 27,* 314–323.

Klein, H. B., & Moses, N. (1999). *Intervention planning for chil-dren with communication disorders.* Boston, MA: Allyn and Bacon.

Kleinow, J., & Smith, A. (2000). Influences of length and syntac-tic complexity on the speech motor stability of the fluent speech of adults who stutter. *Journal of Speech, Language, and Hearing Research, 43,* 548–559.

Knock, T., Ballard, K. J., Robin, D. A., & Schmidt, R. A. (2000). Influence of order of stimulus presentation on speech motor learning: A principled approach to treatment for apraxia of speech. *Aphasiology, 14*(5/6), 653–668.

Kochkin, S. (2002). MarkTrak V: Why my hearing aids are in the drawer: The consumer perspective. *Hearing Journal, 53,* 34–42.

Kochkin, S. (2008). MarkTrak VII: Hearing loss population tops 31 million people. *Hearing Review, 12,* 16–29.

Koman, L. A., Smith, B. P., & Shilt, J. S. (2004). Cerebral palsy. *The Lancet, 363,* 1619–1631.

Konst, E. M., Rietveld, T., Peters, H. F. M., & Prahl-Andersen, B. (2003). Phonological development of toddlers with unilat-eral cleft lip and palate who were treated with and without infant orthopedics: A randomized clinical trial. *Cleft Palate-Craniofacial Journal, 40,* 32–39.

Kopun, J., & Stelmachowicz, P. (1998). Perceived communica-tion difficulties of children with hearing loss. *American Journal of Audiology, 7,* 30–38.

Krebs, N. F. (1999). Gastrointestinal problems and disorders. In D. B. Kessler & P. Dawson (Eds.), *Failure to thrive and pediatric undernutrition: A transdisciplinary approach* (pp. 215–226). Baltimore, MD: Paul H. Brookes.

Kuban, K. C., & Leviton, A. (1994). Cerebral palsy. *New England Journal of Medicine, 330*(3), 188–195.

Kuder, S. (1997). *Teaching students with language and commu-nication disabilites.* Boston: Allyn & Bacon.

Kwiatkowski, J., & Shriberg, L. D. (1993). Speech normalization in developmental phonological disorders: A retrospective study of capability-focus theory. *Language, Speech, and Hearing Services in Schools, 24,* 10–18.

Ladefoged, P. (2001). *A course in phonetics* (4th ed.). Fort Worth: Harcourt Brace Jovanovich College Publishers.

Laing, S. P., & Kamhi, A. (2003). Alternative assessment of lan-guage and literacy in culturally and linguistically diverse populations. *Language, Speech, and Hearing Services in Schools, 34,* 44–55.

Landry, S. H., Miller-Loncar, C. L., Smith, K. E., & Swank, P. R. (1997). Predicting cognitive-language and social growth curves from early maternal behaviors in children at varying degrees of biological risk. *Developmental Psychology, 33,* 1040–1053.

Laurent Clerk National Deaf Education Center. (2007). *Deaf children with multiple disabilities.* Retrieved February 1, 2008, from http://clerccenter.gallaudet.edu/infotogo/141.html.

Laws, G., & Bishop, D. V. M. (2003). A comparison of language abilities in adolescents with Down syndrome and children with specific language impairment. *Journal of Speech, Language, and Hearing Research, 46,* 1324–1339.

Lazarus, C., & Logemann, J. A. (1987). Swallowing disorders in closed head trauma patients. *Archives of Physical Medicine and Rehabilitation, 68,* 79–84.

Leach, J. M., Scarborough, H. S., & Rescorla, L. (2003). Late-emerging reading disabilities. *Journal of Educational Psychology, 95,* 211–224.

Lee, L., Stemple, J. C., & Glaze, L. (2003). *Your child's voice.* Gainesville, FL: Communicaire Publishing.

Leikin, M. (2002). Processing syntactic functions of words in normal and dyslexic readers. *Journal of Psycholinguistic Research, 31,* 145–163.

Lemons, J. A., Baur, C. R., Oh, W., et al. (2001). Very low birth weight outcomes of the National Institute of Child Health and Human Development Neonatal Research Network, January 1995 through December 1996. *Pediatrics, 107*(1), E1.

Leonard, L. B. (2000). *Children with specific language impair-ment.* Cambridge, MA: MIT Press.

Levelt, W. J. M. (1999). Producing spoken language: A blueprint of the speaker. In P. Hagoort & C. M. Brown (Eds.), *The neurocognition of language* (pp. 94–122). Oxford: Oxford University Press.

Levelt, W. J. M., Roelofs, A., & Meyer, A. S. (1999). A theory of lexical access in speech production. *Behavioral and Brain Sciences, 22,* 122–140.

Levisohn, L., Cronin-Golomb, A., & Schmahmann, J. D. (2000). Cerebellar cognitive affective syndrome in a paediatric population. *Brain, 123,* 1041–1050.

Lewis, B. A., Freebairn, L. A., Hansen, A. J., Iyengar, S. K., & Taylor, H. G. (2004). School-age follow-up of children with childhood apraxia of speech. *Language, Speech, and Hearing Services in Schools, 35,* 122–140.

Lewis, M. S., Crandell, C. C., Valente, M., Enrietto, J., Kreisman, N. V., Kreisman, B. M., & Bancroft, L. (2003). Study measures impact of hearing aids plus FM on the quality of life in older adults. *Hearing Journal, 56,* 30–33.

Liberman, A. M. (1998). When theories of speech meet the real world. *Journal of Psycholinguistic Research, 27,* 111–122.

Liégeois, F., Connelly, A., Cross, J. H., Boyd, S. G., Gadian, D. G., Vargha-Khadem, F., et al. (2004). Language reorganization in children with early onset lesions of the left hemisphere: An fMRI study. *Brain, 127,* 1229–1236.

Light, J. (1988). Interaction involving individuals using augmenta-tive and alternative communication systems: State of the art and future directions. *Augmentative and Alternative Communication, 4,* 66–82.

Light, J. C. (2003). Shattering the silence: Development of com-municative competence by individuals who use AAC. In J. C. Light, D. R. Beukelman, & J. Reichle (Eds.), *Communica-tive competence for individuals who use ACC: From research to effective practice* (pp. 3–38). Baltimore, MD: Brookes Publishing.

Light, J. C., & Kent-Walsch, J. (2003, May 27). Fostering emer-gent literacy for children who require AAC. *The ASHA Leader, 8,* 4–5, 28–29.

Light, J., & McNaughton, D. (2007). *Evidence-based literacy intervention for individuals who require AAC.* Seminar presentation at the annual meeting of the American Speech-Language-Hearing Association, Boston, MA.

Light, J., McNaughton, D., Jansen, J., Kristiansen, L., May, J., Miller, L., et al. (2005, November). *Maximizing the literacy skills of individuals who require AAC*. Seminar presentation at the annual meeting of the American Speech-Language-Hearing Association, San Diego, CA.

Lim, J., Lim, S., Choi, S., Kim, J., Kim, K., & Choi, H. (2007). Clinical characteristics and voice analysis of patients with mutational dysphonia: Clinical significance of diplophonia and closed quotients. *Journal of Voice, 21,* 12–19.

Lincoln, M., & Onslow, M. (1997). Long-term outcome of early intervention for stuttering. *American Journal of Speech-Language Pathology, 6,* 51–58.

Lincoln, M., Onslow, M., Lewis, C., & Wilson, L. (1996). A clinical trial of an operant treatment for school-age children who stutter. *American Journal of Speech-Language Pathology, 5,* 73–85.

Lindgren, S. D., De Renzi, E., & Richman, L. C. (1985). Cross-national comparisons of developmental dyslexia in Italy and the United States. *Child Development, 56,* 1404–1417.

Ling, D. (2001). Speech development for children who are hearing impaired. In R. H. Hull (Ed.), *Aural rehabilitation: Serving children and adults* (pp. 145–167). Canada: Singular.

Linscheid, T. R. (1992). Eating problems in children. In C. E. Walker & M. C. Roberts (Eds.), *Handbook of clinical child psychology* (2d ed., pp. 451–473). New York: John Wiley & Sons.

Locke, J. L. (1993). *The child's path to spoken language.* Cambridge, MA: Harvard University Press.

Lof, G. L. (2004). What does the research report about non-speech oral motor exercises and the treatment of speech sound disorders? Retrieved March 10, 2004, from www.apraxia-kids.org/faqs/responsefromlof.html.

Logemann, J. (1998). *Evaluation and treatment of swallowing disorders* (2d ed.). Austin, TX: Pro-Ed.

Logemann, J. (1983). *Evaluation and treatment of swallowing disorders.* Austin, TX: Pro-Ed.

Logemann, J., Gensler, G., Robbins, J., Lindblad, L., Brandt, D., et al. (2008). A randomized study of three interventions for aspiration of thin liquids in patients with dementia or Parkinson's disease. *Journal of Speech, Language, and Hearing Research, 51,*173–183.

Lord, C., & Risi, S. (2000). Diagnosis of autism spectrum disorders in young children. In A. M. Wetherby & B. M. Prizant (Eds.), *Autism spectrum disorders: A transactional developmental perspective* (pp. 149–172). Baltimore, MD: Paul H. Brookes.

Lovering, J. S., & Percy, M. (2007). Down syndrome. In I. Brown and M. Percy (Eds.), *A comprehensive guide to intellectual and developmental disabilities* (pp. 149–172). Baltimore, MD: Paul H. Brookes.

Love, R. J. (1992). *Childhood motor speech disability.* New York: Macmillan.

Luetke-Stahlman, B., & Nielson, D. (2003). The contribution of phonological awareness and receptive and expressive English to the reading ability of deaf students with varying degrees of exposure to accurate English. *Journal of Deaf Studies & Deaf Education, 8,* 464–484.

Lyon, G. R., Shaywitz, S. E., & Shaywitz, B. A. (2003). A definition of dyslexia. *Annals of Dyslexia, 53,* 1–14.

Maas, E., Barlow, J. A., Robin, D. A., & Shapiro, L. P. (2002). Treatment of sound production errors in aphasia and apraxia of speech: Effects of phonology complexity. *Aphasiology, 16,* 609–622.

Maas, E., Robin, D. A., Austermann Hula, S. N., Freedman, S. E., Wulf, G., Ballard, K. J., & Schmidt, R. A. (2008a). Principles of motor learning in treatment of motor speech motor disorders. *American Journal of Speech-Language Pathology, 17,* 277–298.

Maas, E., Robin, D. A., Wright, D. L., & Ballard, K. J. (2008b). Motor programming in apraxia of speech. *Brain and Language, 106,* 107–118.

MacDorman, M. F., Minino, A. M., Strobino, D. M., & Guyer, B. (2002). Annual summary of vital statistics—2001. *Pediatrics, 112,* 1037–1052.

Mackey, L. E., Morgan, A. S., & Bernstein, B. A. (1999). Swallowing disorders in severe brain injury: Risk factors affecting return to oral intake. *Archives of Physical Medicine and Rehabilitation, 80,* 365–371.

Maclean, L. K., & Cripe, J. J. (1997). The effectiveness of early intervention for children with communication disorders. In M. Gualnick (Ed.), *The effectiveness of early intervention.* Baltimore, MD: Paul H. Brookes.

MacWhinney, B. (1996). The CHILDS system. *American Journal of Speech-Language Pathology, 5,* 5–14

Madsen, K. M., Hviid, A., Vestergaard, M., Schendel, D., Wohlfahrt, J., Thorsen, P., Olsen, J., & Melbye, M. (2002). A population-based study of measles, mumps, and rubella vaccination and autism. *New England Journal of Medicine, 347*(19), 1477–1482.

Magnusson, E., & Naucler, K. (1993). The development of linguistic awareness in language-disordered children. *First Language, 13,* 93–111.

Malkus, D., Booth, B., & Kodimer, C. (1980). *Rehabilitation of the head-injured adult: Comprehensive cognitive management.* Downey, CA: Professional Staff Association of Rancho Los Amigos Hospital.

Mander, R., Wilton, K., Townsend, M., & Thompson, P. (1995). Personal computers and process writing: A written language intervention for deaf children. *British Journal of Educational Psychology, 65,* 441–453.

Mann, G., Hankey, G. J., & Cameron, D. (1999). Swallowing function after stroke: Prognosis and prognostic factors at six months. *Stroke, 30,* 744–748.

Månsson, H. (2000). Childhood stuttering: Incidence and development. *Journal of Fluency Disorders, 25,* 47–57.

Marieb, E. (2005). *Essentials of human anatomy and physiology* (8th ed.). San Francisco, CA: Benjamin Cummings.

Martin, F. (1994). *Introduction to audiology* (5th ed.). Englewood Cliffs, NJ: Prentice Hall.

Martin, F., & Greer Clark, J. (2002). *Introduction to audiology* (8th ed.). Boston, MA: Allyn & Bacon.

Martino, R., Pron, G., & Diamant, N. (2000). Screening for oropharyngeal dysphagia in stroke: Insufficient evidence for guidelines. *Dysphagia, 15,* 19–30.

Mashima, P. A., Birkmire-Peters, D. P., Symes, M. J., Holtel, M. R., Burgess, L. P., & Peters, L. J. (2003). Telehealth: Voice therapy using telecommunications technology. *American Journal of Speech-Language Pathology, 12,* 432–439.

Massagli, T. L., Fann, J. R., Burington, B. E., Jaffe, K. M., Katon, W. J., & Thompson, R. S. (2004). Psychiatric illness after mild traumatic brain injury in children. *Archives of Physical Medicine and Rehabilitation, 85,* 1428–1434.

Max, L., & Gracco, V. (2005). Coordination of oral and laryngeal movements in the perceptually fluent speech of adults who stutter. *Journal of Speech, Language, and Hearing Research, 48,* 524–542.

May, P. A., & Gossage, J. P. (2001). Estimating the prevalence of fetal alcohol syndrome: A summary. *Alcohol Research & Health, 25,* 159–167.

McAuliffe, M. J., & Ward, E. C. (2006). The use of electropalatography in the assessment and treatment of acquired motor speech disorders in adults: Current knowledge and future directions. *NeuroRehabilitation, 21,* 189–203.

McCauley, R. J., & Swisher, L. (1984). Psychometric review of language and articulation tests for preschool children. *Journal of Speech and Hearing Disorders, 49,* 34–42.

McClean, M. D., & Runyan, C. M. (2000). Variations in the relative speeds of orofacial structures with stuttering severity. *Journal of Speech, Language, and Hearing Research, 43,* 1524–1531.

McClincy, M. P., Lovell, M. R., Pardini, J., Collins, M. W., & Spoke, M. K. (2006). Recovery from sports concussion in high school and college athletes. *Brain Injury, 20*(1), 33–39.

McConnel, F. M., Cerenko, D., Jackson, R. T., & Guffin, T. N. (1988). Timing of major events of pharyngeal swallowing. *Archives of Otolaryngology—Head and Neck Surgery, 21,* 625–635.

McCrea, M., Hammeke, T., Olsen, G., Leo, P., & Guskiewicz, K. (2004). Unreported concussion in high school football players: Implications for prevention. *Clinical Journal of Sports Medicine, 14,* 13–17.

McDonald, E. T. (1987). *Treating cerebral palsy: For clinicians by clinicians.* Austin, TX: Pro-Ed.

McGregor, K. K. (1997). The nature of word-finding errors of preschoolers with and without word-finding deficits. *Journal of Speech, Language, and Hearing Research, 40,* 1232–1244.

McGregor, K. K., Friedman, R. M., Reilly, R. M., & Newman, R. M. (2002). Semantic representations and naming in young children. *Journal of Speech, Language, and Hearing Research, 45,* 332–346.

McGregor, K. K., & Leonard, L. B. (1995). Intervention for word-finding deficits in children. In M. Fey, J. Windsor, & S. Warren (Eds.), *Language intervention: Preschool though the elementary years* (pp. 85–105). Baltimore: Paul H. Brookes.

McGuire, R., Lorang, T., & Hoffman, J. (2006, November). Speech sound disorders in children: Low-cost speech analysis software as a clinical biofeedback tool. Presentation to the American Speech-Language-Hearing Association Annual Convention, Miami Beach, FL.

McKelvey, M., Dietz, A., Hux, K., Weissling, K., & Beukelman, D. (2007). Performance of a person with chronic aphasia using visual scene display prototype. *Journal of Medical Speech Language Pathology, 15,* 305–317.

McNeil, M. R., Doyle, P. J., & Wambaugh, J. (2000). Apraxia of speech: A treatable disorder of motor planning and programming. In S. E. Nadeau, L. J. Gonzalez-Rothi, & B. Crosson (Eds.), *Aphasia and language. Theory to practice* (pp. 221–226). New York: The Guilford Press.

McNeil, M. R., Odell, K. H., Miller, S. B., & Hunter, L. (1995). Consistency, variability, and target approximation for successive speech repetitions among apraxic, conduction aphasic, and ataxic dysarthric speakers. *Clinical Aphasiology, 23,* 39–55.

McNeil, M. R., Robin, D. A., & Schmidt, R. A. (1997). Apraxia of speech: Definition, differentiation, and treatment. In M. R. McNeil (Ed.), *Clinical management of sensorimotor speech disorders* (pp. 311–344). New York: Thieme.

McNeil, M. R., Weismer, G. Addams, S., & Mulligan, M. (1990). Oral structure non-speech motor control in normal, dysarthic aphasic and apraxic speakers: Isometric force and static position control. *Journal of Speech and Hearing Research, 33,* 255–268.

Menyuk, P., Chesnick, M., Liebergott, J. W., Korngold, B., D'Agostino, R., & Belander, A. (1991). Predicting reading problems in at-risk children. *Journal of Speech and Hearing Research, 34,* 893–903.

Merati, A. L., Shemirani, N., Smith, T. L., & Toohill, R. J. (2006). Changing trends in the nature of vocal fold motion impairment. *American Journal of Otolaryngology—Head and Neck Medicine and Surgery, 27,* 106–108.

Mehr, A. S. (2005). *Understanding your audiogram.* Reston, VA: American Academy of Audiology. Retrieved January 10, 2005, from www.audiology.org/consumer/guides/uya.php.

Mercer, C. (1997). *Students with learning disabilities* (5th ed.). Columbus, OH: Prentice Hall.

Merritt, D., Barton, J., & Culatta, B. (1998). Instructional discourse: A framework for learning. In D. D. Merritt & B. Culatta (Eds.), *Language intervention in the classroom* (pp. 143–174). San Diego, CA: Singular Publishing.

Merritt, D., Culatta, B., & Trostle, S. (1998). Narratives: Implementing a discourse framework. In D. D. Merritt & B. Culatta (Eds.), *Language intervention in the classroom* (pp. 277–330). San Diego, CA: Singular Publishing.

Merzenich, M. M., Jenkins, W. M., Johnston, P., Schreiner, C., Miller, S. L., & Tallal, P. (1996). Temporal processing deficits of language-learning impaired children ameliorated by training. *Science, 271,* 77–81.

Meyerhoff, W. L., & Rice, D. H. (1992). *Otolaryngology—Head and neck surgery.* Philadelphia: W. B. Saunders.

Miccio, A. W. (2002). Clinical problem solving: Assessment of phonological disorders. *American Journal of Speech-Language Pathology, 11,* 221–229.

Miccio, A. W., Yont, K. M., Clemons, H. L., & Vernon-Feagans, L. (2002). Otitis media and the acquisition of consonants. In F. Windsor, M. L. Kelly, & N. Hewlett (Eds.), *Investigations in clinical phonetics and linguistics* (pp. 429–436). Mahwah, NJ: Lawrence Erlbaum.

Miceli, G., Benvegnú, B., Capasso, R., & Caramazza, A. (1997). The independence of phonological and orthographic lexical forms: Evidence from aphasia. *Cognitive Neuropsychology, 14,* 35–69.

Mildner, V., Stankovic, D., & Petkovic. (2005). The relationship between active hand and ear advantage in the native and foreign language. *Brian and Cognition, 57,* 158–161.

Miles, S., & Bernstein Ratner, N. (2001). Parental language input to children at stuttering onset. *Journal of Speech, Language, and Hearing Research, 44,* 1116–1130.

Miller, E. K. (2000). The prefrontal cortex and cognitive control. *Nature reviews: Neuroscience, 1,* 59–65.

Miller, E. K. (2000). The prefrontal cortex and cognitive control. *Nature Reviews: Neuroscience, 1,* 59–65.

Miller, J. F., & Chapman, R. (1981). The relation between age and mean length of utterance in morphemes. *Journal of Speech and Hearing Research, 24,* 154–161.

Mohr, P. E., Feldman, J. J., Dunbar, J. L., McConkey-Robbins, A., Niparko, J. K., Rittenhouse, R. K., & Skinner, M. W. (2000). The societal costs of severe to profound hearing loss in the United States. *International Journal of Technology Assessment in Health Care, 16,* 1120–1135.

Montgomery, A. A., & Houston, T. (2000). The hearing-impaired adult: Management of communication deficits and tinnitus. In J. G. Alpiner & P. A. McCarthy (Eds.), *Rehabilitative audiology: Children and adults* (pp. 337–401). Baltimore: Lippincott Williams & Wilkins.

Montgomery, J. (2002). Examining the nature of lexical processing in children with specific language impairment: A temporal processing or processing capacity deficit? *Applied Psycholinguistics, 23,* 447–470.

Morgan, A. S., & Mackey, L. E. (1999). Causes and complications associated with swallowing disorders in traumatic brain injury. *Journal of Head Trauma Rehabilitation, 14,* 454–461.

Mori, K. (1999). Vocal fold nodules in children: Preferable therapy. *International Journal of Pediatric Otorhinolaryngology, 49,* S303–306.

Moriarty, B. C., & Gillon, G. T. (2006). Phonological awareness intervention for children with childhood apraxia of speech. *International Journal of Language and Communication Disorders, 41,* 713–734.

Morris, R. J., Brown, W. S., Hicks, D. M., & Howell, E. (1995). Phonational profiles of male trained singers and nonsingers. *Journal of Voice, 9*(2), 142–148.

Moskovsky, C. (2001). *The critical period hypothesis revisited.* Paper presented at the 2001 Conference of the Australian Linguistic Society. Abstract retrieved November 12, 2003, from http://linguistics.anu.edu.au/ALS2001/proceedings .html.

Mundy, P., Fox, N., & Card, J. (2003). EEG coherence, joint attention and language development in the second year. *Developmental Science, 6,* 48–54.

Münte, T. F., Altenmüller, E., & Jäncke, L. (2002). The musician's brain as a model of neuroplasticity. *Nature Reviews: Neuroscience, 3,* 473–478.

Murdoch, B. E., & Goozée, J. V. (2003). EMA analysis of tongue function in children with dysarthria following traumatic brain injury. *Brain Injury, 17,* 79–93.

Murdoch, B. E., Thompson, E. C., & Theodoros, D. G. (1997). Spastic dysarthria. In M. R. McNeil (Ed.), *Clinical management of sensorimotor speech disorders* (pp. 287–310). New York: Thieme.

Murry, T., & Carrau, R. L. (2001). *Clinical manual for swallowing disorders.* San Diego, CA: Singular.

Murry, T., & Woodson, G. E. (1995). Combined-modality treatment of adductor spasmodic dysphonia with botulinum toxin and voice therapy. *Journal of Voice, 9*(4), 460–465.

Mysak, E. D. (1989). *Pathology of the speech system: A system approach to organic speech disorders* (2d ed.). Springfield, IL: Charles C. Thomas.

Nakajima, N., Inoue, M., & Sakai, Y. (2005). Contralateral pharyngeal paralysis caused by medial medullary infarction. *Journal of Neurology, Neurosurgery, and Psychiatry, 76,* 1292–1293.

Nathan, L., Stackhouse, J., Goulandris, N., & Snowling, M. A. (2004). The development of early literacy skills among children with speech difficulties: A test of the "critical age hypothesis." *Journal of Speech, Language, and Hearing Research, 47,* 377–391.

Nation, K., & Snowling, M. J. (1999). Developmental differences in sensitivity to semantic relations among good and poor comprehenders: Evidence from semantic priming. *Cognition, 70,* B1–B13.

National Academy of Sciences. (1989). *Recommended dietary allowances* (9th ed.). Washington, DC: National Research Council, Food and Nutrition Board.

National Assessment of Adult Literacy (2003). NAAL Fact Sheet: Overview. Washington, DC: National Center for Education Statistics.

National Cancer Institute. (2008). *Cancer stat fact sheets.* Bethesda, MD: Author.

National Center for Education Statistics. (2004). *English language learner students in the U.S. public schools: 1993 and 2000.* Washington, DC: Author (document NCES 2004-035).

National Center for Education Statistics. (2005). *NAEP 2004 trends in academic progress: Three decades of student performance in reading and mathematics: Findings in brief* (NCES 2005-463). U.S. Department of Education, Institute of Education Sciences, National Center for Education Statistics. Washington, DC: Government Printing Office.

National Center for Education Statistics. (2008). *Fast facts.* Retrieved June 1, 2008, from http://nces.ed.gov/fastfacts/ display .asp?id=64.

National Center for Voice and Speech. (2004). Voice production tutorial. Available at www.ncvs.org/ncvs/tutorials/voicprod/ tutorial/quality.html.

National Early Literacy Panel. (NELP; 2004, November). *The National Early Literacy Panel: A research synthesis on early literacy development.* Paper presented at the annual meeting of the National Association of Early Childhood Specialists/ SDE, Anaheim, CA.

National Health Interview Survey, 2002 [Computer file]. Hyattsville, MD: U.S. Dept. of Health and Human Services, National Center for Health Statistics [producer], 2002.

National High School Center. (2007). *High school dropout: A quick stats fact sheet.* Washington, DC: National High School Center, American Institutes for Research.

National Institute on Deafness and Other Communication Disorders. (2003). *Auditory processing disorder in children: What does it mean?* NIH Publication No. 01-4949. Retrieved September 14, 2003, from www.nidcd.nih.gov/health/voice/ auditory.asp.

National Institute on Deafness and Other Communication Disorders. (2003). *Traumatic brain injury: Cognitive and communication disorders.* Retrieved from www.nidcd. nih.gov/health/voice/tbrain.asp.

National Institute on Deafness and Other Communication Disorders. (2006). *Statistics on voice, speech, and language.* Retrieved from www.nidcd.nih.gov/health/statistics/ vsl.asp#2.

National Institute of Dental and Craniofacial Research. (2003). Oral-systemic health connection. Retrieved from www.nidr.nidr.nih.gov/spectrum/NIDCR2/2menu.htm.

National Institutes of Health. (1993, March 1–3). *Early identification of hearing impairment in infants and young children.* NIH Consensus Statement Online. Retrieved March 1, 2008, from http://consensus.nih.gov/1993/1993 HearingInfantsChildren092html.htm.

National Institutes of Health. (2000). Phenylketonuria: Screening and management. *NIH Consensus Statement Online, 17*(3), 1–27.

National Institutes of Health. (2002). *Stuttering* (NIH Pub. No. 97-4232). Bethesda, MD: Author.

National Institute of Neurological Disorders and Stroke. (2006). Autism fact sheet. (NIH Publication No. 06-1877). Retrieved

February 11, 2008, from www.hinds.nih.gov/disorders/dementias/dementia.htm.

National Institute of Neurological Disorders and Stroke. (2008). NINDS stroke information page. Retrieved February 11, 2008, from www.ninds.nih.gov/disorders/autism/autism.htm.

National Public Radio. (2007, February 28, *Morning Edition*). Interview with Bob and Lee Woodruff. Retrieved from www.npr.org/templates/story/story.php?storyId=7618702#7619075.

National Reading Panel. (2000). *Teaching children to read: An evidence-based assessment of the scientific research literature on reading and its implications for reading instruction: Report of the subgroups* (NIH Publication No. 00-4754). Washington, DC: National Institutes of Health and National Institute of Child Health and Human Development.

Nelson, L. (1985). Language formulation related to dysfluency and stuttering. In *Stuttering therapy: Prevention and intervention with children*. Memphis, TN: Stuttering Foundation of America.

Nelson, M. A., & Hodge, M. M. (2000). Effects of facial paralysis and audiovisual information on stop place identification. *Journal of Speech, Language, and Hearing Research, 43,* 158–171.

Nelson, N. W. (1998). *Childhood language disorders in context: Infancy through adolescence* (2d ed.). Boston: Allyn and Bacon.

Newman, C. W., Hug, G. A., Jacobson, G. P., & Sandridge, S. A. (1997). Perceived hearing handicap of patients with unilateral or mild hearing loss. *Annals of Otolaryngology, Rhinology, and Laryngology, 106,* 210–214.

Newman, C. W., & Sandridge, S. A. (2004). Hearing loss is often undiscovered, but screening is easy. *Cleveland Clinic Journal of Medicine, 71,* 225–232.

Nicely, P., Tamis-LeMonda, C. S., & Bornstein, M. H. (1999). Mothers' attuned responses to infant affect expressivity promote earlier achievement of language milestones. *Infant Behavior and Development, 22,* 557–568.

Niemier, J. P., Burnett, D. M., & Whitaker, D. A. (2003). Cultural competence in the multidisciplinary rehabilitation setting: Are we falling short of meeting needs? *Archives of Physical Medicine and Rehabilitation, 84*(8), 1240–1245.

Nijland, L., Maassen, B., Van der Meulen, S., Gabreëls, F., Kraaimaat, F. W., & Schreuder, R. (2002). Coarticulation patterns in children with developmental apraxia of speech. *Clinical Linguistics & Phonetics, 16*(6), 461–483.

Nilsson, H., Ekberg, O., Olsson, R., & Hindfelt, B. (1996). Quantitative assessment of oral and pharyngeal function in Parkinson's disease. *Dysphagia, 11,* 274–275.

Nippold, M. A. (1990). Concomitant speech and language disorders in stuttering children: A critique of the literature. *Journal of Speech and Hearing Disorders, 55,* 51–60.

Nippold, M. A. (1998). *Later language development: The school age and adolescent years*. Austin, TX: Pro-Ed.

Nippold, M. A. (2000). Language development during the adolescent years: Aspects of pragmatics, syntax, and semantics. *Topics in Language Disorders, 20,* 15–28.

Nippold, M. A. (2001). Phonological disorders and stuttering in children: What is the frequency of co-occurrence? *Clinical Linguistics and Phonetics, 15,* 219–228.

Nippold, M. A. (2007). *Later language development: School age children, adolescents, and young adults*. Austin, TX: Pro-Ed.

Nishimura, K., Satoh, T., Maesawa, C, Ishijima, K., & Sato, H. (2007). Giant cell tumor of the larynx: A case report and review of the literature. *American Journal of Otolaryngology—Head and Neck Medicine and Surgery, 28,* 436–440.

Nishio, M., & Niimi, S. (2006). Comparison of speaking rate, articulation rate, and alternating motion rate in dysarthic speakers. *Folia Phoniatrica et Logopaedica, 58,* 114–131.

Niskar, A. S., Kieszak, S. M., Holmes, A., Estaban, E., Rubin, C., & Brody, D. J. (1998). Prevalence of hearing loss among children 6 to 19 years of age: The third national health and nutrition examination survey. *Journal of the American Medical Association, 14,* 1071–1075.

Nittrouer, S. (1996). The relation between speech perception and phonemic awareness: Evidence from low-SES children and children with chronic OM. *Journal of Speech and Hearing Research, 39,* 1059–1070.

Nittrouer, S. (1999). Do temporal processing deficits cause phonological processing problems? *Journal of Speech, Language, and Hearing Research, 42,* 925–942.

Northern, J., & Downs, M. (1991). *Hearing in children* (4th ed.), Baltimore, MD: Williams and Wilkins.

Nuss, R. C., Hillman, R. E., & Eavey, R. D. (1996). Office and operative diagnostic techniques: The pediatric patient and the use of videolaryngoscopy. In M. P. Fried (Ed.), *The larynx: A multidisciplinary approach* (2d ed., pp. 65–74). Baltimore, MD: Mosby.

Odderson, M. D., Keaton, J. C., & McKenna, B. S. (1995). Swallow management in patients on an acute stroke pathway: Quality is cost effective. *Archives of Physical Medicine and Rehabilitation, 76,* 1130–1133.

O'Donoghue, C. R., & Dudding, C. C. (2004). Mirror writing following left hemisphere stroke: A case study. *Journal of Medical Speech-Language Pathology, 12*(3), 117–122.

Oetting, J., Rice, M., & Swank, L. (1995). Quick Incidental Learning (QUIL) of words by school-age children with and without SLI. *Journal of Speech and Hearing Research, 38,* 434–445.

Ogar, J., Willock, S., Baldo, J., Wilkins, D., Ludy, C., & Dronkers, N. (2006). Clinical and anatomical correlates apraxia of speech. *Brain and Language, 97,* 343–350.

Okie, S. (2005). Traumatic brain injury in the war zone. *New England Journal of Medicine, 352,* 2043–2047.

Oller, D. K. (1980). The emergence of speech sounds in infancy. In G. Yeni-Komshian, J. A. Kavanagh, & C. A. Ferguson (Eds.), *Child phonology: Vol. 1. Production* (pp. 93–112). New York: Academic Press.

Onslow, M., Andrews, C., & Lincoln, M. (1994). A control/experimental trial of an operant treatment for early stuttering. *Journal of Speech and Hearing Research, 37,* 1244–1259.

Orenstein, S. R. (1994). Gastroesophageal reflux disease. *Seminars in Gastrointestinal Disease, 5,* 2–14.

Owens, R. E., Jr. (2001). *Language development: An introduction* (5th ed.). Needham Heights, MA: Allyn & Bacon.

Ozer, C., Ozer, F., Sener, M., & Yavuz, H. (2007). A forgotten gauze pack in the nasopharynx: An unfortunate complication of adenotonsillectomy. *American Journal of Otolaryngology—Head and Neck Medicine Surgery, 28,* 191–193.

Pakulski, L. A., & Hinkle, A. (2003). Patient perception of aural rehabilitation. Poster presented at the Ohio Speech-Language-Hearing Association, Columbus, OH.

Palmer, E. P. (1979). Language dysfunction in cerebrovascular disease. *Primary Care, 6*(4), 827–842.

Pankratz, M. E., Plante, E., Vance, R., & Insalaco, D. (2007). The diagnostic and predictive validity of *The Renfew Bus Story*. *Language, Speech, and Hearing Services in Schools, 38*(4), 390–399.

Paradise, J. L., Rockette, H. E., Colborn, D. K., Bernard, B. S., Smith, C. G., Kurs-Lasky, M., & Janosky, J. E. (1999). Otitis media in 2253 Pittsburgh-area infants: Prevalence and risk factors during the first two years of life. *Pediatrics, 103*(3), 670–672.

Parette, P., & Huer, M. B. (2002). Working with Asian American families whose children have augmentative and alternative communication needs. *Journal of Special Education Technology, 17*(4), 5–13.

Parette, P., Huer, M. B., & Wyatt, T. A. (2002). Young African American children with disabilities and augmentative and alternative communication issues. *Early Childhood Education Journal, 29*(3), 201–207.

Patel, R. (2003). Acoustic characteristics of the question-statement contrast in severe dysarthria due to cerebral palsy. *Journal of Speech, Language, and Hearing Research, 46,* 1401–1415.

Patel, R., & Salata, A. (2006). Using computer games to mediate caregiver-child communication for children with severe dysarthria. *Journal of Medical Speech-Language Pathology, 14,* 279–284.

Paulesu, E., Démonet, J., Fazio, F., McCrory, E., Chanoine, V., et al. (2001). Dyslexia: Cultural diversity and biological unit. *Science, 291,* 2165–2167.

Pauloski, B. R., Rademaker, A. W., Logmann, J. A., Stein, D., Beery, Q., Newman, L., et al. (2000). Pretreatment swallowing function in patients with head and neck cancer. *Head and Neck, 22,* 474–482.

Paul, R. (1995). *Language disorders from infancy through adolescence: Assessment and intervention.* St. Louis, MO: Mosby-Year Book, Inc.

Paul, R. (1996). Clinical implications of the natural history of slow expressive language development. *American Journal of Speech-Language Pathology, 5,* 5–21.

Paul, R. (1998). *Literacy and deafness: The development of reading, writing, and literate thought.* Needham Heights, MA: Allyn & Bacon.

Paul, R. (2001). *Language disorders from infancy through adolescence: Assessment and intervention* (2d ed.). St. Louis, MO: Mosby.

Paul, R. (2002). *Language disorders from infancy through adolescence: Assessment and intervention* (3rd ed.). Baltimore, MD: Mosby.

Paul, R., Cohen, D. J., Breg, W. R., Watson, M., & Herman, S. (1984). Fragile X syndrome: Its relations to speech and language disorders. *Journal of Speech and Hearing Disorders, 49,* 328–332.

Pellowski, M. W., & Conture, E. G. (2002). Characteristics of speech disfluency and stuttering behaviors in 3- and 4-year-old children. *Journal of Speech, Language, and Hearing Research, 45,* 20–34.

Peña, E., Iglesias, A., & Lidz, C. S. (2001). Reducing test bias through dynamic assessment of children's word learning ability. *American Journal of Speech-Language Pathology, 10,* 138–154.

Perfetti, C. A. (1999). Comprehending written language: A blueprint of the reader. In P. Hagoort & C. Brown (Eds.), *Neurocognition of language processing* (pp. 167–208). Oxford University Press.

Perkell, J. S., Cohen, M. J., Svirsky, M. A., Matthies, M. L., Garabieta, I., & Jackson, M. T. T. (1992). Electromagnetic midsagittal articulometer systems for transducing speech articulatory movements. *Journal of the Acoustical Society of America, 92*(6), 3078–3096.

Perkell, J. S., Guenther, F. H., Lane, H., Matthies, M. L., Perrier, P., Vick, J., Wilhelms-Tricarico, R., & Zandipour, M. (2000). A theory of speech motor control and supporting data from speakers with normal hearing and profound hearing loss. *Journal of Phonetics, 28,* 233–272.

Perlman, A. L., & Christensen, J. (1997). Topographic and functional anatomy of the swallowing structures. In A. L. Perlman & K. S. Schulze-Delrieu (Eds.), *Deglutition and its disorders: Anatomy, physiology, clinical diagnosis, and management* (pp. 15–42). San Diego, CA: Singular.

Perry, A., Dunlap, G., & Black, A. (2007). Autism and related disabilities. In I. Brown & M. Percy (Eds.), *A comprehensive guide to intellectual and developmental disabilities* (pp. 149–172). Baltimore, MD: Paul H. Brookes.

Peterson, C., Jesso, B., & McCabe, A. (1999). Encouraging narratives in preschoolers: An intervention study. *Journal of Child Language, 26,* 49–67.

Peters, T. J., & Guitar, B. (1991). *Stuttering: An integrated approach to its nature and treatment.* Baltimore: Williams & Wilkins.

Petitto, L. A., Holowka, S., Sergio, L. E., & Ostry, S. (2001). Language rhythms in baby hand movements. *Nature, 413,* 35–36.

Philips, B. J., & Ruscello, D. (1998). *Differential diagnosis in speech-language pathology.* Boston, MA: Butterworth-Heinemann.

Piasta, S. B., & Wagner, R. K. (2008). Dyslexia: Identification and classification. In E. L. Girgorenko & A. J. Naples, *Single-word reading: Behavioral and biological perspectives* (pp. 309–326). New York: Lawrence Erlbaum Associates.

Pimental, P. A., & Kinsbury, N. A. (1989). *Mini inventory of right brain injury.* Austin, TX: Pro-Ed.

Pinker, S. (1994). *The language instinct.* NY: Harper-Collins.

Pinker, S. (1999). *Words and rules.* New York: Basic Books.

Pore, S. G., & Reed, K. L. (1999). *Quick reference to speech-language pathology.* Gaithersburg, MD: Aspen.

Portnoy, R. A., & Aronson, A. E. (1982). Diadochokinetic syllable rate and regularity in normal and in spastic and ataxic dysarthric subjects. *Journal of Speech and Hearing Disorders, 47,* 324–328.

Preminger, J. (2003). Should significant others be encouraged to join adult group audiologic rehabilitation classes? *Journal of the American Academy of Audiology, 14,* 545–555.

Prendergrast, S., & Kelley, L. (2002). Aural rehabilitation services: Survey reports who offers which ones and how often. *Hearing Journal, 55,* 30–35.

Purdy, S. C., Farrington, D. R., Moran, C. A., Chard, L. L., & Hodgson, S. (2002). A parent questionnaire to evaluate children's auditory behavior in everyday life (ABEL). *American Journal of Audiology, 11,* 72–82.

Purdy, S. C., Moran, C. A., Chard, L., & Hodgson, S. A. (2002). Auditory behavior in everyday life. *American Journal of Audiology, 11,* 82.

Qadeer, M. A., Colabianchi, N., Strome, M., & Vaezi, M. (2006). Gastroesophageal reflux and laryngeal cancer: Causation or association? *American Journal of Otolaryngology—Head and Neck Medicine and Surgery, 27,* 119–128.

Raitano, N. A., Pennington, B. F., Tunick, R. A., Boada, R., & Shriberg, L. D. (2004). Pre-literacy skills of subgroups of children with speech sound disorders. *Journal of Child Psychology and Psychiatry, 45,* 821–835.

Ramig, L. O., Countryman, S., Thompson, L. L., & Horii, Y. (1995). Comparison of two forms of intensive speech treatment for Parkinson disease. *Journal of Speech and Hearing Research, 38,* 1232–1251.

Ramig, L. O., & Dromey, C. (1996). Aerodynamic mechanisms underlying treatment-related changes in vocal intensity in patients with Parkinson disease. *Journal of Speech and Hearing Research, 39,* 798–807.

Ramig, L. O., Pawlas, A. A., & Countryman, C. (1995). *The Lee Silverman Voice Treatment (LSVT). A practical guide to treatment of the voice and speech disorders in Parkinson disease.* Iowa City, IA: National Center for Voice and Speech.

Ramig, L. O., Sapir, S., Fox, C., & Countryman, S. (2001). Changes in vocal loudness following intensive voice treatment (LSVT®) in individuals with Parkinson's disease: A comparison with untreated patients and normal age-matched controls. *Movement Disorders, 16,* 79–83.

Ramig, L. O., & Verdolini, K. (1998). Treatment efficacy: Voice disorders. *Journal of Speech, Language, and Hearing Research, 41,* S101–S116.

Ramig, P. R., & Bennett, E. M. (1995). Working with 7- to 12-year-old children who stutter: Ideas for intervention in the public schools. *Language, Speech, and Hearing Services in Schools, 26,* 138–150.

Ramsay, M., Gisel, E. G., & Boutry, M. (1993). Non-organic failure to thrive: Growth failure secondary to feeding-skills disorder. *Developmental Medicine and Child Neurology, 35,* 285–297.

RAND Reading Study Group. (Chair: Snow, C.). (2002). *Reading for understanding: Toward an R&D program in reading comprehension.* Santa Monica, CA: RAND.

Rao, P. R. (1994). The aphasia syndromes: Localization and classification. *Topics in Stroke Rehabilitation, 1*(2), 1–13.

Raphael, L. J., Borden, G. J., & Harris, K. S. (2007). *Speech science primer: Physiology, acoustics, and perception of speech.* Baltimore, MD: Lippincott, Williams, & Wilkins.

Ratner, V. L., & Harris, L. R. (1994). *Understanding language disorders: The impact on learning.* Eau Claire, WI: Thinking Publications.

Rawson, M. (1986). The Orton Trail: 1896–1986. *Annals of Dyslexia, 37,* 36–48.

Raymer, A. M. (2001). Acquired language disorders. *Topics in Language Disorders, 21*(3), 42–59.

Reau, N. R., Senturia, Y. D., Lebailly, S. A., & Christoffel, K. K. (1996). Infant and toddler feeding patterns and problems: Normative data and a new direction. *Journal of Developmental and Behavioral Pediatrics, 17,* 149–153.

Redmond, S., & Rice, M. L. (1998). The socioemotional behaviors of children with SLI: Social adaptation or social deviance? *Journal of Speech, Language, and Hearing Research, 41,* 688–700.

Reilly, S., Skuse, D. H., & Poblete, X. (1996). The prevalence of feeding problems in pre-school children with cerebral palsy. *Journal of Pediatrics, 129,* 877–882.

Renout, K. A., Leeper, H. A., Bandur, D. L., & Hudson, A. J. (1995) Vocal fold diadochokinetic function of individuals with amyotrophic lateral sclerosis. *American Journal of Speech-Language Pathology, 4,* 73–79.

Rescorla, L. (1980). Overextension in early language development. *Journal of Child Language, 7,* 321–335.

Rescorla, L. (2002). Language and reading outcomes to age 9 in late-talking toddlers. *Journal of Speech, Language, and Hearing Research, 45,* 360–371.

Rescorla, L., & Achenbach, T. M. (2002). Use of the Language Development Survey (LDS) in a national probability sample of children 18 to 35 months old. *Journal of Speech, Language, and Hearing Research, 45,* 733–743.

Rescorla, L., Roberts, J., & Dahlsgaard, K. (1997). Late talkers at 2: Outcome at age 3. *Journal of Speech, Language, and Hearing Research, 40,* 556–566.

Restrepo, M. A., & Silverman, S. W. (2001). Validity of the Spanish Preschool Language Scale-3 for use with bilingual children. *American Journal of Speech-Language Pathology, 10,* 382–393.

Reynolds, A. J., Temple, J. A., Robertson, D. L., & Mann, E. A. (2001). Long-term effects of an early childhood intervention on educational achievement and juvenile arrest: A 15-year follow-up of low-income children in public schools. *Journal of American Medical Association, 285,* 2239–2346.

Rice, M. L. (1996). *Toward a genetics of language.* Mahwah, NJ: Lawrence Erlbaum.

Rice, M. L., Haney, K. R., & Wexler, K. (1998). Family histories of children with SLI who show extended optional infinitives. *Journal of Speech, Language, and Hearing Research, 41,* 419–432.

Richardson, J. S., & Morgan, R. F. (1994). *Reading to learn in the content areas.* Belmont, CA: Wadsworth.

Rickett, D. (1998). *Review: Sandler should have punted "Waterboy."* Retrieved June 15, 2004, from www.cnn.com/SHOWBIZ/Movies/9811/13/review.waterboy/.

Riley, G. (1972). A stuttering severity instrument for children and adults. *Journal of Speech and Hearing Disorders, 37,* 314–322.

Riley, G., Maguire, G., Franklin, D., & Ortiz, T. (2001). Medical perspectives in the treatment of stuttering. *Contemporary Issues in Communication Science and Disorders, 28,* 104–110.

Rini, D. L., & Hindenlang, J. (2007). Family-centered practice. In R. Paul & P. W. Cascella (Eds.), *Introduction to clinical methods in communication disorders* (2d ed., pp. 321–338). Baltimore, MD: Paul H. Brookes.

Risjord, C., Wilkinson, J., & Stark, M. (2000). *Instruction manual for braille transcribing* (4th ed.). Washington, DC: National Library of Congress, National Library Service for the Blind and Physically Handicapped.

Rivara, F. P. (1994). Epidemiology and prevention of pediatric traumatic brain injury. *Pediatric Annals, 23,* 12–17.

Robbins, A. M., Koch, D. B., Osberger, M. J., & Zimmerman-Philips, S. (2004). Effect of age at cochlear implantation on auditory skill development in infants and toddlers. *Archives of Otolaryngology—Head & Neck Surgery, 130,* 570–574.

Robb, M. P., & Smith, A. B. (2002). Fundamental frequency onset and offset behavior: A comparative study of children and adults. *Journal of Speech, Language, and Hearing Research, 45,* 446–456.

Roberts, J. E., Burchinal, M. R., & Zeisel, S. A. (2002). Otitis media in early childhood in relation to children's school-age language and academic skills. *Pediatrics 110*(4), 1–11.

Roberts, J., Jurgerns, J., & Burchinal, M. (2005). The role of home literacy practices in preschool children's language and emergent literacy skills. *Journal of Speech, Language, and Hearing Research, 48,* 345–359.

Roberts, J. E., Wallace, I. F., & Henderson, F. W. (1997). *Otitis media in young children. Medical, developmental, and educational considerations.* Baltimore: Paul H. Brookes Publishing Co.

Roberts, K. (1997). A preliminary account of the effect of otitis media on the 15-month-olds' categorization and some implications for early language learning. *Journal of Speech, Language, and Hearing Research, 40,* 508–518.

Roberts, P. (2001). Aphasia assessment and treatment for bilingual and culturally diverse patients. In R. Chapey (Ed.), *Language intervention strategies in aphasia and related communication disorders* (pp. 208–232). Philadelphia: Lippincott, Williams & Wilkins.

Robertson, C., & Salter, W. (1995). *Phonological Awareness Test.* East Moline, IL: LinguiSystems.

Robey, R. R. (1998a). The effectiveness of group treatments for aphasia: A meta-analysis. *Hearsay, 12*(1), 5–9.

Robey, R. R. (1998b). A meta-analysis of clinical outcomes in the treatment of aphasia. *Journal of Speech, Language, and Hearing Research, 41,* 172–187.

Robin, D. A., Jacks, A., & Ramage, A. (2008). The neural substrates of apraxia of speech as uncovered by brain imaging: A critical review. In R. J. Ingham (Ed.), *Neuroimaging in Communication Sciences and Disorders.* San Diego, CA: Plural Publishing.

Rodriguez, B. L., & Olswang, L. B. (2003). Mexican-American and Anglo-American mothers' beliefs and values about child rearing, education, and language impairment. *American Journal of Speech-Language Pathology, 12,* 452–462.

Rood, D. S., & Taylor, A. R. (1996). *Handbook of North American Indians* (vol. 17; Languages). Washington, DC: The Smithsonian Institution.

Rosenbeck, J. C., LaPointe, L. L., & Wertz, R. T. (1989). *Aphasia: A clinical approach.* Austin, TX: Pro-Ed.

Rosenbeck, J. C., Robbins, J. A., Roecker, E. B., Coyle, J. L., & Wood, J. L. (1996). A penetration-aspiration scale. *Dysphagia, 11,* 93–98.

Rosenberg, S., & Abbeduto, L. (1993). *Language and communication in mental retardation.* Hillsdale, NJ: Lawrence Erlbaum.

Rosen, D. C., & Sataloff, R. T. (1997). *Psychology of voice disorders.* San Diego, CA: Singular Publishing Group, Inc.

Ross, D. G. (1996). *Ross information processing assessment* (2d ed.). Austin, TX: Pro-Ed.

Rossetti, L. M. (2001). *Communication intervention: Birth to three* (3d ed.). Albany, NY: Delmar.

Roth, C. (2008, October). Mechanisms and sequelae of blast injuries. *Perspectives on Neurophysiology and Neurogenic Speech and Language Disorders, 17*(3), 20–24.

Roth, C., Aronson, A., & Davis, L. (1989). Clinical studies in psychogenic stuttering of adult onset. *Journal of Speech and Hearing Disorders, 54,* 634–646.

Roth, F., & Paul, R. (2007). Communication intervention: Principles and procedures. In R. Paul & P. Cascella (Eds.), *Introduction to clinical methods in communication disorders* (2d ed., pp. 157–178). Baltimore, MD: Paul H. Brookes.

Roth, F. P., Speece, D. L., & Cooper, D. H. (2002). A longitudinal analysis of the connection between oral language and early reading. *Journal of Educational Research, 95,* 259–272.

Roy, N., Merrill, R. M., Thibeault, S., Parsa, R. A., Gray, S. D., & Smith, E. M. (2004). Prevalence of voice disorders in teachers and the general population. *Journal of Speech, Language, and Hearing Research, 47,* 281–293.

Rueda, R., & Windmuller, M. P. (2006). English language learners, LD, and overrepresentation. *Journal of Learning Disabilities, 39,* 99–107.

Russell, A., Penny, L., & Pemberton, C. (1995). Speaking fundamental frequency changes over time in women: A longitudinal study. *Journal of Speech and Hearing Research, 38,* 101–109.

Russell, N. K. (1993). Educational considerations in traumatic brain injury: The role of the speech-language pathologist. *Language, Speech, and Hearing Services in Schools, 24,* 67–75.

Rustin, L., & Cook, F. (1995). Parental involvement in the treatment of stuttering. *Language, Speech, and Hearing Services in Schools, 26,* 127–137.

Rutter, M., Caspi, A., Fergusson, D., et al. (2004). Sex differences in developmental reading disability: New findings from four epidemiological studies. *Journal of the American Medical Association, 291,* 2007–2012.

Rvachew, S. (2007). Phonological processing and reading in children with speech sound disorders. *American Journal of Speech-Language Pathology, 16,* 260–270.

Rvachew, S., Rafaat, S., & Martin, M. (1999). Stimulability, speech perception skills, and the treatment of phonological disorders. *American Journal of Speech-Language Pathology, 8,* 33–43.

Sala, E., Laine, A., Simberg S., Pentti, J., & Suonpaa, J. (2001). The prevalence of voice disorders among day care center teachers compared with nurses: A questionnaire and clinical study. *Journal of Voice, 15,* 413–423.

Sambunaris, A., & Hyde, T. M. (1994). Stroke-related aphasia mistaken for psychotic speech: Two case reports. *Journal of Geriatric Psychiatry and Neurology, 7*(3), 144–147.

Sander, E. K. (1972). When are speech sounds learned? *Journal of Speech and Hearing Disorders, 37,* 55–63.

Sapienza, C. M., Ruddy, B. H., & Baker, S. (2004). Laryngeal structure and function in the pediatric larynx: Clinical applications. *Language, Speech, and Hearing Services in Schools, 35,* 299–307.

Satter, E. M. (1996). *Feeding with love and good sense: Training manual for the VISIONS workshop* (pp. 49–51). Madison, WI: Ellen Satter Institute.

Satter, E. M. (1999). *Secrets of feeding a healthy family.* Madison, WI: Ellen Satter Institute.

Scanlon, D. M., & Vellutino, F. R. (1997). A comparison of the instructional backgrounds and cognitive profiles of poorer, average, and good readers who were initially identified as at risk for reading failures. *Scientific Studies of Reading, 1*(3), 191–215.

Scarborough, H. (1990). Very early language deficits in dyslexic children. *Child Development, 61,* 1728–1734.

Scarborough, H. S. (2000). Connecting early language and literacy to later reading (dis)abilities: Evidence, theory, and practice. In S. B. Neuman & D. K. Dickinson (Eds.), *Handbook of early literacy research* (pp. 97–110). New York: Guilford Press.

Schauster, H., & Dwyer, J. (1996). Transition from tube feedings to feeding by mouth in children: Preventing eating dysfunction. *Journal of American Dietetic Association, 96,* 277–281.

Scheetz, N. A. (2001). *Orientation to deafness* (2d ed.). Needham Heights, MA: Allyn & Bacon.

Schleper, D. R. (1995). Reading to deaf children: Learning from deaf adults. *Perspectives in Education and Deafness, 13,* 4–8.

Schmahmann, J. D., & Sherman, J. C. (1998). The cerebellar cognitive affective syndrome. *Brain, 121,* 561–579.

Schmidt-Luggen, A. (2005). Pharmacology update: Dementia. *National Conference of Gerontological Nurse Practitioners, 26,* 94.

Schmidt, R. A. (1975). A schema theory of discrete motor skill learning. *Psychological Review, 82*(4), 225–260.

Schmidt, R. A., & Bjork, R. A. (1992). New conceptualizations of practice: Common principles in three paradigms suggest new concepts for training. *Psychological Science, 3*(4), 207–217.

Schmidt, R. A., & Lee, T. D. (1999). *Motor control and learning: A behavioral emphasis* (3d ed.). Champaign, IL: Human Kinetics.

Schmidt, R. A., & Lee, T. D. (2005). *Motor control and learning: A behavioral emphasis* (4th ed.). Champaign, IL: Human Kinetics.

Schneider, P., Scherg, M., Dosh, G., Specht, H., Gutschalk, A., & Rupp, A. (2002). Morphology of Heschl's gyrus reflects enhanced activation in the auditory cortex of musicians. *Nature Neuroscience, 5,* 688–694.

Schneider, P., Slumming, V., Roberts, N., Scherg, M., Goebel, R., Specht, H. J., et al. (2005). Structural and functional asymmetry of lateral Heschl's gyrus reflects pitch perception preference. *Nature Neuroscience, 8,* 1241–1247.

Schow, R., Balsara, N., Smedley, T., & Whitcomb, C. (1993). Aural rehabilitation by ASHA audiologists: 1980–1990. *American Journal of Audiology, 2,* 28–37.

Schow, R. L. (2001). A standardized AR battery for dispensers is proposed. *Hearing Journal, 54,* 10–20.

Schow, R. L., Seikel, J. A., Chermak, G. D., & Berent, M. (2000). Central auditory processes and test measures: ASHA 1996 revisited. *American Journal of Audiology, 9,* 159–189.

Schuele, C. M., & Hadley, P. A. (1999). Potential advantages of introducing specific language impairment to families. *American Journal of Speech-Language Pathology, 8,* 11–22.

Schulze-Delrieu, K. S., & Miller, R. M. (1997). Clinical assessment of dysphagia. In A. L. Perlman & K. S. Schulze-Delrieu (Eds.), *Deglutition and its disorders: Anatomy, physiology, clinical diagnosis, and management* (pp. 125–152). San Diego, CA: Singular Publishing.

Schurr, M. J., Ebner, K. A., Maser, A. L., Sperling, K. B., Helgerson, R. B., & Harms, B. (1999). Formal swallowing evaluation and therapy after traumatic brain injury improves dysphagia outcomes. *Journal of Trauma, 46,* 817–821.

Seale, J. M. (2007). *Quantitative differences in the conversational performance of people with severe aphasia using three types of visual screen displays on speech generating devices.* Unpublished master's thesis, Duquesne University: Pittsburg, Pennsylvania.

Sears, H. (2003). Average brain weights. Retrieved November 2003, from www.sc.edu/union/Sears/brain/htm.

Secord, W. A., & Wiig, E. H. (2003). *Practical performance assessment.* Sedona, AZ: Red Rock Education Publication, Inc.

Seddoh, S. A. K., & Robin, D. A. (2001). Neurogenic disorders of prosody. In D. Vogel & M. Cannito (Eds.), *Treating disordered speech motor control: For clinicians by clinicians* (2d ed., pp. 277–320). Austin, TX: Pro-Ed.

Seddoh, S. A. K., Robin, D. A., Sim, H. S., Hageman, C., Moon, J. B., & Folkins, J. W. (1996). Speech timing in apraxia of speech versus conduction aphasia. *Journal of Speech and Hearing Research, 39,* 590–603.

Seery, C. H. (2005). Differential diagnosis of stuttering for forensic purposes. *American Journal of Speech-Language Pathology, 14,* 284–297.

Seidman, M. D., Ridder, D. D., Elisevich, K., Bowyer, S. M., Darrat, L., et al. (2008). Direct electrical stimulation of Heschl's gyrus for tinnitus treatment. *Laryngoscope, 118,* 491–500.

Semrud-Clikeman, M., Guy, K., Griffin, J. D., & Hynd, G. W. (2000). Rapid naming deficits in children and adolescents with reading disabilities and attention deficit hyperactivity disorder. *Brain and Language, 74,* 70–83.

Shaiman, S., & Gracco, V. L. (2002). Task-specific sensorimotor interactions in speech production. *Experimental Brain Research, 146,* 411–418.

Shapiro, L., Swinney, D., & Borsky, S. (1998). *Assessment in speech-language pathology: A resource manual* (2d ed.). San Diego, CA: Singular Publishing.

Sharma, A., Tobey, E., Dorman, M., Bharadwaj, S., Martin, K., Gilley, P., & Kunkel, F. (2004). Central auditory maturation and babbling development in infants with cochlear implants. *Archives of Otolaryngology—Head & Neck Surgery, 130,* 511–516.

Shaywitz, B. A., Shaywitz, S. E., & Fletcher, J. M. (1992). The Yale center for the study of learning and attention disorders. *Learning Disabilities, 3,* 1–12.

Shaywitz, S. (2003). *Overcoming dyslexia.* New York: Knopf.

Shaywitz, S., & Shaywitz, B. (2005). Dyslexia (specific reading disability). *Biological Psychiatry, 57,* 1301–1309.

Shaywitz, S., Shaywitz, B., Fletcher, J. M., & Escobar, M. (1990). Prevalence of reading disability in boys and girls: Results of the Connecticut Longitudinal Study. *Journal of the American Medical Association, 264,* 998–1002.

Shea, C. H., Lai, Q., Black, C., & Park, J. H. (2000). Spacing practice sessions across days benefits the learning of motor skills. *Human Movement Science, 19,* 737–760.

Shea, C. H., Lai, Q., Wright, D. L., Immink, M., & Black, C. (2001). Consistent and variable practice conditions: Effects on relative and absolute timing. *Journal of Motor Behavior, 33*(2), 139–152.

Shea, C. H., & Wulf, G. (2005). Schema theory: A critical appraisal and reevaluation. *Journal of Motor Behavior, 37,* 85–101.

Shea, J. B., & Morgan, R. L. (1979). Contextual inference effects on the acquisition, retention, and transfer of motor skill. *Journal of Experimental Psychology: Human Learning & Memory, 5,* 179–187.

Shipley, K. G., & McAfee, J. G. (1998). *Assessment in speech-language pathology: A resource manual* (2d ed.). San Diego, CA: Singular Publishing.

Shriberg, L. (1997). Developmental phonological disorders: One or many? In B. W. Hodson & M. L. Edwards (Eds.), *Perspectives in applied phonology* (pp. 105–131). Gaithersburg, MD: Aspen Publishers.

Shriberg, L. D. (in press). Childhood speech sound disorders: From post-behaviorism to the postgenomic era. In R. Paul & P. Flipsen (Eds.), *Speech sound disorders in children: Essays in honor of Lawrence D. Shriberg.* San Diego, CA: Plural Publishing, Inc.

Shriberg, L. D., Austin, D., Lewis, B. A., McSweeney, J. L., & Wilson, D. L. (1997a). The Speech Disorders Classification System (SDCS): Extensions and lifespan reference data. *Journal of Speech-Language-Hearing Research, 40,* 723–740.

Shriberg, L. D., Austin, D., Lewis, B. A., McSweeney, J. L., & Wilson, D. L. (1997b). The percentage of consonants correct (PCC) metric: Extensions and reliability data. *Journal of Speech-Language-Hearing Research, 40,* 708–722.

Shriberg, L. D., Campbell, T. F., Karlsson, H. B., Brown, R. L., McSweeney, J. L., & Nadler, C. J. (2003). A diagnostic marker for childhood apraxia of speech: The lexical stress ratio. *Clinical Linguistics & Phonetics, 17,* 549–574.

Shriberg, L., Flipsen, P., Thielke, H., Kwiatkowski, J., Kertoy, M. K., Katcher, M., et al. (2000). Risk for speech disorder associated with early recurrent otitis media with effusion: Two retrospective studies. *Journal of Speech, Language, and Hearing Research, 43,* 79–99.

Shriberg, L. D., Flipsen, P., Kwiatkowski, J., & McSweeny, J. L. (2003). A diagnostic marker for speech delay associated with otitis media with effusion: The intelligibility-speech gap. *Clinical Linguistics and Phonetics, 17,* 507–528.

Shriberg, L. D., Gruber, F. A., & Kwiatkowski, J. (1994). Developmental phonological disorders III: Long-term speech-sound normalization. *Journal of Speech and Hearing Research, 37,* 1151–1177.

Shriberg, L. D., Kent, R. D., Karlsson, H. B., McSweeney, J. L., Nadler, C. J., & Brown, R. L. (2003). A diagnostic marker for speech delay associated with otitis media with effusion: Backing of obstruents. *Clinical Linguistics and Phonetics, 17,* 529–547.

Shriberg, L. D., & Kwiatkowski, J. (1994). Developmental phonological disorders I: A clinical profile. *Journal of Speech and Hearing Research, 37,* 1100–1126.

Shriberg, L. D., Kwiatkowski, J., & Gruber, F. A. (1994). Developmental phonological disorders II: Short-term speech-sound normalization. *Journal of Speech and Hearing Research, 37,* 1127–1150.

Shriberg, L. D., Lewis, B. A., Tomblin, J. B., McSweeny, J. L., Karlsson, H. B., & Scheer, A. R. (2005). Toward diagnostic and phenotype markers for genetically transmitted speech delay. *Journal of Speech, Language, and Hearing Research, 48,* 834–852.

Shriberg, L. D., Tomblin, J. B., & McSweeney, J. L. (1999). Prevalence of speech delay in 6-year-old children with comorbidity with language impairment. *Journal of Speech, Language, and Hearing Research, 42,* 1461–1481.

Shuster, L. I., & Wambaugh, J. L. (2003). Consistency of speech sound errors in apraxia of speech accompanied by aphasia. Poster presented at the Clinical Aphasiology Conference, Orca's Island, WA.

Sicher, H., & DuBrul, E. L. (1975). *Oral anatomy* (6th ed.). St. Louis: Mosby.

Simmons-Mackie, N., Elman, R., Holland, A., Damico, J. (2007). Management of discourse in group therapy for aphasia. *Topics in Language Disorders, 27,* 5–23.

Skibbe, L., Justice, L. M., Zucker, T., & McGinty, A. (2008). Relations among maternal literacy beliefs, home literacy practices, and the emergent literacy skills of preschoolers with specific language impairment. *Early Education and Development, 19,* 68–88.

Simser, J. (1995, October). *Assessment and goal setting.* Paper presented at the Natural Communication—Auditory Verbal International Conference. Cuyahoga Falls, OH.

Siren, K. (2004). Cleft lip and palate. In L. Schoeonbrodt (Ed.), *Childhood communication disorders: Organic bases* (pp. 187–228). Clifton Park, NY: Delmar Learning.

Smith, A. (2006). Speech motor development: Integrating muscles, movements, and linguistic units. *Journal of Communication Disorders, 39,* 331–349.

Smith, A., Denny, M., Shaffer, L. A., Kelly, E. M., & Hirano, M. (1996). Activity of intrinsic laryngeal muscles in fluent and disfluent speech. *Journal of Speech and Hearing Research, 39,* 329–348.

Smith, A., & Goffman, L. (1998). Stability and patterning of speech movement sequences in children and adults. *Journal of Speech, Language, and Hearing Research, 41,* 18–31.

Smith, A. J., Geruschat, D., & Huebner, K. M. (2004). Policy to practice: Teachers' and administrators' views on curricular access by students with low vision. *Journal of Visual Impairment and Blindness, 98,* 612–628.

Smith, A., & Zelaznik, H. N. (2004). Development of functional synergies for speech motor coordination in childhood and adolescence. *Developmental Psychobiology, 45,* 22–33.

Smith, B. C., & Pederson, A. L. (1990, September/October). Nutrition focus: Tube feeding update. *Nutrition for Children with Special Health Care Needs, 5*(5), 1–5.

Snow, C., Burns, M. S., & Griffin, P. (Eds.). (1998). *Preventing reading difficulties in young children.* Washington, DC: National Academy Press.

Society for Neuroscience. (2004). *Hearing loss: Making a difference today.* Washington, DC: Author.

Solomon, N. P., & Charron, S. (1998). Speech breathing in able-bodied children and children with cerebral palsy: A review of literature and implications for clinical intervention. *American Journal of Speech-Language Pathology, 7*(2), 61–78.

Solomon, N. P., McKee, A. S., & Garcia-Barry, S. (2001). Intensive voice treatment and respiration treatment for hypokinetic-spastic dysarthia after traumatic brain injury. *American Journal of Speech-Language Pathology, 10,* 51–64.

Soto, G., Blake Huer, M., & Taylor, O. (1997). Multicultural issues. In L. L. Lloyd, D. R. Fuller, & H. H. Arvidson (Eds.), *Augmentative and alternative communication: A handbook of principles and practices* (pp. 406–413). Needham Heights, MA: Allyn & Bacon.

Spafford, C. A., & Grosser, G. S. (2005). *Dyslexia and reading difficulties* (2d ed.). Boston: Allyn & Bacon.

Spielman, J., Ramig, L. O., Mahler, L., Halpern, A., & Gavin, W. J. (2007). Effects of an extended version of the Lee Silverman Voice Treatment on voice and speech in Parkinson's disease. *American Journal of Speech-Language Pathology, 16,* 95–107.

Square, P. A., Darley, F. L., & Sommers, R. K. (1982). An analysis of the productive errors made by aparactic speakers with differing loci of lesions. In R. Brookshire (Ed.), *Clinical aphasiology conference proceedings* (pp. 245–250). BRK Publishers.

Stackhouse, J., & Snowling, M. J. (1992). Barriers to literacy development in two cases of developmental verbal dyspraxia. *Cognitive Neuropsychology, 9,* 273–299.

Stager, C. L., & Werker, J. F. (1997). Infants listen for more phonetic detail in speech perception than in word-learning tasks. *Nature, 388,* 381–382.

Stanovich, K. E. (1991). Discrepancy definition of reading disability: Has intelligence led us astray? *Reading Research Quarterly, 26,* 7–29.

Stanovich, K. E. (2000). *Progress in understanding reading: Scientific foundations and new frontiers.* New York: Guilford Press.

Stanovich, K. E., & Siegel, L. S. (1994). Phenotypic performance profile of children with reading disabilities: A regression-based test of the phonological-core variable-difference model. *Journal of Educational Psychology, 86,* 24–53.

Stanton-Chapman, T. L., Justice, L. M., Skibbe, L. E., & Grant, S. L. (2007). Social and behavioral characteristics of preschoolers with specific language impairment. *Topics in Early Childhood Special Education, 27,* 98–109.

Stemple, J. C., Glaze, L. E., & Gerdeman, B. K. (1995). *Clinical voice pathology: Theory and management* (2d ed.). San Diego, CA: Singular Publishing.

Stevenson, R. D., & Allaire, J. H. (1991). The development of normal feeding and swallowing. *Pediatric Clinics of North America, 38,* 1439–1453.

Stika, C. J., Ross, M., & Cuevas, C. (2002). Hearing aid services and satisfaction: The consumer viewpoint. *Hearing Loss, 23*(3), 25–31.

St. Louis, K. O., & Myers, F. L. (1995). Clinical management of cluttering. *Language, Speech, and Hearing Services in Schools, 26,* 187–195.

Stoel-Gammon, C., & Dunn, C. (1985). *Normal and disordered phonology in children.* Austin, TX: Pro-Ed.

Storch, S. A., & Whitehurst, G. J. (2002). Oral language and code-related precursors to reading: Evidence from a longitudinal structural model. *Developmental Psychology, 38,* 934–947.

Storkel, H. L., & Morrisette, M. L. (2002). The lexicon and phonology: Interactions in language acquisition. *Language, Speech, and Hearing Services in Schools, 33,* 24–37.

Stothard, S. E., Snowling, M. J., Bishop, D. V. M., Chipchase, B. B., & Kaplan, C. A. (1998). Language-impaired preschoolers: A follow-up into adolescence. *Journal of Speech, Language, and Hearing Research, 41,* 407–418.

Strand, E. A., Buder, E. H., Yorkston, K. M., & Ramig, L. O. (1994). Differential phonatory characteristics of four women with amyotrophic lateral sclerosis. *Journal of Voice, 8,* 327–339.

Strand, E. A., Stoeckel, R., & Baas, B. (2006). Treatment of severe childhood apraxia of speech: A treatment efficacy study. *Journal of Medical Speech-Language Pathology, 14*(4), 297–307.

Strom, K. E. (2001). The HR 2000 dispenser survey. *The Hearing Review, 8*(6), 20–42.

Stroudley, J., & Walsh, M. (1991). Radiological assessment of dysphagia in Parkinson's disease. *The British Journal of Radiology, 64,* 890–893.

Stuttering Foundation of America. (2004). *Famous people who stutter.* Retrieved June 10, 2004, from www.stutteringhelp.org/celebrit.htm.

Surveillance, Epidemiology, and End Results (SEER) Program (www.seer.cancer.gov) SEER* Stat Database: Incidence—SEER 9 Regs Public-Use, Nov 2003 Sub (1973–2001), National Cancer Institute, DCCPS, Surveillance Research Program, Cancer Statistics Branch, released April 2004, based on the November 2003 submission.

Svirsky, M. A. (2003, November 13–15). Outcomes of pediatric and cochlear implantation as a function of age at implant. Paper presented at the annual convention of the American Speech-Language-Hearing Association, Chicago.

Swinnen, S., Schmidt, R. A., Nicholson, D. E, & Shapiro, D. C. (1990). Information feedback for skill acquisition: Instantaneous knowledge of results degrades learning. *Journal of Experimental Psychology: Learning, Memory, and Cognition, 16,* 706–716.

Taft, M. (1991). *Reading and the mental lexicon.* Hove, UK: Lawrence Erlbaum.

Talavage, T. M., Sereno, M. I., Melcher, J. R., Ledden, P. J., Rosen, B. R., & Dale, A. M. (2004). Tonopic organization in human auditory cortex reveled by progressions of frequency sensitivity. *Journal of Neurophysiology, 91,* 1282–1296.

Tamis-LeMonda, C. S., Bornstein, M., & Baumwell, L. (2001). Maternal responsiveness and children's achievement of language milestones. *Child Development, 72,* 748–767.

Taylor, G. R. (2001). *Educational interventions and services for children with exceptionalities.* Springfield, IL: Charles C. Thomas.

Teasdale, G., & Jennett, B. (1974). Assessment of coma and impaired consciousness. *Lancet, 2,* 81–84.

Thal, D., & Tobias, S. (1992). Communicative gestures in children with delayed onset of oral expressive vocabulary. *Journal of Speech and Hearing Research, 35,* 1281–1289.

Thompson, C. K., Ballard, K. J., & Shapiro, L. P. (1998). Role of syntactic complexity in training Wh-movement structures in agrammatic aphasia: Optimal order for promoting generalization. *Journal of the International Neuropsychological Society, 4,* 661–674.

Thompson, C. K., & Robin, D. A. (1993). Developmental dysarthria. In G. Blanken, J. Dittmann, H. Grimm, J. C. Marshall, & C. W. Wallesch (Eds.), *Linguistic disorders and pathologies. An International handbook* (pp. 834–858). Berlin: Walter de Gruyter.

Threats, T. T. (2006). Towards an international framework for communication disorders: Use of the ICF. *Journal of Communication Disorders, 39,* 251–265.

Throneburg, R. N., Calvert, L. K., Sturm, J. J., Paramboukas, A. A., & Paul, P. J. (2000). A comparison of service delivery models: Effects of curricular vocabulary skills in the school setting. *American Journal of Speech-Language Pathology, 9,* 10–20.

Thurman, D. J., Alverson, C., Dunn, K. A., Guerrero, J., & Sniezek, J. E. (1999). Traumatic brain injury in the United States: A public health perspective. *Journal of Head Trauma Rehabilitation, 14,* 602–615.

Titze, I. R. (1994). *Principles of voice production.* Englewood Cliffs, NJ: Prentice Hall.

Tomblin, J. B. (1989). Familial concentration of developmental language impairment. *Journal of Speech and Hearing Disorders, 54,* 287–295.

Tomblin, J. B., Barker, B. A., Spencer, L. J., Zhang, X., & Gantz, B. J. (2005). The effect of age at cochlear implant initial simulation on expressive language growth in infants and toddlers. *Journal of Speech, Language and Hearing Research, 48,* 853–867.

Tomblin, J. B., Records, N. L., Buckwalter, P., Zhang, X., Smith, E., & O'Brien, M. (1997). Prevalence of specific language impairment in kindergarten children. *Journal of Speech, Language, and Hearing Research, 40,* 1245–1260.

Toohill, R., & Kuhn, P. (1997). Role of refluxed acid in pathogenesis of laryngeal disorders. *American Journal of Medicine, 103,* 100S–106S. (Supplement for the symposium on gastroesophageal reflux disease).

Torgesen, J. (1993). Variations of theory in learning disabilities. In G. R. Lyon, D. B. Gray, J. F. Kavanagh, & N. A. Krasnegor (Eds.), *Better understanding learning disabilities* (pp. 153–170). Baltimore, MD: Paul H. Brookes.

Torgesen, J. K. (2003, December). *Operationalizing the response to intervention model to identify children with* learning disabilities: Specific issues with older children. Paper presented at the National Research Center on Learning Disabilities Responsiveness-to-Intervention Symposium, Kansas City, MO.

Torgesen, J. K. (2004). Lessons learned from research on interventions for students who have difficulty learning to read. In P. McCardle & V. Chhabra (Eds.), *The voice of evidence in reading research.* Baltimore, MD: Paul H. Brookes.

Torgesen, J. K., Al Otaiba, S., & Grek, K. L. (2005). Assessment and instruction for phonemic awareness and word recognition skills. In H. W. Catts & A. G. Kamhi (Eds.), *Language and reading disabilities* (pp. 127–156). Boston: Allyn & Bacon.

Torgesen, J. K., Wagner, R., Rashotte, C. A., Lindamood, P., Rose, E., Conway, T., & Garvan, C. (1999). Preventing reading failure in young children with phonological processing disabilities: Group and individual responses to instruction. *Journal of Educational Psychology, 91,* 579–593.

Torres, L. Y., & Sirbegovic, D. J. (2004). Clinical benefits of the Passy-Muir tracheostomy and ventilator speaking valves in the NICU. *Neonatal Intensive Care, 17*(4), 20–23.

Tourville, J. A., Reilly, K. J., & Guenther, F. H. (2008). Neural mechanisms underlying auditory feedback control of speech. *NeuroImage, 39,* 1429–1443.

Traxler, C. B. (2000). *The Stanford Achievement Test,* 9th edition: National pastime and performance standards for deaf and hard-of-hearing students. *Journal of Deaf Studies and Deaf Education, 5*(43), 337–348.

Tremblay, K., & Cunningham, L. (2002). Is there a genetic link between noise-induced and age-related hearing loss? *Audiology Today, 14,* 21.

Trenholm, B., & Mirenda, P. (2006). Home and community literacy experiences of individuals with Down syndrome. *Down Syndrome Research and Practice, 10,* 30–40.

Trychin, S. (2002). *Living with hearing loss workbook.* Erie, PA: Author. Obtained November 2004, from the American Speech-Language-Hearing Association annual conference, Chicago.

Turkstra, L. S. (1999). Language testing in adolescence with brain injury: A consideration of the CELF-3. *Language, Speech, and Hearing Services in Schools, 30,* 132–140.

Tye-Murray, N. (2000). The child who has severe or profound hearing loss. In J. B. Tomblin, H. L. Morris, & D. C. Spriestersbach (Eds.), *Diagnosis in speech-language pathology* (2d ed.). San Diego, CA: Singular.

Tye-Murray, N. (2004). *Foundations of aural rehabilitation* (2d ed.). San Diego, CA: Singular Publishing.

Tyler, A. A., Lewis, K. E., Haskill, A., & Tolbert, L. C. (2002). Efficacy and cross-domain effects of a morphosyntax and a phonology intervention. *Language, Speech, and Hearing Services in Schools, 33,* 52–66.

Tyler, A. A., Lewis, K. E., Haskill, A., & Tolbert, L. C. (2003). Outcomes of different speech and language goal attack strategies. *Journal of Speech, Language, and Hearing Research, 46,* 1077–1094.

U.S. Bureau of Labor Statistics. (2008). *Occupational outlook handbook, 2008–2009 edition.* Washington, DC: Author. Retrieved from www.bls.gov/oco/home.htm.

U.S. Census Bureau. (2003). *Language use and English-speaking ability: 2000.* Washington, DC: Author.

U.S. Department of Education. (2001). *Twenty-third annual report to Congress on the implementation of the Individuals with Disabilities Education Act.* Washington, DC: Author.

U.S. Department of Education. (2002). *Twenty-fourth annual report to Congress on implementation of Individuals with Disabilities Act (IDEA).* Washington, DC: Government Printing Office.

U.S. Department of Education. (2003). *Twenty-fifth annual report to Congress on the implementation of the Individuals with Disabilities Education Act.* Washington, DC: Author.

U.S. Department of Education, National Center for Education Statistics. (2003). *Nation's report card.* Washington, DC: Author.

U.S. Department of Education, National Center for Education Statistics. (2006). *Public elementary and secondary students, staff, schools, and school districts: School year 2003–04* (NCES 2006-307).

U.S. Department of Health and Human Services. (1999). *Traumatic brain injury in the United States: A report to Congress.* Washington, DC: Author.

U.S. Department of Health and Human Services. (2000). *Healthy People 2010: Vol. II* (2d ed.). *Objective for improving health* (Part B: Focus areas 15–28). Washington, DC: Author.

U.S. Department of Health and Human Services. (2005). *Quick guide to health literacy.* Washington, DC: Author. Retrieved February 2, 2008, from www.health.gov/communication/literacy/quickguide/.

Van Bergeijk, W. A., Pierce, J. R., & David, E. E. (1960). *Waves and the ear.* New York: Doubleday.

VanBiervliet, A., & Parette, H. (2002). Development and evaluation of the families, cultures, and Augmentative and Alternative Communication (AAC) multimedia program. *Disability and Rehabilitation, 24,* 131–143.

Van der Bijl, C., Alant, E., & Lloyd, L. (2005). A comparison of two strategies of sight word instruction in children with mental disability. *Research in Developmental Disabilities, 27,* 43–55.

Van Der Lely, H. K. J., & Stollwerck, L. (1996). A grammatical specific language impairment in children: An autosomal dominant inheritance? *Brain and Language, 52,* 484–504.

Van de Sandt-Koenderman, W. M. E., Wiegers, J., Wielaet, S. M., Duivenvoorden, H. J., & Ribbers, G. M. (2007). High-tech AAC and severe aphasia: Candidacy for TouchSpeak (TS). *Aphasiology, 21*(5), 459–474.

van Kleeck, A., Vander Woude, J., & Hammett, L. (2006). Fostering literal and inferential language skills in Head Start preschoolers with language impairment using scripted book-sharing discussions. *American Journal of Speech-Language Pathology, 15,* 85–95.

Van Lieshout, P. H. H. M., Bose, A., Square, P. A., & Steele, C. M. (2007). Speech motor control in fluent and dysfluent speech production of an individual with apraxia of speech and Broca's aphasia. *Clinical Linguistics & Phonetics, 21,* 159–188.

Van Lieshout, P. H. H. M., Hulstijn, W., & Peters, H. F. M. (1996). From planning to articulation: What differentiates a person who stutters from a person who does not stutter? *Journal of Speech and Hearing Research, 39*(3), 546–564.

Van Mourik, M., Catsman-Berrevoets, C. E., Paquier, P. F., Yousef-Bak, E., & Van Dongen, H. R. (1997). Acquired childhood dysarthria: Review of its clinical presentation. *Pediatric Neurology, 17,* 299–307.

Van Riper, C. (1963). *Speech correction: Principles and methods* (4th ed.). Englewood Cliffs, NJ: Prentice Hall.

Van Riper, C. (1973). *The treatment of stuttering.* Upper Saddle River, NJ: Prentice Hall.

Van Riper, C. (1982). *The nature of stuttering* (2d ed.). Upper Saddle River, NJ: Prentice Hall.

Vanryckeghem, M., & Brutten, G. J. (1997). The speech-associated attitude of children who do and do not stutter and the differential effect of age. *American Journal of Speech-Language Pathology, 6,* 67–73.

Vellutino, F. R., Scanlon, D. M., & Lyon, G. R. (2000). Differentiating between difficult-to-remediate and readily remediate poor readers: More evidence against the IQ achievement discrepancy definition of reading disability. *Journal of Learning Disabilities, 33,* 223–238.

Vellutino, F. R., Scanlon, D. M., Pratt, A., Chen, R., & Dencklea, M. B. (1996). Cognitive profiles of difficult-to-remediate and readily remediated poor readers: Early intervention as a vehicle for distinguishing between cognitive and experiential deficits as basic causes of specific reading disability. *Journal of Educational Psychology, 88*(4), 601–638.

Vellutino, F. R., Scanlon, D. M., Small, S., & Fanuele, D. P. (2006). Response to intervention as a vehicle for distinguishing between children with and without reading disabilities: Evidence for the role of kindergarten and first-grade interventions. *Journal of Learning Disabilities, 39,* 157–169.

Ventry, I., & Weinstein, B. (1982). The hearing handicap inventory for the elderly, a new tool. *Ear and Hearing, 3,* 128–134.

Verdolini, K. (2000). Voice disorders. In J. B. Tomblin, H. L. Morris, & D. C. Spriestersbach (Eds.), *Diagnosis in speech-language pathology* (2d ed., pp. 233–280). San Diego, CA: Singular.

Vihman, M. M. (2004). Early phonological development. In J. E. Bernthal & N. W. Bankson (Eds.), *Articulation and phonological disorders* (5th ed.). Boston: Allyn & Bacon.

Vihman, M. M., & Greenlee, M. (1987). Individual differences in phonological development: Ages one and three years. *Journal of Speech and Hearing Research, 30,* 503–521.

Voice Disorders Special Interest Division. (2002). Consensus auditory-perceptual evaluation of voice [Assessment Tool]. Rockville, MD: American Speech-Language-Hearing Association, Voice Disorders Special Interest Division.

von Leden, H. (1985). Vocal nodules in children. *Ear Nose Throat Journal, 64*(10), 473–480.

Wada, H., Nakjoh, K., Satoh-Nakagawa, T., Suzuki, T., Ohrui, T., Arai, H., et al. (2001). Risk factors of aspiration pneumonia in Alzheimer's disease patients. *Gerontology, 47,* 271–276.

Wagner, C. W. (1996). Speech rehabilitation following total laryngectomy. In M. P. Fried (Ed.), *The larynx: A multidisciplinary approach* (2d ed., pp. 611–629). Baltimore, MD: Mosby.

Wagner, R. K., Torgesen, J. K., & Rashotte, C. A. (1999). *Comprehensive test of phonological processing.* Austin, TX: Pro-Ed.

Wambaugh, J. L., Duffy, J. R., McNeil, M. R., Robin, D. A., & Rogers, M. A. (2006). Treatment guidelines for acquired apraxia of speech: A synthesis and evaluation of the evidence. *Journal of Medical Speech Language Pathology, 14*(2), xv–xxxiii.

Wambaugh, J. L., Martinez, A. L., McNeil, M. R., & Rogers, M. A. (1999). Sound production treatment for apraxia of speech: Overgeneralization and maintenance effects. *Aphasiology, 13*(9–11), 821–837.

Wambaugh, J. L., & Nessler, C. (2004). Modification of sound production treatment for apraxia of speech: Acquisition and generalization effects. *Aphasiology, 18,* 407–427.

Wambaugh, J. L., West, J. E., & Doyle, P. J. (1998). Treatment for apraxia of speech: Effects of targeting sound groups. *Aphasiology, 12*(7/8), 731–743.

Wang, Y. T., Kent, R. D., Duffy, J. R., & Thomas, J. E. (2005). Dysarthria associated with traumatic brain injury: Speaking rate and emphatic stress. *Journal of Communication Disorders, 38,* 231–260.

Watkins, K. E., Vargha-Khadem, F., Ashburner, J., Paddingham, R. R., Connelly, A., Friston, K. J., et al. (2002). MRI analysis of an inherited speech and language disorder: Structural brain abnormalities. *Brain, 125,* 465–478.

Watkins, R., & Rice, M. L. (Eds.). (1994). *Specific language impairments in children.* Baltimore, MD: Brookes Publishing Co.

Watkins, R., Rice, M., & Molz, C. (1993). Verb use by language-impaired and normally developing children. *First Language, 37,* 133–143.

Watkins, R. V., & Johnson, B. W. (2004). Language abilities in children who stutter: Toward improved research and clinical applications. *Language, Speech, and Hearing Services in Schools, 35,* 82–89.

Watkins, R. V., Yairi, E., & Ambrose, N. G. (1999). Early childhood stuttering III: Initial status of expressive language abilities. *Journal of Speech, Language, and Hearing Research, 42,* 1125–1135.

Watson, P. J., Ciccia, A. H., & Weismer, G. (2003). The relation of lung volume initiation to selected acoustic properties of speech. *Journal of the Acoustic Society of America, 113*(5), 2812–2819.

Watt, N., Wetherby, A., & Shumway, S. (2006). Prelinguistic predictors of language outcomes at 3 years of age. *Journal of Speech, Language, and Hearing Research, 49,* 1224–1237.

Watterson, T., Hansen-Magorian, H. J., & McFarlane, S. C. (1990). A demographic description of laryngeal contact ulcer patients. *Journal of Voice, 4,* 71–75.

Wehler, C. A., Scott, R. A., & Anderson, J. J. (1991). *A survey of childhood hunger in the United States.* Washington, DC: Food Research and Action Center.

Weinstein, B. E. (2000). *Geriatric audiology.* New York: Thieme.

Werker, J. F., & Tees, R. C. (2002). Cross-language speech perception: Evidence for perceptual reorganization during the first year of life. *Infant Behavior and Development, 25,* 121–133.

Werker, J. F., & Tess, R. C. (2005). Speech perception as a window for understanding plasticity and commitment in language systems of the brain. *Developmental Psychobiology, 46,* 233–251.

Westby, C. (1980). Assessment of cognitive and language abilities through play. *Language, Speech, and Hearing Services in Schools, 11,* 155–168.

Westby, C. E. (1985). Learning to talk—Talking to learn: Oral-literate language differences. In C. S. Simon (Ed.), *Communication skills in classroom success: Assessment and therapy methodologies for language-learning disabled students* (pp. 181–213). San Diego, CA: College-Hill Press.

Westby, C. (2000). Multicultural issues in speech and language assessment. In J. B. Tomblin, H. L. Morris, & D. C. Spriestersbach (Eds.), *Diagnosis in speech-language pathology* (2d ed., pp. 35–61). San Diego, CA: Singular.

Westby, C. (2005). Assessing and remediating text comprehension problems. In H. W. Catts & A. G. Kahmi (Eds.), *Language and reading disabilities* (2d ed., pp. 157–232). Boston: Allyn & Bacon.

Westby, C. E. (1991). Learning to talk—Talking to learn: Oral-literate language differences. In C. S. Simon (Ed.), *Communication skills classroom success: Assessment and therapy methodologies for language and learning disabled students.* Eau Claire, WI: Thinking Publications.

Wetherby, A., & Prizant, B. (1993). *Communication and symbolic behavior scales* (1st normed ed.). Baltimore: Brookes.

Wetherby, A., Prizant, B., & Schuler, A. (2000). Understanding the nature of communication and language impairments. In A. Wetherby & B. Prizant (Eds.), *Autism spectrum disorders: A transactional developmental perspective* (pp. 109–142). Baltimore, MD: Paul H. Brookes.

Whitehurst, G. J., & Lonigan, C. J. (1998). Child development and emergent literacy. *Child Development, 69,* 848–872.

Widerstrom, A. H. (2005). *Achieving learning goals through play: Teaching young children with special needs* (2d ed.). Baltimore, MD: Paul H. Brookes.

Wilbarger, P., & Wilbarger, J. (1991). *Sensory defensiveness in children: An intervention guide for parents and other care-takers.* Santa Barbara, CA: Avanti Educational Programs.

Wilcox, M. J., Kouri, T. A., & Caswell, S. B. (1991). Early language intervention: A comparison of classroom and individual treatment. *American Journal of Speech-Language Pathology, 1,* 49–60.

Wilkins, D. P. (2003). *Psycholinguistic considerations in representation selection for communicative interaction: Why it is that interactions are impaired, not individuals.* Paper presented at the meeting of the Department of Special Education and Communicative Disorders, San Francisco State University, San Francisco, CA.

Williams, A. L. (1993). Phonological reorganization: A qualitative measure of phonological improvement. *American Journal of Speech-Language Pathology, 2,* 44–51.

Williams, A. L. (2000). Multiple oppositions: Theoretical foundations for an alternative contrastive intervention approach. *American Journal of Speech-Language Pathology, 9,* 282–288.

Williams, A. L. (2002). Epilogue: Perspectives in the assessment of children's speech. *American Journal of Speech-Language Pathology, 11,* 259–263.

Williams, A. L. (2005). A model and structure for phonological intervention. In A. Kamhi and K. Pollack (Eds.), *Phonological disorders in children: Clinical decision making in assessment and intervention* (pp. 189–200). Baltimore, MD: Paul H. Brookes.

Williams, A. L. (2006). *Sound contrasts in phonology: User's manual.* Eau Claire, WI: Thinking Publications.

Williams, L., & Elbert, M. (2003). A prospective longitudinal study of phonological development in late talkers. *Language, Speech, and Hearing Services in Schools, 34,* 138–153.

Williams, L. (2008). Personal communication, March 3, 2008.

Wilson Jones, M., Morgan, E., Shelton, J. E., & Thorogood, C. (2007). Cerebral palsy: Introduction and diagnosis (Part I). *Journal of Pediatric Health Care 21*(3), 146–152.

Wilson, W. J., & Herbstein, N. (2003). The role of music intensity in aerobics: Implications for hearing conservation. *Journal of the American Academy of Audiology, 14,* 29–38.

Wingate, M. (1976). *Stuttering theory and treatment.* New York: Irvington Publishers.

Wingate, M. E. (2001). SLD is not stuttering [Letter to the editor]. *Journal of Speech, Language, and Hearing Research, 44,* 381–383.

Winkworth, A. L., Davis, P. J., Adams, R. D., & Ellis, E. (1995). Breathing patterns during spontaneous speech. *Journal of Speech and Hearing Research, 38,* 124–144.

Wit, J., Maassen, B., Gabreëls, F. J. M., & Thoonen, G. (1993). Maximum performance test in children with developmental spastic dysarthria. *Journal of Speech and Hearing Research, 36,* 452–459.

Wolf, M., & Bowers, P. (1999). The "Double-Deficit Hypothesis" for the developmental dyslexias. *Journal of Educational Psychology, 91,* 1–24.

Woodcock, R. (1987). *Woodcock reading mastery tests—revised.* Circle Pines, MN: American Guidance Service.

World Health Organization. (2001). *International classification of functioning, disability and health (ICF).* Geneva: Author.

World Health Organization. (2002). Towards a common language for functioning, disability, and health: The international classification of functioning, disability and health. Retrieved August 22, 2007, from www.who.int/classifications/icf/site/beginners/bg.pdf.

Wright, D. L., Black, C. B., Immink, M. A., Brueckner, S., & Magnuson, C. (2004). Long-term motor programming improvements occur via concatenating movement sequences during random but not blocked practice. *Journal of Motor Behavior, 36*(1), 39–50.

Wulf, G., McConnel, N., Gärtner, M., & Schwarz, A. (2002). Enhancing the learning of sport skills through external-focus feedback. *Journal of Motor Behavior, 34,* 171–182.

Wulf, G., Schmidt, R. A., & Deubel, H. (1993). Reduced frequency feedback enhances generalized motor program learning but not parameterization learning. *Journal of Experimental Psychology: Learning, Memory, and Cognition, 19*(5), 1134–1150.

Wulf, G., & Shea, C. H. (2004). Understanding the role of augmented feedback: The good, the bad, and the ugly. In A. M. Williams & N. J. Hodges (Eds.), *Skill acquisition in sport: Research, theory and practice* (pp. 121–144). London: Routledge.

Yairi, E., & Ambrose, N. (1999). Early childhood stuttering: I. Persistency and recovery rates. *Journal of Speech, Language, and Hearing Research, 42,* 1097–1112.

Yairi, E., Ambrose, N., & Cox, N. (1996). Genetics of stuttering: A critical review. *Journal of Speech and Hearing Research, 39,* 771–784.

Yairi, E., Ambrose, N., & Niermann, R. (1993). The early months of stuttering: A developmental study. *Journal of Speech, Language, and Hearing Research, 36,* 521–528.

Yamamoto, L., & Magalong, E. (2003). Outcome measures in stroke. *Critical Care Nursing Quarterly, 26*(4), 283–293.

Yaruss, J. S. (1997). Clinical measurement of stuttering behaviors. *Contemporary Issues in Communication Science and Disorders, 24,* 33–44.

Yaruss, J. S., Coleman, C., & Hammer, D. (2006). Treatment for preschool children who stutter: Description and preliminary evaluation of a family-focused treatment approach. *Language, Speech, and Hearing Services in Schools, 37,* 118–136.

Yaruss, J. S., & Gabel, R. (2005). *The National Stuttering Association's position on the SpeechEasy and other assistive devices.* New York: National Stuttering Association. Retrieved February 20, 2008, from www.nsastutter.org/material/index. php?matid=328.

Yaruss, J. S., LaSalle, L. R., & Conture, E. G. (1998). Evaluating stuttering in young children: Diagnostic data. *American Journal of Speech-Language Pathology, 7*(4), 62–76.

Yoos, H. L., Kitzman, H., & Cole, R. (1999). Family routines and the feeding process. In D. B. Kessler & P. Dawson (Eds.), *Failure to thrive and pediatric undernutrition: A transdisciplinary approach* (pp. 375–384). Baltimore, MD: Paul H. Brookes.

Yorkston, K. M., Beukelman, D. R., Strand, E., & Bell, K. R. (1999). *Clinical management of motor speech disorders in children and adults.* Boston, MA: Little Brown.

Yorkston, K. M., Miller, R. M., & Strand, E. A. (2004). *Management of speech and swallowing in degenerative diseases.* Austin, TX: Pro-Ed.

Yorkston, K. M., Miller, R. M., & Strand, E. E. (2004). *Management of speech and swallowing in degeneration diseases* (2d ed.) Austin, TX: Pro-Ed.

Yoshinaga-Itano, C. (2003). From screening to early identification and intervention: Discovering predictors to successful outcomes for children with significant hearing loss. *Journal of Deaf Studies and Deaf Education, 8,* 11–30.

Yoshinaga-Itano, C., Sedey, A., Coulter, D., & Mehl, A. (1998). Language of early- and later-identified children with hearing loss. *Pediatrics, 100,* 135–164.

Yuan, W., Holland, S. K., Cecil, K. M., Dietrich, K. N., Wessel, S. D., Altye, M., et al. (2006). The impact of early childhood lead exposure on brain organization: A functional magnetic resonance imaging study of language function. *Pediatrics, 118,* 971–977.

Zackheim, C. T., & Conture, E. (2003). Childhood stuttering and speech disfluencies in relation to children's mean length of utterance: A preliminary study. *Journal of Fluency Disorders, 28,* 115–141.

Zatorre, R. J., & Penhume, V. G. (2001). Spatial location after excision of human auditory cortex. *The Journal of Neuroscience, 21,* 6321–6328.

Zebrowski, P. M. (1994). Duration of sound prolongation and sound/syllable repetition in children who stutter: Preliminary observations. *Journal of Speech and Hearing Research, 37,* 254–263.

Zebrowski, P. M. (1997). Assisting young children who stutter and their families: Defining the role of the speech-language pathologist. *American Journal of Speech-Language Pathology, 6*(2), 19–28.

Zebrowski, P. M. (2000). Stuttering. In J. B. Tomblin, H. L. Morris, & D. C. Spriestersbach (Eds.), *Diagnosis in speech-language pathology* (2d ed., pp. 199–232). San Diego, CA: Singular.

Zemlin, W. R. (1997). *Speech and hearing science: Anatomy and physiology* (4th ed.). Englewood Cliffs, NJ: Prentice Hall.

Zick, R., & Olsen, J. (2002). Voice recognition software versus a traditional transcription service for physician charting in the ED. *American Journal of Emergency Medicine, 19,* 295–298.

NAME INDEX

SUBJECT INDEX